GW01607364

# —BEST OF—
# BURNETT

*Compiled by*

DR. H.L. CHITKARA

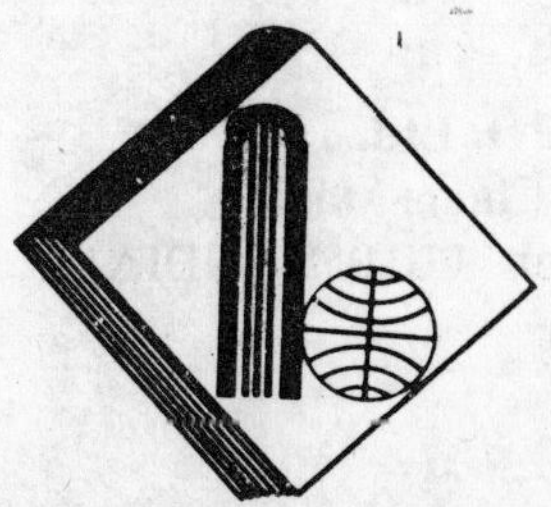

**B. Jain Publishers (P) Ltd.**
New Delhi - 110 055

*Printed in India*

*Price* : Rs. 150.00

*First Edition* : 1992
**Reprint** : 1994



*Published by* :

**B. Jain Publishers Pvt. Ltd.**
1921, Street No. 10, Chuna Mandi,
Paharganj, New Delhi - 110 055 (INDIA)

*Printed at* :

**J.J. Offset Printers**
Kishan Kunj, Delhi - 110 092

ISBN 81-7021-204-9
***BOOK CODE B-3656***

# CONTENTS



## Indices to sub-entries



## THE MAIN TEXT

# Preface

The great thing about Burnett is that he is eminently readable and that his books are still around, in India.

Reasonably small in size and on various topics, these can be read for pleasure and profit. You read one, and would like to read another. I personally found that all the Burnett's titles were not available all the time, and one had to wait for reprinting of one or the other. I thought bringing them together in one place would ensure their availability, and lend them a longer lease of life. Another thing which I concluded was that the text material of the books was made up of three components, namely, his observations; notes on medicines and therapeutics; and narratives of case-reports. These could well be divided into 3 parts.

These two considerations are the reason for bringing out this new compilation and in the present form.

From a distance of about a 100 years, and in the absence of a good homoeopathic library, it was very difficult to piece together an account of Burnett's life and work. Taking a cue from the list of references appended to an article written by Francis Treuherz, I wrote to him for help. He responded by sending a copy of the biography of Dr Burnett's daughter, entitled Ivy When Young — The Early Life of I. Compton Burnett (1884-1919). This Volume One of a two part biography written by Hilary Spurling was first published in 1974, the copy lent me was a revised edition, published in 1983 by Allison Busby, London. Ivy Compton Burnett deserved a biography because she became a renowned novelist of her time and was royally honoured with the title of Dame. This book born out of painstaking research and made up of a number of bits of authentic informaiton gives the genealogical tree of the Burnetts, about 3 to 4 generations back, and devotes whole chapters on Ivys parents and their family. It is from this volume that I have drawn all the factual details, which in some points are corrections even on Dr Clarkes work, the *Life and Work of Dr James Compton-Burnett*, now out of print. Spurling's biography of I. Compton Burnett makes delightful reading and gives a very vivid and often panoramic account of the times and background including the medical *milieu* in which Dr Burnett lived. In fact, this biographer has gone so far as to carefully analyse the make-up of some of the characters in Ivy's novels, which it is thought, gives clue to some of the characteristics of members of Ivy's intimate circle, including her parents.

The short write-up on the factual details of Dr Burnett's life presented in this work is quite bare and stark as compared to the colourful and lively accounts written by Spurling, the reading of which I recommend strangly to the readers if they are interested to delve deeper.

I have tried to collect all the available Burrnett's titles for this compilation. The materia medica notes and case-reports (Parts II and III of this compilation) are almost complete reproductions from originals but selections of observations (as per my personal perceptions and evaluation) are considerably trimmed versions of his elaborate *obiter dicta*.

The German and French portions (not accompanied by English translation) from Burnett's writings have been left out for the purpose of the present work.

I am greatly indebted to Francis Treuherz, editor of *The Homeopath* for his voluntarily lending me his personal copy of Ivy Burentt's biography, and to its author and publishers for my having made use of the facts recorded therein.

I am grateful to my friend BP Rao who stood by me through all the mishaps, which dogged the process of typesetting. It was he who helped in the retrieval and the reconstruction of the manuscript resulting from virus damage and loss of mss files as also in seeing the proofs. Again he very thoughtfully made out an *Index of the Remedies* as also *Indices to the sub-entries*, a sort of detailed *contents*, subjoined before the main text. The typesetters are to be congratulated for their patience in the face of the hinderances, and for having finally completed their part of the work over a period of two years.

B-1/24, Malviya Nagar
New Delhi-110017
*1 May, 1992*

**H.L. Chitkara**

**Postscript :**
After I had finished writing the above as a final act of exorcising the magnificent obsession of completing this assignment out of my system, I read through one of the treatises of Burnett again. I confess, compared to the beauty, the wholeness and the brilliance of Burnett's individual works, my exercise of trifurcating his works to the present shape appears to be a cruel dissection amounting to mutilation, like the action of a botanist who smothers the fragrance, the colours and the wholesomeness of a flower in pursuit of his studies. As an expiation, I earnestly request the readers to go through at least one whole title of Burnett, in order to taste the real flavour.

# JAMES COMPTON BURNETT (1840-1901)
## Life and Constribution to Homoepathy

Homoepathy was brought to Britain by Dr Frederic Quin (of mysterious parentage) in 1832. He become the first president of the British Homoepathic Society, founded in 1844. This Society became the Faculty of Homoeopathy in 1950. A support body for homoeopathy, The British Homoeopathic Association, was formed in 1947, which collected funds for establishing the first Homoeopathic Hospital in UK. It opened in 1849 in Golden Square, Soho. Ten years later, the Hospital was moved to three houses in Great Ormond Street and the present Royal London Homoeopathic Hospital stands on that site.

Dr Samuel Hahnemann died in 1843. JM Honingberger, a Bulgarian geologist, traveller and adventurer was the first to prescribe Homoeopathic medicines in India. He treated Maharaja Ranjit Singh at Lahore in 1839.

Dr James Compton Burnett was born at Redlynch near Salisbury in England on 21 July 1840, to Charles Compton Burnett and Agnes (nee Wilson). Dr Burnett died at the age of 60. After the death of his first wife, he married again. He had six children from his first wife and seven from the second wife. One son died young. Of the 12 children who survived him, one was killed on the front in the First World War; three committed suicide. Two of his four sons made brief childless marriages; his eight daughters remained unmarried. So that, he had no further descendants. Only his fourth daughter Ivy became renowned for her novels. She was honoured with the title of Dame.

The family name Burnett was a fairly common name of Scottish origin. The addition of the word Compton in the family name dated back to an event when one of the ancestors in the family married one Miss Compton who was supposed to have brought a substantial loan from her father to her bridegroom.

### Early Years and Education

His father Charles who had been on the move, changing jobs all his life, appears to have been a farm-labourer in the early part of James boyhood. James spent the early years in the country. He was a dreamy child, tall and sturdy, dark eyed, dark hair and clear-skinned, fond of exploring the woods and always thoughtful beyond his years. Later on, he attained the size and weight which was above average and looked quite burly and broad-faced as can be seen from his portrait.

When he was 10 or 11, his father moved to Southampton to set up shop there. Times were hard and James, who had always wanted to become a doctor, had ordinary education, leaving school at 16. Not much is known of his further formal education. He is supposed to have left for the continent travelling in France and other places. He was fond of philology and became fluent in French and German. Around 1865, he was in Vienna to attend the medical school there. Tuition in Vienna was free, and this served him well. He is said to have spent an extra two years studying anatomy, because he liked it and acquitted himself well in it. He returned to enroll at Glasgow Medical School where he was permitted to take his M.B. in one year instead of the usual three or four years.

After graduation in 1872, he took a post at the Barnhill Parochial Hospital and Asylum in Glasgow. It was here in this hospital that he was converted to homoeopathy at the suggestion of his friend Alfred Hawkes of the Royal Infirmary. His M.D. Thesis at the end of his internship at Barnhill was rejected for being heretically homoeopathic. A second thesis was accepted in 1876.

**Marriage & Professional Advance**

Early in 1874, Dr Burnett found an opening in Chester. He is reported to have been treating patients in a dispensary owned by a homoeopathic chemist named Edward Thomas who was himself interested in veterinary homoeopathy. Edward Thomas' son John and brother Henry became homoeopathic physicians. Burnett had his lodging near Henry's.

Dr Burnett began paying court to Edward Thomas's daughter, Agnes. They were married on 6 July 1874. Within a few months of his marriage, Dr Burnett moved to Liverpool where he set up practice. he prospered there from the start, and began a stiff programme of scientific research, reading of papers to the homoeopathic society and writing in medical journals. His fame spread fast, as is borne by the testimony of his clinical records narrated in his books. He left Liverpool for London a few months before he became the Editor of the *Homoeopathic World* in 1879. His practice flourished. He acquired a large house in the country and himself travelled daily to London for his practice. It was in this country house that his wife, after bearing him the sixth child died in child-birth on 8 Sep 1882.

**Second Marriage**

After about one year of his first wife's death, Dr Burnett married Katherine Rees aged 27, daughter of an Alderman and a prominent citizen of Dover. In fact, she had initially gone to consult him for an illness. The story of that case is narrated as Reason No 26 in his book, "Fifty Reasons for being a Homoeopath" (Case no 194 in part 3 of this book). He describes her as unusually beautiful and sweet, and called her as "love of his life". Dr Burnett again moved and settled his family in a larger country-house at Hove, and himself hired Iodgings in a London hotel from where he commuted to his clinic daily, returning home twice a week. Probably he suffered from Angina Pectoris; he died suddenly of heart failure at his hotel lodgings on 01 Apr 1901.

**The person and the physician**

Dr J H Clarke who wrote the *Life and Work of James Compton Burnett* considered him to be "one of the most remarkable Healers of modern times". The Westminister Gazette wrote, "his was one of the largest consulting practices in London." The monthly *Homoeopathic Review* wrote in an obituary, "He was a remarkably strong character, usually of a rugged, massive type, straight-forward and direct to a degree." The *American Homoeopathist* wrote, "He was simply a grand man, a lover of his kind, a faithful physician, the impersonation of kindness and sweetness."

He was a man of practical action, "that if you want a roasted pigeon for dinner, you must procure the pigeon, roast it; it will not fall ready roasted into your month."

**Conversion to Homoeopathy**

The episode connected with his conversion to homoeopathy is narrated by him at length as Reason No 1 in his book, *Homoeopathic Treatment or Fifty Reasons for Being a Homoeopath* which together with the details of the treatment of his own case (given as Reason No 2 *ibid*), have been taken out from part III of this book and reproduced here to high light these important landmarks in his life.

1. A NUMBER of years ago, on a dull, dreary afternoon, which I had partly occupied at B-Hospital with writing death certificates, I suddenly rose and felt something come over me for the fiftieth time at that period. I hardly know what, but it grew essentially out of my unsatisfactory clinical results. I had been an enthusiastic student of medicine originally, but an arrantly sceptic professor quite knocked the bottom out of all my faith in physic, while overmuch hospital work and responsibilities, grave beyond my age and experience, had squeezed a good deal of the enthusiasm out of me. After pacing up and down the surgery, I threw myself back into my chair and dreamily thought myself back to the green fields and the early birds nesting and fishing days of my childhood. Just then a corpse was carried by the surgery window, and I turned to the old dispenser and enquired in a petulant tone, "Tim, who's that dead now?" "Little Georgie, Sir."

Now little Georgie was a waif who belonged to nobody, and we had liked him and had kept him about in odd beds, as one might keep a pet animal. Everybody liked little Geogie; the most hardened old pauper would do him a good turn, and no one was ever more truly regretted than he.

It all came about in this way: One day I wanted a bed for an acute case, and I ordered little Georgie out of his bed in a warm, snug corner to another that was in front of a cold window; he went to it, caught cold, had pleurisy, and Tims reply gives the result.

Said I to myself: If I could only have stopped the initial fever that followed the chill by the window, Georgie had probably lived. But three medical men besides myself had treated Georgie—all in unison—and all hospital men; still pleurisy followed the febricula, dropsy followed the pleurisy, and poor little Geogrie died. Old Tim was a hardned man and I never saw him show any feeling or sentiment of any kind, or regret anybody's death, but I verily believe he was very near dropping just one wee tear over Georgie's memory, for I noticed that his attention was needlessly and unwontedly fixed on the surface of the bottles he was washing. Be that as it may, Georgie was no more, and I FELT SURE THAT HE NEED NOT HAVE DIED, and this consciousness nearly pressed me down into the earth.

That evening a medical friend from the Royal Infirmary turned up to dinner with me, and I told him of my trouble and of my half determination to go to America and turn farmer: at least I should be able to lead a wholesome natural life.

He persuaded me to study Homoeopathy first, and refute it, or, if apparently true, to try it in the hospital.

After many doubts and fears—very much as if I were contemplating a crime—I procured Hughes' *Pharmacodynamics* and *Therapeutics*, which my friend said were a good introduction to Homoeopathy.

I mastered their main points in a week or two, and came from a consideration of these to the conclusion either that Homoeopathy was a very grand thing indeed, or this Dr. Hunghes must be a very big... No, the word is unparliamentary. You dont like the word—? Well, I do, it expresses my meaning to a T; on such an important subject there is for me no middle way. It must be either good clear Gods truth, or black lying. A fool the man could not possibly be, since it would be quite impossible for a fool to write the books. And as he seemed to speak so eloquently from a noble soul, it lifted me right out of the slough of despond—for a little while, but then came a reaction; had I not often tried vaunted specifics and plans of treatment, and been direfully disappointed? So my old scepsis took possession of me. "What," said I, "can such things be?" No, impossible. I had been nurtured in the schools, and had there been taught by good men and true that Homoeopathy was therapeutic Nihilism. No, I could not be a homoeopath; I would try the thing at the bedside, prove it to be a lying sham, and expose it to an admiring profession!

I was full of febricula on account of Georgie's fate, so studied the say of the homoeopaths thereon, and found that they claimed to cut short simple fever with *Aconite*. Ah, thought I, if that be true, *Aconite* would have saved little Georgie if given in time at the very onset.

Well, feverish colds and chills were common enough just then, and I had, moreover, a ward where children thus taken ill were put till their diseases had declared themselves, and they were drafted off to the various wards, for that purpose provided, with pneumonic, pleurisy, rheumatism, gastritis, measles, as the case might be.

I had some of Fleming's *Tincture of Aconite* in my surgery, and of this I put a few drops into a large bottle of water and gave it to the nurse of said childrens ward, with instructions to administer of it to all the cases of the one side of the ward as soon as they were brought in. Those on the other side were not to have the Aconitic solution, but were to be treated in the authorized orthodox way, as was theretofore customary. At my next morning visit I found nearly all the youngsters on the *Aconite* side feverless, and mostly at play in their beds. But one had the measles, and had to be sent to the proper ward. I found *Aconite* did not cure measles. The others remained a day or two, and were then returned whence they had originally come.

Those on the non-*Aconite* orthodox side were worse, or about the same and had to be sent into hospital—mostly with localized inflammations, or catarrhs, measles, etc.

And so it went on day after day, day after day those that got *Aconite* were generally convalescent in twenty four or forty-eight hours, except in the comparatively seldom cases where the seemingly simple chill was the prodromal stage of a specific disease such as measles, scarlatina, rheumatic fever: these were barely influenced by the *Aconite*. But the great bulk of the cases were all genuine chills, and the *Aconite* cured the greater part right off, though the little folks were usually pale, and had perspired, as I subsequently learned, needlessly much.

I had told the nurse nothing about the contents of my big bottle, but she soon baptized it" Dr. Burnett's Fever Bottle."

For a little while I was simply dumbfounded, and I spent much of my nights studying Homoeopathy : I had no time during the day.

One day I was unable to go my usual rounds through the wards; in fact, I think I was absent two days — from Saturday till Tuesday — and on entering the said children's ward the next time in the early morning, the nurse seemed rather quiet, and informed me, with a certain forced dutifulness that all the cases might, she thought, be dismissed.

" Indeed," said I, "how's that?"

"Well, doctor, as you did not come round on Sunday and yesterday, I gave your fever medicine to them all; and indeed, I had not the heart to see you go on with your cruel experiments any longer: you are like all the young doctors that come here—you are only trying experiments!"

I merely said "Very well, nurse; give the medicine in future to all that come in." This was done till I left the place, and the result of this *Aconite* medication for chills and febricula was usually rapid defervescence, followed by convalescence. But when the stomach was much involved, I at times found the *Aconite* useless, unless vomiting occurred, and so in such case I administered a mild emetic, whereupon defervescence at once set in, and, though a homoeopath now for a good many years, I still think a mild emetic the right treatment when the stomach is laden and cannot unburden itself by natural vomit.

But still this is only by the way : I enter into all these preliminary, incidental and concomitant circumstances merely to put you on the same ground whereon I myself stand; they are not essential, for they only lead to this: *Aconitum* in febricula was, and is, my first reason for being a homoeopath.

Have you as good a reason for being a "regular" ?

2. When I was a lad I had pleurisy of the left side, and, with the help of a village apothecary, and half-a-hogshead of mixture, nearly died, though not quite. From that time on I had a dull, uneasy sensation in my side, about which I consulted many eminent physicians in various parts of Europe, but no one could help me. All agreed that it was an old adhesive something between the visceral and costal layers of the pleura, *but no one of my many eminent advisers could cure it*. And yet my faith in them was big enough to remove mountains. So faith as a remedy did no good.

When orthodox medicine proved unhelpful, I went to the hydropaths (they were called "quacks" then !) and had it hot, and cold, and long; but they also did me no good. Packs cold, and the reverse; cold compresses worn for months together; sleeping in wet sheets; no end of sweatings—Turkish and Russian—all left my old pleuritic trouble in *status quo ante*.

The grape cure; the bread-and-wine cure, did no better. Nor did diet and change help me.

However, when I was studying what the peculiar people called homoeopaths have to say about their *Bryonia alba*, and its affinity for serous membranes, I — what ? — abused them and called them quacks? No! — I bought some *Bryonia alba*, and took it as they recommended, and in a fortnight my side was well, and has never troubled me since !

He had his first lessons in homoeopathy from reading Dr. Hughes' two books - *Manual of Pharmacodynamics* and *Manual of Therapeutics*. For clinical study, he got the opportunity when he moved to Chester near Liverpool, and could attend the clinic of Dr John Drysdale.

## Dr Burnett's Contemporaries

The professional contemporaries of Dr Burnett in England included Richard Hughes, Alfred Hawkes, J Drysdale, RE Dudgeon, JP Dake, AC Pope, J H Clarke and RT Cooper.

Richard Hughes was the more towering among these. At that time, as always the homoeopathic profession was split into two factions. Of the two, one came to be led by Burnett with his group of friends including Clarke, the other by the more influential Richard Hughes. Burnett had learnt his first lessons in homoeopathy from the two books of Hughes, *A Manual of Pharmacodynamics* which Burnett called "homoeopathic milk for allopathic babes" and *A Manual of Therapeutics*. Hughes believed in the totality of symptons as a primary rule of homoeopathy but his whole outlook was dominated by a concern to make homoeopathy more acceptable to the allopathic physicians. With this end in view, and under the auspices of the British Homoeopathic Society and the American Institute of Homoeopathy, Hughes undertook to rewrite the Homoeopathic Materia Medica, limiting the proved symptoms to those which were elicited by medicines not beyond the 6th potency, and further those which were elicited from not less than two provers. Again clinical symptoms (which were confirmations of the efficacy of the drug in patients, yet not appearing in the provings) were completely eliminated and symptoms observed in toxicological and poisoning from the drugs were specially included. In other words, it was meant to be a sort of a physiological Materia Medica and was called *A Cyclopaedia of Drug Pathogenesy*. With the assistance of some of the contemporaries named above, and other American counterparts, it was completed in 4 volumes. Burnett denounced this outlook and strategy as timidly conventional and dangerously restricted.

Dr J H Clarke first became attracted to Dr Hughes. In fact Hughes appointed him as Assistant Editor of the *British Journal of Homoeopathy*. But in the course of two years, Clarke went over to the side of Burnett and became one of his greatest admirers. He was the one who wrote the *Life and Work of Dr James Compton Burnett* soon after Burnett's death. Just six months earlier in 1900, Clarke had completed and published his *Dictionary of Practical Materia Medica* in three volumes. It is ironic that while the much toted scientific works of Dr Hughes including his *Cyclopaedia of Drug Pathogeney* have gone into oblivion, Clarke's Dictionary is one of the most popular reference books extant today in the homoeopathic world, and Burnetts anecdotal tracts and booklets are still encountered on bookshelves.

As has been mentioned earlier, Alfred Hawkes was the friend who introduced homoeopathy to Dr. Burnett. He along with Dr Clarke and Dr Burnett attended the clinic of Dr Drysdale at Liverpool. It was to him that Burnett dedicated his *tour de force, Homoeopathic Treatment or Fifty Reasons for Being a Homoeopath*.

Dr John Drysdale of Liverpool was the Founder Editor of the *British Journal of Homoeopathy*. When Burnett started attending his clinic, Drysdale was in his late fifties. He had qualified at Edinburgh and had spent many years in medical schools in the continent before settling in Liverpool. He was instrumental in founding the Liverpool Homoeopathic Society and his clinic attraced a group of many enthusiastic homoeopathic including J H Clarke and Alfred Hawkes.

## Cooper Club

Dr Burnett, Dr Clarke, Dr Robert Cooper and Dr Thomas Skinner formed a group and they used to meet in a dining club on week day evenings in London to discuss the problems of therapeutics and medical politics. The group became known as the Cooper Club. When Dr Clarke wrote his *Dictionary of Homoeopathic Materia Medica*, he incorporated the conclusions of the discussions held in the Club meetings in his own books. The abbreviations "B" and "RTC" used as references in some of the symptoms recorded by Clarke refer to Burnett and RT Cooper. Clarke's *Dictionary* therefore clarified some of the points made in Burnett's books. In fact as Francis Treuherz pointed out in one of his articles, some of Burnett's one liners finished up in Clarke's *Clinical Repertory*.

**Contribution to Homoeopathy**

Homoeopaths in Britain were a small persecuted sect, generally looked down upon by the orthodox medicine. Doctors and eminent patients shunned any connections with homoeopathy. Professional medical associations of the orthodox medicine specifically prohibited their members to consult with, or, even to meet socially, homoeopathic practitioners. The allopathic chemists refused to stock and dispense homoeopathic medicines or even to sell homoeopathic literature. In the face of such hostile conditions, Dr Burnetts decision to go over to homoeopathy was a brave one indeed. He knew the adversities and disparities he would have to contend with, for he wrote, "the social value of surgery is a baronetcy, the social value of homoeopathy is slander and contempt".

Far from being an apologetic adherent to homoeopathy, Burnett was quite aggressive, pugnacious and often acerbic.

In the very first issue of the *Homoeopathic World* under his editorship, he held forth a tirade against the medical establishment and wrote, "We are free men and we refuse to allow our right to free thought and free action, to be trampled under foot by any earthly powers whatsoever. It is useless to prate about peace, there is no peace but the peace of the manacled and the fettered."

He waged a regular war with the *Lancet*. "The Egyptians worship their leeks and onions, in fact grew their gods in their own gardens, and British surgeons worship their *Lancet*, of course bound by their religious vows."

Burnett struck an original line of therapeutics in homoeopathy which he called *organopathy*, and registered signal success through it. Many other practitioners have followed in his trail and this line of treatment is still around a hundred years after his death. He made a number of provings like *Bacillinum, Cundurango, Ceanothus*, etc. and added clinical symptoms of many others like *Jaborandi, Juglans Cinerea, Quercus, Levico, Brassica Murialic, Bursa Pastoris, Urtica Urens*, etc. A very large number of such remedies used by him successfully are still in vogue in the hands of homoeopathic practitioners throughtout the world and are credited with success.

He was also one of the first to stress the importance of nosodes, beginning with his own *Bacillinum*. He was a man of vision and by the sheer theoretical reasoning based on his insight into anatomy and physiology, he was able to make inroads in the treatment of such congenital diseased conditions as harelip, cleft palate, and again problems like cataract, etc. In this way, he showed a new line of research which however has not been followed up by his successors.

Not the least of his contributions are his writings in the form of his articles published in medical and homoeopathic journals of his time, and as an Editor of the *Homoeopathic World* and the 26 books which he wrote.

However in his crusade against the allopathic way, Dr Burnett had no misgivings about the odds he was fighting against. He chose the following words from Bolingbroke (King Henry IV) for inscription as an epigraph on the inner title page of his book *Homoeopathic Treatment or 50 Reasons for Being a Homoeopath*.

"It may sound oddly, but it is true, in many cases, that if men had learned less, their way to knowledge would be shorter and easier. It is indeed shorter and easier to proceed from ignorance to knowledge than from error. They who are in the last must unlearn before they can learn to any good purpose; and the first parts of this double task is not, in many respects, the least difficult; for which reason it is seldom undertaken."

**Homoeopathic Treatment or Fifty Reasons for Being a Homoeopathy**

By the nature of the special creed, homoeopathy and homoeopaths have always been on the defensive. All apostles of homoeopathy, following Hahnemann, have made affirmations of their faith by epistemological writings of their credo. It has almost been a liturgical exercise on their part. Burnetts contribution was *Homoeopathic Treatment or Fifty Reasons for Being a Homoeopath*. It came about this way. There was a Member of British parlimament, a patron of homoeopathy and a friend of Dr Burnett whose nephew had recently graduated in medicine. The uncle wanted to convince the youngman about the virtues of this science and arranged a dinner for the three for this purpose. The young doctor was brash enough to call Burnett a quack. Dr Burnett was stung to the quick and took upon himself to rebut the charge. He wrote out 50 letters to the youngman as a series of arguments, which were later on compiled in a book form and called *Homoeopathic Treatment or Fifty Reasons for Being a Homoeopath*. The book is a delectable assortment of cases ( a few being repetitions from his other published works) duly included in Part III of this book, except the first two which have been cited above in this writeup. Although these and other cases seem dated by todays sophisticated parlance, these were indeed bold and masterly strokes of argument at that time.

This one book sums up and exemplifies many of the traits of Dr Burnett's personality. his style of writing and the large affluent clientele in his practice.

**Burnett's Success as a Homoeopath**

From his own reading and perhaps by intuition, Burnett based his homoeopathic practice on a different and individual line which he called *organopathy*. He was however very clear and unambiguous and honestly convinced about the correctness of his stand *vis-a-vis* classical homoeopathy. He has explained his stand and principles many times in his books.

*"I would summarize the whole thing thus : Where the organ-ailing is primary to the organ, use organ remedies in little material doses frequently repeated; where the organ-ailing is of piece pathologically with that of the organism, use the homoeopathic simillimum in high potency infrequently repeated."*

*"I do not regard organopathy as something outside of homoeopathy, but as being embraced by and included in it, though not identical or co-extensive with it. I would say — Organopathy is homoeopathy in the first degree. And finally, I would emphasize the fact that where the homoeopathic simillimal agent covering the totality of the symptoms, and also the underlying pathologic process causing such symptoms, can be found, there organopathy either has no raison d'etre at all, or it is of only temporary service to ease an organ in distress."*

*"Finally, I am very far from supposing that in the vast majority of cases, an organ disease exists primarily and permanently by itself independently of the organism; on the contrary, I know well from close observation of nature that the part and the whole are commonly qualitatively the same."*

He was the chief proponent and pioneer exponent of this form of homoeopathy which can be termed as specific therapy. Many others have since followed in his trail with great success. Till date, this form of homoeopathic treatment is quite popular, even amongst the elite practitioners who when finding it quite difficult to arrive at the simillimum and its uncertainty in the course of treatment often resort to adjustments in the form of the organ remedies. Burnett was however quite clear about the value of classical homoeopathy and the limitations of his organ remedies. He likened the utilisation of subjective symptoms for arriving at the prescription to the reading of a text by spelling out each word. For instance, if we have to read the text, "the quick brown fox jumps over the lazy little dog" and we do it by loudly spelling out each word, letter by letter, such as T-H-E the, Q-U-I-C-K quick and so on, it would obviously be very tedious as well as tardy and not perhaps leading to a meaningful result in any way, he argued.

"This is true always in the use of organ-remedies for organ-diseases; unless the ailment is primary to the organ acted upon by the organ-remedy, we only attain transitory relief."

Although many of his cases took a lot of time, from three to four years of treatment, his specific therapy did a lot of good to the patients. It will be seen that he took up mostly those cases which are generally considered beyond the reach of medicine or which are considered purely surgical. For instance, Cataract, Fistula, Gout, Tumours, Stunted children, enlarged Tonsils, Consumption (at that time there were no antibiotics), harelip, cleft palate etc. He maintained a meticulous record of all his cases and his books mirror his therapeutic skills in his clinical practice almost in entirety. No other practitioner has done that. Even in Hahnemann's writings, there are barely about 10 to 12 case records published so far.

To crown it all, with his detailed knowledge of human anatomy and physiology, and without the aid of subsequently invented, diagnostic tests, he was a diagnostician par excellence.

# LIST OF BURNETT'S BOOKS

The list of his books with the year of first publication is as under :

1. 1879-1885 : Editor, The Homoeopathic World.
2. 1878 : Natrum Muriaticum; as test of the Doctrine of Drug Dynamisation.
3. 1879 : Gold as a Remedy in Disease.
4. 1880 : On the Prevention of Hare-lip, Cleftpalate, and other Congenital Defects.
5. 1880 : Ecce Medicus, or Hahneman as a Man and as a Physician and the Lessons of his Life.
6. 1880 : Curability of Cataract with Medicines.
7. 1880 : Diseases of the Veins.
8. 1882 : Supersalinity of the Blood; an Accelerator of Senility and Cause of Cataract.
9. 1882 : Valvular Disease of the Heart.
10. 1886 : Diseases of the Skin.
11. 1887 : Diseases of the Spleen.
12. 1888 : Fifty Reasons for being a Homoeopath.
13. 1888 : Fevers and Blood Poisoning, and their Treatment, with Special Reference to the Use of Pyrogenium.
14. 1888 : Tumours of the Breast.
15. 1889 : Neuralgia, its causes and its remedies.
16. 1889 : Cataract : Nature, Causes and cure.
17. 1890 : Five Years (Later Edition, Eight Years) Experience in the Crue of Consumption by its own Virus (Bacillinum).
18. 1890 : On Fistula, and its Cure by Medicines.
19. 1891 : Greater Diseases of the Liver.
20. 1892 : Ringworm, Constitutional Nature and Cure.
21. 1892 : Vaccinosis and its Cure by Thuja; with remarks on Homoeoprophylaxis.
22. 1893 : Curability of Tumours by Medicines.
23. 1895 : Gout and its Cure.
24. 1895 : Delicate, Backward, Puny and Stunted Children.
25. 1896 : Organ Diseases of Women.
26. 1898 : The Change of Life in Women, and the Ills and Ailings Incident Thereto.
27. 1901 : Enlarged Tonsils Cured by Medicines.

It may be mentioned that No. 5 of the above list, "Ecce Medicus" constituted Dr. Burnett's Hahnemann Oration for the year 1880. This was during the active career of a London School of Homoeoapthy, Dr. Burnett holding for a brief period the lecturership of Materia Medica in succession to Dr. Hughes.

# THUS SPAKE BURNETT

Burnett was quite aware of the many thorny problems besetting the corpus of homoeopathy, not a few of which are still around. His views regarding many such questions sound refreshingly modern, besides being insightful and prophetic in some ways. He was a master of the English expression and used it to good advantage. That he was incisive and acerbic is quite understandable considering the times and the hositility which homoeopathy has had the honour to live with all along. Infrequently, we come across sparrks of his wit and wisdom and irony in his writings. He called the allopaths "our friends, the enemy".

## Medicine and Surgery

Knife-men — our surgical carpenters are waxing bolder and bolder every day, and the very excellences of aseptic and anaesthetic surgery are fast running legitimate medicine to the ground and with it our common humanity.

Years ago, I was the means of converting an allopathic medical man to Homoeopathy; he came over bag and baggage at considerable pecuniary loss; he subsequently caught the itch, and placed himself under my care, and he remained faithfully under my care for over a year, and I totally failed to cure him, whereupon he exclaimed to me, "I cannot stand it any longer, I shall go mad; look what an awful state I am in." He then gave up Homoeopathy and everything connected with it.

The lady was, however, very patient, and went on with my treatmentt, feeding principally on hope; but hope, though not a bad auxilliary, is no remedy for tumours or skin diseases.

## The Ideal Medicine

My ideal of medicine is rather that which tends to its own elimination, i.e., the more it advances, the nearer it comes to its own destruction, and hence, preventive should have the highest rank.

I do not hold it to be right to try experiments from mere curiosity.

Perfection is unattainable except in effort, and finality is ultramundane.

The limits of the curable and of the incurable are not represented by any fixed lines; what is incurable today may be curable tomorrow, and what we all of this generation deem incurable may be considered very amenable to treatment in the next generation.

## Psora

The psora of the homoeopaths seems somehow true, but it has no proper beginning, no definite course, and ends in pathological chaos.

Have I then hit upon a solution of the psora-problem, No; but if we cannot break the whole faggot, we may per chance break one stick of it.

## Scabies

You cannot cure the itch by dynamic medication, and you must therefore kill the acari; they should be killed on the spot, the sooner the better; you cannot kill acari with dynamic remedies, and they should be killed at once.

## Douches

I hold very strong opinions on the question of intro-vaginal injections; they are altogether damnable and pernicious, shallow in conception, wrong in theory, and harmful in practice.

## Potencies

The degree of homoeopathicity conditions the degree of potency, the greater the degree of homoeopathicity the greater (higher) the potency and conversely.

Giving crude drugs does not necessarily exclude homoeopathicity of drug to disease, and the mere fact of giving high dilutions never was Homoeopathy and never will be. Hahnemann was an omnidilutionist, and gave low dilutions, although it is quite true that he subsequently gave much higher dilutions the preference.

I find myself often unable to cure simple organ diseases with dilutions; but I also find myself unable to cure the great constitutional diseases with organ remedies, and from very close observation, and not a little experience, I maintain that the organopathy of Rademacher (i.e., of Paracelsus) is just elementary homoeopathy, the degree of similitude being very small, wherefore small material doses are needed in fairly frequent repetition. As the degree of similitude increases so must the dose of the remedy be lessened.

## Pathological and Homoeopathy

The future of medicine — belongs to homoeopathic pathologists, and to really cure the great diseases (with a pathologicao-anatomical basis) we MUST HAVE remedies homoeopathic to such morbid anatomy, at any rate in its earlier stages.

## Nosodes

That zoic remedies constitute the field of promise, for the further development of progressive scientific homoeopathy, I am beginning clearly to see, though only through the gate ajar, but I live in hope of more light.

## Correlating Skin Diseases with Internal Diseases

In the near future, I hope we may have some definite conception of the correspondences that undoubtedly exist between certain regions of the body surface and the internal organs, independently of general organismic interdependence, and then we shall, perhaps, be able to see why certain cutaneous diseases affect certain parts preferntially, and also why, when these diseases are driven in whence they came, by external means, certain internal organs have to bear the brunt of it.

## Rheumatism and Tonsils

The statement that rheumatic fever has been known to follow tonsilitis — that is true enough. The inference usually drawn is that had there been no tonsils there would have been no rheumatic fever. I read the phenomena the other way. Had the tonsils been stronger and more adequate, they would have borne the whole burden of the rheumatism, and there would have been no fever. It is highly probable that minor degrees of rheumatism are arrested by the tonsils, and there dealt with, and that their function is very largely vicarious, protective of the organism and its parts.

## Rabies and Sexual Mania

The sufferings of the celibate state, notably in women, are at times amenable to the benign influence of lyssinum and to this I was partly led by a consideration of the prime cause of rabies, viz., pent-up sexual longings.

## Neurosis

Probably few practitioners of experience will deny that we are living in an age of neurosis, where neuralgia is becoming more and more prevalent, and I am strongly of opinion that tea, coffee, tobacco, alcohol, wear and tear and worry, are essential causal factors.

## Cancer and Insanity

I have come to the conclusion, from a good many observations and therapeutic trials, that genuine insanity is cancer of mind. By cancer of mind, I mean simply that if the ailing fix upon, say, the breast, we have simply cancer of the breast, whereas if it fix upon mind organ, we have what we commonly call insanity.

(A century after Burnett wrote this, a modern radiation oncologist and therapist, Dr Carl Simonton, has this to say, "The role of illness as "problem solver" has been a major insight for me. People often find it impossible to resolve stressful problems in a healthy way and therefore choose, consciously or unconsciously to get sick as a way out. What intrigues me about mental illness is that most mental illnesses tend to exclude malignancy. For instance, it is essentially unheard of for catatonic schizophrenic to develop cancer. A person may develop cancer or catatonic schizophrenia but wont do both.... They are mutually exclusive." The **Uncommon Wisdom** by *Fritjof Capra*)

### Burnett and Hahnemann

*It is bemusing to notice that the life courses of both Burnett and Hahnemann resembled in some points. Both came from a comparatively poorer background. Hahnemann was the son of a porcelain painter, Burnett son of a farm-labourer. Both had flair for languages. Hahnemann was a linguist, well-versed in a number of languages including Greek and Latin. Burnett also had love of language and early in his life toyed with the idea of becoming a phisiologist. He was well-versed in German and French which he learnt at first hand during the years of his stay in the continent. Hahnemann scoured extensively into the medical literature of his predecesors, Burnett read specially Rademacher and Paracelsus and professed to have based his particular approach to homoeopathy termed organopathy on the teachings and principles of these two masters. Both Hahnemann and Burnett studied medicine at Vienna. The first theses for M.D. in both cases were rejected by the University authorities because of their being pro-homoeopathy. Both married twice, both being happy in their second marriage. Both had their successful practice, Hahnemann in his old age, Burnett from very early years of his practice. Both were staunch and forthright in championing the cause of homoeopathy and specially harsh on pseudo-homoeopaths.*

# Indices to Sub-entries

## Part I — Observations : General and Clinical

Page

## Part II — Materia Medica Notes and Therapeutics

# Part III — Case Reports

**Reference Code**

References at the end of excerpts, including case-reports, are cited in Roman and Arabic figures : the first indicates title of the book listed against it as per the above list, the second i.e. figure in Arabic denotes the page number of that book.

For instance, the first paragraph on page 11 of this compilation, with the caption, Child - Bearing No Disease has the reference (XXIV 5) cited at the end. This means that this extract has been taken from page 5 of the book, "The Change of Life in Women" listed at serial No XXIV of the above list.

Available books of Burnett are in various page sizes, printed by off-set process in India from out of the original publications. References to page numbers have been listed on *as-is-where-is* basis.

Part I

# Observations : General and Clinical

## Acute Diseases — Sequelae

Now the effect of acute diseases on the economy are known to last a very long time; how long does not appear to be determinable. (XX 215)

## Allopathy

Allopathy is in an advanced stage of senile decay, from which there is no recovery, and the sooner the general break-up comes, the better for mankind. (XXII 78)

### Allopathic Poachings

Our friends, the enemy, can never rise to the height of our simple therapeutic law, and yet the crumbs that fall from our table the greatest of them do not disdain. (XIV 120)

### Allopathic Practice and Homoeopathy

Now, the fates are distinctly unkind to our allopathic friends who had begun to score one by their cure of myxoedema with thyroid glands added to the food of the sufferers : the place of the atrophied thyroid being supplied by the thyroid food, and here comes experimental science and shews that the thyroid feeding in the long run contingently produces atrophy and not only atrophy, but complete atrophy of the healthy parts of the thyroid gland. So that in future the dose of the thyroid extract must be lessened because this new therapeutic acquisition of allopathy over which we homoeopaths had certainly become not a little jealous, is after all not only pure homoeopathy but its symptomatic and pathologic homoeopathicity is demonstrated already for us in their own laboratories. Now our allopathic friends must do as they did in regard to tuberculinum , *viz* : admit the efficacy of small doses and with it the truth of the homoeopathic law, or officially drop the thyroid business, as they did with tuberculinum.(XVII 14)

## Anaemia — Vaccinosis and Gonorrhoea

Beyond any question there is a form of leucocytosis that is surely and rapidly cured by iron, a remedy which the Paracelsists considered *universal, i.e.,* affecting that which is common to the whole economy (the microcosm), and not having any particular affinity for any one of the organs of the body above another. It follows, therefore, that from Hohenheim's standpoint iron would be no remedy for leucocythaemia splenica unless the disease was one of the entire organism (or its blood), and, indeed, iron is no remedy in leucocythaemia splenica; and regard the therapeutic uselessness of iron in a bad form of anaemia as a first step to diagnostic differentiation of the *kind* of leucocytosis one is dealing with. Nevertheless, good authorities claim that iron will reduce the spleen, but this may be by reason of its unquestioned action on blood. I have found it of considerable therapeutic advantage to regard leucocythaemia as being causally connected (often - remotely) with vaccinosis and gonorrhoea — to me a great clinical fact, but on which I have here nothing further to say. And, indeed, *cui bono?* The world that would not listen to Autenrieth, Hahnemann, Grauvogl, Wolff, H. Goullon, and others, would also not listen to me.
Well, we can wait; and since the spleen, on which I have been here already too discursive, is the *organon risus* of the ancients, I must keep my own funcionally intact. (X 63)

## Angina — Fag and Shock

The Modes of Thought in Therapeutics : The modes of thought in medicine are very important, as they condition the mode of treatment :

those who think surgically treat surgically, even when they administer drugs. We are taught to regard angina as a pure neuralgia, or as a spasm, or as having atheroma of the coronary artery, and all three.
Fag is a potent factor in angina, and so is wounded pride and nerve shock. Not infrequently, fag and shock combine to produce it. Take the case of the late Sir Morton Peto, who did great things and many, and lived to be wounded to the quick in his pride as a financial giant : he had angina pectoris from the two factors combined. (XIV 166)

**Angina Pectoris**

But angina pectoris can but rarely be cured with one remedy; there is often a constitutional taint lying behind and beyond the cardiac symptoms. (II 119)

One can hardly have to deal with a more formidable affection than *Angina pectoris*, and in its treatment Homoeopathy can do great things. It is, however, a mighty mistake to treat the cases all alike, as quite a number of different diseases give rise to the usual anginal symptoms; the cases must be diagnostically and therapeutically differentiated if they are to be really *cured*.(XI 68)

Angina pectoris is much more frequent in men than in women — at least that is my experience. In women, it is often from oligohaemia, and only occasionally from psychic cause, though a priori one would expect the very reverse to be the case; tear-shedding (blessed gift!), I believe, prevents it. That grief-tears are very poisonous appears pretty certain. "Dry" grief is justly in evil repute. The commoner case of angina pectoris in women seem allied to asthma, or are synalgias from disturbances in the liver, stomach, or spleen.

Angina pectoris is mostly met with in its severer forms in men of doughty deeds and power, as it were as the physical impress of their deed-rich lives. Luther suffered from angina pectoris, and no wonder. Athletes are apt to get it in later life : this is about equal to chronic traumatism, but acute traumatism will also cause it. Hence, it is that *Arnica montana* and *Bellis perennis* are so frequently indicated in its treatment, where the trauma has not set up an actual lesion. The anti-traumatics are a very real help, and so is *Aconite*.

When the heart itself and the great blood vessels have been duly considered, the abdominal organs immediately under the diaphragm should be critically mustered, for they very often encroach upon the heart's playroom (liver, spleen, distended stomach, and duodenum), and in such cases it is manifestly useless to treat the heart itself, because it may be quite equal to the work normally required of it when there is no obstruction, but yet cries out in agony when obsturctions under the diaphragm are superadded. Just as a horse may be equal to dragging a heavily laden wagon along a smooth road, but put a stone or a brickbat before one of the wheels and the case is altered.

"When I walk or hurry, particularly after a meal," causes us to think of the heart as a muscular pump, and to wonder whether the pump-organ is itself at fault, or its valves, or the suction-force, or whether there is any obstruction in the way. When this is done with a little care and thought and circumspection, we become aware that though angina pectoris is often purely a neuralgia cordis, yet it is at least as often a synalgia, having its starting point in obstructions. And here it must be manifested that the therapeutic indication is to get rid of the obstruction. Hepatics, pancreatics, and splenics here come into play with immense advantage. Of course, an ideal master in therapeutics, who can spot the *simillimum* to the entire case, will not need these little organopathic side helps; but, speaking for myself, I cannot do without them : they help me, and I praise them. Organ interacts with the organism as its environment, besides having its life in common with the organism. Else I cannot understand why it is that a given organ will go on, so to speak, jibbing and kicking till the appropriate organ remedy has been given, after which the organ will jog along happily and comfortably, and will then react to systemic remedies which before were without effect. This view of individual life of each organ has received a very remarkable corroboration from the researches of Brown-Sequard, as also by the latest teachings of physiology in regard to the use of the thyroid. When angina pectoris is due to organic change in the heart's own substance or in its own arteries, metals and minerals will come into play, such as *Aurum*, *Mercurius*, *Vanadium*, *Arsenicum*, *Phosphorus*, etc. Where the circulation has become impossible of being adequate, I have made three or four very remarkable cures, the most striking of which I will now shortly relate as perhaps unique.(XIV 148)

## Assessment in Private Practice

This is the usual thing. People will not be at the trouble of seeing the doctor as soon as they are better, they seem not to understand any interest one feels in the case. We can only make periodical reliable examinations of patients in a hospital; in private practice it is extremely difficult, as all practitioners know to their chagrin. (X 18)

## Biochemistry

However, I would not appear to be ungrateful to friend Schussler for I have learned much from his writings, beginning at the time when he was — what I think he still cannot help being — Schusslerism notwithstanding — a homoeopath! His work confirms my long since formed opinion that heresy and schism are the grandest means of human progress, and, when the prayer against these comes in, I commonly remain — silent! (XX 99)

## Blood Count

By the way not so long ago, they were very great at blood-corpuscle counting in splenic tumefaction; strange to say that also did not cure anybody, and the blood-cell counting is going ... out of fashion; in fact is almost as much out of date as the crinoline. (XX 221)

## Breast Feeding and Mother's Health

Personally, were I a woman with a baby, I would suckle it from purely selfish motives, merely to departure my own blood and organism, for woman who has a family and does not suckle her offspring, is drawing a bill on the future of her organism which she is likely to be either unable to meet at all or to do so with great difficulty. Mother Nature suffers no tampering with her provisions; with her it simply and emphatically, Obey; or suffer disease or extinction. (XIII 43)

## Cancer — Medicinal Approach

Very notable surgeons, fellows of the Royal Society, and others are at times condescendingly hopeful that we look forward to the day when "a remedy for cancer will be discovered." Whatever knowledge such people possess, or do not possess, there are two things of which they know nothing real, *viz.*, cancer, and the modes of action of remedies in cancer and cancerous diseases. (XX 285)

You might as well try to grow potatoes in a field consisting of one chemical element instead of ordinary humus; or live in the hope of some day being able to win a long and very difficult game of chess by making "one" move all by itself.

This running after a remedy for any disease of complex nature is simple ignorance of fundamental principles and bars the road of progress. (XX 286)

Cancer is a chain of links, and each kind has links of different nature and each link is a biological process. And you are going to alter all that with "a" remedy? It is absolutely unthinkable, and has no parallel in physio-biological phenomena. (XX 287)

## Case Taking — The Last Expressions

Just as postscripts are said to contain the real *raison d'etre* of a given epistle, so the parting observation of a patient often throws a strong light on a case. (IX 99)

## Cataract — Aetiology

But, leaving for the present the origin of the capsule undecided, we are in no doubt of the epidermoid nature of the lens, and also in no doubt of the endothelial nature of the intercapsular cells.

From which we may deduce the general statement that the drugs that affect the epidermis and epithelial structures specifically will also be our remedies in some of the abnormalities of the nutrition of the lens, and therefore in some forms of cataract.

From the *albuminous nature* of the lens we may deduce *the general statement that substances which in the living body enter into combination with the albumen to form albuminates, will likewise be remedies in certain forms of cataract.* (V 7)

**— Causes**

Some of the most frequent causes of cataract are, in my opinion, gout, rheumatism, rheumatic gout and syphilis, and here what benefits the gout or rheumatism will tend to better the cataract.

But my limits will not admit of my dealing with all the causes of cataract, and I therefore propose to confine myself more particularly to three that have hitherto been brought before the profession, and to which I attach very great importance. I refer to :

(a) Salt,
(b) Sugar, and
(c) Hard Water.

I have watched cataract cases with great care for some years, and I am perpared to maintain that the most frequent causes of cataract are the use of much *salt*, or of much *sugar*, or of *hard water*; very frequently we find all three causes operating at the same time in the same individual. (V 30)

**— Curability**

In a little monograph I have sought to defend the thesis that cataract can be often cured, and still oftener ameliorated, by the aid of medicines given internally. The bulk of the profession, of course, ignore the thing entirely. That I expected. A few of the more enlightened welcomed the little book as an honest attempt — as an imperfect, but solid beginning. Yet others shook their heads in good old-fashioned honest doubt, and muttered something about "mistaken diagnosis"; and this not without a chuckle at their own superior powers in this regard.

Since the publication of "Curability of Cataract with Medicines", I have continued my humble efforts in the same line, sneers and jibes notwithstanding. I have only treated a very few cases, partly because I do not care to begin unless a patient is willing, if necessary, to go on for a year or two, and this most of them decline.

It is wonder people are very incredulous about the possibility of modifying the stroma of an opaque lens; for it is indeed very difficult, and I fail myself but too often, yet by no means always, and I consider the future of the question very hopeful. (XI 50)

To me an opaque lens exising by itself in an otherwise healthy body is inconceivable, except from trauma, or from mal-development, or from obstructed nutrition; but given a normally developed lens, not mechanically or chemically injured, it cannot of itself become opaque unless from some other part of the organism. It is barely possible to have a sclerosis of the lens and a supple elastic condition of the other parts of the economy. In a word, the sclerotic change in the lens is of a piece with the state of the other tissues of the same individual at the same time.(V 29)

**Facts and Opinions concerning the Curability of Cataract from General Medical Literature** : I may begin by saying that the great mass of oculists utterly ridicule the idea of curing cataract with medicines; they nearly all forget that no number of negative facts can do away with one single positive fact. Moreover, they appear to ignore the very important point that they are incompetent to judge of the subject. Why? *Because they (as a rule) never try to cure cataract with medicines.* If they were to do this in a careful, persevering, scientific way, for a sufficient length of time, with a sufficient variety and number of cases, then they could give an opinion on the subject that would be worth having. But this they have not done. I give them all honour for their surgical knowledge and operative skill, but I cannot see what they can possibly know about the curability of cataract with medicines, since they do not try to cure it medicinally. That they should just give — *solatii causa* — a tonic, or a bitter, or a little mercury (or *much* of it for the matter of that!) or iodine, cannot reasonably be called a fair trial. (V 15)

*"We are, however, certain that by a careful selection of drugs according to the homoeopathic law, and by continuing the use for a long period, we may succeed, in a large proportion of cases, in checking the progress of the disease, and are enabled to clear up a portion of the diffuse haziness, thus improving vision to a certain extent.* But after degeneration of the lens fibres has taken place, no remedy will be found of avail in restoring its lost transparency and improving the sight. We must then - providing the vision is seriously impaired and it is senile or hard cataract - wait until it has become mature, when the lens should be extracted. (V 64)

**— A cutaneous affection**

Dr.Bernard also notes that in several of the cases, habitual perspiration reappears, or a cutaneous eruption either appears or reappears.

Need we any further proof that cataract is a *cutaneous* affection. (V 75)

**— Diabetes**

When a patient comes to you, and you find the lenses opaque, the skin dry, the quantity of urine excreted large, the thirst great, and the specific gravity of the urine much increased — say 1040 or 1045 — then you test the urine, and find it is full of sugar, you say your patient has diabetic character. (V 34)

**— Holistic Treatment**

"If, therefore, one part of the body is diseased, we must not direct our treatment to it solely, and use what is called local treatment alone. We must act on the whole constitution in the same way as we would direct our attention to the whole tree when it bears decayed fruit. In this case, and for this very simple reason, it is not only advisable, but necessary, to have internal treatment, and this way of attending to disease will prevent many a failure, and the harm which might ensue from local treatment. In a case of cataract, therefore, the whole constitution must be acted upon, as in all diseases. Our *Materia Medica* has many a remedy against such a state." (V 51)

**— Prevention**

The Prevention of Cataract : The above has doubtless already wearied you, and hence it is fortunate that what I have further to say may be epitomized in a few words. In view of these facts, I am in the habit of suggesting to persons suffering from cataract that they would do well to reduce their consumption of salt and salted provisions, as well as that of sugar, to a minimum, because both in excess can produce cataract. Also that hard *water* is to be equally avoided; and if *soft* water cannot be got, the expressed juices of succulent fruits in a fresh state can more than take its place. (V 37)

**— Salt**

When too much salt is ingested, the blood becomes supersaline; when the blood is supersaline, its specific gravity is raised, and the lens is deprived of its natural condition as a transparent body — in fact, it becomes opaque. If this condition of the blood continues for any lengthened period, the lens must necessarily degenerate, and the cataractous state becomes permanent. (V 33)

**— Sugar Consumption**

The diabetic cataract is not due to a primary disease of the lens; it is not due to the hepatic or neural lesion underlying the disease, known to us as diabetes; it is due to the presence of sugar in the blood of the diabetic patient.

When sugar is put into the circulation of animals, it produces cataract in just the same way as does the saccharine blood of the diabetic.

In like manner, when a person habitually partakes of sugar in considerable quantities, cataract may ensue as a direct physical effect thereof.

If you doubt this proposition, just question your cataract patients closely, and I believe you will soon come over to my view.

Of course, it is not maintained that every large sugar consumer must necessarily develop a cataract; no, but let a person with some morbid proclivity partake of a great deal of sugar as a general thing, and let a surplus of this ingested sugar course about in his blood for a lengthened period, then it must be obvious that such a person *must* suffer from *sugar poisoning;* the sugar in his blood *must* develop its physiological effects, one of which is the formation of cataract. (V 35)

## Cervical Glands and Surgery

This we see every day in regard to strumous glands in the necks of young children which it is the fashion to cut out "to save the constitution and prevent ugly scars." It does neither; but, on the contrary, tends to wreck the constitution, and the scars left by operations are worse than those from natural suppuration, in so far as they show more. And why? Because when these strumous glands are cut out there is loss of gland and of connective tissue, so that the environment of the gland sinks in, whereas when the gland suppurates naturally (under the influence of adequate constitutional treatment, be it remembered) there is hyperplasia of areolar tissue to fill up the gap, and in the end the scar is much less noticeable than that left by excision. (XXIII 142)

## Child Bearing No Disease

In my opinicn, it is very rare for a woman to die of child-bearing, though deaths in childbed are not uncommon; at any rate I have rarely known a woman die "of" childbed : in childbed, yes.

The most common causes of childbed mortality are certainly inflammation and haemorrhage.

Haemorrhage, is, most usually, due either to a consumptive taint of the individual expressed in the pelvic parts, or to other locally expressed diseases, and is no necessary part of child-bearing. That is to say, child-bearing is, in the normal and under healthy conditions, a healthy thing, fraught with absolutely no danger whatever to the parturient person, all danger is from the abnormal. A distinguished lady journlist wrote not long since that a woman "descended into the valley of the shadow of death in order to bear a child!"

What ineffable twaddle! (XXIV 5)

## Children — Delicate etc.

We say of certain children that they are delicate, backward, peculiar, odd, stunted, puny, and the like, without being able exactly to state what disease they are suffering from. The development of a given child receives a shock from a fall or fright; or its further growth is arrested by some acute disease, such as measles or influenza; or a child is glum, taciturn, excitable, or what not, and yet people hardly know what is wrong or how to set about putting the wrong right. Again, some children do not see, hear, or speak properly; or they are unclean in their habits, wet their clothes or their beds, and cannot be taught nice, sweet ways like their fellows. (XXII, Foreword)

### — Treatment

The ordinary treatment of delicate and backward children may be compared to sowing the seed in unprepared ground which is not scientific, and is also inadequate; whereas I advocate the plan of preparing the ground, of first putting the actual wrong right at the very start, so that thc particular state which causes us to affirm of a given child that he or she is delicate or backward, glum or excited, may disappear, and give place to the normal, so far as that may be possible in any given case.

I regard mental backwardnesses as of physical cause and origin, and I say that the *first step* to be taken is to alter this physical cause of the abnormality, and *then* to go on to the teaching; whereas the poor delicate or backward ones either lie hopelessly fallow, or are worried and crammed with what little they can take in, resulting often in but a poor return for all the trouble taken in their behalf. (XXII 2)

Cure the constitutional wrong as *soon* as possible, as thus growth comes AFTER the cure, and then natural growth may result in complete normality. For, when in the case of arrested or retarded development the hindrance is medicinally removed before growth is over, we get results veritably marvellous, as some of my herein narrated cases (Part III) will show.

The point bears reiterating. A given individual does not thrive because of a constitutional disease or taint blocking the way; now, remove the block by the right constitutional remedies, and then normal developmental power is restored, and said individual starts off growing, and the backwardnesses disappear. (XXII 6)

**— Glumness : A Taciturn Boy**

There is a certain type of child — more frequently boys than girls — who hang their heads and who will not willingly answer questions put to them, and who will not talk if they can help it. (XXII 44)

**— Treatment, Diet and Air**

The grandest results in the treatment of backward children are obtainable when the constitutional bars to physical and mental completion are medicinally removed, and THEN the full effects of food and air crown the edifice. I do not mean that food and fresh air are at any time unimportant, but what I do maintain is that disease taints in children are NOT curable by ANY AIR or ANY DIET whatever. The power of the organism to resist them may, however, be much increased.(XXII 65)

**— Incontinence of Urine Considered as Retarded Development**

For some time now I have regarded wetting the bed in children who have attained a certain age as retarded or arrested development about the sphincter region of the bladder. (XXII 122)

The question of bed-wetting in children is very much more important than the inexperienced might imagine; the unfortunate sufferers feel very much humiliated, and their moral tone is distinctly lowered by the habit. A few cases are very easily cured with almost any well-chosen remedy, but where the case withstands domestic allopathy, domestic homoeopathy, local allopathy, and local homoeopathy and consultants of all sorts (as in this case), it is best to take a wide aetiological survey of the case, and treat it as arrested or retarded development.(XXII 124)

**— Moral Obliquity in Children**

We are all too much disposed to regard moral deviations in children ( and in adults, too, for the matter of that) as something separate and apart from any physical basis.

What can minister to a mind diseased?

Remedies homoeopathically adapted to each individual case can.

How do I know?

Because I have done it myself any time and oft during the last twenty years.

And it is not even difficult, given a knowledge of homoeopathy and of pharmaco-dynamics, with a little knowledge of diagnostics and physiology. Of course, the more one knows the more one can do, as in all other branches of applied knowledge.

Most people one meets with in daily life can play at whist more or less — mostly less. There is whist and whist; likewise there is homoeopathy and homoeopathy.

The mental and moral balance in children when disturbed is *so disturbed mentally and physically,* and, if we keep this well before our minds, we can restore such disturbed balance just as readily as we can cure any other disease. (XXII 141)

**— Treatment Oil Massage**

As I have mostly used homoeopathic remedies as well as the inrubbings of sweet oil, it is not easy for me to *prove* that any good is derivable from such inrubbings; but I affirm from experience, that children of puny growth are much helped and improved in their development thereby.

In the case of twins it is very well-known that one of the twin is apt to be by much the smaller, and this wee one's hold of life is not grêat. It was once my lot to be called in to advise in regard to such a tiny mite, the stronger of the two being a fine specimen, and, in the opinion of the family doctor, fit to take its chance on the bottle, — the babies bottle, — a bottle, by the way , that claims *more* victims than that other bottle we know of. Well, I had a wet nurse

for my almost infinitesimal charge, and had him rubbed* with warm salad oil, and kept for long in old oiled flannel, and now he is a fine yongman, — so I am informed by his mother, though I have never since seen him, - - at present serving in the Cape Mounted Police. His strong twin brother died in infancy of marasm, as I am told on the same authority. Here I can ony affirm — I cannot prove — that the wee mite's life was saved by the wee rubbings of oil, though at first he was too weak to take the breast. (XXII 9)
At first it was really more dabbing than rubbing.

**— Treatment, Post-Natural Growth**

In my introductory remarks I have laid great stress on the desirability of beginning the curative treatment as early as possible; this needs no further insisting upon. But it is curious to note that in the case of blighted and arrested growth the *period of growth* seems pushed out rather than irretrievably gone by, — a certain amount of growth being possible even at middle life. This post-natural growth is presumably pent-up developmental power liberated by the treatment. Thus a patient of mine had hardly any beard on one side of his face, but a fair quantity on the other. After a course of treatment by me, the failing beard grew, although patient was past forty years of age. Evidently the *power to grow* was present all the time, but was, so to speak, locked up, much as we may suppose is the case with people's wisdom teeth, which come at such different ages that it is difficult to say when they are really due. (XXII 15)

## Chronic Diseases — Series of Medicines

From these considerations it is manifest that there are cases that cannot possibly be cured by one remedy and in as much as the symptoms form part respectively of groups of different causations, covering the totality of all the symptoms present in the patient would be a useless and fruitless task. Hence it is that Rademacherian organ-testing helps me so much in my every-day practical clinical life; for, if I cure an organ with its *Appropriatum Paracelsi,* and certain symptoms go while others remain I am enabled slowly to unravel the most complex groups of symptoms and finally find a simile or even the simillimum of the ground-evil.(XVII 63)

## Clinical Symptoms

For clinical purposes these experiments teach us too little; we require less acute cases not carried quite so far. For the pathology of the dead-house is not the pathology that we meet with at the bedside, any more than the pretty sights we see *en route* to Paris are those that delight us when we get there. (II 85)

## Congenital Defects and Diseases

I think it will be conceded that it is at least highly probable that the preventive treatment of congenital deformities and defects may be undertaken with good chances of success, and I venture to submit that this corner of the field of practical medicine is well worthy the attention and skill of all physicians, and also of all well-wishers of the race, lay as well as medical.

It will be of surpassing interest to the individuals and families more immediately interested, through having undesirable family proclivities. There is here great scope for the tissue remedies, especially when dynamized, as it is likely to be qualitatively changed nutritive building material that is required.

No doubt, the various cases of congenital defect and deformity differ essentially in their natures, and will require accordingly different remedial or preventive treatment.

This immense field lies fallow ready for the tilling talents of willing workers. (III 119)

## Constitutional Disease — Its Treatment

Where a case is of deep-going constitutional nature, it can only be cured by a series of remedies; and when the thing is cured, it is further of only historic interest. It is very difficult to say exactly how much of the curing was done by each separate medicine here. (XXV 39)

## Consumption — Conclusions

I will make a few brief remarks in the form of general explanatory propositions :

1. The virus of the consumptive process itself — here termed variously *the* virus, the bacillic virus, etc. — cures promptly the incipient stages of tubercular consumption in all parts — brain, lungs, skin, joints, etc.
2. The virus is to be administered by the mouth in what the homoeopaths call high potencies.
3. The doses must *not* be too frequently administered; one dose every sixth to tenth day is my own practical rule.
4. Low dilutions are inadmissible; myself I have never gone below the thirtieth centesimal potency, and as I have known even this to give rise to grave constitutional disturbances, I now very rarely go below the one-hundredth centesimal potency.
5. At a given stage of the consumptive process the virus is no longer a cure, but I have not been able to determine the precise stage at which it ceases to act curatively.
6. In as much as the disease which the virus cures is similar to the one producible by a full dose of the virus itself, it follows that the action is homoeopathic, and the remedy the homoeopathic pathologic simillimum of the to-be-cured disease.
7. Theoretically the stage at which the virus ceases to be of any use is, I think, where the disease has become aggressively-infective in quantity, or bulk, *and where homoeopathicity merges into identity.* Assuming that the bacilli at a given stage of the malady become in quantity aggressively infective, we can readily see that a dynamic simillimum must get, so to speak, swamped, and therefore become inoperative. Hence, if it is to cure it must act before the bacilli are numerous enough to get the mastery. Hence also it is not the chronicity or age of the consumption that determines our point, but the *degree of intensity*; a new case may be incurable by it, while a very old one may be quickly and completely cured by it.
8. The power of resistance of the organism in consumption is of the highest importance, as may be seen from the very numerous cures of consumption, wrought by very numerous medicines, by able men of all therapeutic views, by climate, by foods such as cod-liver oil, suet and milk, rum and milk, by calcifying remedies such as the salts of lime, by oil, frictions, etc., etc., and therefore the use of the bacillic virus excludes none of these, but on the contrary, the virus might become the remedy *after* other more or less helpful means,

even after it had been administered in vain previously. For if the body can be increased in healthy bulk, and the power of resistance of the organism augmented, the extreme point of the homoeopathic action of the virus would be pushed further out. (XVIA 118)

Let, therefore, the consumptive beware lest they undervalue the great helps of the past in the cure of consumption, which are the common property of all thoughtful medical men of all shades of views therapeutic, and not rush after the mad notion that *any* remedy can neutralize an unhealthy life or foul air, or counteract carping cares, or supply food and drink, or stamp out the footprints of the Nemesis of physical and psychic wrongs. (XVI 124)

**Consumptiveness and Consequences**

Persons with a strain in their constitutions are very prone to sunstroke, typhoid fever, and in later life to softening of the brain. (XXIII 127)

## Contraception — The Nemesis of Physical Wrong-doing

During the past twenty years the number of cases in which married women prevent conception is steadily on the increase; their many dodges in attaining this end need not be dwelt upon, but the almost uniform results are the following :

1. The breasts shrivel, and in extreme cases almost disappear : the erstwhile fine bust, the shapely breasts shrink into shocking ugliness.
2. The great female characteristics diminish, and the individual is apt to become hairy in the face and elsewhere, while the rotundity of limb is a thing of the past : the limbs are often scraggy and thin, or, if obese, flabby and old.
3. The nerves are greatly affected, there is almost always neurasthenia, and the once sweet woman becomes irritable and cross and miserable.
4. Spinal irritation is very common.
5. The uterus is the greatest sufferer of all: it has been cheated, and resents the wrong done to it with terrible vigour: it becomes enlarged, hard and gristly, and is not infrequently the seat of tumours

of various kinds. And no woman with such a womb is, or can be, other than miserable and discontented, and very frequently there is morning sickness analogous to that of pregnancy, with no end of other dyspeptic troubles. (XXIII 21)

"Be fruitful, and multiply, replenish the earth." This command may possibly be out-of-date, but this one thing I do know for very sure, that old Mother Nature wipes us all out without mercy when we disobey her laws: here, at any rate, the fittest survive. (XXIII 24)

In my judgment, a young woman who does not wish to bear a family should not get married at all. I know some goody-goody couples who are joined together, not in holy wedlock at all, but . . . "We live, and always have lived ever since our marriage, just like brother and sister." Some of them teach in the Sunday School, and do what they are pleased to call "the work of the Lord," particularly when it is taking the chair, or otherwise or elsewhere, but anyway always to the fore. Child-bearing and home duties are shirked by these unwholesome byproducts of civilization. They have their reward: Nature wipes them out herself, and labels them for the ultimate sorting, "Depart from me, I know ye not." (XXIII 26)

## Convincing the Unconvinced

The frankness and honesty of one's allopathic colleagues are wonderful articles. However, they have, as usual, had to munch the leek. Their great pity is that so much energy should be used up by us medical reformers merely to keep on our feet. We boast a good deal of our advanced state of culture and civilisation, but will some one explain to me how it is that many of even the most wonderfully cultured and most highly educated people of the day seem absolutely incapable of differentiating between self-denying, not to say heroic, medical reformers and persons who sell nostrums. In practical medicine this is *crux* indeed. But the world was ever thus. (XIII 53)

## The Curable and Homoeopathy

You will perhaps say that this *aphonia* case is also not a mortal malady. Will you once for all disabuse your mind of the very vulgar professional and popular error, according to which the homoeopaths are said to claim to cure the incurable! Just note, at least for *your own information*, that the homoeopaths make no such claim; what they say is this : Homoeopathy cures what can be cured much better than any other system of medicine hitherto made known to the world. The homoeopaths do not maintain that other systems are valueless, or that the homoeopathic system is faultless, only that thus far in the art-treatment of disease by remedies, Homoeopathy, by very long odds, beats all the records. Do you see?

Be that as it may, I trust that curing an old case of singers aphonia with *Arnica* is a fairly sound reason for being a homoeopath; any way it is my *thirteenth*.

P.S. — When I say that Homoeopathy does not claim to cure the incurable, that leaves the question of curability an open one; Homoeopathy does not accept anything as incurable because certain physicians who are "regular" declare it to be so. Incapacity to cure does not render the uncured incurable. Kindly take a mental note of this, because what you "regulars" consider incurable may, or may not, be so considered by the homoeopaths. My old pleuritis trouble was declared and proved to be incurable by and for the entire family, and yet the *Bryonia alba* of the homoeopaths cured it! (XI 23)

## Curable and Incurable

The limits of the curable and of the incurable are not represented by any fixed lines. What is incurable today may be curable tomorrow; and what we all of this generation deem incurable may be considered very amenable to treatment in the next generation. (XI 45)

### Curable and Medicable

I understand by "medicable" and "medicability" not quite the same as "curable" and "curability".

*Medicable*, for me, is that which may be treated by medicaments (remedies, medicines) with a fair prospect of being ameliorated or cured thereby, and *medicability* is the substantive formed therefrom. I have never seen these words used in English, but adopt and adapt them from *medicable* and *medicabilite,* which I have observed here and there in French works. (XX 44)

**Cure — Time Factor**

I have noticed that the longer it takes to cure a tumour by medicines the less people esteem it; and, indeed, that from their standpoint is natural enough, for the simple and sufficient reason that they have not enough knowledge to form a correct judgment. Still the gentleman referred to had been to Oxford, and thus runs his creed :

"My name is Blow-it,
And whatever KNOWLEDGE, I know it.
I'm master of New College;
And what I don't know isn't KNOWLEDGE." (XX 61)

**Cure — What it is?**

'Let me know what you mean by cure. Do you mean to alter the diseased state of the parts, or do you mean by your medicine to remove the parts diseased?' 'I mean to destroy them', he replied. 'Well, then, that is nothing more than I or any other surgeon can do with less pain to the patient.' (XX 128)

**Curing — Trying and Pretending**

Trying to cure what is commonly held to be incurable is a laudable ambition, and by no means the same thing as pretending to cure, though unhappily for medical progress "trying" is commonly confounded with "pretending."

If you try and fail, you are laughed at; if you try and succeed, you are hated; I have experienced both, and so speak feelingly. (XX 45)

## Dermatology

If the position which I take up be the true one, skin doctors are working great evil in the world, and sadly need enlightening; while, on the other hand, if they are right, and their almost universally accepted views and practice are sound and in accordance with the facts of disease, then I must be in the wrong, and wrong should everywhere be crushed like a nut under a steam-hammer. Dermatologists ! I ask no mercy, as I give no quarter. (IX 119)

## Diet — Value of Fruits in Gout

*Is Fruit Good or Bad For the Gouty?*

I have myself cured gout over and over again with grapes taken in bulk; and several of my patients, who were formerly sorely plagued with gout, have entirely ceased to be troubled so long as they have partaken freely of grapes.

I may say the same of oranges. In fact, my standing advice to my gouty friends runs thus : Eat plenty of fresh, ripe, uncooked fruit, and drink plenty of fresh cold water.

It is in this wise : fresh fruits stir up the gout and often render its manifestations more active : but, at the same time, its tendency is to diminish gout, and, finally, to get rid of it. in some cases, altogether.

A *very* little fruit, in a very gouty individual who is unaccustomed to it, will punish the patient very severely, as the numberless stories related by the gouty amply testify.

Fruit does not produce gout, it stirs it up and drives it out; fruit does not produce eczema, it stirs it up and drives it out; and, pray, where is it safest to have gout and eczema? Surely not inside. (XXI 130)

### — Value of Vegetables and Fruit in Health

*Do vegetables and Fruit Conduce to Longevity?*

I am much disposed to answer this question in the affirmative, though my experience and knowledge are not sufficient to supply me with facts and arguments to prove the proposition. (XXI 134)

That the tissues of those who eat neither fruits nor vegetables show grave signs of senility already at or about middle life is, for me, almost beyond question; but whether the want of the vegetable causes the decay, or whether the decay is due to a morbid cause resulting in a dislike for fruits and vegetables, as well as in senility, I am unable to say. (XXI 135)

## Discharges — Their Meaning

*Centrifugal fluxes and discharges should not be lightly stopped.*
*Why* the flux? *Whence* the discharge? Let the questions of the why? and whence? be answered as we go along. Here I merely insist upon the elementary truth that a morbid process having a, perhaps, time-honoured name, may be nevertheless no disease at all, but merely a means of cure set up by nature herself, and that there are diseases which it is disadvantageous or dangerous to cure, that is to cure in the sense in which the verb to cure is commonly used in English by the thoughtless. Of course, to effect a *really* radical cure of any *primary* disease can never be other than a gain to the individual. (XVII 27)

## Disease — Dynamic vs. Material

I will, however, not touch upon this question here, contenting myself with observing that *catching a complaint* in the common and natural order of things, and being *compelled* to take it by the injunction of material quantities of its stuff, are not equivalent by any means, though Pasteur, Koch, and biological experimenters very generally work and write as if they were. And this, indeed, constitutes the weak link in their chain of argument. More particularly is this the case with Koch and his experiments in tuberculosis. (XVIII 45)

The greater the poison the greater the remedy; true, but only homoeopathically. Throw out the homoeopathic law and the high potency, and you are stranded, and your virus is a virus and nothing more; and where is Koch? Stranded just here — at this very point. He casts aside the homoeopathic law, he ignores the possibility of the action of high potencies, and tries nevertheless to cure with likes or identicals, and he fails; and he not only fails to cure, but he kills as do all who follow him, as he and their own published results clearly testify. (XVIII 47)

### Disease and Heredity

No matter what part of a parent is weak or diseased, of that weakness or disease the child will partake. The child is specially made from the mother. If the paternal element is strong, it takes hold strongly upon the maternal, but what the mother has not, that she cannot give. If she has weak lungs or liver, fragile bones, here child has the same in greater or less degree. (XIII 39)

**— Incurable Disease and Incurable Stage**

It is extremely important to carefully differentiate between an incurable disease and the incurable stage of a perfectly curable complaint. People will say, of course it is, but is it not a fact that new therapeutic measures are commonly tried in the last hopeless stages of disease, and even then often clumsily and unwillingly? (XX 11)

**Disease and its Causes**

The study of disease and its causes is the study of the human race, its passion, its sins, crimes, sorrows, and agonies. (XIII 39)

**Disease and Personal and Family History**

***Diagnosis and Prognosis***

The fundamental idea underlying this little work ("The change of life in woman") is that an absolutely healthy woman changes without any ills or ailings whatever, and therefore a normal woman, married or maiden, who has no disease or disease taint, has nothing to fear from the change of life. The period will cease as it began, almost imperceptibly; it just leaves off, and there is an end of it.

But unfortunately, very few women are truly free from disease and taintless; no doubt there are such, but these do not throng our consulting rooms. A medical man is hardly a fair judge of the number of really normal persons, for the very sufficient reason that such individuals need no physician, and rarely come to him. There is, however, a large class of people whom I would designate as *more than healthy, i.e.*, whatever may be wrong with them, they are loud and voluble in persistently declaring that they are *always quite well and wonderfully healthy*, and all their ancestors from Noah on have been perfectly well and quite free from any disease. So far as they will confess they are, in regard to health, absolutely holy. The wise practical physician knows at once that this is all fudge, and gives no credence to their statements; on the contrary, he at once suspects that the most grave constitutional disease lurks behind in these health-holy boasters, whose statements are commonly entirely mendacious. A gentleman once brought his little daughter to me suffering from scrofulous ophthalmia, and, said he, she has had it over a year, and I cannot understand it, as we are all so healthy, and my father lived to be nearly ninety. Now I happened to know from the old gentleman himself, who was formerly my patient, that though he himself did indeed live to be nearly ninety years of age, still all his very numerous brothers and sisters died young of tuberculosis in one form or another.

*Bacillinum* cured the scrofulous ophthalmia in three months, and the fond father commented on the cure thus : "I knew there could not be very much the matter, as we are so healthy, and my father lived to nearly ninety."

A young lady was recently brought by her mother to me for haemorrhage of the lungs, and was thought to be doomed to die of phthisis of the lungs, two physicians of repute having given this prognosis. Said I, "What sort of health-histories have your people; is there any consumption in your family?"

"Oh, no! We are all wonderfully healthy; there was never any consumption in *our* family."

The true history being, as I happened to know, this — Her own mother died of cancer of the bowels; her eldest brother has asthma; her father had haemorrhage of the lungs as young man; her third brother died of rapid phthisis; her eldest sister died of tuberculosis of the pelvic organs; her second sister has very severe eczema and disfiguring rheumatoid arthritis; her third sister is actually under my treatment for tumour of the breast with deeply retracted nipple; while her youngest brother is suffering from a huge lipoma.

So much for this example of the wonderfully healthy ones.

However, given a really pure blooded normal woman, I contend that the change of life is purely negative process in a pathological sense.

Why, then, do we think and speak of the change of life almost as if it were of necessity a dangerous, mysterious period that all women do and should dread?

The reason is that most women are not quite normal, and their abnormalities are for the most part inherent diseases that may be observed in them any time from puberty to menopause and afterwards. As before observed, the cessation of the monthly PURIFICATION fully explains the whole series of morbid phenomena. Take any half-dozen cases of ill-health at the change of life and you will readily trace the troubles back often even to the period of dentition, and almost always to the comencement of the period. I constantly trace such climacteric troubles to gout, rheumatism, cancer, consumption, and venereal affections from a parent down through the daugher's life. Thus consumptiveness will show itself at puberty as painful and excessive, or deficient menstruation, and ending as cancer at the change of life - cancer and consumption often alternating in succeeding generations; a small patch of eczema at puberty not infrequently means scirrhus at the menopause. As I have before pointed out in "Tumours of the Breast", the various tumours of the breast commonly have their seat of origin in the womb or ovaries; and holding this view, I have succeeded from time to time in curing very many such tumours in women at all periods of life, and notably at the change of life. Thus recently the Baroness X, telegraphed to me from the Hague that her doctors there had diagnosed Interstitial Mastitis of her right breast, and urged an immediate operation. I wired back forbidding the operation, saying that medicines would cure it. Her laydyship appeared in my consulting room two or three days thereafter, and I found the diagnosis correct — the right pretty uniformly infiltrated and hard. Under *Scirrhinum* C. the breast became quite normal within two months; but it then became manifest that the real origin of the trouble still persisted, and lay in the pelvic organs, and this pelvic root trouble I am now treating. I can afford to forgive certain insolent remarks of a very prominent medical brother at the Hague; he knows no better, and what he does not know of interstitial mastitits is not knowledge. What on earth is the use of ablating a breast for a swelling that has its root-life in the female pelvic organs? (XXIV )

**The Product of Disease**

My standpoint is that a tumour is the product of the organism, and to be really cured the power to produce the same must be eliminated, got rid of; cutting it off merely rids the organism of the product, leaving the producing power where it was before, often the operative interference acting like pruning a vine; *i.e.*, the tumour-producing power is increased, and the fatal issue is brought nearer. The following case brings well into relief what I mean : Miss X., aet. 49, still regular, came under my care on July 31, 1893. *Formerly had had eczema,* was cured in a fortnight by an ointment; several years later — June, 1885 — a tumour was excised from her left breast; said tumour recurred in the same breast and was, July, 1887, again removed together with the whole breast; then a tumour came in the right breast and in January, 1888, the tumour and whole right breast were removed by a very neat operation. She came to me for a recurrence of the process in the middle of the scar of the right side with a good deal of inflammation. The treatment lasted four years, *ending during the course of the cure in eczema,* and patient is actually in better health than ever before in her life and has now begun life anew as an amateur artist. The eczema is also well. What I am here concerned to demonstrate is not how this particular case was cured, but to make manifest that a tumour is really a vital growth arising from disease in the individual and is not itself the disease at all; the initial and subsequent eczemas and the tumours being one and the same thing; *i.e.*, the *products* of the disease. (XX 5)

## Douches — An Evil

The talk about personal cleanliness and comfort is mere moonshine : all mucous membranes are self - cleansing, and the use of injections, far from being sweet and clean, is in fact a dirty proceeding. Why, the epithelial cells are being constantly cast off with all the impurities clinging to them, and extruded from the body, and exquisitely clean brand new cells are left behind — the tubings of the human body are living tissue, not drain-pipes. Who cleans the lining membrane of the faeces-carrying gut? It is self-cleansing, and so is the lining membrance of the vagina. Well do I know that practically all the gynaecologists of the civilised world tell their lady patients to use vaginal injections for purposes of cleanliness : the error of this teaching is stupendous, and fraught with untold evil consequences, and nasty and vulgar to boot. Am I conscious of the terrible opposition my thus expressed view of the perniciousness of the practice of using vaginal injections will call forth? (XXIV 9)

## Drug Action — Similarity and Range

We thus find that a drug, to really cure a disease, must affect the same or similar part as the disease; it must affect it in a similar manner, and moreover the range of drug-action must be co-extensive with the disease-action. (XX 33)

### Drug Dynamization

The writer has long been cast about on a sea of doubt and perplexity with regard to this doctrine of drug dynamization; he has frequently listened to the arguments brought forward for and against it , and frequently himself joined in ridiculing it, constantly feeling himself *unable to believe it possible* that the remedial potentiality of a given drug could be increased by any process of subdivision whatever, in fact, by any process whatsoever. The question is constantly presenting itself to one's mind thus : can the billionth of a grain be potentially more than a grain? and the ready answer willingly follows — impossible. It may be conceded that the doctrine of drug dynamization is *a priori,* absurd : so is homoeopathy. How can a drug that causes diarrhoea cure diarrhoea? Surely, it must make it worse. What, castor oil for an alvine flux? Clearly it cannot cure it. Yet experiment shows that what causes diarrhoea *does* indeed cure diarrhoea; like *does* cure like whether we believe it or not; and hence, what is *a priori* absurd, may be a *posteriori* true. We are all very apt to lose sight of the fact that our beliefs have nothing to do with truth. Truth is truth whether it be believed or not. The born blind may not believe in the existence of the sunlight because he does not see it. Sound is absurd to the deaf.

The existence of the word paradox shows that things apparently absurd and untrue may yet be true in fact.

However, there is this to be well considered. In the drug treatment of disease we have to deal with conditions and not with entities, and it is not paradoxical to suppose that two like and equal forces may neutralize one another. Two equal showers of rain will make the ground wetter than one, but a pair of scales weighed down with a one-grain weight is restored to equilibrium by the addition of another one-grain weight on the other side; it is similar in its action, and like in its power, only it works at the other end of the beam. Here the state of equipoise is brought about by similar means that are also equal : rest results from two motions.

Those ignorant of homoeopathy laugh at it; the writer went through this laughing stage of ignorance, but did not find it very blissful, and so constrained to put the doctrine of similars to the test of scientific experiment, and found it a true one of great practical value. Almost all homoeopaths have come that way. Hence disbelieving a thing does not disprove it.

Those ignorant of the doctrine of drug dynamization in truly scientific practice, laugh at it; so did the writer, and that in very good company; but finding that Hahnemann spoke truly in regard to drug action, he thought that circumstance some slight presumptive evidence in favour of his other doctrine that remedial power is developed and increased in a drug by trituration and succussion.

Therefore, he put the theory to the test of careful clinical experiment with the result that he has passed considerably beyond the laughing stage. The results obtained from clinical experiments ought to satisfy the most critical mind, if not blinded with prejudice, for they constitute the only scientific method of settling the question at all either one way or the other.

But it is much easier to satisfy one's mind about the truth, or otherwise, of homoeopathy than about the truth or falseness of the theory of potentizing drugs.

Expediency and policy can have no weight with us; if the Hahnemannian doctrine of drug dynamization be, as it is averred on competent authority, a great stumbling-block to the profession and a hindrance to the spread of the major doctrine of similars, we can only regret it, but must proceed, and also insist upon it before the whole world, in the path of truth seeking *coute qui coute*. What can be more beautiful than truth for its own sake? (XVIII 7)

## Dysmenorrhŏea not Normal

I hold that every woman who suffers from dysmenorrhoea is, so far, abnormal and ailing in some particular; it may not be much, but pain at the period is not normal. (XXIV 6)

## Evil Habits

I am very strongly of opinion that evil habits in the young are of physical origin and nature, and that they can be cured by medicines, if physicians will take the trouble. (XXII 134)

## Excreta Inimical to the Excretant

The emanation of organisms are noxious and obnoxious to the self-same organisms. Any one can notice that where horses and cows graze in the same meadow the horses will nibble off the grass close to cow-dung but not near their own, and conversely the cows will eat the grass close to horse-dung, and even push it away with their mouths without evincing the slightest objection.

All creatures abhor their own dejecta. Even the "dirty pig" is *very* sty-clean if he has the chance, and evidently on the same principle, while he has no objection whatever to the dejecta of other animals.

The emanations from living organisms are very evidently hurtful to themselves, and, if sufficiently concentrated, more or less deadly, and it seems probable that the fungi come in and thrive thereon to the advantage of the organisms, tending at any rate to postpone the fatal issue; organic remains and emanations constitute the pabulum of the fungi. Of course, the fungi must follow the ordinary law of Nature, and they in their turn must succumb to their own products.

Nature does not tolerate any dead thing, for as soon as there is any dead thing present new life starts therein forthwith. How far fungal products poison the hosts of the fungi is worthy of study and thought, and will in the future loom large into therapeutics.

It seems to me that those children who are suffering from ringworm are in better health with their ringworm than they are when the ringworm fungi are killed off by local measures. My own observations on this part of the subject are as yet too few for me to be able to form a positive opinion, but as far as they do go they tend to the conclusion that serious ill-health often dates from the time when they are cured of ringworm, *i.e.*, from the time when the fungi were locally more or less destroyed from the surface.

Just as the fungal disease of hollyhocks was most virulent where they were crowded, so is the fungal disease ringworm in most evil report in schools, or, in other words, where the children are numerous and close together. School-masters and school-surgeons are very positive about ringworm having been "imported into the *schools*" by a boy coming from his home, but my own experience goes to show that as a rule ringworm is bred in the schools and is exported thence into the families. Not only so, but it is large families that supply us with specimens of ringwormy children more frequently than small ones, and it is the large schools that suffer most. At least so it appears to me from my only moderately numerous observations.

And in regard to tuberculosis we find this behaves similarly, and it is certainly true that where numerous human beings house together in closed apartments, there anthropotoxine is generated, and the bacillus of tuberculosis finds its cradle and home. (XVIII 108)

## Exploring the Dark

I have always tried at least to strike a match in any dark corner where medical mysteries midst ghostly terrors most abound; and although the illumination emanating from one solitary match is not exactly blinding, still it is more helpful than utter darkness. (XXIV Foreword)

## Eye Doctors

Is it not a sad thought that the great army of eye-doctors are to a man nothing but mechanicians; and what is still sadder, they do not even aim at being anything else. (XXII 106)

## Fasting

Of course, no one questions that we all can get rid of our tissues by starvation. The art is to *keep* plenty of good tissues, and therewith remain in good health and vigour. I have tried many dietetic experiments on myself, and thus have often lessened and increased my bulk almost at will, and what I have invariably found is this : you cannot make *big* fire with a *small* quantity of fuel; that is impossible. Consume, as a general thing, very little, and you can only spend a very little in energy; you cannot get much out of little. Of course, you may get too bulky, and thus waste much energy in mere locomotion. That is a question of being overweighted; and when some of this overweight is got rid of by diet, there is, apparently, more energy developed on less food, but this is only apparent and not real. For here we have two factors to consider — *First*, the overweight is lessened, and less energy is required for locomotion; and, *secondly*, the overweight that is got rid of must be *added* to the food taken, inasmuch as the dieted individual has himself consumed a portion of himself : his organism has used up some of its stored fat. But, if the diminished import of food be continued too long, deterioration and debility must ensue. This is where the fallacy comes in stored food is used, and so the quantity of fuel is not less, whereas the bulk to be carried is less, and so the initial state of the spare diet process is very commonly accompanied by a feeling of well-being and lightness; they feel so much lighter, and get about so much more easily. Of course, they do. But as soon as the stored-up food is gone, weakness supervenes if a too spare diet be persisted in. Therefore, in all dieting we must stop a little before the fatty reserve store is all used up; for if we go on we just consume ourselves and as far as this goes it is death. This brings us along to the question of diet in gout and diet for the fat. Fat people are not necessarily gouty, and gouty people are not necessarily fat : still gout and obesity touch one another so closely that they in a certain number of cases, are not easily separated in practice. (XXI 108)

## Favus — Local Disease

### Case of Generalized Favus

If there be any one disease of the skin more than another to which one might accord the quality of being *local* and *external*, it is certainly *Favus*. (IX 95)

## Fistula and Lime-water Application

For the relief of the pain of acute gatherings I have very great confidence in lime-water rags. I have often felt very thankful to this excellent practical tip that I first learned of Dr. George Wyld, of London. (XVI 16)

### — and Liquor

I will here interpolate the remark that whisky often causes itchings at the seat at night, and then the cure consists in leaving off the whisky. (XVI 47)

### — and Other Organs

Certainly there are liver-fistulas, *i.e.* fistulas of hepatic origin, and here the liver must be cured or the fistulas cannot be. Certainly there are lung-fistulas, *i.e.*, fistulas of pulmonary origin. Here the lungs must be first cured, or the sequel brings constituitional retribution; here we must be especially beware of operations, for if this kind of fistula be forcibly closed, phthisis comes soon.

Certainly there are spleen fistulas, or fistulas of splenic origin. (XVI 80)

According to my views, almost every fistula has a cause more or less remote from the fistula proper; we might almost compare the fistula to the crater of a volcano. (XVI 82)

**— and Skin**

Still, you will generally notice that persons with fistula have a more or less unhealthy skin, which is cheesy, greasy, spotty, pimply, or dirty looking, and they are also commonly anaemic. (XVI 12)

**— Constitutional Cause**

It has, however, long been contended by able medical thinkers that the fistular process is the local expression of a constitutional cause, and that the true philosophical and scientific way of treating fistula is to remove the said constitutional cause, and then the fistula will heal of itself with little or no local aid at all. (XVI 2)

Here I would like to ask the fistula cutters how it is that (the fistula being, as they contend, of local origin and nature), I ask, how is it that when they fail to force the healing-up process, they then say that the *fistula* will *not* heal ! Leucorrhoea is a constitutional disorder; so is fistula; and they are not infrequently of absolutely identical nature and significance, though, of course, they just as often differ so much that they have nothing in common but their ill fate of constituting the happy hunting ground of specialists "of the world worldly, of the earth earthy". (XVI 61)

But the pre-fistular abscess differs widely from the two kinds of abscess just mentioned. It is not a stasis-abscess, for *its* stasis is a means to an end, the means being to mortify a bit of tissue to form an outlet; and the end being the detrusion of *not* a simple innocuous thing or substance, but some *organismic morbid product* that is being daily and hourly produced, and therefore needs daily and hourly discharge, in fact a constantly open issue, which a fistula in my opinion often is. If I am correct in this view, it must follow that a fistula should not be made to heal up by any and every local means, but the fistula-patient should be cured by internal constitutional treatment. (XVI 75)

**— Individualization and Surgery**

I am quite satisfied that there is fistula and fistula, — that it must, in fact, be looked upon as a generic term for several constitutional complaints of a totally different nature, and that surgery of all and every kind is absolutely inadequate to cope with these various constitutional states grouped together under the conventional term fistula. (XVI 10)

I lost all my allopathic friends when I threw in my lot with the peculiar therapeutic people called homoeopaths, and have learned to do without them in my strong consciousness of right. Now I am beginning to learn to do without my chirurgical friends just because I can do without them, and so they cease to love me as of yore. Well, well, the pretty elastic ligature of my friends for *fistula-in-ano* is no more a cure for the fistular disease than is a catheter for the sclerosed state of the urethra, which we commonly call stricture. (XVI 23)

People with fistula are not well, else they would not have fistula, and my own idea is that having one's cut for fistula is not a sign of courage, and still less of intelligence. (XVI 24)

The writer says that when the case came into his hands, and examination revealed what he expected, viz. fistula. *Hamamelis* I was prescribed, and shortly the case was cured. Now, what do we gain by the statement that *Hamamelis* is good for fistula-in-ano? And shall we prescribe it for every such pathological condition? I cannot see that we add in the slightest degree to our knowledge of therapeutics by such generalization, and if we expect *Hamamelis* to cure every case of fistula-in-ano we shall be sadly disappointed. A patient presents himself to us suffering from headache, and states that it is made much *worse* from motion; now, when we hear this key-note, we must not feel satisfied that *Bryonia* is the remedy from this characteristic symptom, for whoever prescribes upon one subjective symptom will find himself as much mistaken, many times, as the man who prescribes upon one objective symptom, or the morbid anatomy and pathological show alone, regardless of the others, instead of the totality of the symptoms. (XVI 32)

**— and Surgery**

In fact, in really dyscratic cases of fistula, the surgeon's knife is of no more use than the north wind. And, indeed, how should it be possible for local work to cure a constitutional ailment, which fistula undoubtedly is nine times out of every ten? (XVI 5)

On May 22, 1882, a married London merchant, thirty seven years of age, called to consult me in regard to recurrent fistula and circumanal abscess. He related to me that eighteen months previously he got an abscess at the seat, which his surgeon lanced and treated, and in the end pronounced as cured. Cured it was, in the surgeon's opinion; he was quite honest in this expressed opinion, but you might as well say that when you have plucked the apple-trees in the autumn, you have cured the said apple-trees of apple-bearing, for, although the surgeon had "cured" the abscess he had not cured the patient of his power to produce more fistula-leading abscesses, inasmuch as the disease had returned each subsequent spring and fall. And this is really the point I am contending for *viz* : The abscess at the seat with its sequential fistula is not disease in its real essence, but only its local expression in the anal region. (XVI 8)

**— A Tubercular Diathesis**

In my opinion, fistula, wherever situated, is almost tubercular alone, or tubercular and something else. It also frequently happens that oophoritis is likewise of tubercular quality, with or without a superadded gleety quality. (XXIII 136)

**-- Tuberculous Fistula by Infection**

A certain number of cases of anal fistula in middle-aged, highly-nourished men come under my observation, and I have been struck with the fact that their wives had either died of, or were suffering from consumption.

I imagine that the fistula represents, in such cases, an infection from a consumptive wife communicated to the husband in the intimate relations of married life. I commend the subject to the consideration of my colleagues.

They simply maintain a tuberculous sore — the fistula-in-ano.

I take it that the infection is truly tuberculous in the bacillary sense, but the soil is not fit; the consitututional power is too great to allow of the develpment of general tuberculosis. (XVI 51)

## Food and Work

In considering the question of diet we rarely find people take due cognizance of the mode of life of the individual who is to be fed, and yet in the case of horses, for instance, every horse-keeper feeds his horses according to what he expects them to do. I formerly, very frequently, went to a country house, four miles from the railway station, to see a patient suffering from a grave malady. For some weeks the ordinary carriage horses were sent to take me to the patient's abode, and so long as this was the case the hills offered no impediment, and I found myself transported rapidly; and this was very satisfactory to me, for doctor's time is his capital. Patient's malady was, as before stated, a grave one, and his belongings were very anxious to get me to the house as quickly as possible, so good-conditioned horses were put in to the carriage. But after a while the patient got better, and then I found that a fat old pony was sent to the station to meet me, and it took us nearly an hour to reach the squire's mansion. On the way back to the station I inquired of the coachman how it was that "Shaggy" seemed so pumped out with such a short journey. Said he : "Well, you see, Sir, she is out at grass in the home-park, and gets no oats or dry food at all."

Now, the coachman's explanation of "Shaggy's" weakness gives us the clue to what I desire to say in regard to diet in general. When anyone asks — What am I to eat and drink? The answer must duly reckon with the mode of life of the questioner, and the amout of work which is required of him. As a rule, no work whatever was required of "Shaggy" : She just ran about in the home-park, thriving beautifully on grass and water and on this diet she seemed exceedingly happy and plump and sleek, and when spoken to would gallop away in fine style, the picture of health, strength, and happiness. Yet a three or four miles run, in a very light cart, was a severe trial for "Shaggy". It is not different with human beings; if they do nothing but just loll about — turned out to grass, so to speak — bread and water, with fruit and vegetables, amply suffice; but if they work, they need the equivalent of oats and dry food. I am here not giving expression to mere theory, for I have tried numerous experiments on my own person and proved the point over and over again; and I emphatically affirm that you cannot get much work out of little food, any more than you can make a very big fire with a very little fuel. Whether the authority be Salisbury, Canterbury, or York, I care not; you cannot get much work out of a spare diet.(XXI 111)

## Full Stomach — Mild Genesis

I still think a mild emetic the right treatment when the stomach is laden and cannot unburden itself by natural vomit. (XI 10)

## Generation and Sin

I never could understand why almost everything connected with generation seems to suggest sin to almost all of us. Surely we are not entirely right here; however, I am not dealing with dogma, but with problems in practical medicine, and I regard the task I had set myself as finished. (XXII 152)

## Genius Has No Gender

### Girls and Boys

The same thing applies to the question of the relative powers of girls and boys, and most of what is commonly said on this point is nothing but weak twaddle. Only the Almighty can make a New Woman. Put broadly, up to the age of puberty, the girl, all other things being equal, beats the boy; with puberty the damsel throws away every month a vast amount of fluid power in the order of Nature. Let us call this *pelvic power*. Assuming the girl to be the superior of the boy up to the pelvic power stage — which, indeed, anyone can observe for himself, in his own sphere, — but once arrived at the stage of pelvic power, and the damsel is left behind in her lesson by her brother in the natural order of things, or else the girl's brain saps the pelvis of its power, when she will also lose in the race with the boy, because he will be physically well, while she, with disordered pelvic life, must necessarily be in ill-health more or less. The whole thing is a mere question of quantity of energy. If it were otherwise, the girl would be able to buy lollypops with her penny and yet keep her penny; while the boy, having spent his penny, would be penniless. You cannot spend your penny and have it.

The New Woman is only possible in a novel, not in Nature. The intellectual Sandow is also impossible, and for the same reason; too much on one side of the scales conditions too little on the other. I have very many times watched the careers of exceedingly studious girls who spent the great mass of their power in mental work, and in every case the pelvic power decreased in even pace with the expenditure of mental power. Not one exception to this have I ever seen, and all the lady students of the higher grades whom it has been my duty to professionally advise were suffering in regard to their pelvic lives and power. I have sat at the foot of Nature a good many years, and I give as my opinion that to be a mother in its best sense is the biggest thing on earth, and comes nearer the Creator's work than anything else under heaven; to be a learned girl or woman graduate is a very good and respectable thing enough, and twelve of them make a dozen.

At the same time, genius has no gender: it can be in a female or in a male, as the case may be. (XXII 89)

## Good Intentions

But good intentions are not necessarily of any service; when the blind lead the blind and both fall into the ditch together, the good intentions of the blind leader avail nothing. (XX 60)

## Gout — Aetiology

I have held with Eisemann, Hahnemann, Grauvogl, Wolf, Goullon, these twenty years, and I will just say here that I believe the malady in question has a very decided influence on the organism, being contingently capable of generating a constitutional state which cannot be distinguished from the uric acid diathesis. My conception of the thing is that the gonococcic virus so poisons the organism that acid dypepsia is set up, and then we have what cannot be distinguished from the uric acid diathesis. So often have I seen this state set up in the wake of the gonorrhoeal infection, that I have almost come to the conclusion that the typical gouty attack is a child of gonorrhoea. Thus I explain to myself the curious fact that it is principally men who get the typical gouty attack. And it is in this line of thought that I have met with my greatest success in the medical eradication of the uric acid diathesis. But this is a subject by itself which I may one day work out; however, in case I should not do so, let my advice to the initiated be to this effect — Regard the uric acid diathesis as originating (at least very frequently) in the Tripperseuche, and in its medicinal treatment stick to the antisycotics, and always remember its autopoison in very high potency at considerable intervals. Let it be well understood that I am here speaking of the uric acid diathesis, and not of the uric acid deposits. It is of the very highest importance always to keep in one's mind the diathesis separate from the gouty attack and the gouty tophi. The homoeopathicity of the remedy to the diathesis is mainly historic; the homoeopathicity of the remedy to the attack is mainly present and actual. It is just because these two are considered together that the homoeopathic literature of gout is so poor. And that others have thought of the sycotic nature of arthritis may be inferred from the fact that *Thuja occidentalis* has been recommended as an anti-arthritic; but clearly it was so recommended for the arthritic dyspepsia, and not for the arthritic attack; and hence we are not surprised to find that, having used it in the attacks without benefit, they have written off Thuja as useless in gout. In the attacks it is indeed useless; in the arthritic dyspepsia it is a princely remedy. (XX 138)

**— and Alcohol**

"Oh! I see you are a *Scotch*-whisky doctor. It seems to me that the only difference between you gout doctors lies in the kind of whisky you order; you order Scotch, and Dr.Moore used to order Irish. I often tell papa that if I were he I would drink both, and then he would be sure to be right."(XXI 2)

1. People who have descended from ancestors long accustomed to the use of stimulants generation after generation, these need stimulants in their debilitating illness, and therefore in their attacks of gout. They also need a certain amount of building up. If they are dieted too severely and deprived of their alcoholic stimulants they get weaker and weaker, and their gout gets the entire mastery; whereas with a sustaining diet and a reasonable amount of stimulant, they get well and thrive on their ancestral constitutional basis.
2. In certain brain-workers (and in their immediate descendants) whose nervous systems are exhausted, if you take away their stimulants they are apt to fare very badly. (XXI 7)

**— Exhaustion**

So I conclude that food and stimulants *per se* are not necessarily the cause of gouty attacks. The thing presents itself to my mind thus — Just as in the case of a smoky chimney almost any kind of fuel will fill the room with smoke, so in gout almost any kind of food will produce gout; but the real fault lies, not in the fuel, but in the chimney; not in the food, but in the organism.

I call these cases of gout *Exhaustion Gout*, and certainly they need stimulants. (XXI 9)

**Surfeit Gout :** I call surfeit gout that which is *Curable* by abstemiousness either as regards food or stimulants, or both. In such cases I have known an attack of gout to be brought on by a single bottle of beer or a pint of even the driest champagne, and on one occasion from eating goose-berries; in such cases all alcoholic stimulants, and certain foods, yet in different degrees, act like oil on a fire; they set up a blaze.

In exhaustion gout alcoholic stimulants act like oil on troubled waters : they calm the waves. (XXI 12)

Taken in its simple elementary forms, we may regard the exhaustion gout and the surfeit gout as respectively inherited or acquired.

In the most simple form the hereditarily gouty may get gout on almost any diet. Surfeit gout is self-produced by excessive input or inadequate output; too much is put in, too little is put out, and hence the ureal smoke and soot which is the gouty product. A gouty father begets a child while he is actively gouty; like begets like, and hence the offspring is of necessity gouty on any diet whatsoever; such children pass grit and gravel as soon as they get away from the pure milk diet. A milk cure for gout echoes all down through time. But active, middle-aged men in the full swing of daily life commonly find a milk diet inadequate if they keep at work. "It does not seem to satisfy me," say they, or "even when I am full of milk I seem to be empty." The fact is, milk is good for the very young — calves and babes. (XXI 15)

**— and Offspring**

In other words, rearing children require a very differnt regimen and dietary to what experience may find best for maintaining gouty adults. (XXI 14)

**— and Ordinary Homoeopathic Treatment**

Now, so long as I kept to the ordinarily commended homoeopathic remedies for gout, so long were my results mostly only tedious recoveries; cures they could not be fairly called. (XXI 26)

**— and Spleen and Faulty Excretion**

*The gouty product is the uric smoke and soot of the human economy* — that is, the pure paroxysmal affection commonly manifesting itself as podagra, and more or less in many varieties of goutinesss.

Where the renal excretion is such that some of the uric matter (Urea, uric acid, urate of sodium) remains in the blood, it is deposited in certain of the tissues, and when it culminates in, say, the big toe, we get the classic gouty attack.

In other words, gout, for me, is ureal poisoning.

I grant that the uric acid produces the sufferings, but I maintain that the *disease gout* is that which produces the uric acid — in fact, the Paracelsic motto on my title-page expresses exactly my philosophy.

It seems to me, further, that gout stands in some relation to the spleen as well as to the kidneys and sweat glands. It does not appear to me that gout has so much to do with the liver or its functions, and stirring up the liver to increased action and purging the bowels do not, so far as I have been able to discover, aid in the very least in the cure of gout, acute or chronic, unless a primary liver affection be its prime cause in the organopathic sense.

Moreover, it is by no means an uncommon thing for very gouty people to suffer from habitual looseness of the bowels, and yet the gout does not diminish. On the other hand, as before remarked, I am strongly of opinion that the spleen is very intimately concerned in the production of gout.

And this I believe to be due to the fact that gout is very difficult to cure dynamically, because we have behind the symptoms the uric deposits; and remedies that are homoeopathic to the symptoms of the gouty patients from the deposits are not necessarily homoeopathic to the state productive of such deposits; and it must be manifest that remedies, to be really curative of arthritis, must be homoeopathic to the state productive of such deposits of urates within the tissues. It is not enough to cure the symptoms due to the urates : to be the remedy of the case, not only the uric deposits must be included within the simillimum, but the state which produces such deposits. (XXI 19)

The gouty individual is like a smoky chimney : his organism does the carrying-off imperfectly, and as in the case of the smoky chimney it does not suffice to get the sweeps, but the services of a chimney-doctor are needed to remedy the defect, so in the gouty person this uric acid may be got rid of by *Gichtwasser, alkalies, Piperazine* or *Urtica,* but the real cure has not been effected; the smoke and soot only have been cleared away, the products are gone, the power of further production remains; only the sweep has done his work not the chimney doctor; he it is whose services have now to be invoked. (XXI 67)

**— Arthritic Nature**

When we say "gout" we really mean that the individual lives goutily, whether such individual gets attacks of gout or not; thus the child of a gouty father may teethe goutily and have gouty urticaria, and here the gouty quality cannot be eliminated by gum-lancing or soothing ointments.

Assuming that both parents of a given individual are pronouncedly gouty, how should the offspring be other than gouty? In the painful menstruation of young ladies I have over and over again cured the dysmenorrhoea by treating the painful affection as of gouty quality — in fact, as gout. It would be better to restrict the term gout to the form of disease that occurs in attacks of paroxysmal arthritis, and use the word goutiness to designate the more or less hereditary quality of the constitutional crasis. In fact, I would use the words goutiness and gout to indicate the same relation which consumptiveness bears to consumption. But in this matter of terminology custom will fix our words for us, no matter what we say or do. (XXI 17)

Dr. Holtz* maintains that the fever of gout, as observed by him in hundreds of cases, rarely exceeds about half a degree, whereas the fever of rheumatism commonly runs high, and this he regards as an essential difference between the two processes. This is, no doubt, correct : still there *is some* fever, and at times there are distinct rigors. There is often, as Tanner points out, uneasiness in the left rib region, with inability to lie on that side, so that, with this symptom added, I think I may fairly claim that *Urtica* is a true simile to gout. It has :

1. Fever, heat and cold, flushes.
2. Passages of grit and gravel.
3. Uneasiness of left rib region.
4. Great restlessness. (XXI 75)

**— The Acute Attack**

In genuine gout we have to deal with the *attack* : this is the mountain of difficulty. (XXI 28)

**— Treatment : Uric Acid and Alkali**

It is not possible to cure the uric acid diathesis with alkalies, in as much as the alkalescence thus produced is only the chemical, and not vital; as for the alkalescence thus set up, to be rendered permanent it is requisite to continue unceasingly the input of alkalies. (XXI 61)

It must, therefore, be manifested that the mineral water, the alkaline treatment of gout (and the piperazine cure must be reckoned to the alkaline) is a cure, more or less, of the *gouty products*, but has little or no influence upon the gout disease itself in the sense of the uric acid

* Das. Wesen und die hygienische Behandlung der Gicht Detmold, 1894.

diathesis. The products are got rid of; *the power of producing* remains unimpaired. The grit, gravel, tophi and, with *piperazine,* perhaps even calculi, can be eliminated by the chemical treatment, but the diathesis remains untouched. (XXI 64)

**Differences between the Cure of the Gouty State by Mineral Water and Alkalies and by Homoeopathic Remedies :** Essentially, the cure of the gouty state by mineral waters and alkalies is mainly chemical, *viz.,* they set up a condition of alkalescence, and the uric concretions are thus rendered soluble, and the mass of fluid drunk washes them out, while in the homoeopathic treatment the *organism itself becomes its own sweep and turns them out,* In the former case the urine becomes clear, while under the homoeopathic action of the remedies the urine becomes *dark* and *visibly charged with gravel.* Only in the case of large portions of gravel, and in the case of actual calculi, does the *Piperazine* and *Gichtwasser* treatment seem to me to be preferable, inasmuch as in this latter case the organism itself cannot possibly do the work until the concretions have been dissolved. (XXI 68)

**— True Treatment**

In a given case of gout the symptoms are not those of the individual himself, but of the gouty matter, of its material presence in the individual: the pain, the swelling, the redness, the tenderness, the fever, the restlessness— these are produced by the gouty material, which we see from the fact that they disappear as soon as this material is washed out; so that what we require are remedies that are homoeopathic to the state of the patient which preceded the gouty deposit into the tissues, inclusive of these deposits. In fact, the pathology of gout must be considered, in prescribing adequately, homoeopathically. Our anti-arthritic remedies must be capable of producing a state that leads upto a deposit of gouty material, and not be merely homoeopathic to the symptoms produced by the material itself. The process, together with the product, must be within the pathogenesis, or else a real totality of the symptoms is not obtained. In fine, the gouty material is the *stop-spot* of the action of the remedies thus far mostly employed in the homoeopathic treatment of gout. I have been severely taken to task for claiming that *pathology must be considered in a homoeopathic prescription in order to ascertain the* **Stop-spot** *of the action of each remedy,* but I beg these esteemed colleagues to note that I did not say *morbid anatomy,* but *pathology,* two widely different things. Morbid anatomy we study in the deadhouse; that may or may not have to be considered as throwing some light on a given subject, but pathology is the doctrine of the disease in the living — the actual pathic biology of the diseased individual, which *ends* where the morbid anatomy *begins*. (XXI 71)

**— Two Phases**

For the successful treatment of gout it is necessary to have a clear idea of what constitutes its various parts; notably must we differentiate between its pre-deposit symptoms and its post-deposit symptoms, for much of the want of success in its cure is due to a mixing-up of the two sets of symptoms. The symptoms that precede and lead upto the uric acid retentions in the blood are a series by themselves; those due to the uric acid in the blood and which lead up to the gouty deposit as an attack, or as chronic deposits, are a second series. The former really spell arthritic cacopepsia, while the latter are synonymous with uric acid poisoning; in the one we deal with the producing power, in the other with the product. (XXI Preface)

## Grand Diseases and Grand Remedies

As I often say .. . *aux grands maux les grands remedies*. Such pop-guns as *Nux vomica* or *Pulsatilla* or *Subnitrate of Bismuth* will not cure tumours of the stomach, and hence if they are to be cured we must bring out bigger guns, and the zoic remedies are the very biggest guns of all beyond compare. (XX 196)

## Haematocele and Haemorrhoids — Constitutional

In cases of considerable extravasations of blood, such as this case of peri-uterine haematocele, the condition must be first tackled from the constitutional standpoint. The same reasoning applies to constitutional haemorrhoids : it is inadequate to treat the varicosis till the constitutional taint has been cured. (XX 106)

## Haemorrhoids and Surgery

As a matter of fact, piles can no more be *radically* cured by surgical operation than can a hole in the roof of a house be cured by catching the infalling rain in a bucket.

I have never met with a case of uncomplicated haemorrhoids (I would not deny that more experienced men may have) but could be cured by one, or all, of the follwing measures — *viz.*, diet, rest, *posture*, and medicines internally and topically.

Topical applications are absolutely needful in *very extreme* cases in which the bowel is protruded very much and the atony of the part is so extreme that the very hypostasis becomes a source of danger and a part of the tumour being thus practically outside the organism. But very few appreciate the value of *posture*.

I find many homoeopaths even never attempt the medicinal cure of piles. How wrong and unfair is this to the patient, and, moreover, how cruel! Unhappily, too many medical men "finish their education" when they get their sheep skins; others again use practical medicine as a milch cow and spend all their spare time on a hobby. (II 108)

### — Constitutional Disease

There is no such a thing as primary piles — they are all either hypostatico-obstructive or merely obstructive, or from pressure from above, or from constitutional ailments, which, all lumped together, constitute the haemorrhoidal diathesis, notably of German authors.

The frequent haemorrhages from the haemorrhoids are, in my judgment, all of constitutional origin, and constitutional treatment will cure such, but the constitutional cause must be got rid of before a radical cure can be effected either of the haemorrhoids or of the haemorrhoidal bleedings. (VI 17)

### Haemorrhoid Surgery and Cataract

To begin with traumatism is *admitted* when it arises from *contre-temps* in obstetric practice, and no one of experience will be disposed to deny it when ascribed to blows, falls, railway accidents, and the like. This is so well recognised in homoeopathic practice that many successful cures have been wrought by falling back on the traumatic etiology of, may be, twenty or more years ago.

What made me *first* think about it was the very frequent observation, in taking the cases of cataract patients, that *operations for piles* were so often a part of their life history. It could not be accident or mere coincidence, I thought; if *mere* coincidence, it is, to my mind, very strange. (VI 43)

**— Surgical Treatment — Sequelae**

In my own practical experience I trace cases of diabetes and cataract to the surgical traumatism inflicted in operation for piles. But more of this anon. (VI 28)

**— Treatment**

Then again, all aperients must be *absolutely* forbidden; this is of prime importance, and if a patient (the case being a bad one) will not absolutely give in on this point, I invariably decline the case. There is nothing for it but this. Of course, the diet must be modified accordingly. The physician who allows aperients *cannot* CURE bad piles, though he *treats* them with all the skill of Hippocrates, Galen, Sydenham, and Hahnemann combined. Why? Because the peristaltic action set up by the aperient acts from above downwards, and therefore increases the haemorrhoidal mischief mechanically, to begin with, and then by increasing the active congestion, and finally making the hypostasis worse than ever.

Furthermore, it is almost of equal importance *to forbid the patient to go to stool until he postively cannot hold out any longer;* that is of course, in very severe cases. Why? Because haemorrhoidal sufferers have often a knack of *pressing* at stool as if they were parturient; the abdominal press acts upon the whole contents of the belly, and thus the pressure *from above* brought to bear upon the piles will do more harm in a few moments than the best directed efforts of any physician can mend by the time another stool takes place.

It is simply not possible to cure *very severe cases* unless aperients be *totally* abandoned, and unless *all use of the abdominal* pressure for the time, given up. (VI 88)

Heart affections; imperfect aeration of the blood; liver affections; congestions in the portal system of veins; enlarged spleen; abdominal tumours; great accumulation of fat in the omentum, or of faeces in the intestines; in fact, anything that disturbs the reflux of blood to the right heart, vena cava inferior, vena portae, tends to hypostatic hyperaemia of the haemorrhoidal veins. The successful treatment of piles involves an accurate appreciation of the topography and of the anatomical relations from the midriff to the pelvic outlet as first groundwork, and then a consideration of the etiology of each case. (VI 152)

Some cases of piles depend upon a disturbance in the brain, others upon a spinal affection, especially about the *cauda equina*. Some are due to a liver complaint, and some to portal congestion; others, again, are connected with a disturbance around the neck of the bladder, the prostate, the spermatic veins, the uterus, the ovaries; or they may arise from chronic constipation, or be due to a really local cause in the rectum itself, mere proctostasis, or be merely a topic expression of general varicosis. Then again, the lungs and the rectum are often in wondrous sympathy with one another. So each case has to be looked at all round, as to the other constituent organs and parts of the same economy. Then there are various nosological forms that complicate piles : pregnancy, phthisis, gout, general plethora, cephalic congestion with threatened apoplexy (how often does apoplexy follow a wrong treatment of piles !) heart affection, and syphilis. Syphilitic haemorrhoids are at times the most painful of any, and the pain is often an inch or two above the sphincter.

But, with all the varieties, there is always one prominent and distressing condition, viz. : HYPOSTASIS. in other words, much of the distress is due to the hypostatic congestion, and this it is that an operation gets rid of, and nothing else; only, with the operation, not only is the bath emptied, but the baby has been forgotten, and poured out with it.

I have adopted the very simple plan of *raising the buttocks above the horizontal*, by means of various little mechanical contrivances improvised at the time, according to the circumstances of the patient; two or three pillows serve the purpose. Every one is familiar with the contrivances for raising the heads of sick people; well, I just reverse the process and raise the lower part of the trunk, and this is a great help in very severe cases. (VI 98)

**— Treatment Local**

Of course, it will be objected that as I used *Hamamelis* externally, and *Aloes* internally, I do not know how much of the curative action is due to each respectively. This I grant, and the scientific value of the prescription is thereby lessened, no doubt. The gentleman was away from home at the time at the seaside for his holidays, and this prescription was forwarded to him by post. (VI 92)

## Hahnemann

But some have naughty notions of free thought in matters medical, and, to use an inelegant expression, chew their own cuds, and these do read Hahnemann. (II 31)

### — and Hughes

I should not thus take upon myself to correct Dr.Hughes, for I owe my conviction of the truth of Homoeopathy largely to a perusal of his beautifully written and most erudite works, and I shall never be able to pay this great debt; but as he corrects his master, Hahnemann, I may perhaps be fairly forgiven for correcting mine. For my part, I find Hahnemann so reliable and so exact that if my observations and his do not tally, I look again and am convinced of my error. (II 30)

### — and Paracelsus

Hahnemannic medicine in its pristine purity is based on pure pharmaco-dynamics; it is in fact therapeutically applied pharmaco-dynamics; its first and deepest ground-work being the principle that given drugs affect given organs (parts) by self-elective preference. Therefore up to this point Paracelsic medicine and Hahnemannic medicine coincide. (XX 19)

### — and Rademacher

I sometimes regret that the disciples of Hahnemann and those of Rademacher became so closely assimilated, for it seems to me that drug provings are not everything, and I cannot help thinking that had the Rademacherians kept by themselves, they would have taught us much of the higher physiology of the various organs that we still have to learn. *And I am bound to say that some of the organ remedies of Rademacher possess a direct healing power over organ diseases that their provings in no way explain.* Perhaps further knowledge will throw light on this; we must accept the fact, and wait for the explanation.

In daily life we make certain acquaintances with our fellow-beings, and some of these pass out of sight for a time, or for ever. Months or years roll by, and we meet with some of them again, and as so-and-so is with us, we introduce our friend to him, remarking that we have known him ever since a certain memorable event. We find that with a physician diseases and drugs stand out as so many individual acquaintances along the path of his professional life; if he meet a congenial brother chip he will very soon run off the first subject of conversation and begin to "talk shop". Most people will join in a very hearty condemnation of "talking shop", but, nevertheless, the genuine man will not be long with you before you can form a pretty correct opinion of his walk in life. Let two medicoes meet for a little soical chat, and you will not have to wait long for the sign of the leech. And why should it be otherwise? Do we really expect a plant-loving botanist to prefer astronomy as a subject of conversation? (X 8)

Rademacher's organopathy (that an otherwise able modern writer appropriates with child-like *naivete* ) is no more and no less than the homoeopathic specificity of seat, with just a dash of a mystic psychic something in the several organs; if we set aside this little particular soul for each organ, it is only local affinity, or elective affinity. And it is quite true in nature, and the mind that cannot, or will not, recognize it, is wanting in catholicity of perception; and *in practice will often go a mile when three paces would have reached the goal.* Whatever else *Cantharis* may be, it is first and foremost a kidney medicine; *whatever else Digitalis may be, it is primarily a heart medicine,* and let *Belladonna* be what it may, it is before all things an artery medicine, and just in this sense *Ceanothus Americanus* is a spleen medicine. (X 12)

**—, Glory of**

It is the great glory of Hahnemann to have introduced the systematic study of the effects of drugs in the healthy subject into medicine, thereby laying the very foundation of *any* system of Scientific Medicine. This is now admitted on all sides, except that every little chanticleer gets the credit of it rather than Hahnemann. The world is not yet capable of appreciating the herculean labours of this great teacher. The day will come when the *Hahnemannian Oration* will be the rendezvous of all that is great and good in the medical world. At present his lot is scorn, ridicule, slander, and contempt, and worse than all, *his life labour is daily filched from him by the pygmies of the hour.*

But Nemisis lives, happily, through all time, and may tarry, but will surely overtake them. Awaiting this, it is for the small and persecuted body of the disciples of Hahnemann to follow in his wake, fearing neither ridicule, slander, nor hatred. (II 26)

**Hahnemannian Provings**

As far as my reading carries me, a better or more reliable provers committee never existed for working out the pathogenesis of any drug whatsoever. Complete it is not, neither is it, or could it then be, perfect. We miss the use of the ophthalmoscope to interpret the eye symptoms; of the stethoscope for the investigation of the heart and lungs of the provers, both before, during, and after the provings; the renal secretions were not examined, and the temperature was not taken. Future Regii Professors of Experimental Drug Pathology will fill in the Hahnemannic Cadre, and thus bring it abreast of modern requirements. But even as it is, how immeasurably superior is it to *the cat-dog-and-rabbit crudities of the dominant sect in medicine*, whose one aim would seem to be paralyse and kill countless lower animals to see how much a given drug can do and how soon it can do it. These points have a certain value as giving us a knowledge of the last links in the chains, but what we require for clinical purposes is an accurate knowledge of all that drugs can do on the *hither side* of that stage of absolutely lethal organic change from which no recovery is conceivable. These able and honest men are working hard for the science of the deadhouse, but not for that at the beside. On them the light of the Hahnemannic Law has not yet dawned, and they are still where Haller was. (II 41)

## Harelip Treatment

Now, although I felt the idea of trying to prevent harelip with the help of *specificity of seat* in the ordinary homoeopathic sense unworkable, still this lay in the nature of the case rather than in the nature of thing generally. Thus in those liable to beget offspring with defects or deformities, or displacements of organs, or parts to which we have approved remedies with specific affinities for such organs or parts, we might, and undoubtedly should, find it of eminent service, and also of the careful application of the homoeopathic law of similars; also of the tripartite pathology of Hahnemann; and of the constitutional states of Grauvogl, and, perhaps, even of the *Remedia "universalia* of Rademacher*. (III 111)

---

* *Remedium universale* is not a would-be panacea or cure-all, but one that hypothetically affects the universe of the microcosm, i.e., not an organ.

## Hay Fever

Two or three successive summers must pass before we can rely upon a cured case of hay fever being really cured to return no more. From the remedies I have found useful, and also useless, in the therapeutics of hay fever I have come to the conclusion clinically that what nosologists and clinicians call hay fever includes several aetiologically and pathologically totally different ailments or diseases. In some, I think hay fever very distinctly a manifestation of a phthisical taint — about the others I have not yet made up my mind. The pollen of grasses has the same relationship to hay fever as the north wind has to a phthisical cough — the cough is hardly a north-wind cough in a patholgical sense. (XVI 168)

## Health — Height, Weight and Diet

I go a little out of my way to point out the common fallacy underlying almost all the data given as to what the normal weight of a person of a given height should be. If my reader will consult the tables, he will find that the assumed basis is faulty in a very important particular. Let me explain. Place a dozen persons of a given height — say 5ft. 9in. — side by side in a row, and as they are all the same height, the tops of their heads will be in a line, *but* their hips will be at very different heights. In fact, it will be seen that the height of an individual is no sure guide to his *bulk*, and *therefore not to his weight*. In some a *long neck* makes an inch or more difference, in others it is a very long *thigh bone* that gives the greater height; but in both cases the weight is not determined by the length of the neck or of the legs, but rather by the relative *length of the trunk*.

There are many *big* people who stand at 5 ft. 6 in., and there are a good many *small* people who stand about 6 feet high.

There is a saying amongst the people that little women make the best mothers; but these so-called little women are really *big* women, only they are on *short legs*. When examined very closely I find they are large in the trunk and have fine pelves, while *big* women (so-called) are really smaller in the capacity of their trunks and pelves, and hence less adapted for the duties of motherhood.

The neck carries the head, the legs carry the trunk, and certainly heavy heads and heavy trunks are more safely carried on supports not too long in the perpendicular. This being so, all the data given in our tables of how much you ought to weigh if you are of a given height require to be revised; for any one whose attention has been called to the subject can readily see that there are many little people who are tall, and very many big people who are short. There are, of course, a few people — very few, really — who are both big and tall. As a rule, very tall people are not of great constitutional power, though some tall thin people are *very* tough and wiry, and exceedingly vital.

What have height and weight and their relative merits to do with gout? Just this : every little medico thinks he knows all about the diet suitable for this ailment and that, and is so very sure that a person of a given height should only weigh so much, and that a big gouty individual may be safely and profitably starved till his height and weight proportion tallies with the table published in his text-books, but which tables are based entirely on false data.

In fine, in judging of the diet suitable to a person, keep in view the amount of work he has to do; and before you determine the proper weight of an individual, do not merely consider his height from crown to sole, but rather have greater regard to the diameters of his trunk.

What first led me, twenty odd years ago, to think more closely of what should be the criterion of a person's weight, was the fact that I have long since come to the conclusion that the big may be short and the tall small. Also that the power of an individual is in proportion, not merely to his height, but to *all* his measurements, and these must be carefully considered before a true conclusion can be arrived at. (XXI 115)

## Herpes — Pain

### The After-Pain of Shingles

As I have before stated, neuralgias offer a good test of the opposing schools of Medicine, and in the treatment of the after-pain of shingles we see the incomparable advantages of homoeopathy. By curing this variety of neuralgia I have over and over again, made notable converts to homoeopathy, — and by curing I do not mean merely lulling the pain temporarily, but its radical and definite extinguishment. It is in the middle-aged and elderely that the after-pain of shingles is so distressing, — often, in fact, little less than terrible. Let us take a very high — perhaps the very highest —allopathic authority on the subject, and his most recent utterances. I refer to Mr.Jonathan Hutchinson, late President of the Royal College of Surgeons. It will be observed that Mr. Hutchinson does not for one moment entertain the idea that what he fails to cure could possibly be cured by anyone else. (XIV 132)

## High and Low Dilutions

I have satisfied myself that Hahnemann's doctrine of drug dynamization is true and capable of scientific experimental demonstration. I honour the high dilutionist as a true physician, and can but pity the arrogance of a crude materialist who denies ability and scientific attainments to high dilutionists because they are high dilutionists.

On the other hand, I cannot but feel that the high dilutionists are very much to blame in their self-assumed isolation. It savours too much of pharisaism.

Militant Homoeopathy wants all her adherents, and has a right to their allegiance. Do not let us delude ourselves. Giving crude drugs does not necessarily exclude homoeopathicity of drug to disease, and the mere fact of giving high dilutions never was Homoeopathy and never will be. Hahnemann was an omnidilutionist, and gave low dilutions, although it is quite true that he subsequently gave much higher dilutions the preference. (II 134)

### High Dilutions

By the way, the great objectors to the use of *Bacillinum* and the like for the most part declare that the higher dilutions contain *none of the drug*; but as I use these zoic medicines *only* in high dilutions they are objecting to ... nothing, and this on their own shewing! Either the higher dilutions contain of the essence of the drug, or they do not; if they do not the names they go by must be a matter of total indifference. If higher dilutions contain none of the original drug it must follow that *Pulsatilla* CC., *Bacillinum* CC., and *Syphilinum* CC., and *Broomhandle* CC. are one and the same thing, viz : a wee quantity of sugar of milk.

In what university did these sapient objectors learn their logic? (XX 173)

### High Potency and Pathology

I learned the lesson that the pathologic similimum of a disease must be administered in high potency and infrequently. Moreover, the worse the case the higher must be the potency as a rule. (XVI 209)

### Homoeopathic Remedy, A Stimulus

Remedies do not cure directly at all, but through the organic processes of nature. It is exceedingly difficult to fix the mind on how and why of a given cure if of chronic nature, becuase after the medicinal stimulus has been given, we must bide a wee till nature mothers the action caused by the stimulus. (XXV 17)

**Homoeopathic Milk for Allopathic Babes**

"A Manual of Pharmacodynamics", that was a new revelation to me in so many ways. It has been called "Homoeopathic Milk for Allopathic Babes"; it would be a good thing for the world if the allopaths would but partake freely of this precious milk. However, there is one condition absolutely necessary to its digestibility, viz., the allopathic babe must have a clean tongue, and a stomach that calls loudly for healthy therapeutic food, or it will disagree with him. For, if his tongue be coated with crass prejudice, and his stomach gorged with medical conventionalism and scholasticism, he will be unable to take it up or assimilate it. And if he cannot bear the milk, how is he to partake of the more solid food of the "Organon". (VI 31)

**Homoeopathic Treatment — Infrequent Dose and Tissue Salts**

The experienced know well what I mean when I speak of the long thin neck of the consumptive and consumptively-disposed, and if they will treat these thin-necked ones as I here relate they wil slowly get a very weighty change. In case it should be lost sight of I would again expressly state that one does of, say, six globules of *Bacillinum* (30, C., CC., or M.) every eight or ten days is enough, because we want not the remedy itself but *its action*, and the action when set up lasts well for a week. And it seems to me that when the *Bacillinum* is too frequently repeated the action of one dose trips up, so to speak, the action of the previously-given dose, and that therefore we get *more* permanent drug-action from *fewer* doses than from the same remedy frequently repeated.

I would also like to repeat what I have before adverted to, viz. : *Bacillinum* will *not* cure vaccinosis, for instance, it works in its own sphere only. Also that the progress is much hastened when tissue salts are given *after* the consumptive state has been cured — thus after the *Bacillinum* had cured Lord X.'s consumptiveness and he was well but *weedy*, *Calc. phos.* 3x followed with very good effect. (XVI A154)

## Homoeopath, the Onus of not Being a

This is my twenty-sixth reason for being a homoeopath, and it alone were amply sufficient; and whether it be God's will that I die to-night, or live for another fifty years, I feel that while I do live I am in duty bound to fight the good fight of Homoeopathy with all the power I possess : were I to do less I should be afraid to die.

Young man, the responsibility of not being a homoeopath is very terrible. (XI 39)

## Homoeopathy

*Like cures like,* no more and no less, whether people have onus enough to see it or not.

Now this Hahnemannian doctrine of similars has been fermenting the medical world for the past eighty years, and although it has not yet leavened the whole lump, it has leavened some small portion, for which humanity has cause to be grateful, and is so, too, as far as light goes. Unhappily, this homoeopathy is nothing like so good as — health! But it comes next to that delightful boon, which most of us throw away when we have it, and then work hard to get it back again. (II 146)

### — and Aggravation

"Well, I find I cure best if I get an aggravation, so that if I do not get any aggravation I conclude I have not got the right remedy for the case; they may laugh at it as much as they like, *but that's what I find*".

We do not often get aggravations in organopathic practice, because the degree of drug-likness to the disease is small; but they do occur at times when there happens to be a great degree of homoeopathicity existing between drug-action and morbid state; and in reading the literature of the organopaths one is stuck with the curious fact that the more experienced they became in applying organ-remedies to organ diseases *the smaller became their doses* : thus Rademacher slowly came down from twenty-five or thirty drops of the ordinary strong tincture to 15, to 12, to 10; aye, even to "one drop well diluted in water!" (XX 209)

**— and Deafness**

Deafness is a very troublesome thing to deal with, but it is worthwhile being a homoeopath, were it only for the power it gives one over deafness. I never could make out what you allopathic fellows did for deafness beyond the everlasting syringing. I have peered about in the aural departments of big hospitals, and read the books of noted aurists, beginning with a namesake of my own, but could never find that they did any real good beyond clearing away mechanical hindrances. And even in Homoeopathy it seems to me that our specialists rely far too much on cutting, scraping, and syringing. (XI 57)

**— and Difficult Cases**

Homoeopathic (and other!) practitioners are often hoodwinked by the personal surroundings of a patient, and to be pitchforked into a nest of unbelivers to cure a desperate case is verily no pleasant position to be in, as any physician of the homoeopathic ilk knows but too well. (XI 54)

**— and Faith Healing**

It is often curiously interesting to notice how a given patient will, during a course of treatment, pick out a particular remedy with almost unfailing certainty, and this always impresses my mind afresh and again, since there is no possibility of doubting the evidence. For where is the "personal magnetism", the "personal equation", here? Where the faith, and where "the influence of mind on matter"?

This patient had powders at different times containing on a number of occasions very infrequent doses of *Bacillinum*. C (in fact, two or three a month), and on other occasions the medicament was *Thuja* 30 or *Sabina* 30 (also three a month) and YET she knew the difference between the powders from their influence, while to look at they were identical. (XXIII 110)

**— and the Homoeopath**

You ask me whether the homoeopaths as a body endorse my views as to the amenability of cataract to medicines?

My answer is that some do and some do not, but that is not material; the task is very difficult, and not within the power of every physician who happens to practise on homoeopathic lines : the higher and highest work of which Homoeopathy is capable depends upon the capacity of the operating clinical artist — i.e. upon the homoeopathic practitioner. *What I claim for Homoeopathy is what I have done with its aid myself*; other physicians will be able to do more, and some less. (XI 48)

**— and Morbid Anatomy**

Homoeopathy must progress on the lines of pathology and morbid anatomy, or it will wane, and study on animals will have to help us. (XVIII)

**— and Numbers**

You ask how it then is that with all the merits which I claim for Homoeopathy, its practitioners should be in "such a contemptible minority in the praofession"? I presume, being in the minority does not necessarily mean to be in the wrong.

I suppose you hold that the world moves? There was a time when those who said so were in the minority, and not very far from the stake if they dared to aver their belief! (XI 27)

**— and Organopathy**

The reason why homoeopathy swallowed up organopathy lies in the fact that homoeopathy *is* organopathy and something else besides, viz. : the differentiating law of similars. (XX 21)

**— and Orthodox Medicine**

Pray understand that I am not in the least desirous of making you, or anybody else, a homoeopath; it makes no difference to truth, it will get on very well without any of you.

Nor do I anticipate any particular good from all this scribbling of my fifty reasons to you; I do it just to substantiate my own position, and slap the jeering ignorance of orthodoxy in the face. (XI 37)

**— and Pathology**

I lay great stress upon these cures of osteomata by Hecla lava because they conclusively demonstrate that the law of similars *is a workable instrument* in the medicinal treatment of tumours; also it shows that the accepted anatomical classification of tumours is *some* help to us. And, moreover, what a vista of therapeutic possibilities this opens up to us! When we know what natural bodies can produce myomata, neuromata, fibromata, lipomata, &c., we shall to some extent have their remedies straight away. (XX 83)

**— and Pathology**

To go no further, I have myself demonstrated that *Natrum Muriat.icum* in dynamic dose is powerfully antidotal of the effects of the same substance in repeated material quantities, and I think conceivable that *silicea* may be a potent causator of cartilaginous and osseous tumour formations. (XX 95)

It is needless to say to the man who has read and understood Hahnemann that the accurate individualization of each case is the true way to wander *always*, but generalizations and pathology must not be neglected, for they are most important in actual practice, and a diagnostic survey of the state of the various organs will be generally necessary. At least, generalizations and pathology are tools *I* cannot do without. It is a silly proceeding to work out an elaborate homoeopathic equation in a case of scurvy for instance, and the practitioner who understands the constitutions of Grauvogl will, all other things being equal, have more success than he who pooh-poohs them. Furthermore, although we certainly cannot cure all that is curable with Dr. Schussler's twelve tissue remedies, yet our knowledge of the spheres of action of these same remedies is vastly enlarged by his original way of working out his deductions. (VI 140)

From this it follows that an accurately correct scientific homoeopathic prescription is only possible in the hands of sound diagnosticians; it is not enough to work out the homoeopathic equation symptomatically; it must be motived, or the homoeopathicity is empirical only. That is to say the *range* of action may be from end to end of the affection, or it may be homoeopathic to, and reach as far as, for instance, the nail in nail-pneumonia, or the microbes in microbic pneumonia.

To the (1) *seat of action*; and the (2) *kind of action*; we have now added the (3) *range of action* of the remedy.

It is a sad reflection upon the scientific spirit of the age that the theory and practice of scientific homoeopathy are not taught by the most able and most accomplished pharmacologists and pathologists honours and money could obtain.

Homoeopathy is not taught at all.
Why?
Just because it is not understood by the common medical unionists, and what *they* do not know is not knowledge. A few of them at times seem to catch hold of its skirts here and there, but as even this constitutes them black-legs one hears no more about it. This the curse of medical priest-craft. (XX 28)
Now, I have a partiality for cases with a good sound pathology that can be seen, felt, cut out, put into the scales and weighed! They seem so much more proof-affording than mere symptoms in given parts, as headache or neuralgia, as these often depart of themselves. (XI 66)

**— and Posology**
Perfectly true; I cannot discuss homoeopathic (or, if you will, *my*) posology with you, but I will give you my rules, viz. : *The dose depends upon the degree of similitude*; the greater the similitude the higher the dilution and the less frequent the administration; the smaller the degree of similitude the lower the dose and the more frequent the repetitions of the dose. My own range of dose is from a few gloubules of the two-hundredth dilution at eight day intervals, down to ten drops of the mother tincure (of weak drugs, of course) four times a day.
The dose is quite often as important as the remedy, and your exclusively low, as well as the exclusively high dilutionists, are only one-eyed practitioners, though of course kings among the blind, i.e. the allopaths.
It is your fault that I have touched upon the vexed question of the dose, that is to Homoeopathy what the everlasting Irish question is in British politics. (XI 30)

**— and Truth**
You complain that I indulge in too much abuse, and that I am unnecessarily pugnacious and offensive. Perhaps so. Did you not have the impertinence to call the homoeopaths quacks ? You who know nothing about what they do! and do not you allopaths, every man of you, go about day by day and slander the homoeopaths!
You allopaths bear false witness against your homoeopathic neighbours every day of your lives — did I not once hear you say to your

aunt at table, "Oh, yes, Auntie, take some of your little homoeopathic pilules, *they won't* hurt!"

You said I must give you my fifty reasons out of my own life's work, as I had promised, or "come down the tree".

Well, I sit firmly on a very big bough of the old tree of truth, and it is not an ignorant allopath who will ever dislodge me. (XI 37)

**— Definition, Widening of**

The practical question with me is this : is it not time to *widen* our definition of homoeopathy in regard to the choice of the remedy, and, while leaving the choice of the remedy according to the totality of the symptoms in full force and dignity, draw into it *all* the aids that may lead to the right choice of the remedies; more particularly the natural history of the morbid processes themselves. (XX 14)

**— High Potencies**

Past experience teaches me, that really radical curing on lines of scientific precision with high homoeopathic potencies is not in harmony with prevailing views, and, therefore, totally incomprehensible and unacceptable to the profession at large, and hardly more acceptable to eight-tenths of the medical men practising homoeopathically. Even the homoeopathic practitioner seems very commonly quite unable to crawl out of his own old ways. Well, medical progress will pass him by and go on.(XVIII 26)

**— Individualisation**

Hence we see that neither Koch's nor any other fluid; neither *Bacillinum* nor any other remedy will, in itself, suffice, in the majority of cases, for the simple reason that each will act only in its own sphere, *i.e.* that to which it is homoeopathic it will cure and naught else. Of course, to a man who really understands Homoeopathy this is self-evident; all the same we are apt to lose sight of it more particularly in the presence of a series of successes, so that unless we are mindful of this, our very successes will in the end land us on the rocks. In fine : remedies cure homoeopathically and not otherwise, and hence a specific is only so far a specific as it is homoeopathic to any given case in its totality - for where there are other pathologic elements in the case the specific *does not cure* these other pathological elements; it is not homoeopathic thereto, and it will, therefore, not cure them, it will only cure *that part* of the case to which it is homoeopathic; the other part, or parts, of the case must be treated by *their* similars. I dwell upon this, and reiterate, because of its essential importance to correct views and successful practice. Thus I would refer to a case, mentioned at the beginning, of syphilis and tuberculosis manifested in a urinary fistula; in this case *Mercurius* and *Bacillinum* in alteration cured the case while neither alone would do so. This *kind* of alteration is, I think, really scientific and sound practice.

So we must always analyse our cases aetiologically and pathologically as well as *individualize them synthetically.*

The neglect of aetiologic diagnostics is indeed a "fatal error". Heresy? *Tant pis.* (XVI A 149)

**— Like a Game of Chess**

Of course a case of tumour that takes four years to cure, and needs a number of remedies to effect that cure, is, particularly to the uninitiated, of no great interest unless the subject is thought out somewhat, but if this be done, it becomes more and more interesting to the student, and the more interesting the more he knows of drugs, drug-action, the phases and causations of disease and of doctrinal pharmacology. A difficult game of chess can only be understood by one who knows chess well, and only a man well-grounded in the science can appreciate a finely played game; to the man who cannot play chess, the grandest game ever played means . . . nothing. (XX 156)

I always feel that unless we can use a series of remedies in very difficult complex cases, such cases will remain forever uncured or, as people usually say, incurable. And the complaint raised against "using so many medicines in a case" is really on a par with a complaint against a difficult game of skill such as chess that it "takes many moves to win". (XX 159)

**— Makes One a Master**

What I mean in my fifth reason requires to be insisted upon a little more, that you may perceive my meaning the more clearly. I said Homoeopathy raises one from the dependent position of a journeyman therapeutist to that of a master. (XI 15)

I have before pointed out to you that I love the grand independence conferred upon me by Homoeopathy : when I have a difficult case

I do not want to slide softly away from responsibility by the support of a consultative old fogey, whose brains have long since gone to sleep and whose *raison d'etre* is only medico-social. I want to cure my patient, and were it only for the mental satisfaction. Now, guided by Homoeopathy, and a wee bit of reasoning power, I can generally do this. (XI 60)

**— Prescribing on Symptoms Alone**

Well, it is very difficult; and symptoms alone do not commonly suffice, and I fancy this is the rock on which they stranded, and still do strand.

I wish to say nothing that is unkind to the absolutely-nothing-but-symptoms men, but their self-sufficiency, when they fondle the symptoms as the in-all and be-all of medicine, is only paralleled by their vulgar imputations of base motives to those who decline to admit that symptoms are other than a means to the end. A grand means, but still only a means : never the goal.

When I brought out my "New Cure of Consumption" I did it because Koch forced my hand, which I had held back for years; my wife often urging me to publish my experience with *Bacillinum* two or three years before Koch's Cure was heard of, but I hesitated, because I felt the world was not ripe for it, and a man with a very large family has no right to court ruin — so I held back. When I did come forward, because of the Koch fever, to vindicate the rights of the homoeopathic school to priority (myself included), I was accused by certain journalistic symptom-hunters of yapping for Kochian loaves and fishes!!!

When I shewed the review to my wife she exclaimed, "What a cruel shame!" But this is only by the way, and only brought in as a parenthesis.

*Que Voulez-vous?* think of the Inquisition in the name of the gentle Jesus of Nazareth.

Our sufferings are but microscopic specks by the side of mountains. and Paracelsus they actually battered to pieces with cudgels, and then made fun of him because, having written on longevity, he died (!) early!

At the same time it is very important to not to under-value symptoms as we cannot get on without them; and the more's the pity. I say this advisedly, because symptomatic equations are very time-devouring, and working at them too much is apt to become stultifying, and I have at times thought, narrows the medical mind —

turning it slowly into something very like a machine. When homoeopathy casts off its swaddling clothes, the subjective symptoms will be to Higher Homoeopathy what spelling is to reading. (XX 178)

**— Ridiculing it**

You say, "Your letters lately would seem to be intended to show how very superior your Homoeopathy is to that of your co-practitioners."

Well, that was certainly not my intention, but rather to show that people's beliefs have often nothing to do with facts; for instance, you allopaths ridicule Homoeopathy, but that system of medicine is true all the same. Many practitioners of Homoeopathy ridicule some of the most brilliant clinical triumphs of the very system they belong to. In both cases the error is the same; they both childishly suppose that *their powers* are the limits of the possible. I was merely trying to show the fallaciousness of their judgment; and this is important, as the greatest enemies of Homoeopathy are often its own weak-kneed or incompetent practitioners. (XI 29)

**— Rule or Law**

***Pro Lege : The Rule of Thumbers***

There is an able and learned faddist, and there are also a certain number of not very learned therapeutists, who maintain that the principle underlying the scientific practice of homoeopathy should be properly designated a *therapeutic "rule"* and not the *"law"* of similars."

At first sight it might and indeed does, appear that the question of whether we say *law* or *rule* is really only a matter of tweedledum and tweedledee. Examined, however, more closely, we shall find that it makes all the difference, for therapeutic rules are alterable and arbitrary, and often entirely unreliable. But homoeopathy in its essential principle is not alterable, arbitrary, or unreliable. If it had been, it would not have withstood the storms and attacks of the past fifty years and more. The practitioners of homoeopathy may later; their policy (if they had any) might alter; they may be greater or fewer in number; they may be honest or dishonest, learned or unlearned, clever or dull, many or few, and even disappear altogether *de facto* or politically, and STILL *homoeopathy in its essential principle remains* purely and simply as a *law of Nature*. If no one ever took remedial substances, which we call remedies, at all, the *law of similars* would still exist, though it would be out of operation. *The law exists quite independently of its operativeness.* America is immortal; rules are very mortal indeed. You can render the law of similars inoperative, but so you can have the law of gravitation or any other law of Nature. *Jaborandi* did not acquire its power to produce diaphoresis when that action was discovered in Paris a few years ago; *Jaborandi* did not acquire its power to reduce and check a diaphoresis when the French physicians first administered it for night-sweats; *Jaborandi* did not acquire its diaphoretic power when it was found out and utilized by man.

Those gentlemen who parade the term *therapeutic rule of similars* have, of course, a perfect right so to do, just as they would have the right to any other therapeutic rule, as, for instance, *the therapeutic rule of thumb.* But their frantic efforts to persuade the medical world that rule is the correct designation for the principle of homoeopathy are beneath contempt.

*God* made the *law* of similars; many physicians all through the ages have had faint glimpses and inklings of this therapeutic law. Hahnemann saw it in the full light of pharmic knowledge, and scientifically and practically demonstrated it, and around this *law* of similars a considerable number of rules have been placed by medical practitioners, some of which I will mention.

The rule of the schools is that homoeopaths (men who found their practice on applied pharmic knowledge based on the law of similars) are to be destroyed, by fair means if possible; if not, then by foul.

The rule of the allopaths is to refuse all dealings with the homoeopaths, except to solicit their alms.

The rule of the Ringerites is to practise the homoeopathy of the books, but not in accordance with the law of similars, but according to the therapeutic rule of thumb; and in this way they can so far satisfy their longings for a better than allopathic therapeusis, and yet keep their share of the loaves and fishes, with the contingent possibility of an odd baronetcy in the dim and distant future. Moreover, Mrs. Grundy visits with the Ringerites.

Finally, there are a few homoeopathic professional sprigs who feel that the one thing that debars them from complete happiness is the *law* of similars. It is just a rule, say they, and not a law at all! Like the Ringerites, they are nothing but rule of thumbers, and FOR THEM there is indeed no law of similars, for the very sufficient reason that *they* have not discovered it. And if any proof were needed that there is *absolutely no law* of therapeutics for these greatly distended *rule of thumbers*, their own therapeutic barrenness would afford it. Wherever the *rule of thumbers* rule, there rule also the surgeon's knife and the hypodermic syringe. (XIV 122)

**— Single vs. Series of Remedies**

You take exception to the *number* of remedies used in my last case, and want to know "which cured the case?"

Will you get a long ladder and put it up against the side of your house, and mount it so as to get into your house by the top window; and when you have safely performed the feat, write and tell me which rung of that ladder enabled you to do it. (XI 53)

I often compare the cure of a difficult case of disease to a game of chess in which you have king, queen, bishops, knights, rooks, and pawns, the various powers of which you must learn before you can play chess. (XI 54)

**— The Grand Therapeutic**

I am not ignorant of the range of the art-cure of disease in the wide literature of the world, and I affirm that outside of Homoeopathy *such* grand therapeutic work has literally and absolutely no existence.

Should it be the will of the Most High that I live on in my present vigour, I shall have yet a great deal more to say to the world in regard to Homoeopathy and other views of curative medicine; if not, then let these *Fifty Reasons* be my legacy to my country and to my fellowmen the world over. I say this because I intend to publish them, omitting, of course, all recognizable reference to your individuality. And of you personally I have very small hope, for well do I know that though one rose from the dead yet would you allopaths *not* believe in any, and therefore not in my "Fifty Reasons for Being a Homoeopath". (XI 72)

**— The Law**

I have it from you that *Arnica* causes erysipelas; I will not doubt *your* statement; you may now take it from me that *Arnica* cures erysipelas, and this I offer you as my fourteenth reason for being a homoeopath. *You* know the bad character of *Arnica* in that it is apt to *cause* erysipelas; *I* tell you of its good fame, viz. that it possesses the power of curing erysipelas, and the intellectual link that completes the little chain is the law of likes that God put into the mind of one Samuel to explain to the world.

You need not be so angry at my last reason; *I* did not make *Arnica* grow in the world; *I* did not endow it with the power of causing erysipelas; and *I* did not discover the therapeutic law in question; I just use this law in order to cure my patients, even as I use the useful invention known as a spoon wherewith to partake of my broth. With me it is merely a means to an end; there is no hocus-pocus about it. (XI 24)

**— The Little David**

My dear allopathic *confrere*, WHY are you so very simple that you leave us homoeopaths with this enormous advantage over the best of you? Any little homoeopathic David can overcome the greatest allopathic giant if he will only keep to his Materia Medica, *and the directions of Hahnemann*. And the good thing lies so near, and is so constantly thrown at you. If we homoeopaths were only to make a secret of our art, you would petition the Government to purchase it of us! (XI 46)

**— The Mighty Weapon**

It is unfortunate for the progress and extension of Scientific Medicines, — and by Scientific Medicine I mean no more and no less than Homoeopathy — it is unfortunate, I say, that our surgeons are so clever with their hands, for they do their work for the most part so well, so neatly, so painlessly, that medical men have come to rely more and more upon the knife, to the almost total exclusion of the more gentle, more humane, and more rational treatment with medicines.

The medical profession at large condemn homoeopathy, — they know nothing about it. There was a time when I also condemned it, — I also then knew nothing about it; but now, having studied it and practised it, my airy contempt has given place to humble-minded thankfulness, and I maintain that homoeopathy — real scientific homoeopathy — is the most mighty weapon against any disease known to mankind. It is in the hope that others may share in this knowledge that I send these pages to the press. (XVI Preface)

**— Proven Fact**

Had the Medicina Hahnemannica not been based upon a law demonstrable by pure scientific experiment, it would have been long since extinct except as an historic expression. But the law sticks fast, and there is no removing it — be you symptomatiker or specifiker, allopath or eclectic. That *opium* in due dose constipates has been proved : it is admitted. That *opium* in refracted dose opens the bowels has been proved : it is admitted.

That the kind of constipation which *opium* produces is similar to the kind of constipation which it does away with has been proved : it is admitted. (XX 22)

**— Symptom Covering**

***Stop-Spot of the Action***

The *stop-spot* of the action of a remedy is that spot in the morbid process beyond which it cannot go. Thus in the treatment of nail-pneumonia by phosphorus, the action of the phosphorus is spent or stopped at the spot where the nail is; the nail is its *stop-spot*. In microbic pneumonia the stop-spot is where the microbes are operative.

We have, therefore, in the range of drug-action to consider whether it is co-extensive with the range of the disease-action, and so reaching to the end, having been coincident from start to goal, or whether it only goes a part of the way. If it only goes a part of the way I call the place where it ceases the *stop-spot*, or the spot where the action is stopped or becomes spent.

A consideration of this is highly important, because finding out the stop-spot in the range of action of any given remedy will enable us to winnow the wheat of real cures from the chaff of pseudo-cures.

The contention that the disease is *all* expressed in the symptoms is one to which I cannot assent, because it is not true : it may be, or it may *not* be. It is *not enough* to cover the totality of the symptoms; for when this has been done we are only half way, we have then to ask these questions : what is the real nature, the natural history, the pathology of the malady under consideration? What caused it? Is the cause still there or has it gone? Is the *drug* chosen *capable* of producing a real disease like the one before us? In fact : is it *really* homoeopathic to the morbid process — coincident — adequate — reaching from beginning to end? *If not, we are on the wrong scent if we are to really cure and not merely palliate.* (XX 30)

To speak of the "all-sufficiency of symptoms" is to mislead some, to disgust others; and in general it effectively dams the stream of homoeopathic progress. (XX 42)

**— Treated with Disdain**

Here the eminent specialist treated the very idea of homoeopathic remedies having any good effect in such cases as utter non-sense. For all that the girl's father quite cured her with globules of *Sepia*. And how could the mighty gynaecologist know the effects of homoeopathic medicines since he had never tried them? The opinions of allopaths or the value of homoeopathy are nothing but spiteful splutter : vulgar and nasty. (XXIII 11)

**— What Good is it in Tumour-Curing**

There are many thousands of more or less learned medicos — in fact, the vast majority of *the* profession, who "don't believe in homoeopathy at all, you know". I have heard it called by many names; some of which are "nonsense made difficult". (That's what I used to call it!!) "Therapeutic nihilism,"(von Schroff); "the negation of science in therapeutics;" "the deathbed of diagnostics;" "old women's plaything;" "d — quackery;" "a trade-mark for the unsuccessful;" "an advertising medium;" "the invention of a German quack who sold pnoeum at a high price, which pnoeum' was borax."

Perhaps the wittiest I ever heard was ... "Homoeopathy! my dear madam — yes, I know what Homoeopathy is; it is — nothing!" and lately I was reading a smart pamphlet in which the author thus burst forth into eloquence :

"The medical world was at this time governed by Theory, Empiricism, Authority, and Speculation. The majority of practitioners blindly followed the authority of the past, and bled and dosed by the book, or adopted some strange theory. For example : Doctor Letsom, a practitioner of standing in London, read a paper to the Medical Society of that city in 1783, recommending lizards for the cure of cancer and other diseases. Well may the following lines be attributed to him. He is made to say :

*"When patients come to I,*
*I physics, bleeds and sweats'em.*
*And if they choose to die,*
*What's that to I, I lets'em.*

A good illustration of the speculative tendency may be found in the theory formed by Hahnemann, at the close of the last century. He ignored all previous medical knowledge; denied the existence of any curative power in the system; that any knowledge of anatomy; physiology, pathological anatomy, diagnosis, or the investigation of the nature of disease, was necessary to the physician, and claimed that symptoms alone should be treated, and that the more the medicine was diluted the greater its power over disease."

So if calling bad names would kill, we should not have to expect much help from homoeopathy in tumour-curing, or in anything else, for it would be dead.

"What do you think of these apples, Sir?"

"Don't know; let me eat a few and I'll tell you." So let us take a bite or two at the homoeopathic apple and see what it is like.

Homoeopathy says that those natural bodies called drugs that will cause morbid symptoms, will cure morbid symptoms thereunto similar; and to find out what drugs can do therapeutically, we must try them on healthy people to find out. But where are the healthy people to be had, who will eat drugs long enough and in quantities large enough to grow tumours in their bodily parts? — clearly they are not forthcoming.

This has rendered homoeopathy almost helpless in medicinal tumour-curing, but all the same the chapter of accidents proves theoretically its absolute soundness, as does also pure symptomatic treatment without any regard to morbid anatomy at all. It has been proved that the homoeopathic treatment of symptoms does sometimes result in the cure of the tumour causing such symptoms; thus *Colocynth* given for its pains has several times cured, not only such pains, but also the entire state, tumour and all. (XX 70)

— **Why Sneered at?** : I often wonder in this age of science that its scientific spirit so much neglects the scientific therapeutics of Samuel Hahnemann, particularly as Hahnemann has been so long dead. It cannot now make any difference to him! And faith! It makes no difference to me either.

Then why do I stand up for homoeopathy so persistently if it makes no difference to me?

Why, indeed?

Only one reason.

And what might that one reason be? Shall I confess, or let the black secret die with me?

Just this : *Homoeopathy is true, that's all.*

And if true, why do people sneer at it?

Fools always do sneer at what they do not understand. (XVII 170)

## Homoeoprophylaxis

### Some Remarks on Homoeoprophylaxis

In the April number, 1884, of the *Homoeopathic World*, there appeared the following communication to the Editor :

### Dr. Skinner on M. Pasteur's Homoeopathy

Dear Sir, — If the italicised is not Homoeopathy, what is it?

Thos. Skinner, M.D.

25 Somerset St., W., Feb. 27, 1884.

M. Pasteur's Experiments

M.Pasteur made an interesting communication to the Paris Academy of Sciences on Monday in relation to canine madness. His experiments had shown him that an injection in the region of the skull of the virus of rabies always produced the malady in an acute form, but that an injection in the veins only occasionally had acute results, being often followed by chronic affection only, without barking or ferocity. If a dog were inoculated with fragments of marrow or of nerve taken from a mad dog, the disease would be communicated. *M. Pasteur further stated that he had rendered twenty dogs proof against the disease by inoculating them with other virus than the virus of rabies.* Fowls and pigeons, injected with the latter became affected, but soon recovered spontaneously.

"If the italicised is not Homoeopathy, what is it?" Just so, *what* is it?

I think a little reflection will show that it belongs in the sphere of preventive medicine, and is not homoeopathy, i.e., it is an extension of the principle of similars to the prevention of disease.

Many other ardent homoeopaths besides Dr. Skinner have claimed that vaccination is a proof of the truth of homoeopathy; that it is, in fact, part and parcel of it. Evidently this is from the want of a little thought on the subject, since it must be manifest that such is quite impossible, for the simple reason that homoepathy is a system of *curing* — *similia similibus curentur* — whereas vaccination is not a *curative* measure at all, but a *preventive* one. And since prevention is, admittedly, *better* than cure, it must follow that it cannot be the *same*; therefore, vaccination is not homoeopathy, though I shall suggest that it might fitly be termed *Homoeoprophylaxis,* in as much as vaccinia and variola are similar pustular diseases, and the former being preventive of the latter, it may be in obedience to the principle — LIKE PREVENTS LIKE. Being a question of prophylaxis, it cannot be classed in *any* system of *cure*. And that likes *are* prevented by likes, *I* could adduce very many examples to show, did the narrow limits of this little treatise admit of it. Here it must suffice to differentiate between homoeopathy and homoeoprophylaxis, and to endeavour in a very general way to study a little the true nature of the latter as exemplified in vaccination and analogous facts such as Pasteur's inoculations.

Giving a variolous patient vaccine pus, or lymph (*vaccininum*), wherewith *to cure* his small-pox, that is homoeopathy, and we have ample testimony that it will thus act if given in refracted dose, and thus acting, it can hardly be other than homoeopathic in such action. The law of similars is the groundwork of both; in the one case to prevent, and in the other to cure. (XIX 83)

Strewn about in literature there are examples of small-dose homoeoprophylaxis; see Hahnemann's little essay on *Belladonna*, for example, at the very birth of Hahnemannian homoeopathy.

Then vaccine "lymph" — pus — has been dynamized *more homoeopathico* and given as a prophylactic against small-pox in epidemic times, and apparently with effect. *Thuja Occidentalis* has been used in like manner by more than one homoeopathic practitioner, and they claim that it is effective. The eminent Dr. David Wilson, of London, has, I hear, long used *Thuja*, in dynamic dose, as a sure preventive of variola.

Speaking for myself, I have for the last nine years been in the habit of using vaccine matter, in the thirtieth homoeopathic centesimal potency, whenever small-pox was about, and I have thus far not seen any one so treated get variola.

Dr. Massoto inoculated the diphtheritic exudation in an epidemic of diphtheira, and that with success.

It seems to me that the requirement of the age is to *systematize* the prevention of disease according to the law of similars, AND IN DYNAMIC DOSE. Clearly the dynamic dose is ESSENTIAL, or at any rate the very small dose, for otherwise the homoeoprophylactic aggravation would be a serious detriment in every way. It is easy to see that M. Pasteur and his fellow-workers are sailing down straight on this rock, whereon they are sure to suffer shipwreck. (XIX 104)

As a last word I would put in a plea for homoeoprophylactic vaccination, or what might be termed homoeopathic vaccination. That is to say, the vaccine matter is to be prepared as a homoeopathic remedy, and to be given by the mouth, in dynamic dose as the homoeoprophylactic. Pasteur's attenuating it by poisoning a series of animals is a very serious proceeding; an ordinary vial will do just as well if only attentuation is wanted. It is with virus thus attenuated that I used to treat myself when I was attending small-pox instead of being re-vaccinated. I used to treat my family and others with whom I was compelled to associate in the same way. None of us ever took small-pox. (XIX 110)

In regard to homoeoprophylaxis, I have here and there been written to know if I recommend any special mode of applying the law of similars to the prevention of disease. I should like here to briefly answer the question as falling well within the scope of our inquiry.

Does *Belladonna* — the red-rash-producing *Belladonna* — really prevent the evolution of the red-rash-producing virus of scarlatina? The question has been kicking about Europe for the past hundred years, and is mostly rejected of men of science, and yet I more than once raised the ire of our late (alas! that it should be late) friend, Dr. John Drysdale of Liverpool, for calling in question this prophylactic virtue of *Belladonna*. Drysdale thoroughly believed it after forty years of practice behind his back, and yet Drysdale found it very, very difficult to believe anything unless supported by very much evidence indeed - I, too, require a good deal of evidence before I *inwardly* believe. And though I have also used *Belladonna* in this sense, and very often seeming success, yet I somehow would like a *little* more positive proof!

*It seems so hard to believe it, and yet we cannot disbelieve it*. When it comes to animal viruses it is easier, of acceptance even *a priori*. And then comes the question of *how long the preventive* power of — say vaccininum against vaccinia, or against variola, would be likely to last? For it, too, must be a constantly decreasing quantity just as any other force-effect. And with the data from the work of the Pasteurians we do not know what to do : are the various viruses as passed through diverse animals still the same in a diluted form, or all different but allied bodies, and, if allied, how? (XIX 111)

**Homoeoprophylaxis — Nature of**

**Nature of Homoeoprophylaxis** : The *prevention* of disease according to the law of similar — homoeoprophylaxis - is still struggling with its swaddling clothes, but we may reflect on the following :

Two similar diseases will affect the organism similarly : they will affect the same parts, organs or tissues, and in a like manner.

If we call the two diseases *a* and *b*, and organism O, then if *a* fall upon O, and affect it positively (positive effect = *c*), this effect of *a* upon O, *c* will be like the effect of *b* (=*d*), for *a* and *b* are alike.

Now, if we admit that the similarity between *a* and *b* is enough to render them effectively equal, potentially congruent, then we should say $a = b$, and therefore $c = d$. Consequently $O + a = O + b$, and $O + c = O + d$.

That is the question for the solution of which we must appeal to scientific experiment, both at the bedside and in the laboratory, as well as to abstract reasoning.

It has frequently appeared to the writer that *time* and *quantity* (dose), are not duly reckoned with in the question of the efficacy or inefficacy of Jennerian vaccination; and Pasteur seems also to lose sight of both factors in his own experiments. The great mass of medical men firmly believe that vaccination protects against variola; and, that vaccinia and variola *are* ALIKE is quite certain; it is only the *degree* of the likeness that can be subject of dispute, for both are pyrexial pustular diseases.

Statistics of a number of years, nevertheless, shew that variola is in the aggregate, about as deadly as ever, allowing for a natural decrease of its vis by age; this cannot be controverted, so much must be conceded to the anti-vaccinators.

And yet, given groups of individuals are evidently protected *for the time* from variola by vaccination, and the more recent the vaccinia the greater the temporary protection, *provided the effect of the vaccination be not too great, in which case there will be a homoeoprophylactic aggravation, and then there will not only be no protective power, but on the contrary the vaccinate will be predisposed to it, i.e.*, instead of a positive and a negative eliminating one another we shall have two positives to be added together.

Let us express the difference between a vaccinated and an unvaccinated individual by the algebraic quantity $x$. Now, what is the nature of $x$? Is it positive or negative? *Quoad* perfect health it is negative, but *quoad* the organismic individual it is positive, if a diseased condition can be said to be a positive one.

To begin with, it is inconceivable that $x$ should be a CONSTANT FACTOR, which is evidently the general assumption; it must be an always lessening quantity, and $x$ might thus be initially congruent with variola, while it may at any subsequent point be incongruent. This really expresses the sum of human experience on the question of the efficacy or inefficacy of Jennerian vaccination, though it is not apprehended; whence the cry for re-vaccination *coup sur coup* on the one hand, and the want of faith in vaccination on the other, both positions being readily comprehensible if the effect of vaccination be recognised as an *inconstant* factor.

And from these considerations it must be manifest that the protection afforded by vaccination will be different in different individuals, and diminishingly different in the same individual, and always growing less and less until it is *nil*. Thus *x* might to-day be preventively equal to variola in an endemic form, but not equal to it in epidemic form. In other words the protection afforded by *x* is relative and contingent. Moreover, if the vaccinosis be too great, *i.e.*, too powerfully diseasing, it not only does not protect, but must actually add fuel to the flames.

We thus appear to arrive at the conclusion that vaccination does relatively and contingently protect from small-pox as a disease, but nevertheless, the mortality from small-pox remains in the aggregate the same, but in a greater percentage. That is to say, fewer people probably get small-pox, but the absolute number of deaths is not affected, or is greater.

In pro-vaccinational and anti-vaccinational literature, *morbility* and *mortality* are commonly confounded together. We have no means of knowing how many people *get* small-pox, either absolutely or porportionately, we, only know how many *die* of it. Therefore *all* the vaccination statistics are wide off the mark except perhaps those in certain hospitals. The pro-vaccinators maintain that vaccination protects from variola because they see that, as a general rule, the vaccinated do not get small-pox. The anti-vaccinists say, "Oh! but a good many of your vaccinated persons *do* get small-pox nevertheless, and the mortality from small-pox is as great as ever, or greater than ever!" Both sides are honest; both are apparently dealing with facts; both are striving after truth, and collectively they expend enough human energy to enrich a nation or colonize a continent. Where then is the missing link?

On the other hand it has been often noticed that a healthy person gets variola soon after vaccination, which to my mind militates in no wise against a belief in the protective power of vaccination, but is to be interpreted as meaning that the vaccinial infection was more than enough; just the same as a *little Aconite* will *lessen* feverishness, while *much Aconite* will make the feverishness worse.

Continuing now to let *x* stand for the difference between a vaccinate and a non-vaccinate, we must keep well before our minds that *x* represents the remaining effects of a disease — vaccionosis — and this is *not* a constant quantity; in an otherwise healthy person it must be continually growing less and less, and finally become extinct. Therefore, in order to determine whether vaccination protects against variola or not, we must first have the date of the vaccination in each case of varioloid or small-pox in the vaccinate. Were a considerable number of such cases tabulated we might arrive at some idea as to how long a given vaccination continues to affect the individual sufficiently for the vaccinosis to leave no room for variola, provided always that the vaccination were unipotential. (XIX 81)

## Hydrocephalitis

We have all met with cases of oddly-shaped more or less piled-up or bulging-out heads, and these people really bear about with them a cephalic misshapenness (perhaps very trifling, but still peculiar) as the permanent expression of the hydrocephalic states of their early lives. Such people are frequently gifted, their children are very delicate and apt to die of consumption; and although they have grown out of their hydrocephalus and may be gifted and distinguished members of society, they generally suffer more or less in various ways; they are apt to be a bit peculiar in their sexual spheres and their ways — glum sort of folks, by no means excelling in amiability. (XVI A 178)

## Ignorance and Error

It seems to me that *Aconite* and *Bryonia* alone, if we studied and rightly used, would convert the whole world to Homoeopathy, at least I see no escape for any honest *un*prejudiced man.

But prejudice is well-nigh almighty. As Bolingbroke says, "It may sound oddly, but it is true, in many cases, that if men had learned less, their way to knowledge would be shorter and easier. It is, indeed, shorter and easier to proceed from ignorance to knowledge than from error. They who are in the last must unlearn before they can learn to any good purpose; and the first part of this double task is not in many respects the least difficult, for which reason it is seldom undertaken." (XI 13)

## Illness and Vanity

People who are sick of some chronic disease and are given over to their fate by those who ought at least to have the courage of hopefulness, find not infrequently their greatest enemies in their nearest relations, who resent efforts at cure. These Job's comforters seem to regard determined efforts to cure their friends as personal insults.

This phenomenon I have observed so often that I have wondered what the explanation thereof might be : in ultimate analysis it would seem to be human vanity. *They* have pronounced the case hopeless, and therefore it is so and not otherwise. (XVII 131)

## Improvement of Human Race, Factors for

When a good gardener puts seed into the soil, he takes care that it shall be supplied with whatever experience teaches him is conducive to its development and growth; he does so because he knows that the future plant can be thus modified while still in Nature's earthly womb; indeed, we may say the plant never gets beyond this stage of dependency, as it lacks locomotive power.

We all know how chemistry has been successfully applied to scientific agriculture; and any Hodge looking at a poor crop of wheat in a field will be shrewd enough to surmise that the manuring or tilling had been neglected. He knows full well from what he sees in his own cottage plot that the well-dunged, carefully tended portions bear the best crops, and that what grows in this plot is not so readily affected by disease and drought by reason of its more sturdy growth.

Any country schoolboy knows that the poorest apples are on the neglected trees of hedgerows and of neglected grazed orchards, while the fine juicy ones are within the well kept garden.

Who has not noticed the scraggy, stunted appearance of the calves born of the kine that are turned out to common or forest after they cease to give milk? The future mother-cows lead a hard life and get but poor sustenance, and their offspring are proportaionately undersized and ill-conditioned, and have an ancient, wizened appearance generally.

Similarly, in the human subject, the child of the well-fed, well-worked, cheerful, happy woman, living in a sunlit airy habitation, is at birth the finest specimen of its kind.

On the other hand, what a miserable sight do the new-born babes of our courts and alleys, and of the pampered, tight-laced, high-heeled, lazy, lounging carriage-possessing women of the higher classes present! The extremes meet; the poor blanched creature, half starved, over-worked, shut up in some close, sunless dwelling, brings forth fruit very like that of her pale-faced, over-fed, under-worked, sofa-loving sister of the mansion and of the palace.

And nature is inexorable; look at our bills of infantile mortality if you do not believe it. It is well so; God ordained in his undeviating laws that the fittest should survive, and they do.

Clearly, then, *we may take it for granted that the development of the fruit within the womb can be modified for good and for ill.*

We need not mince the matter; the future human being is made up of four principal factors. First, the maternal ovum; secondly, the spermatozoon of the father, which requires, thirdly, a suitable soil for its development and growth. The womb is this suitable soil. These three factors being given, the blood of the mother supplies the fourth.

In the entire plant and animal world, the choice of the seed and soil lies more or less within ken and control, and faulty specimens get a short shrift, while the more fit are allowed to multiply; or in a wild state the weak are crowded out by the strong, and thus the fittest survive.

In our stock-breeding, the bovine and ovine species are well weeded of their faulty and diseased specimens by the butcher. That innocent individual, called the butcher, purchases the rickety or scrofulous calf of the honest farmer, and John Bull enjoys his *Kalbfleisch* through the Norman medium of veal. Thus nature cares for the survival of the fittest of the bovine species.

With the human species it is very different; faulty specimens of man may not be annihilated for the bettering of the race, and civilized life tends to the protection and fostering of the physically faulty, and hence to the deterioration of the race. This is one great reason why civilization tends to the destruction of society through a gradual deterioration of the race by the preservation of the weak from destruction under the reign of law, and by the collateral power of wealth.

In a savage state the weakling goes to the wall; in a civilized state he may be very rich, and of ancient lineage, and then it becomes most important, from the particular standpoint, that he should be married and beget offspring. This ramifies all up and down the various social strata. So in the end the barbarians are strong, and then numerous, and then they break in upon a highly civilized community, and a reconstruction of society ensues.

It remains to be seen whether science and art will in the future be able to save civilized society from being overwhelmed by savage hordes.

The true source of national greatness is large families of healthy children; these are the only true "fruits of philosophy". Those other "fruits of philosophy" are rotten at the core, and, like all rottenness, lead by the shortest road to annihilation, having here, however, a preliminary stage of bondage and servitude to the seed of the truly philosophically fruitful.

Surely it would be a strange philosophy that came in the mouths of ranting demagogues; fruit is the means of reproduction; *Dawn of Destruction* is what they mean.

Mankind is moved to marriage from purely selfish motives; the pairing takes place for almost every reason except for the physical bettering of the race. No doubt it is well so; the production of the most massive members, or of the biggest brains, can hardly be the chief end of man. (III 102)

## Incurable and Difficult Cases — A Clue

My own plan in difficult cases that seem so hopeless is to lay firmly hold of *some point* that may serve as a reasonable therapeutic starting point whence to carry out a cure. (XX 105)

In difficult, chronic, complicated cases of disease you require not a remedy but a ladder (series) of remedies, not one of which can of itself effect the cure, but each of which works cure-*wards*, their cumulative action eventuating in a cure — THAT *is how I cure cataract*, and many other chronic diseases that are currently held to be incurable by most men of all shades of the therapeutic opinion. I regard this power of utilising a long series of remedies for the cure of difficult chronic cases as only second in importance to the law of cure itself. I originally learned the thing in conversation with Dr. Drysdale, of Liverpool, though not formulated by him, and I doubt if Dr. Drysdale ever did formulate it. In my own mind I call it the *ladder of remedies plan*. It is what I often heard Dr. Drysdale call "a course of medicines". (XX 113)

## Insanity and Cancer

**Genuine Insanity : Its True Nature :** What is it? I have come to the conclusion, from a good many observations and therapeutic trials, that Genuine Insanity is Cancer of Mind. By cancer of the mind I mean simply that if the ailing fix itself upon, say, the breast, we have simply cancer of the breast, whereas if it fix upon the mind-organ, we have what we commonly call insanity; this I only name parenthetically, and reserve its elaboration for a future occasion, — to dwell upon the fascinating subject now and here would lead me too far away from my present task, which deals with the ailments of the climaxis. (XXIV 42)

**Insanity — Treatment**

We see that Homoeopathy patiently applied *can* minister to a mind diseased, only there is no specific for an abstraction bearing a name as if it were a tangible entity that had got into a wrong place, and needed only to be seized by "a cure" and ousted from its place. Strictly speaking we cannot cure diseases at all. We can, however, cure people whose states and conditions bear man-given names, such as insanity, hyperaesthesia, a cold, rheumatism, or what not. It lies in the nature of things that we should think and talk of diseases as entities, and just as every baby gets a name, so does every disease.

The foregoing case I call "Climacteric Insanity", but other nosologists might prefer another name.

But, doctor, you use such a lot of remedies; who is to know now how to cure "Climacteric Insanity"? Quite so. I once played a game of chess all night, and I really could not say which move won the game, or which portion of the night's work caused the fever that set in next day.

"That's a long ladder you have got there, Carter."

"Yes, sir, it is; but you see your house is so high!" (XXIV 45)

## Internal Affections and Outward Manifestations

Striking instances of internal affections being cured by some outward other acute manifestation constantly recur in medical literature. (IX 19)

## Jenner Vaccine and its Efficacy

Assuming that vaccination does protect, relatively and contigently, what do we pay for the protection, not in money, but in vaccinial morbidity, or vaccinosis?

It seems to me probable that ordinary Jennerian vaccination is not efficiently protective in those whose proneness to catch small-pox is very great, while it *is* efficiently protective where the proneness to catch small-pox is less. (XIX 99)

My line of argument here stands thus : Vaccination is preventive of small-pox when the proneness to catch it is small ; and when the proneness to catch it is small, those who do get small-pox do *not* die of it, therefore vaccination affects the *morbility* rather than the *mortality* of small-pox. I refer to ordinary Jennerian vaccination, and not to microposic homoeoprophylaxis.

If I am right then we can affirm on aprioristic grounds that ordinary microposic vaccination will diminish morbility but *increase* the mortality, *i.e.*, fewer will get it, but more will die : the mortality will be greater.

How so?

Vaccination is a homoeoprophylactic diseasing measure : one disease is given to prevent a like one — vaccinia to prevent variola. If the diseasing process of vaccination fail to protect, then the vaccinated person will be *more* likely to die because there is the homoeoprophylactic *aggravation* : the two diseases combine to kill the patient just the same as too much of the homoeopathic remedy will aggravate the disease to which it is highly homoeopathic — with perhaps, the like result.

This is manifest, for in vaccinating a person we are *diseasing* him; we communicate vaccinosis to him; if he, in addition to the vaccinosis, now get small-pox, he is more likely to die the worse he has the vaccinosis. If $y$ represents the prospective mortality of the unvaccinated, and $x$ the difference between the vaccinated and the unvaccinated, *i.e.*, vaccinosis, then the chances of dying of the vaccinated person who gets small-pox are $y + x$.

Against the hypothesis that vaccination may be protective in some cases (relatively and contingently), and add fuel to the flames in others, *i.e.*, decrease the morbility and increase the mortality. Against this hypothesis it will be objected that the mortality is much greater in variola than it is in varioloid. This, I submit, proves nothing, because the unvaccinated belong almost exclusively to the social residuum in whom all diseases are relatively very fatal. Vaccination has been *comme il faut* now for many years, and hence almost everybody who is anybody has been vaccinated. Nearly all the anti-vaccinists have themselves been vaccinated. Now that the mental *elite* of the world are rising against vaccination, I venture to foretell that in the future the mortality in *their* unvaccinated offspring will be very small; probably only those who inherit the PURULENT DIATHESIS will die, and many of these would be saved if homoeopathically handled, or homoeoprophylactically vaccinated in refracted dose. (XIX 100)

## Kidney Diseases and Wens

These wens are very curious things, and to me biologically decidedly puzzling. For instance, why does kidney-disease follow their forcible removal? Why are their owners so prone to pains, and paresis? At present I am studying a number of them with much interest; and although I not infrequently cure them, still I cannot say I understand them. Sebaceous cysts from occluded outlets of the sebaceous follicles are only the dry bones of the thing. (XX 237)

## Leucorrhoea — Its Significance

Leucorrhoea is a catarrh differing very much in pathological quality in different cases; there is not one substantive disease called leucorrhoea, but the thing is commonly of a depurative nature and stopping it by local measures is a wrong proceeding. Leucorrhoea may in many ways be compared to eczema of the skin, for eczema is also a catarrh, often of a depurative nature, and treating eczema by local remedies, unguents, and lotions is equally a wrong proceeding. (XXIV 13)

**Is Leucorrhoea a disease** : Yes, certainly, just the same as pain — only forcibly drying it up is no more a cure than lulling pain with *opium*. I do not consider the leucorrhoea sign of health, and so I do not let it alone. (XXIV 14)

### — and Spleen

I have elsewhere maintained that leucorrhoea is frequently connected with the spleen.

The leucorrhoea I regarded as from this spleen enlargement, and I also thought the varicosic tumour was likewise due to the state of the spleen. (XXIII 68)

### — and Tuberculosis

Leucorrhoea is often a manifestation of a tubercular constitution, and when suppressed leads to graver developments of the same diathesis. And surely if leucorrhoea is sometimes a manifestation of a tubercular diathesis, it is not the leucorrhoea which is primary, but the tuberculosis, which is the real disease, and the leucorrhoea is secondary to it, and its existence constitutes in the main an oulet for morbid matter or disease-stuff of some kind. These are not fanciful pictures, but based on facts from my own experience, and they may be seen in my (and anyone else's) clinical work any day and almost any hour. (XXIV 12)

## Life is What Remains

We must remember that what we call life is to each individual of us a varying quantity, according to our respective ages, and at 78 life to this lady *is what remains to come after 78*! (IX 126)

### Life, Death and Disease

Life is just change. Nature knows no dead material, for the grave of one organism is the birthplace of many more; the animal lives on the vegetal, and man lives on them both. *En revanche* man decays and dies, and vegetal and animal again swarm into being in his remains. Verily, an awful contemplation, but so it indubitably is. Then there is another death in the form of emanations; our very breath is death in a certain sense. The products of any assembly of organisms at a given stage of intensity poison and kill their producers, they getting diseases constituting their ante-mortal stage. It is just the same throughout Nature and with all degenera and species. It is the degree of concentration that is really determinative. (XVIII 101)

## Liver and Cheerfulness

The fact is, our brightness and chatty sunniness in our social life do verily depend much upon the liver. (XVII 118)

### — and Skin

The "Sternal Patch". One often meets with liver affections connected with cutaneous manifestations. I would like particularly to refer to a patch of eruption of skin covering the lower part of the sternum which I have several times found co-exist with heart disease and swelling of the left lobe of the liver. In my case-takings, I call it the "sternal patch". (XVII 66)

Of course, a good complexion means health, more or less, but the liver is very specially involved in producing a clean skin and clear complexion; and I propose by-and-by to dilate upon this point somewhat, as I consider it important. (XVII 105)

**—, Brain and Skin**

People have certain preconceived ideas of diseases : if they know you are suffering from "liver," they smile; if you have anything wrong with your brain, rendering you insane or vicious, they are afraid of you and lock you up in an asylum; if you have anything wrong with your skin, they shun and despise you, little weening that the same or a like morbid essentiality may be at the bottom of them all. And hence, when questioned about their "skin", people not infrequently stop short of all the truth. (IX 73)

## Local Diseases

Gout in the eye is as much as gout in the big toe, and tuberculosis in the ovaries is as much phthisis as phthisis pulmonalis, and requires the same qualitative treatment as set forth in my *New Cure of Consumption*. (XXIII 138)

## Low Potencies

I have occasionally found the third decimal dilution answer better than the thirtieth (of *Thuja*).

But this is not the point of my thesis, for this case was evidently cured by the low dilution, and when the low dilutions cure, and cure promptly, even though not very agreeably, but well, it cannot be necessary to go up any higher, especially as one's faith is sufficiently on the stretch without it. (XIV 49)

## Man and Environment

That man acts upon his environment has been well demonstrated by the changes that have been wrought in physical nature in the United States, Canada and Australia since they have become inhabited. The differences in the American, Canadian, and Australian shew clearly that nature reacts back on man who is moulded and formed by his climate. I am personally acquainted with a gentleman, now resident in London, who at twenty years of age left England for Eastern Euope, and there remained till he was thirty years of age when he returned to this country. When he went he had an abundance of light curly hair. On his return his hair was abundant and curly but nearly *black*, so that his own mother did not know him and his own brother who went on board the steamer by which this gentlemen returned and hunted for him amongst the passengers entirely failed to recognize him though he stood close by him for some time, he was looking for a light-haired man. After ten years further residence in England his hair had almost returned to its original light colour. (XVII 1)

## Marasmus and Eczema

One meets not infrequently with bad cases of eczema in babies that are apt to end in marasmus and death : the eruption in such cases is almost all over the body, wetting, more particularly in certain more or less circumscribed patches, and driving the poor little patients almost mad with irritation, particularly at night. (IX 154)

## Marriage Counselling

To pretend to inaugurate marriage on racial or scientific grounds is crooked; and although the good old institution known as the family doctor may now and then be asked about the physical desirability of a given projected union, still this very rare, and when it occurs it usually serves as a cover for other and occult reasons. Therefore, the physician's *role* begins later on. We all know what it usually is. (III 106)

## Materia Medica, Study of

Would that we homoeopaths kept closer to our study of the Materia Medica Pura, and spent less of our valuable time and talents in internecine squabbles about the precious dose and the eternal name of the school. (II 124)

## Medicine : a fresh approach

No doubt some bacteriologist will cultivate, some fine day, the germs of the ringworm, and astound the world with his subcutaneous injections. It is well that medical men should approach each subject from a different standpoint as they serve to correct one another. (XVI A 115)

### — and Surgery

One very great drawback to the medicinal treatment of so-called surgical complaints is its difficulty as compared with their knife-work, and then any one can appreciate a clever operator, but very few can appreciate the best work of the real physician, of which the effects can only be seen after many days. (V 56)

### — extending its domain

It might be as well, perhaps, to say that I lay no claim to any *special* knowledge of the diseases of the eye in general, or of those of the lens, or of its capsule in particular; at the same time I am not one of those physicians who consider ophthalmology as lying with out their province and within that of the ophthalmic surgeon *only*. On the contrary, I consider that the *duty of the true physician consists in constantly seeking to limit the domain of the surgeon by extending that of the physician*. The treatment of cataract concerns, first, the physician, and failing him, the surgeon. (V 87)

### — giving it a chance

At any rate, let us give *medicines* a full and fair trial and in the end humanity and science must be the gainers. A cataract cannot be operated on until it is ripe; then why not try the medicinal treatment during the ripening process? (V 88)

**— Minister or Master**

**Is The Physician Nature's Master or Servant?** Many have been the discussions in the history of medicine as to whether the physician should be the minister or master of nature; it seems to me that *he should be both.*

It occurs to me that the physician is in much the *same position as a gardener*, who, for instance, wants to grow apples. Only nature can grow apples; but then it is crab apples that she grows unaidedly, not edible apples. No gardener can grow apples or crabs of himself, that has to be done by nature herself organically. But although no gardener can grow either crabs or apples of himself, yet, guided by human wit and experience, the gardener can compel nature to grow apples of the finest sorts and varieties; he need not ask nature's permission at all, he merely arranges nature's forces so that she produces the apples required.

This, I take it, is the true position of the physician. *It is only nature that can heal anything really, and yet nature cannot heal many things at all till the physician gardener arranges her forces, so as to compel nature to grow apples in lieu of crabs*; the physician's position is like an apple grower's further, in that nature requires *time* to grow apples; so also is it with nature's healing ways, nature requires time; and any attempt to cure in less time than she needs for her organic processes results in failure — absolute failure.

The element time in the cure of disease is not sufficiently considered either by medical men or by their patients.

These remarks are introductory to a short consideration of the treatment of chronic tubercular processes by *Bacillinum*, etc., so as to find out the direction of nature's way.

Whenever we have chronic ailments to cure, it is necessary to pause a wee bit and think, and we soon see that *the duration of the treatment must be proportionate to the time required by nature to effect her organic processes*, the sum of which makes up the cure. (XXV 17)

**— the old silly teaching**

IN human life we have our favourites; we have them in our families, and in therapeutics I have a great fondness for certain remedies, one of which is GOLD.

The allopaths say Gold is no medicine at all, because it is an insoluble metal! That's what the best Professors of Materia Medica taught me; it is fundamentally false all the same!

Oh, the silly, silly things they teach one at the schools! What a frightful heap of old fossil beliefs! (XI 69)

**— vs. Surgery**

There are eye surgeons in plenty, and not a few of them are men of the highest attainments; we want some good eye *physicians*, NOT specialists but medical practitioners, who can focus their energies upon a small part of the human economy without ever for a moment forgetting that *the part is qualitatively* the *whole*, and conversely. We should then make rapid strides in norrowing the limits of the supposedly incurable. To have one's ailments cured surgically is good, but to have them cured medicinally is better. (V 90)

## Menopausal ailments

**Change of Life in Women; Its Ills and Ailings.** Of course we do not expect to find any virus-disease from without as peculiar to the change of Life. The English name — change of life — is singularly appropriate : it is what its name implies and nothing more. The woman who is really in sound health — *i.e.*, of good constitution — is quite as well at and after the change as before. A good constitution does not then become bad. It is, as it were, sleeping dogs that then wake up to bark and bite; hence it is that we must early look to the principle of heredity to get correct and helpful views of the troubles that beset a woman at the change, notably where they have lain more or less latent prior thereto. Manifestations of gout and rheumatism are most common. **Goutiness — Arthritism.** Like begets like, which no one can gainsay; but as two beget one, we have a third entity whose qualities are not absolutely apparent. When we learn to read, and come across a new word, we spell it; so it is with the hereditariness of disease. I have occupied myself a good deal with this question and hope to say my say thereon in due course. Here I must confine myself to its bearing on the subject matter of this book.

The offspring of a gouty parent must be gouty more or less, unless indeed the one of the twin completely neutralises the other, which is conceivable, but not probable. The girl that comes of a gouty father will teethe goutily; she will menstruate goutily; and at and after the change of life her ills and ailings will be gouty.

Many times I have remembered this point in the trouble of dentition with much advantage. Even in using the Repertory it throws a valuable side-light on the case, and helps. My two big guns in gouty menopause are — *Bursa Pastoris Q and Pulsatilla Q*). The similitude is very small; the dose must therefore be material, a few drops of the tincture; and on the treatment of gout I may fairly refer to my own monograph on the subject, in which what I know of gout may be found. *Bursa pastoris Q*, ten drops in a teaspoonful of warm water at bedtime, is a very frequently indicated remedy in gouty ladies at the change of life. The gouty diathesis must be treated on its own merits in a woman just the same as in a man. (XXIV 31)

**— and Cataract**

**Post-climacteric Cataract.** There are many kinds of cataract in quality and in causation — even senile cataract is of different pathology in different cases.

In spite of jibes and jeers, sneers and snubs from many very superior persons whose world is spectacles, I still maintain that many cases of cataract can be cured by medicines.

Difficult task? Oh, yes, very; but difficult does not spell impossible. Cataract in women at and after the change of life is, probably, the least difficult of any to cure with medicines. My plan is to subject patients to, say, a given constitutional course of treatment by high dilutions, and when this seems to have done all that can be achieved, I put patients on small material doses of uterine remedies, principally *Pulsatilla Q*, from five to ten drop doses once or twice a day. (XXIV 25)

**— and Flushes of heat**

**Heats and Flushes.** One of the most common complaints of women after menopause is *Heats and Flushes*, and the phenomena are very curious and not easily understood. Personally I have never been able to satisfy my mind whether they are morbid or normal; but all things considered, I incline to the view that they are not normal. (XXIV 7)

**— and Health**

The change of life is a perfectly harmless thing in the absolutely healthy, for in itself the Change of Life is absolutely free from morbid sequels in those who are really and truly healthy. Perfectly healthy — really normal — women have no pain at the period, the period is moderate in quantity; there is no pain and no whites, and when the menopause arrives the function ceases almost without the woman's knowledge — she merely knows that the thing has left off, and there is an end of it. That is normality. There are many degrees of ill-health, but the absolutely normal woman is not, by reason, of her sex, a suffering creature at all, either at puberty, or at the menopause, or at any time between ; and not only so, but her health is better than that of the corresponding man, by the very fact that her sex provides her with an automatic depurative overflow for superfluities and impurities; so much is this the case, that many women in a blooming state would, if they were males, be on a much lower scale of health, or not even alive at all. But these, when the menopause comes, lose the manifold advantages of their sex, and descend to the common (male) level. Wherefore a truly normal woman when she passes the menopause enters upon a period of vigorous life in which she manages a good deal more than half creation. A perfectly healthy child has no trouble with his teeth, they are simply found, nobody knows when they come ; even so is the menopause in perfectly healthy women. (XXIV 15)

**— and Leucorrhoea**

**Leucorrhoea in Relation to Menopause.** Ordinary leucorrhoea ceases with the period to which it very commonly stands in relationship. Where the whites persist after the change of life, we must regard it as the expression of a morbid constitutinal state, and very often of positive womb diseases. And as leucorrhoea usually ceases with the period, the organism is also thereby robbed of a constitutional outlet for many morbid products. This may not be Orthodox Doctrine in the schools, but it is certainly the doctrine of Nature, as any clear unbiased observer may see for himself. The practice of using injections for the whites is utterly bad, a downright sin against Nature's ways.

The presistence of leucorrhoea after the menopause is of considerable import, and certainly betokens positive disease of the womb (or ovaries), and the same may be said of the swelling of her breasts, for breast in an appendix to the womb, and ever under its influence and domination. Whenever there is anything wrong with the breasts I direct my attention straightway to the womb, for it is in the womb, respectively the ovaries, that the ailing is surely primarily located.

When I speak of leucorrhea I mean leucorrhoea and not gonorrhoea. This latter is a dirty disease introduced from without and not from the constitution, and should be killed *in situ* the sooner the better, if possible. I hold the same of the acarus disease — the pure itch — the nasty little acari are from without, and should be slain. (XXIV 36)

**— Days of Reckoning**

**Nature's Days of Wrath and Vengeance.** So long as the menses offer an outlet for disease products and disease germs, so long is the organism of the woman kept free for the time being : but neither primary nor what I would term "echoic" diseases are thereby cured, and we may very aptly compare the state to that of baling-out a leaky ship; if the baling-out process be adequate the navigation of the leaky ship is not greatly interfered with, but if the baling-out is less than the leakage the water accumulates and in time sinks the ship. Precisely so it is with the diseases of menstruating women; during the period of active menstruation the baling-out of disease elements by the female organism is commonly adequate, and the woman lives on fairly well; she is indeed a leaky vessel constitutionally, but the leakage of the month is baled out, so to speak, with every menstruation. And just as with the leaky vessel, the time of the ultimate sinking comes on by degrees not all at once; so, as the menopause begins to cast its shadows before it, we see symptoms in our patients of defective depuration in the form of "spasms," dyspepsia, rheumatoid arthritis, uterine trouble, tumours, eczema, asthma, cancer. Let any physician listen attentively and sympathetically to the health-histories of a few scores of ladies in their sufferings at the change of life, and carefully note all their historic points, and he will find that the troubles *at* the change of life are not *of* the same but far anterior to it : the ills and ailings incident to the change of life in women date from, often, far back in their lives, or in the lives of their parents, and are, as it were, the stems, branches, leaves, flowers and fruits of the long-gone-before. This in a general way, I will come to the concrete anon; here I merely desire to state in general terms the ground-thought that many of the ailments at and after the menopause seem to me to be, so to speak, nature's wreakings of wrathful vengeance for persistent disobedience during the previous course of the life, and by Nature I mean the laws of nature in accordance with which we do not reap oats when we sowed barley. What evidence of this can I bring? (XXIV 9)

**—, Tumour of Breast at the**

It is very instructive to note the beginnings of tumours principally in the breasts and womb as the change of life *is looming*, but has not yet arrived. I read it thus : The pre-existent constitutional taint that heretofore has overflowed and sailed off in the menstrual flux no longer does so completely, and hence the organism has to deposit what has remained behind somewhere, and this constitutes the beginning of many of the tumours. Of course the causation may not be *merely* a lack of elimination by way of the period, but it is seemingly so to a large extent. (XXIV 15)

## Menorrhagia and Rheumatoid Arthritis

Just as pain at the period proclaims that something is wrong, so does an excess of the flow, in an even louder tone. I have noticed many, many times that whenever a woman has persistently suffered from excessive menstruation, the change of life rarely fails to disclose the cause ; for, as the flow diminishes, so, in equal pace, do some other constitutional ailings crop up. A very common thing is rheumatoid arthritis, expressed as swelling of the bones of the fingers. (XXIV 6)

## Menses & Longevity

*With the monthly period the woman throws away her disease elements and products, her monthly period is a monthly purification.*

Has any one ever seen a normally menstruating woman in an acute attack of gout of the classic variety? I never have; clearly the gout is cast out menstraully. And so we observe that *menstrually active* woman have — apart from their own peculiar ailings — by far fewer diseases than the corresponding man. So much is this the case, that women commonly live longer than men, and this I attribute to their power of monthly purification, to a very large extent. (XXIV 5)

## Motherhood

I have long considered that being a mother is about the biggest thing on earth, but on this point all women do not agree; some willingly face death without daunt in order to become a mother. (XXIII 12)

## Muscle Power and Brain power

Muscle-power is gained by muscular exercise; brain-power is gained by brain exercise. And if the brain is in a morbid state, the malady from which it is suffering must be cured, whereafter the brain may be cured, where after the brain may be safely exercised and thereby strengthened. Muscle-exercise does not directly strengthen the brain, neither does brain-exercise strengthen the muscles : due exercise of each duly develops each; over-exercise of either is at the cost of the other. A given organism can produce only so much and no more. Great brain-workers are not muscular; great muscle-workers are not at the same time capable of great brain work; it is impossible, all cackle to the contrary notwithstanding.

It is of prime importance to keep the foregoing lesson well in mind. I say *great* brain-workers cannot at the same time be *great* muscle-workers. It is not maintained that an individual of great muscular power may not at the same time be a big-brained highly intellectual person. What I maintain is that I never yet met a person who excelled in both. (XXII 86)

## Myopia and Glasses

If we want to get good muscles, we exercise them. No one denies that: and yet when we put spectacles on young children we are in very deed denying it to a very large extent.

I have over and over again cured strabismus or squint with medicines,sometimes with *Gelsemium* 6 alone. Myopia should not be treated with spectacles at all until all the possibilities of medicines, eye-exercises, and growth have been exhausted. Then, but not till then, should spectacles or folders be had recourse to. I am in the habit of putting aside all spectacles worn by little children, and putting them instead upon a course of medicinal treatment, and the result most commonly is that such spectacles can in the end be dispensed with more or less. We must remember that spectacles have no beneficial influence upon the nutrition or health of the eye. Indeed, quite the contrary; they are a mighty boon in certain irremediable defects, but they mend nothing. Thereapeutically they may be compared to crutches or a wooden leg. The eyes must be thought of and regarded as living organs of the body susceptible to organic improvement and growth; they are not merely optic instruments.

Spectacles come in for the organically irremediable; but to start children in life with spectacles without first trying to mend their ocular defects vitally is hardly worthy of really scientific physicians. A truism? Quite so, but bespectacled children are all over the place nevertheless, and practically no one ever tries to cure eyes. (XXII 110)

If you want to make a weak arm strong, do you order it to be carried in a sling? The boy's general nutrition was poor, his glands were indurated and enlarged, his limbs thin, his abdomen distended, and the state of his eyes was of a piece with that of the rest of his organism. I ordered his spectacles to be removed, and treated his entire being with remedies, and in time he improved in health, he grew stronger in *all* his organs and parts, and his eyes grew and improved in like manner, so that now he has no need of spectacles whatever, and I see no reason to suppose that he ever will need any. (XXII 104)

## Neuralgia : and Homoeopathy

If there is anything in this earth-life of ours that is hard to bear, surely it is *neuralgia*. And if there is anything in this world that can cure — I do not mean relieve, lull, dull, deaden, or kill, but *cure* really cure neuralgia, that thing is homoeopathy.

If the world at large had the very faintest idea of the immense range of homoeopathically chosen remedies in the treatment of neuralgia (as in so many other affections). the aggregate of human suffering would very surely be by far less than it is, and it is in the hope that pain-bearing humanity may learn that I want also to teach that neuralgia is not only, as a rule, radically, curable by properly chosen remedies, but that the curing of the neuralgia by the right remedy (or remedies) is a cure of the internal cause of said neuralgia, and therefore a cure of the organismic self of the individual. (XIV (PREFACE)

### — and Materia Morbus

I do *not* maintain that neuralgia is a strictly scientific term, inasmuch as I hold that *every* neuralgia has a positive pathology if we only knew it, for our not knowing the *materies morbi* does not get rid of its presence. (XIV 2)

**— Treatment with Higher potencies**

I will not quote the whole case, although it tallies with my own views, that neuralgias yield best to higher dillutions. (XIV 33)

## Nutrition and Medicine

To draw a line of demarcation between the nutritional and medicinal treatment is not now possible. Undoubtedly some cases will require nutritional treatment solely; others will require medicinal treatment directed to the mother's constitutional crasis; in others, again, a debilitated generative sphere may claim attention. Or a presumable taint in the marital product may call for the principal intra-uterine therapeutic endeavours. (III 120)

## Ophthalmologist — no grudging

But ever since Helmholz invented the ophthalmoscope, in 1851, the ophthalmologists have been busier than bees in the instrumental investigation of the eye; and now, as a well-known oculist later informed the writer, they count over three thousand diseases of the eye. Such is the simplicity of science. I am dealing here with only one of these diseases, and that will leave two thousand nine hundred and ninety-nine for the ophthalmic surgeons : hence they ought not to complain of this little poaching raid. (V 88)

## Organopathy

The functions of the liver are too large a chapter for me now to touch upon, but the newest data of science in regard to goitre and thyroid feeding bring out into a clear light these points:-

1. That the organ in the organism does indeed possess not only autonomy but hegemony, *i.e.* the organ is an independent state in itself and in and on the organism exercises an important influence.
2. That both a plus and a minus of a given organ results in disease of the organism.
3. That the organ-to-organ homoeopathy of Paracelsus is a scientific fact. (XVII 16)

It is well to realize that an organ remedy while capable of curing an organ-disease, and all the concomitant symptoms which *arise from* the organ-disease, nevertheless can in the nature of things *not* cure the concomitant symptoms in the patient when these symptoms stand in no nexus with such organ-disease. (XVII 61)

In my judgment the full range of the art-cure of disease by remedies used on scientific lines starts from the due recognition of the primary seat of the disease, and of the remedies that electively affect such primary seat. This, I take it, is the homoeopathic specificity of seat. Experience teaches me that if we are to avoid false issues in treatment we must *start* with diagnosing, if possible, *where* the malady is primarily located. At any rate, I find this the *shortest* way to curing. If this be neglected we not infrequently cover and cure the symptoms, leaving the malady itself more or less untouched.

No doubt — and on this I lay some stress-when the symptoms are scientifically (*i.e.* homoeopathically) covered and cured, the disease causing the symptoms is at the same time often radically cured also; but also, and not seldom, the symptoms are got rid of, but the disease remains.

It has been urged that any untrained person can treat homoeopathically by mechanically covering the symptoms; and no doubt, this is, to some extent, true. But such cures are not worth much; they do not reach very far, and are only of practical value when the malady and the symptoms are convertible terms. The simillimum of the symptoms may, *or may not* be the simillimum of the malady; if of latter, we have an ideal therapy beyond which there is nought to be desired; if of the symptoms only, we are apt to keep on curing our patients till they die.

If homoeopathy is to go on advancing we must face the question of *getting behind the symptoms* so that we may not only treat the symptoms homoeopathically, but also the malady in its essence. In other words, it will not suffice to find the simillimum of the symptoms, but that being found, it will be needful to put this pertinent question : Is this symptomatic simillimum also homoeopathic to the anatomical essence of the malady itself?

In the simple and well-defined forms of disease affecting an isolated organ, Paracelsic homoeopathy or organopathy is a very valuable guide to cure, and helps to define the disease and to fix its cure with the *pathologic simile*.

This results from a recognition that certain organs of the body are, as it were, organisms within the organism; minor systems within the general system. They have special individualism, both as to their functions and as to their diseases. Such an organ is the liver. It can be made ill by the organism, but, in its turn, it can make the organism ill. They act and re-act upon one another. Neither can exist without the other.

Certain drugs have been discovered by man, almost in all places and at all times, that have an elective affinity for these organs, and these drugs have some of them received names indicative of their action, hence we have head medicines, spleen medicines, liver medicines.

The cure of organ-disease by organ-remedies is often called organopathy, and this it was that very largely constituted the practice of Paracelsus, and for which he was hounded to death. (XVII 147)

The strength of a chain is equal to that of its *weakest* link, and similarly the value of a person's life may be equal to that of his *weakest* vital organ; here the particular organ is equal in importance to that of the entire organism.

Even where the tissue state of the entire organism is everywhere equally bad, it may be a life-saving act to relieve the particular organ that *first* gives way, so that time may be gained to alter the entire crasis or the quality of the stroma.

Death itself is often at the start in a particular organ, *i.e., local*, and if the part be saved in time life may be preserved. In the acute processes the value of a particular organ strikes one often very forcibly, there may be no need of any constitutional treatment; the one suffering part may be the whole case. And in many chronic cases certain organs claim, and must have, special attention. This is my standpoint in the following pages on DISEASES OF THE SPLEEN. As Forget says,"*Entre la nature medicatrice et la nature homicide il n'y a souvent que l'e paisseur a' une oponevrose.*"

I deem it necessary to guard myself against misapprehension in one or two particulars. In the first place, I understand by organ-remedy *not* a drug that is topically applied to a suffering organ for its physical or chemical effects, but a remedy that has an elective affinity for such organ.

Then I do not put forward organopathy as an idea of my own, or as something new, but as that of Hohenheim, and of his co-doctrinaires, as resusciated, extended, elaborated, and systematized by Rademacher, in the early part of this century. Honour to whom honour is due; poor Hohenheim has been maliciously befouled and meanly robbed long enough, and it is high time he should have the credit of his own genius, as well as of his own folly.

The modern father of organopathy is **Johann Gottfried Rademacher,** who was born on the 4th of August, 1772, and died on the 9th of February, 1850. His great life-work bears this title : **"RECHTFERTIGUNG der von den Gelehrten misskannnten verstandersrechten ERFAHRUNGSHEILLEHERE, der ALTEN SCHEIDEKUNSTIGEN GEHEIMAERZTE, und treue Mittheilung des Ergebnisses einer 25-jahrigen Erprobung dieser Lehre am Krankenbette, von Johann Gottfried Rademacher".**

The preface to the 1st edition is dated 1st April, 1841.

This is the work I so often refer to herein, and from which I translate the part on diseases of the spleen, though slightly condensed.

Further, I do not regard organopathy as something outside of homoeopathy, but as being embraced by and included in it, though not identical or co-extensive with it. I would say — *Organopathy is homoepathy in the first degree.* And finally, I would emphasize the fact, that where the homoepathic simillimal agent covering the totality of the symptoms, *and also the underlying pathologic process causing such symptoms,* can be found, there organopathy either has no *raison d'etre* at all, or it is of only temporary service to ease an organ in distress.

It it be asked, What is here meant by ORGANOPATHY? my reply is, that organopathy is the specific local action of drugs on particular parts or organs, as first systematized by Rademacher in the early part of this century. It is thus, a very convenient term in therapeutics as well as in aetiology and pathology. In pathology the term organopathy has long been in general use, particularly on the continent of Europe. The French understand by *Organopathie* an organ disease, and as such it is an accepted term in pathology. The same is true of *Crganleiden* in the German language. All this by the way.

But the real father of organopathy in essence and substance is Hohenheim, an eminent and learned physician commonly called Paracelsus, for proof of which see his works, and hereafter in this little volume on *Diseases of the Spleen,* if space permits. Organopathy is *included in* the wider generalization known as homoeopathy;

Homeoeopathy may be said to be based upon organopathy, for a drug to cure the heart of its disease specifically must necessarily affect the heart in *some* manner. But the homoeopath specializes, and says further : The drug that is to cure the heart must affect the heart, certainly, that is one of the foundations of our whole therapeutic edifice, but that is not enough; the nosological organopathy and the therapeutic organopathy must be and are *similar*. And inasmuch as we can know disease only by its subjective and objective symptoms (its language), it follows that the two organopathies must be symptomatically alike, though possibly antipathic in their *mode* of action as against one another.

I am not maintaining that treating an organ affection by an organ remedy after the manner of Hohenheim, Rademacher, and their respective co-doctrinaires, will stand as a medical system sufficient in itself, but that it is eminently workable, and is largely of the nature of *elementary homoeopathy*, is, in fact, specificity of seat.

Finally, I am very far from supposing that in the vast majority of cases an organ disease exists primarily and permanently by itself independently of the organism; on the contrary, I know well from close observation of nature that the part and the whole are commonly qualitatively the same. The organ which, to my mind, is the most systemic is the skin; and, on the other hand, the spleen has clearly a very distinct life of its own, and its own sufferings may be, and are well pronounced.

Whether any particular value is to be attached to the doctrine lately proclaimed by certain clearseeing people that the spleen is the storehouse of vital energy I am unable to say; but I am much struck with the teaching of Rademacher, that a very large percentage of dropsies are curable by spleen remedies.

I beg no one of my readers will confound what I here say with *local treatment* of disease. I am thinking and writing about *self-elective specific treatment, not local treatment*.

The whole organism may suffer, or a part of it, and when such part or organ is wrong in its life and being, it generally speaks and lets its owner know, and that in its own way. The altered state of the organ sometimes produces a sense of tightness, or fulness, or pain in its own immediate vicinity; at other times, it expresses itself vicariously through another neighboring or distant organ. First come first served is a good maxim, and is generally acted upon also in diagnostics. If a man coughs, his lungs are wrong; if he gets palpitation, his heart is at fault, always to the extent of being the seat of the symptom, though not necessarily its primary one, for the symptom COUGH, PALPITATION, may arise from the prompting of another organ or part either near or distant. In other words, an organ may speak out complainingly, either because it is wrong itself — *organopathically*; or it may be moved to express itself on behalf, or at the instigation of another organ — *synorganopathically*; or of the entire organism — *holopathically.* (X 2)

**— and constitutional ailments**

In the case of organ remedies, small material doses act best, — indeed brilliantly; such remedies also need to be repeated at short intervals. On the contrary organ hypertrophies from constitutional causes are not curable by organ remedies at all until the constitutional disease has been cured by infrequently repeated high dilutions of the remedies closely homoeopathic thereto.

Some of the critics have suggested that the use of organ remedies by me, learned largely from Rademacher, constitutes a falling away from my faith in homoeopathy, and one writer speaks of Rademacher as "Dr. Burnett's new love." As a matter of fact my acquaintance with the works of Rademacher and with those of Hahnemann fall within a year of each other, and the standpoint of each is true at the bedside. Hahnemann is a hero to me, but so is Rademacher; is Rademacher small because Hahnemann is great?

Now I find myself often unable to cure simple organ diseases with dilutions; but I also find myself unable to cure the great constitutional diseases with organ remedies, and from very close observation, and not a little experience, I maintain that the organopathy of Rademacher (*i.e.,* of Paracelsus) is just elementary homoeopathy, the degree of similitude being very small, wherefore small material doses are needed in fairly frequent repetition. As the degree of similitude increases so must the dose of the remedy be lessened. (XXIII 44)

Not that I claim to hold a brief for homoeopathy; for if homoeopathy be not the very best thing in drug therapeutics, then let it be swept away; only it seems to me that organopathy and elementary homoeopathy are identical, and that the heather for the besom that shall sweep homoeopathy away is not yet planted. "*Shall* we give up the law of homoeopathy and revert to chance again?" So exclaimed one of the reviewers of my "*Diseases of the Liver.*"

Not at all, dear friend; but also do not let us give away so big a bit of the foundations of our homoeopathic house as is included under the term specificity of seat, or organopathy.

Whether it lies within homoeopathy, as I contend, or not, it is true — very true — at the bedside, and that is good enough for me. It will not cure constitutional disease at all whose environment is the macrocosm, but it sets right the relationship of the organ to the microcosm, the organism. (XXIII 59)

**— and Diagnosis**

The aid to a correct diagnosis of a given case afforded by a due regard to the organ, by itself and *quoad* the other organs, and to the organism, is very great; at times a correct diagnosis is, without such appreciation, impossible. Science is constantly adding to our knowledge of the hierarchy of the organs; thus some lately performed experiments by a French observer show that the spleen is of all organs of the body the most highly endowed with oxidizing power, next comes the liver, and in third place only the lungs. (XXIII 65)

**— and Homoeopathy**

This is rarely in accordance with all my experience in the use of organ-remedy, viz., wherever the degree of homoeopathicity is at all pronounced, the dose must be small. In ordinary cases where there is only specificity of seat, i.e., homoeopathicity of the lowest degree, small material doses are the best and the most rapidly curative. (X 65)

I have long maintained that organopathy is elementary homoeopathy — that in the very nature of things, homoeopathy necessarily includes organopathy. (XVII 149)

Here we have a proof for the ten thousandth time that high dilutions do act curatively, and that well-defined characteristic symptoms or keynote can lead to most brilliant cures, and the best of such keynotes is that one can remember them and so save time. The time spent with one's nose in a repertory ought to be saved, if possible. Said a well-known gentleman on entering my consulting room one day; "I say what a lot of repertories you have; I am astonished; I have always understood that you never used repertories, and go in mostly for what you call organ remedies. "Ah", said I, "the repertory is my haven of refuge to which I fly in case of need; the more I know of the diseases themselves the less I need repertories; I live and move and have my medical being in *behind the symptoms,* there lies the future of Higher Homoeopathy : organ-remedies are only the bottom rung of the ladder." (XXIV 51)

At the beginning of narration of the foregoing case(Case 429, Part III — Atheroma of Scalp), I said that homoeopathy, organopathy and zoic medicines all helped in its cure; I do not mean that these are distinct from one another, but I mention them thus separately by name because many homoeopaths do not admit organopathy as an integral part of homoeopathy, while many others pooh-pooh or turn up their superior noses at the use of zoic medicines such as *Bacillinum, Morbillinum, Variolinum.* Whereas I maintain that organopathy is basic elementary homoeopathy leading up to symptomatic differentiation ,and the zoic medicines begin where the ordinary symptomatic differentiation leaves off. In regard to tumour-curing I find that organopathy is very helpful indeed, and with it I often succeed alone without the serious expenditure of time called for in truly differential symptomatic treatment. It saves the physician's time and preserves his mental strength. Its weak point is the relatively uncertain power of organ-medicines over the disposition, it gets rid of the product more effectively than it does with the diathesis. This same weak point, however, exists likewise in purely homoeopathic symptom-covering; in neither case is the neoplastic diathesis materially influenced *unless the degree of homoepathicity* in the drug chosen be very considerable; for looking deeply into the thing makes us aware that it is *not* the mode of choosing a remedy that is of greatest import, *but* the degree of likeness existing between drug-pathogenesy and the natural history of the malady in its anatomical and physiological essence.

This is where the zoic medication *begins* : it hits the diathetic quality as well as the product. Here only higher dilutions at longer intervals are any good, or fuel is added to the flames; whereas in organopathy small material doses act well and suffice, and the doses are repeatedly given with advantage — the greater the degree of homoepathicity the higher the dilution and the longer the interval between the doses. This I have before pointed out in my "Fifty Reasons for Being a Homoeopath," and although it has apparently attracted no notice from critical pens, still herein lies the real solution of the "question of the dose." (XX 205)

**— and Organismic Disease**

The cardinal point in this narration lies in the fact that I did not first give an organ remedy in a small material dose, and why?

Because, though there was an organ disease, it was not primarily a disease of the organ, but one of the organism, and from the organism, though located in the organ as well as in the organism. Organs may be affected in themselves and of themselves, and their ill-influence goes thence into the organism, and in such a case organ remedies are the indicated curative agents.

As the organ is ill of the organism and from the organism, and consentaneously with it, here the primary ailment is organismic, and must be treated with the homoepathic simillimum, which in this case was *Tuberculinum testium*, and, as the curative influence sought for was of a high degree of similitude, a high potency was used, viz., *Tub. t.* C.

And the result? Quick cessation of the urgent symptoms, viz., haemorrhage, and this being thus radically cured, general improvement at once set in. At the bottom of the whole thing lay a tubercular state of the endometrium, manifested by the deeply pigmented state of the anal and vulvar regions, and by the feelably hardened state of the inguinal glands.

In fine, I would summarize the whole thing thus : Where the organ-ailing is primary to the organ, use organ remedies in little material doses frequently repeated; where the organ-ailing is of a piece pathologically with that of the organism, use the homoepathic simillimum in high potency in-frequently repeated. That is how I work, with much satisfaction and delight, at the curative results so obtained. (XXIII 79)

**— and Skin Diseases**

Now the curative sphere of organ-remedies stops *short of blood* diseases; they do *not reach* the diathesis, and they therefore do not cure, *e.g.*, Chronic Skin Diseases; skin diseases are commonly diathesic. (IV 221)

**— and totality**

In *my* judgement they may *all* be included in the word homoeopathy, *but there are some* who dispute this, and say that treatment to be really homoeopathic must be purely and solely according to the totality of the symptoms. Well, I am bound to confess that I am not infrequently unable to cure tumours by choosing the remedies according to the totality of the symptoms as set forth in the provings of the remedies. If others can, let them come forward with their clinical evidence; and, if their results are better than mine, I will sit at their feet; if, however , mine are better than theirs, let them sit at mine; but *facta, non verba.* (XX 13)

**— Historical**

Rademacher, in the early part of this century, re-discovered this *Medicina Paracelsica* and having practised it with much success for many years he taught its precepts and practice with such power that a School of Medicine arose, his disciples bearing the honored name of Rademacherians. With these came into general use the words organ-remedy, organ-disease; the general fact being called organopathy. (XX 18)

**— Its Limitations**

That prince of splenics, *Ceanothus Americanus*, readily cured the splenic engorgement, but did not touch the blood disease which caused it. This is the inherent defect of organopathy, that it is not sufficiently radical in its inceptive action, but the like remark applies to every other pathy more or less, because the primordial cause is more or less elusive, and generally quite beyond positive science, which only admits of what it knows, and will not seek to encompass the unknown by the processes of thinking and reasoning. Because in former times philosophy made science impossible, the votaries of science now round upon philosophy, and sneer it out of view. To trace back proximate effects to remote causes is now ridiculed in medicine because *mere* science is productive of gross-mindedness, incapable of following the *fine* threads of the higher perception. (X 23)

**— Simple diseases**

In the simple diseases of organs and parts, we can get on beautifully well ,and cure our patients with joy and satisfaction , with the aid of the homoeopathic specificity of seat, or organopathy; the quality of the action here is simple, and simple homoeopathicity is enough. (XX 34)

**— Sphere of action**

Clearly organ-remedies restore only tone and equable circulation in most instances but do not alter the organismic quality of the organ, nor do they cure any diathesic quality of the stroma of the organ.

In fine : Where the organ ill comes from the organism and keeps on coming, the organ remedy is capable only of clearing the organ of its organismic soot, so to speak, for the time being; it is only while where the organ ailment is in and of the organ that the organ remedy is adequate. Also where the ailment is in and of the organ it is useless to attempt its cure with high dilutions affecting the whole organism : a localized organ disease calls for a localized organ remedy, just as a general diathesic organismic disease needs the homoeopathic simillimum in some potency sufficiently removed from its materiality. The degree of homoeopathicity conditions the degree of potency, the greater the degree of homoeopathicity the greater (higher) the potency and conversely. Hence it is that I use mother tinctures in the organopathic states and ailments. Thus even in the use of simple organ-remedies of but small pathogenetic powers, yet considerable local affinity, a few drops of the mother tincture may act very perturbingly. (XVII 223)

## Pain — the Warning Signal

Here there was a pain — a *neuralgia* in the heart — and a pain down or up the left arm- a *synalgia*. It might be very difficult to say where the actual primary seat of the angina was. There was pain up or down the left arm, and in the praecordia; so the two would constitute a synalgia, or a pain starting from one place going to another.

The importance of the synalgic conception is considerable in neuralgia, as it bears on the proper treatment of the case; and the more this line of thought is pursued in practical therapeutics the better aid our treatment becomes. The word sympathy expresses etymologically what we often mean, but it is of such frequent use in social and emotional life that it is of hardly any further service in the strict speech of science.

In pubescence, the intimate sympathy between the pubes and the breasts is well known, and in young men mammary synalgias and synaesthesias are not so very uncommon, though they are not severe, like the mastodynias of ladies.

Hence I have often thought that the railings, wailings, and complainings against Providence for allowing *pain* to exist in this world are readily reducible to the ingorance of the wailers. For it needs but a few moments' reflection to see that if we are to possess free sentient life at all, *pain* becomes a natural sequence, and a *beneficent necessity to the end that the pleasure may cease on the higher side of harm, and that the pain may preserve us by its warning.*

Why do we not incontinently plunge our hands into the fire? Because we know that pain would ensue. It is the *pain* (*i.e.,* the certainty of its speedy appearance if we burn ourselves) that keeps us away from the fire, and *hence* we preserve our flesh unimpaired and ourselves intact. If we were without the possibility of painfully feeling too high a temperature, we should not be safely able even to warm our hands at the fireside. Hence I conclude that **WHEREVER THERE IS PAIN THERE MUST BE SOMETHING WRONG. WHY the pain? WHAT the wrong?**

Now what is ever and every-where considered is the ***pain per se***, which is only the message, and in order that the message called pain may not come, the messenger is maltreated or massacred! Witness the injections, the nerve-stretchings, and the nerve cuttings! And yet the poor nerves are commonly but the faithfully warning speakers of the organism speaking at the appointed part which is most likely to lead foolish man to hearken and to understand.

What I here understand by synalgia, *i.e.*, a pain, an *algia* not orginally of the place in which it is felt. (XIV 102)

## Pathological Prescribing

The pathologic simillimum is the furthest point yet reached in drug therapeutics, and embodies a very great and fertile idea. (XXIII 78)

## Perfection, Pursuit of

No doubt it would be better and more instructive if my cases were systematically grouped and classified in some way or another, but I do not seem to know enough to be at present capable of doing this. What I present in this volume is really so new to practical medicine, that I can hardly hope to get beyond the stage of preliminary fragments : some material towards the upbuilding of practical phymatology from the clinical side. I have before to-day quoted the saying of a great French physician, that the pretension of being perfect, and of only furnishing something that is entirely finished, too often results in absolute sterility. I know a very able physician in the north, who years and years ago was in the habit of sketching out to me the way he intended to handle this and that subject, by and by when he could do it perfectly. "I detest the crude things that are published." Phthisis was the subject of which he knows a good deal, and about which he was going to write all these

years since, going to work in a hypothetically perfect way, having at least some approximation to finality, and the style was to be literary, polished, and worthy of the subject and of homoeopathy.
It has not come to pass : it never will, because perfection is unattainable except in effort, and finality is ultramundane.
The man who bakes a few bricks might as well say he will make no bricks till the house is built and roofed in. — But the bricks are needed for the building of the house. (XX 276)

## Phthisis And Popgun stools

The mode of exit of the motion from the bowels in this case was, "pop", as it were out of a popgun; this I have several times noticed. It has often been noted that the phthisical are wonderfully hopeful, but this does not hold good when there is tuberculosis of the brain, but, on the contrary, they are mum, taciturn, sulky, snappish, fretty, irritable, morose, depressed and melancholic, even to insanity. (XVI A 102)

## Physician's Duty

December. — Patient was very ill, and everybody gave her up, excepting myself. I did not see my way out of the wood, but still I hold that the physician who gives up a case before the patient dies is on a par with the soldier who runs away from the enemy. (XVII 190)
This must be always borne in mind in regard to the amenability of tumours, whether benign or cancerous. Nevertheless physicians must be firm and not allow themselves to be sneered or jeered away from their duty, but always *try to cure everything*; I do not mean pretend, but *try*. Many a clinical battle have I fought *and won*, although the winning had been previously proved to be impossible. (XX 12)

### Physician's True Role

Not a few mighty men have expressed the opinion that the proper *role* of the physician is merely to pilot the patient from the sea of sickness into the harbour of health. Still, my own ambition is never satisfied with such a *role*; my constant strivings are ever directed to being the master of disease, and I am not satisfied unless and until I deem myself the victor, always within the limitations of "thus far and no further." (XXI 27)

## Portal congestion and liver

Many of those old chronic cases of "liver" are in reality portal congestion; the sufferers therefrom have generally tried many physicians and many medicines, and get a little relief, but soon are as bad as ever. It is clearly *the liver*, and yet the very best treatment has failed. They have often had the right remedies, but did not take them long enough; in vein affections we have to deal with a *state* that will only yield to well followed up *coup sur coup* treatment. (VI 72)

## Possible and Impossible

Everything is impossible until it is tried. At one time it was impossible to heal an inflammation without blood-letting. (V 56)

## Pregnancy — ailments, troubles of

These are very manifold, according to the constitution of the expectant mother, *and* according to the constitution of the father. This latter may look fanciful, but it is a clinically verifiable fact. Where there is much incovenience it is as well to find out by actual palpation and percussion whether the bowels, kidneys, liver, or spleen are mechanically or functionally at fault.

No case of severe vomiting of preganancy should be given up as hopeless unless *Medorrh.* C. and CC. in very infrequent dose has been tried. In my experience no other *one* remedy meets such a large percentage of these cases curatively.

Why? The history of the affects of the marital urethral lining will not infrequently give the answer : the urethral lips will be found toc red and swollen, and when held apart bridles of sticky mucus testify to the former presence there of *Neisserian cocci.* Of course, there are many other causes of this pregnancy-vomiting and retching, and then other remedies will be needed. (XXIII 97)

## Pretended Non-believers

In defending and fighting for unloved doctrines, I often see these positive refusals to believe SELF-OBSERVED facts, and I marvel at the cowardice of these *pretended* non-believers. I sometimes fancy that the reason lies in the fact of their not being the orginators.

The amount of dense-mindedness and disingenuousness that lies hidden in those WHO HAVE SEEN great homoeopathic cures and still resist the truth, must be immense. Though one rose from the dead they would not believe. Still, perhaps, I ought not to blame them, for it *is* very difficult to believe that medicines can cure tumours; indeed, there was a time when *I could not* have believed the contents of this book. I therefore desire to be charitable to others, being myself a Saulus and a Paulus.. (XIII 5)

## Primary point of Disease

To find the primary starting point of any ailment is of the highest importance, deny it who may. (XXIII 86)

## Prolonged periods

When the period is unduly prolonged, in nine cases out of ten it is no longer an ovulation at all, but there is something wrong with the person, which wrong should be set right in lieu of making efforts to stop off the bleeding. (XXIV 21)

## Provings

It is now admitted on all sides that a true and thorough knowledge of a medicine can be obtained in only one way, viz., *by first testing it on the healthy.*

Why?
Because if you give a sick person, X, a dose of medicine of any kind, and there follow, say, six phenomena, how many and which of these were due to the drug, and how many and which were due to the disease? You cannot tell and therefore you give it to a healthy person to find out. (II 6)

## Pruritus — its treatment

Is the treatment of pruritus by soothing applications efficacious and rational? It is neither. I grant that a little *Calendula* ointment, lanoline, or vaseline, or the like, do ease for the time, and that, perhaps, harmlessly, and that is no small boon, as it allows patients to get to sleep. But when it comes to forcibly lulling sensation of the parts with active sedatives, I believe such a proceeding to be very harmful.

A proper course of homoeopathic treatment commonly suffices for its cure, but not always; there are some obstinate cases that defy all known efforts at cure. The very largest amount of success is obtained when we abstract ourselves from the name of the ailment and study the constitutional bearings of the case, and treat the woman's organism on general principles. Here the Totality of the Symptoms principle works exceedingly well, particularly where the pruritus seems to exist by itself without any diagnosable anatomical pathological basis.

Taken by itself, the most frequently successful remedy in my hands is *Caladium seguinum*, about the fifth dilution. It almost always does some good. *Sepia* comes next, but personally I generally have recourse to nosodes before I can really and radically cure it.

Sometimes the spleen is at fault in pruitus vulvae, and when the irritation is at the seat the liver may require attention. Some people find that pruritus ani will depart when the usual nightcap on retiring for the night is omitted. (XXV 24)

## Pseudo large Stature

Patient was of fine stature — what the French call *large* — of tender fibre, her tissues having large meshes Such people look much more healthy than they really are, and very commonly they are the product of a cross between a powerful individual and a consumptive one; the dash of consumptiveness is shown in their growth-largeness; they are large-celled and lacking in toughness. (XXIII 32)

## Psora — What it means

**The Hahnemannian Doctrine of Psora Re-stated.** The Hahnemannian doctrine of psora as usually comprehended in the ranks of really pure Homoeopathy is so vague and mind-confusing that many of us have never known what to say or think about it. When I first tried to practise homoeopathically I accepted the doctrine of psora purely and simply, and honestly believed that the itch could be, and was commonly cured dynamically by the strict Hahnemannians, and I copied their practice in this regard. Thus I kept a young lady under treatment with antipsorics, and principally with *Sulphur*, high, higher, and right away into the very high, for over a year, and the result? Total failure; and the parents very properly gave me up as inadequate. Patient was quickly cured by a near medical brother with *Sulphur* ointment and soap and water, and I was regarded by those who knew the circumstances as a mere faddist.

I went on for several years believing in and trying to cure the itch with homoeopathic dilutions, and What? I failed practically in every case.

Now the test of all doctrinal medicine must be clinical, and if I cannot cure on the lines of a given doctrine I throw the doctrine overboard. But a man who owes so much to Hahnemann's teachings as I do, hesitate much and long before discarding any of his doctrines. Hence I tried and tried, and failed time after time. Now I will take as an example what I will term *my Doctrine of Ringworm* I say that Ringworm and fungi notwithstanding, is dynamically curable by *Bacillinum*. I cure case after case *almost* always. I say the same of Vaccinosis and its cure by *Thuja* and the like in dynamic dose. Then why cannot I do the same with itch? Well, I cannot, and for me there is an end of it. It is no use to tell me that I fail to cure itch with *Sulphur* 30.C., CC., etc., because I lack in the skill requisite for such work. Well, let us grant that it is lack of skill on my part, then what is the use *to me* of a medical doctrine that is beyond my skill? Just none. The truth, *for me*, is that you cannot kill acari by any dynamic dose of any remedy whatsoever, and hence I have thrown the doctrine overboard.

Then is the teaching altogether false?

I would re-state the doctrine thus : You cannot cure the itch by dynamic medication, and you must therefore kill the acari; they should be killed on the spot, the sooner the better; you cannot kill acari with dynamic remedies, and they should be killed at once. But I am NOT speaking of *its concomitant constitutional eruptions brought forth by the acari*, neither do I say that the acari may not poison the blood — indeed I think they do, and *therefore* they should be sulphured to death instanter. But, and this is very important, if the acari have called forth an eruption from a previously existing internal state, THIS cruption may NOT be got rid of by external remedies. There is the rub. *Da liegt er Hundbegraben* ! It is the fullest results of suppressing the constitutional eruptions that have been *called forth from their internal lurkings* by the acari themselves, or by their poison, that we have to fear. If we watch cases of itch carefully we find that the cases of those of tainted constitutions get quite a number of different kinds of eruptions which were potentially there before they were infected with the acari, and these constitutions have to be mended by proper homoeopathic remedies, and their eruptions may not be driven in, but the acari must be killed by parasiticides. The best men in the homoeopathic ranks should set to work and clear this matter up, as it trammels our progress not a little. Years ago I was the means of converting an allopathic medical man to Homoeopathy ; he came over bag and baggage at considerable pecuniary loss; he subsequently caught the itch, and placed himself under my care, and he remained faithfully under my care for over a year, and I totally failed to cure him, whereupon he exclaimed to me — "I cannot stand it any longer, I shall go mad; look what an awful state I am in." He then gave up Homoeopathy and everything connected with it.

However, Homoeopathy is true, although you cannot kill acari dynamically. I have long been tussling with this question of psora, and this is my solution of it :

The dangerous results from the suppression of true itch are in reality not from the itch itself at all — on the contrary, the acari are poisonous little brutes that should be killed instanter.

These dangerous results are from the driving in of dyscratic eruptions present in the itch-patients, but *not* due *primarily* to the itch itself, but pre-existent in the individuals suffering from the itch, and not infrequently brought out on to the cutaneous surface by the acari or their poison, though not really due thereto.

It is the source of very considerable mental satisfaction to me to have thus solved the question of psora, as now I cure the itch — the acarus disease — as quickly as possible with *Sulphur* ointment and soap and water, regarding it as a dirty parasitic disease impinging *from without* on to the individual but *at the same time* do not suppress any concomitant skin trouble which is *from within* the organism, being there before the itch was caught, though very likely *called forth* by the irritating influence of the acari : that which is from without, is to be cured from without; that which is from within must not be treated from without, but from within. (XX 36)

**Psora — Not clear, but real**

It is due, let us say, to psora, but we have no clear conception of what psora is. Psora needs to be split up into its component parts, no easy task; it roots in the vague, its trunk and boughs run away into anywhere. The psora of the homoeopaths seems somehow true, but it has no proper beginning, no definite course, and ends in pathological chaos. Perhaps we study it in Hahnemann, and in the best writers on the subject, and after doing our best to master it, we rise from our studies with no clear idea, and we finally decide to abandon psora as an intangible myth, and then we proceed with our clinical work; but, before long, we stumble against a very tangible something, and on looking at the stumbling block, we find writ large upon it the word *Psora*! Have I then hit upon a solution of the psora-problem? No; but if we cannot break the whole faggot, we may perchance break one stick of it. (XVIII 9)

## Rectal Symptoms and Head symptoms

I have often been stuck with the grave head symptoms that occur at the same time as rectal troubles and these former are made much worse by surgical interference. (XVI 50)

## Remedies — their Rise and Fall

This is the rock upon which lawless therapy has always stranded; at first a given drug is a "new remedy," then it is a wonderful medicine, and then a universal panacea, then it is not such a very good medicine after all, and finally it is accounted no good at all, is abandoned like an old mine, and venturous spirits set out in quest of another "new remedy.," and so on in a veritable vicious circle. (II 15)

## Repertory — The Final Court of Appeal

The only efficacious plan is to begin by making a diagnosis of the constitutional wrong, and curing that. It may lie in the liver or spleen, or in the kidneys or bowels. The hepatics often render the very greatest aids : *Chelidonium, Chelone, Carduus, Myrica cerifera, Diplotaxis tenuifolia, Cholesterinum;* often pancreatics render eminent services, such as *Iris versicolor, Nux vomica, Pulsatilla, Mercurius, Iodine, Jaborandi,* and *Pilocarpine,* used as they may be called for.

*Bryonia*, too, is often indicated, as also *Sulphur* and *Heparsulphuris*.
We also find, as very frequently indicated, the commoner splenics, such as the already many times mentioned *Urtica urens*, the *Persicaria urens*, the *Rubia tinctoria*, the *Spiritus glandinm quercus*, and the like.
In the renal sphere we may need *Coccus cacti*, *Coccinella*, *Solidago virga aurea*, etc. Going over the notes of some of my cases I find that *Sulphur*, *Thuja*, *Sabina*, *Pulsatilla*, *Bryonia*, *Rhus tox*. *Lycopodium*, and *Antisycotic nosodes* are most commonly to the fore.
But, which of all these?
In ultimate court of appeal there remains the priceless *Repertory* to lead us to the correct choice of the remedy. With me, personally , the *Repertory* has always been my reserve force, to be called out only in case of need; but, for all that, I feel and know full well that, with my *Repertory* in reserve, I am *never* quite beaten.

## Retarded Growth — Treatment

I must demur to the statement that the arrest of development occuring before a certain period necessarily involves the conclusion that treatment in the latter months of gestation would be useless. This is a pure assumption, and based on normal observations. Here we have to do with arrested and *therefore retarded* growth, and hence the nutritional or medicinal treatment should not only be begun early, but continued to the end; and one begun late would still be hopeful of obtaining amelioration, if not of complete normality.

## Retracted Nipples — their significance

The retraction of the nipple is held to be a gravely important symptom in tumours of the breast, but the retracted nipple in young seemingly healthy girls and young women is usually not regarded as of any particular importance; but I have myself come to regard it as indicative of, perhaps latent, womb or ovarian disease; and thus regarding it as of pelvic origin, I have ameliorated a certain number of them and quite cured a few. The curative process is a tedious one, and takes a good deal of time, but it can be done. Whenever there is a retracted nipple, even in the most blooming young woman, there you are sure to find, very likely latent, but still positive disease, that will crop up in the later course of the life of the individual. Just as the milk rises to the breast after childbirth, so do morbid activities rise from the female pelvic organs at the change of life, or before. The retracted nipple in young girls has, I maintain, its place of origin, its primary seat, in the uterus or ovaries, and we do not often notice that the breast that has a retracted nipple is, at the beginning of lactation, the seat of a mammary abscess? Such abscesses are generally either strumous or hereditarily cancerous. I do not mean actually cancer, but merely of a carcinosic quality. I have often heard about the time of the menopause this remark from a lady . . . "I have a lump in my breast; it is the same breast that has the nipple drawn in, and in it I had an abscess when I was nursing my first baby."

Mammary abscesses during lactation should not be backed, but allowed to gather, burst and discharge, and left to go on discharging as long as they will, the child being kept on the sound side, the gathering breast being kept in full function by an exhauster till the abscess has healed, when baby may have both; only the patient should be kept under *Bacillinum* (high) till the fever, which is of the phthisic type, quite disappears and subsequently the lady's health is *better* than before the gestation, and it becomes also subsequently manifest that the abscess was a constitutional depurative effort : hence I encourage the ripening of mammary abscesses and do *not* back them. Sometimes the mammary abscess is of carcinosic quality, when *Scirrah*. C. plays precisely the same role as *Bacillinum* in the strumous form.

## Ringworm — Allopathic Cure And Prevention

What first struck me was the fact, that in a given household infected by ringworm only *some* of the members got the disease, and these were invariably the weaker ones, the weedy, and the unhealthy. I have known households in which rignworm existed in one or two of its members, and although towels, brushes and combs were used almost indiscriminately, still the disease did *not* spread. Conversely I have known others in which only one child would have, perhaps, just one small patch, and in which the greatest care was taken to prevent the thing spreading, yet many of the children finally caught the complaint. (XVIII 30)

### — An internal disease

Well, few need to be told that the task of treating ringworm successfully by external means, *i.e.* killing the fungi, is so unsatisfactory, so uncertain, so tedious, so often an entire failure, that I well understand the state of mind of an eminent London skin specialist, who six weeks ago exclaimed to Lady X., who wished to know *how long* it would be before her little boy would be quite cured of his ringworm, and fit to return to school, "How long? Heaven knows, I don't ; perhaps by the end of next term, I really cannot say!"

RINGWORM IS AN INTERNAL DISEASE *of the organism having for its outward sign the ringworm consisting of fungi thriving in a certain order* : the fungi are the guests of the diseased host; cure the host's diseased state, and the fungus — the ringworm — dies off from lack of a proper medium. Ringworm may be regarded as mould of the skin, analogous to the mould on cheese, bits of bread, oranges, or lemons, and warm moisture favours its development.

You cannot grow a common mushroom except under given conditions, neither can you the trichophyton of ringworm.

The trichophyton is not the disease itself, but its organic scavenger. Cure the internal disease, and this scavenger dies.

In other words, the ringworm fungi cannot live and thrive in really healthy animals, and the ill condition of those that have the disease is not a consequence of the disease, but a necessary antecedent condition of the animals before the trichophyton can thrive.

NOTE WELL : the cure is not only organismic, but *organic; not* chemical, *not* mechanical, *not* local, *not* topic, *not* antiparasitic, but organic, *vital*. The fungi are not attacked, but the "host" of the fungi is healed, and the wee fungi die, and their spores cannot germinate any further in the same soil.

There are two elements in herpes tonsurans to be thus considered : *1st*, the soil-quality; and, *2nd*, the fungi. Every organic thing needs certain conditions of its own life in order to thrive, and what I maintain in regard to ringworm is, that the disease proper is not to be sought in the presence of the fungi, but in that quality of the body which constitutes its fitness for the fungi to develop and thrive. (XVIII 20)

Is Ringworm a Disease Due to Dirt?

No; not one of my cases of the past three or four years was due to dirt, all being members of the higher and upper middle classes, who tub and scrub, perhaps, even too much. (XVIII 82)

**— And Tuberculosis**

This all confirms me in my view, which is the underlying idea of this book, that there is some close relationship between tuberculosis and ringworm, the precise nature of which deserves attention and study. (XVIII 36)

**— True nature**

*"It may be so, I cannot tell, and wouldn't like to say,*
*I don't incline to this or that, nor yet the other way;*
*I can't at any time feel sure, yet hardly like to doubt,*
*And feel I musn't trust to"guess" for fear of being out*
*Not feeling any certainty, I do not like to speak,*
*I don't know what I want to know nor what I ought to seek*
*I never like to venture far for fear of running wide,*
*And I haven't any notion how I ever can decide."*

Of ringworm I hold positively — (I) That it is a constitutional complaint. (2) That it is generated by the together-being of numbers of young people in close spaces *i.e.*, by their personal emanations, or anthropotoxine. (3) That it is so to speak, "subtuberculosis." (4) That it is curable by its pathologic *simillimum,* here termed *Bacillinum,* in high potency, internallly and infrequently administered. (5) That the mycosis is merely the concomitant external manifestation of the disease and not the disease itself. (6) That the external treatment of the disease is irrational, unscientific, and, probably, harmful to the patient. (7) That it is commonly bred in schools. (8) That truly healthy children cannot catch it because the fungus cannot grow upon such. (9) There is, therefore, no reason why a ringworm child should be excluded from school life or the company of its fellows in home life (10) And, finally, that the trichophyton of ringworm is to ringworm what the bacillus of Koch is to tuberculosis, — the trichophyton and the bacillus being, moreover, nearly related to one another. (XVIII 118)

## Simillimum — Varieties

In other words, I maintain that choosing the remedies according to the totality of the symptoms is only *one way of finding the right remedy;* and, moreover, sometimes totally inadequate.

You may *find* the right remedy once in a way according to the old doctrine of signatures; and, even though so found, it acts *homoeopathically*; the way of choosing is poor and crude, but it *is a way*.
You may *find* the right remedy by organ-testing after the manner of Paracelsus, and *the remedy acts homoeopathically* although *found* that way.
You may *find* the right remedy purely hypothetically, after the manner of Von Grauvogl and Schussler, the mode of action remains the same, *i.e.*, homoeopathic.
You may use dynamized salt — *Natrum muriaticum* — to cure marine cachexia, sea-side neuralgia, sea-side headache, and the like, and still the action of the remedy is homoeopathic.
You prove, or assume as pure theory, the double and opposite actions of large and small doses of the same remedy, and treat chronic arsenicism with *Arsenicum*, and it is still homoeopathy. You may theorize clinically as I do in "New Cure of Consumption," and reach no mean degree of success — further than ever before reached, — and I maintain that it is homoeopathy all the time.
The fact is we need any and every way of finding the right remedy; the simple simile, the simple symptomatic simillimum, and the farthest reach of all — the pathologic simillimum; and I maintain that we are still well *within the lines of the homoeopathy that is expansive, progressive, science-fostered, science-fostering, and, world-conquering*. (XX 14) (Homoeopathy larger view)

## The Simile and Simillimum

As far as I could ascertain, the secretions and excretions were not affected in the least degree; the remedial action must, therefore, be considered specific. My conception of the cure is simply this, that the specific *Ceanothus* stimulus persistently applied restored the spleen tissue to the normal. This homoeopathic specificity of seat suffices only in simple local disturbances; it is only a *simile*, not a *simillimum*. (X 29)

## Single and Multi-Remedies

It is no use to urge against the medicinal cure of tumours that so many remedies are often needful : if one remedy will not cure, we must use as many as will and no fewer; such is our art ... difficult and too often complex .... (XX 121)

## Skin and Cataract

The connection of cataract and various skin affections has long been noticed and written about by numerous authors, but the doctrine is not accepted by many. (IX 49)

### — and Heart — Sternal Patch

This vicarious phenomenon between heart and the skin of the thorax I have observed over and over again. So that when an individual has an eruption on his chest, he is not wise to let any skin specialist treat it from the narrow standpoint of the specialist, lest heart disease supervene. See here anent my remarks upon the "Sternal Patch." By the way the "Sternal Patch" is in the lowest third of the sternum, rather to the right : this thoracic pityriasis patch is rather to the left, and just over the arch of the aorta. The "Sternal Patch : is not a brown, so called, liver mark, but an eruption; the importance of this eruption lies, I think, not so much in the kind of eruption as in the fact that when it vanishes from the surface, without being really cured from within, symptoms of heart disease, more or less grave, at once supervene. The more one really studies skin diseases the more one is struck with their *habitats*, which are often constant and characteristic. (IX 145)

### — and Internal Treatment

If lupus is ever to be cured it must be cured by *internal* medication in some *direct* way by a medicament, or by medicaments, standing in *some* relationship to the *whole* lupus process; to pretend to cure it by killing the bacilli is like the grand old way of catching sparrows by putting salt on their tails. (IX 94)

## Skin Diseases

If any one will take the trouble to watch nature's ways — say, in skin diseases — he will see that even where the first origin of the disease is by infection at a given point of the outside, the disease indeed at first marches inwards; but then in the within great battles are fought and many slain, whereupon the organism reacts centrifugally by carrying the dead and dejected inside the camp to a point at the periphery — *i.e.*, she ejects them. (XXV 25)

**— Local Treatment**

And here I may state once far all that I hardly ever order local applications of any sort in cutaneous affections. If in any of my cases herein recited any local applications are used, the fact will be stated; but I believe in no case herein communicated was any local application whatever used, so far as I am aware. (IX 137)

The use of remedies applied as ointments or lotions is absolutely bad; and when I read of the homoeopathic treatment of skin diseases whereby ointments and lotions play a part, my respect for the quality of such treatment is small indeed. It is wonderful how people will cuddle and fondle the ointment pot; and "Regular Medicine" would be indeed badly off without its grease pot and clyster. I often think the use by the homoeopaths of their *Calendula cerate* or ointment comes dangerously near the thin end of the wedge of the vulgarly-conceived putty-and-paint treatment of the medicines of the schools.

It is almost incredible, but the discovery of a new fat for an unguental excipient is an event of the first magnitude in the dermatological world, the vault of whose heaven is still ringing with the echoes of the wonders of vaseline and lanoline. And what does it all amount to? (IX 138)

**— The Course of Treatment**

I deal with the organism, they deal with the parasites. The organism was admittedly improved, the number of parasites demonstrably greater. I claim that the child was visibly getting better. There being more parasites, they considered that she was worse, or at any rate that the ringworm was worse, although the patient was better in herself.

Now, I not only do not claim that the number of parasites and their spores decrease in the beginning of my treatment, what I claim is that *eventually* they go altogether as soon as the organism is normally healthy. Of course, it must be obvious that there would be fewer parasites present on the head while it was being scoured twice a day than while the head was let alone entirely. That the number of the parasites and their spores can be kept down by external parasiticidal treatment I do not for one moment dispute; what I say is, that the parasites themselves are not the disease, but are merely the trichophyton mould living on the surface of a diseased organism; and, further, I incline very strongly to the belief that not only are the fungi harmless to the patient, but probably actually beneficial as organismic scavengers. (IX 176)

**— Treatment**

Gout in the big toe is not a disease of the said toe; acne on the shoulders of young persons is not a disease of the skin of the shoulders; neither is a yellow-coated tongue a disease of the tongue. (XVII)

Ringworm inspires disgust; more or less almost all skin diseases do that, and yet a perfectly clear skin may enclose a very diseased organism, and a skin-diseased person may have a relatively much better constitution, and have all his internal organs in a relatively much better state, his cutaneous manifestations not withstanding. (XVII)

In other words, the disease being of the organism, it is a smaller evil to have it outside on the skin than to have it inside in a given organ. Gouty inflammation of the big toe is one thing; the same process in the stomach, quite another; therefore, the disease being given, it is the stronger person who throws said disease *into* his skin; but that does not make it a disease *of* the skin. (XVII)

**— True Nature**

I take largely the clinical standpoint, and consider the Diseases of the Skin constitutionally. The treatment of skin diseases as merely local affairs concerning the skin only, as is now current with *nearly* all medical men of all schools and all the world over, is, in my opinion, nothing less than a crime against humanity, and eminently characteristic of the cultured shallowness of the medical profession of today.

In these days of "scopes and meters," *thinking*, in the profession, is well-nigh dead. One sees no end of percussing and auscultating : the faintest murmurs, sounds, tinkles, *rales* and *bruits* are well known and learnedly discoursed of, but what of the *curing*? What of the *real* aetiology of the Consumptive process itself? Bacilli. Yes, but what went on before bacillary life became possible? and how are the bacilli to thrive unless the soil be, for them, of the right kind?

I do not maintain that there is no such a thing as a skin disease of a purely local nature, such as common phthiriasis and other parasitic dirt-diseases that impinge upon the skin, but, speaking generally, I do maintain the following points :-

1. That the skin is a very important living ORGAN of the body.
2. That it stands in intimate, though ill-understood, relationship to *all* the internal organs and parts.
3. That its healthiness is conditioned by the general healthiness of the organism — *i.e.*, a healthy skin on an unhealthy body is inconceivable.
4. That, speaking generally, its unhealthiness — its diseases — come from within, sometimes even when they initially impinge upon it from without.
5. That being *biologically within* the organism, being *fed from within*, having its *life from within*, having its *health from within*, and having its *diseases from within*, it must also be treated medicinally *from within*.
6. That skin diseases are most commonly not merely organic, but at the same time organismic, or constitutional.
7. That the skin being an excretory organ, and being spread out all over the organism, is often made use of by Nature to keep the internal organs free from disease.
8. That as each portion of the skin corresponds vitally with some internal organ or part, so the skin disease is often merely the outward expression of internal disease.
9. That, in fine, the generally received *external* treatment of Diseases of the Skin, whether with lotions or ointments or whatsoever else, is demonstrably shallow in conception, wrong in theory, harmful in practice, and therefore inadvisable.

These points embody my views on Diseases of the skin; they guide me in my practice, and I might call upon the dermatologists to refute them, did I not hold them to be absolutely irrefutable.

If disease of the body bubbles up, so to speak, into the skin like water from a spring, to treat this Disease in (of) the skin by washes and ointments, or other outward applications, is really *not* treating the *diseased state* at all, but *only preventing its peripheral* expression. The skin does not live an independent life of itself — hung on, as it were, outside of us — but is of all our organs the most systemic; but what can we expect from an age in which people think they get a beautiful healthy skin from soap, and sound teeth from toothpowder?

The bark of a tree is a very fair analogue of the skin, and when I one day asked my gardener why the bark of a certain apple tree was so knobby, rough, and unhealthy-looking, he replied, "The *roots* have got down on the clay, Sir."
So it is, I opine, when a person's skin becomes diseased. "The roots have got down on the clay." (IX Preface)

**— Correspondence with Specific Organs**

If I have in the foregoing pages succeeded in showing that diseases of the skin are really diseases *of* the system, though on the skin, then my task is accomplished. In the near future I hope we may have some *definite* conception of the correspondences that undoubtedly exist between certain regions of the body surface and the internal organs, independently of general organismic interdependence, and then we shall, perhaps, be able to see why certain cutaneous diseases affect certain parts preferentially, and also why, when these diseases are driven in whence they came, by external means, certain internal organs have to bear the brunt of it. (IX 100)

**— Local Applications**

We have had a vaseline era in dermatology, then came the era of lanoline, and at present we are basking in the full glory of the era of ichthyol, and it is all as inane as we can well imagine. (XXI 158)

## Spleen Diseases — Clinical Picture

People whose spleen is much affected like to lie on their backs, just as do those who have the right lobe of the liver much enlarged, and neither can lie comfortably on their sides. When we further bear in mind that the spleen (so far as we know at present) is neither an excretory nor a secretory organ, it follows that we cannot have any symptoms indicating a disturbance of such like functions. When we further consider that the gall ducts are sometimes sympathetically affected in spleen complaints, with the urine discolored as in gall affections — that, in fact, the *menstrua digestionis* in general are qualitatively altered; and that to fill the cup of difficulties to overfilling, abdominal plethora will simulate painful spleen disease; it is easy to see that the finding of good spleen medicines is, indeed, a very difficult affair.

The states and symptoms that, during my medical career, I have known to arise more or less frequently from spleen affections are the following :

Pain in the stomach (often).
Cough, and that oft, violent, and suffocative.
Bellyache (at times).
Chronic diarrhoea, and rather more frequently.
Constipation.
Asthma (seldom)
Disturbed renal functions and their consequent dropsy.

And with regard to such dropsies, in so far as they are not due to organismic affections, I ascribe, according to a rough calculation, about one-third to the spleen.

In women the spleen affects the womb and the vagina, causing emansion, or excess of the flow, and leucorrhoea. [This I (Burnett) have myself observed very frequently, and also a very distinct sympathy between the male urethra and the spleen, which Rademacher does not appear to have noticed, since probably peccant urethrorrhoea were not very common in a place like Goch.]

Brain affections, such as mania and melancholia, eye diseases, such as diplopia, ambylopia, chronic inflammations, I have seen arise from the liver, but thus far not from the spleen. If I had ever witnessed an epidemic of spleen affections, I should know more about the organ. As it is what I have to say about spleen medicines can only be imperfect. (X 39)

**Sterility and Hysterectomy**

Where childlessness is the malady to be cured, the sterility being due to the womb being thick, heavy, and retroverted, hysterectomy at any rate is no cure. (XXIII 88)

**Sternal Patch and "Liver and Heart"**

**Sarcognomy**. I foretell that, in the future, when the relations of the various cutaneous regions will be recognised as constituting the very base of medical and medicinal diagnosis, this *sternal patch* will be understood to indicate "liver and heart." (IX 62)

**Stop Point**

Now, therefore, if we are to find remedies for such diseases we must, I opine, go in quest of them; we want remedies whose ranges of action shall be equal to and co-extensive with the ranges of action of the diseases.

Thus tuberculosis affects the brain-coverings — so does *belladonna*; here we have specificity of seat, or organopathy — but this does not suffice; the acute tuberculosis flushes the face, causes delirium, dilatation of the pupils, &c.; belladonna also flushes the face, causes delirium, dilatation of the pupils, &c ; and therefore we may say that belladonna and tuberculosis are therapeutically convertible, which is true up to a certain point, *viz.* the stop-point of the tuberculosis action and the stop-point of the belladonna-action do not coincide.

I am going to walk twenty miles to my goal along a given route, my strong friend is going the same route, and thus I shall have a companion, but Amicus only goes twelve miles, and this therefore leaves me eight miles to go alone; and as the danger lies in the last few miles only, the companionship of Amicus in the twelve miles he travels my way is no good to me, as I shall be robbed and killed after he quits me. This is the exact relative position of tuberculosis of the meninges, or hydrocephalus, and belladonna; belladonna is the friend who only goes the first twelve miles of the twenty-mile journey.

We want a twenty-mile remedy, twelve is not enough; for with a twelve-mile remedy we perish.

Far be it from me to undervalue the importance of the symptoms, or to speak lightly of the totality there of as a sure means of finding the remedy in a given case, but be it equally far from me to regard symptoms and covering the totality there of as other than a means to the finding of the remedy; for covering the totality of the symptoms may be, and often is, nothing but scientific palliation.

If the range of action of the remedy be not coincident with the disease itself a real cure does not result, no matter how many symptoms you may silence

I cannot subscribe to the generally accepted view that when you have covered all the symptoms of a case you will necessarily work a real cure; you may do so, or you may only palliate the case; certainly this kind of palliation is scientific and, *pro tanto*, beneficial, but palliation it is and palliation it remains, *e.g.*, Gallstones are not gone when you have laboriously covered the symptoms and thoroughly cured them And so on.

To cure a disease by remedies the remedies must stand in some relationship to the disease-process itself, no matter whether the symptoms reveal the process or not. If the symptoms spell out the morbid process, the symptoms suffice.

To me the physician who never gets beyond the symptoms is like a reader who, in order to read, is always obliged to spell his words.

The disease-processes are in quality zoic; the remedies, to have a range of action equal to the disease-processes, must be likewise zoic (like in quality). That **zoic remedies** constitute the field of promise, for the further development of progressive scientific homoeopathy, I am beginning clearly to see, though only through the gate ajar, but I live in hope of more light. Here let me just say that where zoic remedies are named in this work. they were chosen on a tentatively workable hypothesis of my own, and that although they are often so chosen purely hypothetically, they are no more and no less than homoeopathic remedies, pointing to a great advance in homoeopathy.

Some Hahnemannian reviewers of certain of my writings have said hard things about me, possibly with the good intention of stifling a new heresy. I have nothing to do with any man's subjective opinions; the *future* of medicine — belongs to homoeopathic pathologists, and to really cure the great diseases (with a pathologico-anatomical basis) we MUST HAVE remedies homoeopathic to such morbid anatomy, at any rate in its earlier stages. (XX 35)

## Surgeons — The Mad Persons

Our operating surgeons are mad; the biggest ones are clean mad.

No sooner does a poor woman get a lump in her breast than she is frightened out of her wits by consultations between these eminent and eminently ignorant knife-people, whose diagnositics are confined to feeling, seeing, and the microscope. (XIII 44)

## Surgery and Medicine — The Reward

The social value of these quasicures by the knife is-baronetcy. The social value of medicinal cures of tumours is slander and contempt. (XIII 44)

### Surgical Treatment

A *merely* surgical cure is no *real* cure at all, and in its very nature cannot be radical; better than nothing, no doubt, and often nearly as good as a cure, but still not a healing, in its true sense. (VI 30)

Far be it from me to detract from and honour due to my surgical brethren; nay, I am free to admit that, had my hand possessed the chirurgical cunning that lies in theirs, I should no doubt have also suffered from the surgeon's itch, and I may never have had the *patience* to try medicines as I have done, in the very worst forms of piles and other varicoses, and thus finally triumphed, to my own intense satisfaction. (VI 40)

## Swelling of Lower Extremities

Where the lower extremities are both equally involved, and the hypogastric veins are also dilated, it is often due to indurated abdominal glands. (VI 12)

### Swelling of One Leg and Spleen

The diagnosis of the seat of the dam is of very great importance in these cases. Where one lower extremity is enlarged from perturbed circulation in the deep-lying veins of the limbs, looking like phlegmasia alba dolens, but occurring in the male, and not necessarily with any increase of sensation — the left leg is most commonly involved — the condition would appear to bear some relationship to the spleen, and may, perhaps, be to the spleen what myxoedema is to the thyroid. (VI 14)

## Symptom Covering and Diagnosis

God forbid that I should say one disparaging word about symptomatic treatment as such, for we but too often have only the subjective symptoms to go by, but where an exhaustive physical diagnosis is possible, it should always be made, and should stand in importance far before merely subjective symptoms, as these may be, and often are, consequently in this sense delusive. (X 35)

## Therapeutic Insights

But Nature is not thus childishly constituted; the same substance is either good, bad, or indifferent, according to how it is used, and according to the state of aggregation of its parts.

Two equivalents of hydrogen and one of oxygen, as water, will quench our thirst, act as a solvent to our food, with a few other constituents float about in our bodies as blood. Hail, ice, sleet, and snow are also only hydrogen and oxygen in the same proportion; they are practically only water, just the same as the steam that whirls us along in the train. We are not astonished at these things; the most marvellous things cease to excite wonder after we have grown accustomed to them.

Tell the noble savage that snow, hail, ice, water, and steam are chemically the same, though physically and dynamically so different, and he will not fail to laugh at *your* ignorance! *He* knows better. Tell the mediocre medical mind that common table-salt may be so subdivided by means of friction that it thereby becomes a most powerful and even dangerous drug, and he will not fail to laugh at you! *He* knows better. (II 3)

## The Three in Medicine

For Paracelsus there were only ***three*** universal remedies, and so also for Rademacher and for their followers. Hahnemann has but *three* fundamental morbid states — psora, syphilis, and sycosis. Von Grauvogl has but three constitutions of the body — they might have all been working out the fatherlandish proverb, *Aller guten Dinge sind drei*! (X 11)

## The True Physician

Many very learned physicians do not believe in medicines. Just so; a man may be a splendid mathematician without knowing anything about Latin irregular verbs, and a physician may be very learned and yet know nothing of remedies; whether such a one, however, is *properly* called a physician may be doubted. All knowledge is good; but *the* knowledge that makes the real physician is the knowlege of how to cure. (XXIII 119)

## Tonsils Treatment

**Enlarged Tonsils.** In the medicinal treatment of enlarged tonsils there are two main lines of procedure, and the first is to cure the cause of the enlargement which is commonly not only not attempted, but it is not even thought of. For it must be manifest that to get rid of the cause of the enlargement is the prime consideration. If this be done the enlargements usually disappear — this is the best way. When you cut off a tonsil you certainly get rid of it, so you do if you shrivel it with gland tissue-destroyers, but the perfect cure is where the enlargement disappears under the influence of dynamic remedies, the normal tonsils remain to do the work alloted to them within nature's cycle. (XXV 67)

If we want to be quite successfull in the treatment of enlarged tonsils by medicines, we must look away from the mere tonsils, and remember that although the tonsils are the thing complained of, the constitutional cause of their enlargement is the real disease, and this it is that can *not* be removed by operation. Those who see the mere enlargement, and give remedies for such enlargement merely — those practitioners will mostly fail to cure enlarged tonsils by medicines, and will have much to say of the advantages of their mechanical removal.

It is not at all a bad plan to begin the course of treatment with *Sulphur* 30; after a while follow with *Calcarea carb.* 30; and in the third place give *Thuja occidentalis* 30. Each remedy should have a month or two to develop its action, to do its work.

**Tonsils — What Are they**

**My Private View of them.** There are views private and public, and my private view of the tonsils is as follows :

They are placed on either side of the fauces for the primary purpose of lubricating the food as it passes along, and so prepare it for its passage down the gullet into the stomach proper. That the tonsils actually do lubricate the food can be tested by any one so disposed, unless he has lessened his organic integrity by having them removed, or unless disease has done it for him. A pair of good, healthy, wellformed tonsils is a rare sight indeed, it is quite pretty to see them when normal.

The tonsils lie at the top of the digestive tube, and whenever certain parts or portions of the body have to deal with something harmful, the same is passed along the circulation to the tonsils to be cast out, and the tonsils then act vicariously for said parts from elsewhere. A great advantage in having it cast out at the top of the gullet is that what is cast out at that part may be rolled up in the food and so rendered harmless, and if it is disposed to decay, it is disinfected by the gastric juice. In fact, an evil-disposed particle of anything sent by the economy to the tonsils to be dealt with, has a very poor chance of doing any harm in its journey from throat to anus.

The various ailings of tonsils are for the most part not on their own account, but for and on behalf of the organism or one of its parts. During the past two years I have watched several cases of phthisis *cured* by the tonsils, — that is to say, a series of abscesses formed in the tonsils, each going through the various stages of heat, inflammation, swelling, suppuration, and bursting, and had these degenerative processes been in the lungs or bowels, they would have been of great and serious moment.

But being in the tonsils, they were slowly sacrificed for the organism, and the patients' lives were saved, and also their health. The organism works from its centre towards the periphery and into the tonsils, which cast out. An uninjured tonsil is clothed with epithelial cells, and these form a perfect protection against infection from without. I have never seen any real proof that uninjured tonsils take up disease germs; in fact, I do not believe it, and not only do I not believe the tonsils guilty of carrying in infection from without, but, on the contrary, they are specially arranged to defend themselves and the organism against outside enemies, and all the ailments and diseases that I have ever encountered in the tonsils have come from the within of the organism.

The life and the diseases of the tonsils come from within, and they are but useful servants of the organism, and always at their post.

In curing tonsillary enlargements, it is often necessary to find out the causes of such enlargements. Thus in rheumatic tonsillitis the rheumatic state of the person should be mended, and therewith the tonsillitis. The statement that rheumatic fever has been known to follow tonsillitis — that is true enough. The inference usually drawn is, that had there been no tonsils there would have been no rheumatic fever. I read the phenomena the other way. Had the tonsils been stronger and more adequate, they would have borne the whole burden of the rheumatism, and there would have been no fever. It is highly probable that minor degrees of rheumatism are arrested by the tonsils, and there dealt with, and that their function is very largely vicarious, protective of the organism and its parts. (XXV 53)

**Rheumatic Tonsils.** *Guiacum*, *Phytolacca*, *Salix*, and such anti-rheumatics come into play in the treatment of tonsils whose enlargements are of a rheumatic quality. There seems a disposition to regard the tonsils as the entrance door of the rheumatism into the organism. I am satisfied that this is entirely erroneous, and that, on the contrary, the organism endeavours to eliminate rheumatism from the organism by way of the tonsils, and it seems to me probable that it is when the tonsillary outlet is insufficient that rheumatic fever may result, not from without into the tonsils towards the centre, but from the organism out into the tonsils, to be cast away by the defecatory work of the tonsils.

The more I watch the behaviour of the tonsils, the more I am convinced that they are charged with an excretory, a defecatory function, and that they excrete things out from the organism, casting them out both at the time of swallowing food and also as a kind of lubricating trickle; such excretions pass with or without the food, down the oesophagus like corn down a shute.

Moreover, I think the bulk of the private troubles of the tonsils, *i.e.* their diseases, are vicarious for the mucous lining of the body.

I am satisfied from my observations that the tonsils are capable of sacrificing themselves on the altar of the economy by ulceration, till nearly or quite all the tonsillary tissue is gone.

The extension of phthisis to the organism from the tonsils from the exterior is practically hyperaemia, and then there is a seemingly encapsuled mass, the containing membrane looking like fascia on the surface of the tonsil; it will take first one side and then another, and will repeat itself at intervals over a period of several years, and in the end terminate in the good health of the individual. Whether unaided nature would end by curing the organism with the aid of a series of tonsillary gatherings and dischargings I am unable to say, because I have treated all the cases I have observed with remedies, notably with *Bacillinum* in high dilution. (XXV 73)

In conclusion, I will state as my opinion, based upon clinical facts as I see them in my daily work, that enlarged tonsils can be more or less readily cured by medicines withal the task is often tedious; and moreover, that *the tonsils are important organs of the body, that have as one of their functions the preservation of the life and integrity of the individual.* (XXV 78)

## Totality of Symptoms — Animal Provers

**Pathology and morbid anatomy.** It has often been maintained by the well-meaning in the homoeopathic ranks that animals cannot be used as provers for our remedies. This is no doubt true as regards pure symptomatology, but I am of quite the contrary opinion as regards pathological states : disturbances of nutrition, tissue-change and tumours.

Let me prove this by adducing a case of exostosis cured purely homoeopathically, yet without any regard to symptoms, the choice of the remedy being based upon the morbid anatomy alone. This *proves* that morbid anatomy may be taken as a prescribing basis in medicinal tumour-curing on homoeopathic lines. This point is very important, because many deny it, and maintain that the totality of the symptoms alone must serve as the basis for a truly homoeopathic prescription.

This case also *proves* that *animals* may be utilized as provers : on the basis of morbid anatomy, of course. (XX 76)

## Treating Ill-health and Not Disease

As Brights Disease at any rate cannot be operated upon, it is just as well to let the wens alone, since they are a lesser evil than *Morbus Brightii*. Furthermore, the lady was not *well*, and it was by treating her ill-health that I succeeded in getting rid of the wen. (XX 205)

## Treatment — From Simple to Complex

If we are ever to succeed in veritably curing grave disease by medicines, we must proceed from the simple to the complex; from the benign to the malignant; and it is reasonable to begin with the least difficult, and start at the thing in its very earliest stages, for there comes an incurable *stage* in almost every ailment of a progressive nature. (XX 10)

### Treatment — Many Approaches

It is astonishing how many pegs there are on which therapeutic ideas may be hung : Paracelsus, Hahnemann, Rademacher, Fletcher, Grauvogl, Virchow, Schussler, Guttceit — all help. (VI 139)

## Trigeminal Neuralgia and Hemicrania

Hart says : Neuralgia trigemini is liable to be confounded with rheumatism and hemicrania. From the former it may be distinguished by the character and severity of the pains, by the shortness of the par-

oxysms, and by the attacks being excited by such causes as a sudden jar or touch. From hemicrania it may be known by the transient and darting character of the pains, and by their corresponding accurately with the course and distribution of the nerves. Many cases of hemicrania, however, have their starting point in the supra-orbital branch of the trigeminus; but these, instead of being confined to the trifacial nerve, soon extend over the scalp, and, by involving the sympathetic, give rise to vasomotor and sensory disturbances peculiar to that affection. (XIV 114)
In the former case, as when the disease arises from cold, malarious influences, bad habits, or nervous debility, it will generally yield to the rightly-selected remedy; but when the affection depends upon organic changes, such as tumours, exostoses, and other structural alterations, it is very likely to prove permanent. At best, the patient is apt to suffer more or less from the complaint as long as he lives.
On the subject of treatment the author (*Practice of Medicine*, p. 96) has elsewhere said : "It follows from the purely subjective character and limited range of the symptoms, that the treatment of prosopalgia needs to be conducted with special reference to the cause. Hence it becomes necessary, first of all. to institute a careful scrutiny into the general state of the patient's health, his habits and surroundings, travelling, as it were, beyond the boundaries of the symptomatic indications, in order to ascertain, if possible, the true cause of the malady. In this way the prescriber is enabled to make his anatomical, physiological, and pathological knowledge contribute, not only to the diagnosis, but, in a large proportion of cases, to the cure of this obscure, obstinate, and very painful disease. (XIV 117)

## True Pathy

For my part, I make but one demand of medicine, and one only, viz. that it shall cure! The pathy that will cure is the pathy for me. For of your fairest pathy I can but say —
What care I how fair she be,
If she be not fair to *me*? (XI 11)

## Truth and the Apparent Truth

Truth is not Truth save only to the infinite : to the mind of mortal man Truth is not necessarily Truth, but only that which *appears* to be true.

Hence it is that what is a glorious truth to one man is inglorious nonsense to another, and both individuals may be equally honest of purpose and of like earnestness in their search after Truth.

Minds have their affinities no less than matter, and no one ought, after reflection, to be disappointed to find his own most cherished pursuits contemned and ridiculed by men of other minds. (XIX Preface)

## Tuberculinum and Koch's Vaccine

For them — medical and lay — tuberculinum is tuberculinum whether the matrix substance or a homoeopathic potency, whereas the one is a poison that kills, while the other is a grand harmless remedy, that cures a very dire and fatal disease. (XVIII 48)

So Kochism is dead, as dead as a door-nail. And all because they will not, cannot, accept Hahnemann's dosage.

But Koch's tuberculins will become and remain great homoeopathic remedies. Oh, the irony of the thing! Pretty well all the best work of the orthodox school ends in — what?

In securing the ultimate triumph of homoeopathy. (XIX 124)

## Tuberculosis — And Piles

The phthisical and the phthisically-disposed are very prone to piles, notably those who are dark and dusky; and, indeed, I have often found the piles in such more troublesome and painful than the phthisis proper. (XVI A 166)

### — Signs

**Pelvic Consumptiveness.** Consumptiveness may show itself not merely in the lungs, in the glands, but also in the brain. It shows itself, perhaps almost as frequently, in the pelvic region; as disturbances of the menstrual or sexual functions : in young men as more or less furious incoercible nocturnal emissions, masturbations, or excesses in venery, that if not cured run the sufferer to ground. The excessive fecundity of the tuberculously disposed needs no dwelling upon. The girls develop very quickly and ripen perhaps unduly in the bust. (XVI A 184)

The little son of a distinguished clergyman, two-and-a-half years old, was brought to me on May 9th, 1889, for feverish attacks that were clearly pointing to tuberculosis, evidenced by the strawberry tongue, the indurated glands, and pining state generally. (XVI A 85)
What I regard as tubercular teeth are those — often more or less rudimentary — with holes in their external surface. Whether this is a recognised pathological fact I do not happen to know, perhaps it is not. (XVI A 110)
A little girl of 6 was brought by her mother, Lady X., in the month of August, 1888, for evident symptoms of incipient tubercular disease : restless nights; sleeplessness; grinds her teeth; tendency to diarrhoea; want of appetite; foul breath, notched teeth; pain after food; vomiting of food; indurated glands; strawberry tongue; naughty; very irritable temper; puny growth; very thin. (XVI A 99)

### Tuberculous State

There are certain cases of what may, perhaps, be termed CONSUMPTIVENESS, but where the patients, through being fed largely and richly manage to get stout, even very fat, and who yet are distinctly afflicted with the tuberculour taint, and who in the end get diabetes, or go into common consumption. (XVI A 53)

## Tumours and Cancer and Suppressed Skin Diseases

Quite a number of cases of tumour have their starting point in silenced cutaneous discharges; this is no vague theoretical statement, but a fact in nature which I have oft verified and which is clinically verifiable any day. Many cases of chronic skin-diseases are no more and no less than chronic diffuse cancerosis.
This is one reason why cancer is more common now than formerly, while skin diseases are less common. The ordinary dermatologist works, unwittingly, great evil; and when driving along the Thames Embankment one day, and gazing at Cleopatras Needle, I said to myself — How much mischief did good old Sir Erasmus Wilson work in getting together the money that went to fetch and erect that?
A persisting skin-disease in a really healthy taintless person is a sight I have myself never seen, just as I am not acquainted with any other causeless effect. (XX 166)

**— and Injuries**

No experienced practitioner will deny the important part played by bruises, blows, and falls, in the genesis of tumours and cancer; and hence our anti-traumatics ought to figure much more largely in our therapeutics of growths from blows. (XIII 14)

**— and Post-Operative Treatment**

Where an operation has been performed, constitutional treatment should be begun *at once*, to get at the root of the matter and prevent any further local expression of the disease, by attacking its cause or causes. I say *or causes*, for cancer is not a disease that can produce its like after the manner of, say syphilis or scarlatina, but is essentially a hyperplasia of a degraded type at the end of a chain that has many (causal) links. (XIII 23)

**— and Surgery**

Truth to tell, I am sick and weary of the lying statements that the knife is even any, and least of all the only cure for tumours. Not only does the knife not *cure*, but any one having a tumour or lump cannot, as a rule, take a shorter road to the grave than *via* the knife — that is, unless it be very large, and unless the tendency to its recurrence be outrooted simultaneously with the operation, or soon thereafter.

Oftener than not, cutting out a small tumour is like pruning a vine. Simply because a very considerable number of people with tumours literally die of the doctors opinions, and then what is the use or value of the opinion of a never so eminent a pathologist on a therapeutic point? Just none.

Of course, I know it is said to be very unprofessional to decline an eminent colleague's co-operation in a given case. But I did it for my patients' good, *not* for my own; and moreover, they do the same to me when people want my opinion. (XIII 31)

The surgical removal of tumours seems to me to be unsatisfactory in every important particular.

It only professes to deal with the produce and can never be, even theoretically, a Hunterian cure : the *disposition* is not even aimed at!

The treatment by the actual cautery gets rid of the superficial effect — the product — the cause is not even considered at all. (XX 258)

A human being without ovaries is not a woman at all. Where a lady's breast is removed for a tumour — can that lady be said to be still marriageable?

Hardly. And whether or not how fearfully shocking the mutilation, even to the lady herself. (XX 254)

Thinking the matter over it seemed manifest that if a lump would stay for nine years, there must be an internal cause — disposition — *ever operative,* for if it had not been *continuous* in its operativeness, the lump must have long since disappeared : a causeless lump cannot be. (XX 264)

**— and Vaccinosis**

Amongst the frequent causes of tumours I must, therefore, reckon vaccinosis, and on this subject I would refer the reader to my little treatise entitled *Vaccinosis and its Cure by Thuja etc.,* in which this thesis is to some extent elaborated. Sometimes we have to do *with* trauma upon vaccinosic tissue, and then the just appreciation of the two genetic factors leads to a cure. (XIII 20)

**— and Vitality**

Just because the thing is impossible. And why impossible? Simply because the organism GROWS tumours *vitally,* and anything that is to *cure,* really cure must bring back the *perverted* VITALITY of the part of the normal, and, fortunately, the semeiology and symptomatology of the sufferers, when read in the light of homoeopathy, give us good stout hand-rope to guide us in our search for the right remedies.

If we *reflect* upon the subject, we shall readily come to the conclusion that the attempt to cure tumour by locally-applied absorbents or by operation is like trying to cure an apple-tree of its apples by painting the apples with iodine, or performing an operation on the apple-tree for "apples." (XIII 46)

**— Difficulties in Treatment**

WHY is it that odd cases of tumour have been cured by remedies here and there for many years, notably by homoeopathic practitioners, and yet the systematic medication for tumours is still non-existent? I take it that the difficulties of the task, the complexities of the clinical problems to be solved, the incapacity of mankind to value and understand the work done, all tend to prevent it. And even more still, the venomous hatred of those who can *not*.

But I will imitate the little birds by taking my little notions one stick at a time ... *petit a petit, Poiseau fait sone nid*, which is a process of proved practicability, and I will in like manner endeavour to construct a method of curing tumours with medicines; as it is not absolutely scientific, I cannot present it as a complete and polished whole, with a smoothly euphonious Hellenic name, but what it lacks in science it fully makes up in sense, and so let it be known as my stick-by-stick method.

After all there is nothing positively of saving grace in Hellenic names, as witness the name *Surgeon*, which is indisputably Hellenic, being from Χειρ the hand and εργου work, and hence Χειρουργοξ is a handworker and Χειρουργ*ια* is surgery, or handiwork; and yet notwithstanding this very respectable family history, surgery offers no cure for tumours sufficiently pleasing to my mind for me to be desirous of its aid were I afficted with a tumour in any part of my body. Surgeons may think the cutting-out and cutting-off processes "curing;" I think them a last sad refuge of helplessness. One of the great difficulties in the medicinal treatment of tumours lies in the *kinds* of studies that have been prosecuted in relation to tumours, their aetiology being but scantily considered, while therapeutics is simply scouted.

Hunter, however, knew very well that when he cut out a tumour he had only got rid of the *product* of the disease, not the disease itself. But then Hunter was a thinker; and, instead of being made a baronet, was hounded to death by pettifoggers.

Composed wholly or mostly of, or growing from fibrous tissue, the tumour is called a fibroma; of bone, osteoma; of cartilage, enchondroma; of fat, lipoma — respectively stertoma; of muscle, myoma; of nerve, neuroma; of embryonic fleshy stuff, sarcoma; of glia, glioma; encapsuled, and like a bladder, cystoma; and so on almost endlessly.

Of course, for purposes of classification, as a mere matter of natural history, this positive scientific method is absolutely sound and useful, and biologically even interesting, but for the practical physician (not to mention the patient!) it is at present of but small value. (XX 62)

It does not help the surgeons (though I hope to make it help me a little). And the proof of this lies in the fact that the longer this line of research is continued in, the more diseases we get, and the more doctors mankind needs. The more "omas" we have the more surgeons we want ! To turn human suffering to account for biological research is not my ideal of medicine.

My ideal of medicine is rather that which tends to its own elimination, *i.e.*, the more it advances, the nearer it comes to its own destruction, and hence, preventive medicine should have the highest rank. Fortunately it is just in preventive medicine, in its crudest form, at any rate, that nearly all medical men work, wherefore they deserve well of mankind.

But to return from this wandering at large to my tumours, I would say that though in my judgement lipoma, fibroma, myoma, sarcoma, &c. as designations of tumours are therapeutically so little helpful, still they do, nevertheless, constitute a comparatively fixed basis of classification, and that is something. And even here it is not entirely valueless; the fact is, *all* real knowledge helps.

One reason why tumour-curing by medicines has barely entered upon its baby life, lies in the wholesale and crude way in which the subject has been therapeutically approached; people have sought a *solvent* for tumour generally, but tumours are vital growths, and must be *vitally* approached and regarded. What comes vitally, must go vitally, and therefore gently, painlessly, and comparatively slowly. This slowness is very detrimental to its adoption : I will exemplify — I had cured a lady of a tiny tumour in her nose; she was pleased and grateful, and subsequently brought to me her niece, on whom the doctors were about to operate for a small ovarian tumour; I cured this tumour also, but it occupied two years or thereabouts, and then aunt and niece both persuaded a friend, a lady residing at Sheppards Bush, to come to me. How long did I think it would take to cure her ovarian tumour? At least two years. I prefer the operation said she, that will only take six weeks.

But it took less — she died under or shortly after the operation.

Of such examples I could give so many that I must conclude that the operational statistics I read in the medical journals are made up very hastily.

The same aunt and niece persuaded a lady from Chatham to come to me for a tumour of the breast; the lady's husband declined my treatment, as I thought it would take two years at the very least. She was successfully operated on, and thoroughly cured thereby of her mammary tumour; nine months later, she was again thoroughly cured of another tumour, by a perfectly successful operation, a few months thereafter, she was again successfully operated on for another tumour, and just as she was getting well — she died.

But here the difficulty of finding a remedy which shall be homoeopathic not to the symptoms due to the presence of the tumours, but to their causation — that is to say, to those symptoms which constitute the disease-picture, and which lead up to, and end in the formation of tumours — this difficulty is, in the present state of our knowledge, well-nigh insurmountable; hence I have learned to hang my hat on any peg I could find. And as the chapter of accidents helps us a little, let us start with it.

**— Fatty**

Of all tumours, ivory osteomata and lipomata, and certain cystomata, I find the most difficult to touch.

The fatty tumours seem very indolent, and though I generally get them down about one-half or two-thirds, I do not succeed beyond that. Fatty tumours appear to arise from friction, as in this case from the rubbing of the fleshy thighs against one another — as witness the *lipoma professionale* of certain Russian women. Of course the friction is only the exciting cause, there is the neoplastic disposition behind. They are more common in women than in men, and I know several cases where the exciting cause is evidently due to the friction of the corsets. (XX 305)

**— Living and Old**

One thing I may say — it is quite useless to try to cure *old* tumours either cancerous or benign, unless you are gifted with PATIENCE of no ordinary kind. *Rapid* cures of old tumours by medicines I have never seen, nor do I think such tumours *ever* will be cured *rapidly,* simply because they are *vital* products — THEY ARE LIVING GROWTHS. Nevertheless, some recently-formed tumours do get well in a very few weeks or months. While other require as many years. Speaking broadly, the tumour takes proportionately as long to cure by medicines as it has taken to grow. And hereby is not to be forgotten that a tumour has often existed a long time *before* it is found out. It is equally useless to try to cure tumours by giving drugs with a view of *dissolving* them chemically.

Why?

Because, as just stated, tumours are ALIVE : they are GROWTHS; they come *via vita,* and vitally they must be cured; and for this process time, often much time, is needfull. At least that is my experience, and I therefore specially emphasize the fact, that I know of no short cut to tumour-curing by remedies, and the work must be done by internal remedies.

Nevertheless, externally applied remedies are not to be entirely neglected, *i.e.*, where the growth is for any reason, as it were, *extra-organismic*. Where I use a remedy externally I shall state the fact. (XIII 11)

**— Medical Treatment**

In common with a certain small number of other practitioners of scientific medicine in different parts of the world, I have long been in the habit of treating *tumours* of various parts of the body by medicines, and that with great success. When, a few days since, a young girl, whom I knew, was sent to a hospital for operation for a small mammary tumour that I am quite sure could have been cured by medicines, I felt it to be my imperative duty at once to bring my own views and experience more prominently to the fore, and the more so as our knife-men — *our surgical carpenters* — are waxing bolder and bolder every day, and the very excellences of aseptic and anaesthetic surgery are fast running legitimate medicine to the ground, and with it our common humanity. (XIII)

Often when I have saved a breast, I have vividly before my mind the pregnant exclamation of the lady (*Diary of a Physician*) in regard to her ablated breast — "Ah doctor, but my husband!" A greater reward than to prevent this anguish of soul in some of my sister the world cannot offer me.

I declare that *the knife is no cure for tumours*, and that tumours can be cured by medicines, the requisite knowledge and *patience* being given. In order to be able to excise a tumour successfully, a man must first learn how to do it; it is the work of a skilled mechanic merely, in which there are many masters. In order to be able to cure a tumour by medicines, a man must also first learn how to do it, but it is the work of the patient chess player, in which there are but few masters. Still, without being a master, the art of curing tumours by medicines can — thanks to Hahnemann and others — be learned and practised by all in direct proportion to their ability and industry.

The great art in curing tumours by medicines may be thus summerized — *keep on pegging away*! Only, of course, we must peg away with the right remedies. Any medical person who reads this book attentively will have a good idea of how to set to work. I do not attempt or pretend to be in any sense apologetic or diffident on the question of amenability of tumours to drug treatment, for the good and sufficient reason that I have been curing tumours by remedies for the past dozen years and, therefore, I am discoursing only of what I know and have seen; that I have attained to my present certain position with much difficulty, endless gropings, and, I fear, some bunglings, goes without saying — *Ca va sans dire* in fact.

In like manner I am of opinion that the physician who sets about trying to cure tumours by means of medicines does more service to mankind and to medicine than he who only talks of how to cut them out, and of the microscopic and macroscopic characters and peculiarities of such growths after he has cut them out. Accordingly, I had not been in practice very long before I occupied myself with the question of the curability or noncurability by medicines of quite a number of diseases commonly called incurable, and amongst them *Tumours*. (XIII 2)

A good many years have passed since then, and I have been treating cases of tumour ever since with medicines, whenever I have had the opportunity; and when the patients have been as patient as their physician, have generally succeeded in curing them. (XIII 3)

**— Mode of Treatment**

1. Were I asked to put down shortly my mode of setting about curing a case of tumour when it comes before me for medicinal treatment, I would say : First of all, I begin by remembering Hahnemann's method of case-taking, and follow it partially; I say partially, because *time* is an element of importance nowadays.
2. Then I go over in my mind the various medical doctrines, such as those of psora, syphilis, sycosis, vaccinosis, Grauvoglian constitutions and traumatism, not forgetting all the illnesses and diseases of the patient and any possible bearings of taints and dispositions, hereditary or acquired.
3. I take, then, a purely organopathic survey of the organ or part, and then weigh and balance the various facts which physiology, pharmacology, and pathology tell us about it.

When all this is done, I have usually *at least* one good reason for giving one good remedy which is then ordered, and which commonly teaches me the next step, either because it helps, or behaves indifferently, or otherwise.

Most commonly I find tumours are pathologically *hybrid* in their nature and they will not yield to treatment of a simple nature, *e.g.*, a person of the herpetic diathesis, who suffered much from gastric fever, was then vaccinated, then had much grief and sorrow, and finally had suffered from unrequited affection; and last of all, got a blow on her breast, followed by the formation of tumour, such a person in her very history tells the thoroughly competent therapeutist how to proceed without any symptomatology at all.

It has been urged against the homoeopathic treatment of tumours that as the remedies used have (as a rule) never caused tumours or anything like them, and, moreover, are in all probability quite incapable of doing so, it must follow that there can be no real homoeo-therapeutics of tumours. This little volume is a first part of my practical answer to this objection. It is brought out by itself for the reason already stated in my preface. I hope in a later publication to set forth in a clearer light my reasons for giving the remedies which I have found of greatest use in the treatment of tumours, some of which I have herein already referred to.

What I aim at in this volume is to *prove* that tumours can be truly and genuinely cured by medicines given by the mouth; and if I have proved that, then I have attained my object.

NEVERTHELESS, IN ORDER TO AID any younger practitioners in attempting the internal treatment of tumours, *i.e.*, by remedies, I will just add a list of a few of the most useful medicines for this purpose, giving them alphabetically, with a practical note or two for the uninitiated. For further information, see Hughes' *Pharmacodynamics* last edition, and back numbers of the *British Journal of Homoeopathy*, of the *Monthly Homoeopathic Review*, and of the *Homoeopathic World*. (XIII 64)

**— No Small Disease**

Some ailings are like sparrows; very small arms will suffice to kill them — say hydropathy, or homoeopathic simples, but tumours generally resist small arms. (XX 196)

**— of the Breast — Diet Restrictions**

In case I should subsequently omit to state the fact, I would say that pig-meat, milk, much salt and pepper, are, in my judgement, to be avoided in tumours of the breast. New milk is particularly bad for mammary tumours and inflammations, as also for menstrual troubles. (XIII 11)

**— of the Female Breast — Causes**

Under this heading I desire to make a few cursory yet practical remarks on the causation of mammary tumours in women. To begin with, the tumours in the female breast are very rarely primary to the breasts, but are most commonly produced in the breasts much in the same way that organ is enabled to perform its natural function of suckling the human offspring, *i.e.*, the part is rendered physiologically active from the utero-ovarian sphere. Whether this view of the origin of mammary tumours has ever been promulgated before I do not know, in any case I have it from my own observations in practical life. Usually there is some disease or irritation in the lower part of the body, either arising primarily there or else expressed there holopathically. I will not enter into the details of these causes here, as the subject is too large for my present purpose, which will be sufficiently served if I say that wearing pessaries, making intra-vaginal injections for the purposes of cleanliness or otherwise, or for the cure of mechanical hurts and injuries to the parts, the cautery, genesaic frauds and surrogates, all these may serverally result in the formation of tumours in the ovaries, uterus, or breasts. The point I here insist upon is that mammary tumours do not usually arise from a cause existing primarily in the breasts themselves, but the cause is usually in some other more or less remote part of the organism, most frequently in the ovaries. Or the cause is organismic, and the tumour is the mammary expression of the constitutional condition of the individual.

And even where the tumour arises directly from a knock or blow; or from pressure from the stays, there is usually something the constitutional crasis that favours neoplasms; and it is this something which constitutes the danger to the future integrity of the individual. If I am correct in what I here maintain with regard to the place or real primary origin and causation of tumour in the female breasts, then it must follow that operation can *never* be any *cure* since it is only the product that is operatively got rid of, and not the disease radically. In proof of this, see the number of cases which I relate even in this small volume, in which the disease returned in the other breast after it had been cut out of one. The number of times in which I myself have seen this recurrence of tumours, after they had been got rid of by operation, is so great that I could adduce an absolutely overwhelming chain of evidence to prove this my contention, but I forbear; the fact is patent, and within the experience of all medical men, and, indeed, of almost all ladies of experience who take cognizance of what goes on in their own social circles.

I conclude, therefore, that both theory and experience condemn the use of the knife, which is no cure for tumours. Is an operation, then, absolutely and always useless and damnable? Not quite that, though it is not often needful if the case is taken early, when the tumour is young, as medicines can cure it vitally; BUT when it has become large — very large, broken, granulating, and auto-infective, *then* an operation is called for, but medicinal means should be at once used to prevent recurrence. In the earlier stages operation is damnable and dangerous. (XIII 58)

Now, in the first place, I hold very strongly that mucous surfaces under natural conditions are not intended by nature to be washed, inasmuch as they are self-cleansing, and, in the next place, I maintain that diseases of the mucous membranes are for the most part constitutional, and should not be treated by local applications.

I reason in this way : The mucous membrane is to the inside of the body just what the skin is to its outside, and should be thus regarded physiologically and therapeutically.

Discharges from mucous surfaces are essentially much the same as eruptions on the cutaneous surface, and in the very deed are not infrequently identical.

And then Nature makes use of mucous surfaces from which to discharge peccant matter, of which she wishes to rid the economy. In ladies, the mucous lining of the vagina and of the womb are most convenient for this purpose, and hence the common occurrence of whites, which is its expression. (XIII 60)

Now, just a word or two anent dietetic causes of tunours, and then I have done. In my experience they are — 1. Much meat, notably pig meat; 2. Pepper and salt; 3. Milk; and in regard to this lastnamed, no doubt many will be much amazed at my condemning the use of milk in tumours (particularly in those of the breast), but I do so most emphatically, and that from my own personal experience. Practical men would do well to remember this. (XIII 63)

**— of Breast — True Nature**

The point I claim is that Tumours of the Breast do not commonly arise primarily from the breasts, but from the utero-ovarian sphere, and that therefore it is very poor treatment to excise the fruit while leaving the roots (in the pelvic organs). Whether the excision of the ovaries or uterus will be any good remains to be seen, but I doubt it very much. However, we shall soon have the records of vast numbers of Beatsons operations, so here we leave the question *sub judice*. (XXIV 65)

**— of the Eyelids**

Two or three days after penning the foregoing account of medicinal cures of tumours of the eyelids, I chanced to go to the office of a city solicitor for a matter of legal business. "Ah, doctor," said he, "I have been away for a fortnight from business. I have had an operation on my left eye; just look. I have been at home a fortnight with it since. I had to keep it bound up".

On looking at his *eye* I saw nothing abnormal, and I said, "Your eyes are all right." I then found that he did not differentiate between eye and eyelid, and that he had been operated on for a tiny cystic tumour of the eyelid!

Said he, "Mr. B. did it for me. I am all right now."

The gentleman he referred to is considered, and indeed is one of the first opthalmologists (eyecarpenters) of the day, and the solicitor, I may say, stands well in his own profession; so we may take them both as fair samples of the educated professional classes of to-day. In other words, a layman with a trained mind gets a little lump on his eyelid, FROM INTERNAL CAUSE as I submit. He merely wished it removed with the knife, as if it had dropped from the sky, and had impinged upon his "eye." He goes to an eminent oculist — what more natural? and said oculistic chirurgeon being on the same general educational and physiological level, gains in every way by cutting out the little cyst!

Both the individuals concerned have not the faintest suspicion that they are other than the *creme de la creme* of all that is most advanced in knowledge, and in the very van of progress. They will die in the happy delusion, and their work and names will not be remembered.

Did I try to enlighten my solicitorial friend by explaining that in as much as the said cyst was autochthonous, it ought to have had its existence cut short autochthonously?

Did I explain to him that the cyst was a qualitative outcome of his organismic self and that this self-same microcosmic should have been put right vitally?

Did I? No.

Why? Because you cannot put a large quantity into a small vessel, whether the vessel be called surgeon, solicitor, or beerglass.
Of the tumours of the eyelids, the meibomian cyst is very common, and also very amenable to medicinal means. It will once in a way disappear of itself without any medicines, but not very often; usually it must be got rid of either by operation or medicines. The usual way is to reverse the lid, and make a small incision from the inner lid surface which cover the tumour, and then squeeze out the contents. But "the tumour is liable to recur." says a very experienced operator! Of course it is!
In my opinion, the encysted and other tumours of the eyelids are nearly always of constitutional origin, and must be constituionally cured. (XIII 5)

**— Treatment and Hope**
The lady was, however, very patient, and went on with my treatment, feeding principally on hope; but hope, though not a bad auxilliary, is no remedy for tumours or skin diseases. (XIII 20)

**— Treatment — Lessons**
I have given so many tedious details of this obstinate and difficult case (Case 228, Part III) to illustrate several points as clearly as I am able. In the first place, this case caused me to modify my previously oft-expressed opinion, that when once an operation had taken place, treatment by medicine is useless. I now know that this is not necessarily the case, but that a cure may be obtained even after an operation, and after a recurrence has begun. In the next place I again learn, and continue to insist upon, the importance of dogged perseverance in medicinal treatment. And finally, it confirms my general practice of striking out new therapeutic lines when the old ones do not suffice. (XIII 27)

## Typhoid and Tuberculosis
I have often noticed a proneness to typhoid in those disposed to phthisis. (XX 190)

## Uterus and Breast

The submammary pain — the classic "pain under the left breast," and its equally classic remedy, *Cimicifuga* — indicate a certain relationship between the uterus and upper part of the left side in women. (XXIII 72)

## Vaccination and Hair

Still it might have been so, as the hair is very powerfully influenced by the vaccine poisoning. Thus Kunkel observed both a very weak growth of hair and an excessive growth, especially in wrong places, as effects, he believed, of vaccination. (IX 39)

### — and Prophylaxis

**Wherein Does the Protective Power of Vaccination Consist?** Given a *perfectly healthy* individual who has never been vaccinated. We say to such a one, you must be vaccinated or you are liable to catch small-pox, which is often about. Let us pause to note clearly that the individual thus warned by us as being liable to catch small-pox *is perfectly healthy*. Now let us vaccinate this perfectly healthy person, and, the vaccination succeeding, we say he is henceforth protected from small-pox. That is to say, this thoroughly healthy non-vaccinated person becomes more or less proof against the contagion of small-pox by vaccination, or, at any rate, it is so averred.

It may be safely admitted that no one can be *more* than perfectly healthy, and any modification or altering of perfect health must result in a minus, *i.e., less* than perfect health; and *less* than perfect health must necessarily be disease or ill health of some sort and in some degree.

Hence it follows that the protective power of vaccination is due to a *diseased* state of the body. [See Remarks on Homoeoprophylaxis further on.] (XIX 6)

### — and Skin Diseases

However, by no means must be attributed all skin affection, following closely or remotely in the wake of vaccination to the pathogenetic effect of the vaccine virus itself; it *does* cause numerous skin diseases without a doubt, but it also, and frequently, *rouses latent disease* for which anti-vaccinial treatment will, of course, not suffice. (IX 48)

**— and Styes**

Here it might not be amiss to observe casually that the presence of styes on the eyelids is often, in my opinion, a symptom of vaccinosis. (IX 40)

**— Unsuccessful**

I do not expect many to agree with my theory that, when an individual is unsuccessfully vaccinated, he may have been seriously affected in his health by the reactionless vaccination, perhaps more so than as if it had "taken." But it is a *settled* point with me, and in these cases I find Thuja as promptly efficacious as in the ordinary forms of vaccinosis. (XIX 51)

## Vaccinosis

**Vaccinosis Bars the Way to the Cure of Ringworm.** Some of my readers may know that I have started the theory that ringworm is in its nature of a tuberculosic quality, that the presence of the fungi on an individual is a proof of this, that the presence of ringworm on such an individual is to his (or her) advantage, and that external treatment of ringworm is harmful, and finally I have written a small treatise on the subject of the curability of ringworm by internal constitutional treatment, notably *Bacillinum*. (XIX 79)

**— Forms of**

Vaccinosis shews itself as a formidable acute disease that may terminate fatally, or it may manifest itself as a chronic affection. The ordinary forms of vaccinia must be included under acute vaccinosis. The word Vaccinose (Vaccinosis) is used in the homoeopathic literature of Germany, though hardly generally accepted. So far as I know, it has no place in English literature, either homoeopathic or general, at all. But the literature of anti-vaccinators teems with examples of "ill-effects of vaccination," "consequences of vaccination," and the like. Most of these would fall under the general term vaccinosis, but only in so far as they are due to "pure" vaccine pus. Here let me remark that it is too often lost sight of that "*pure* vaccine lymph" means vaccine pus (matter) and nothing else, just as we would say *pure* consumption, *pure* syphilis, *pure* poison. The general idea is that *pure* vaccine lymph is as harmless as bread and butter. (XIX 7)

**— Latent**

The vaccinate is one who is suffering from vaccinosis; he may not be ill in the ordinary sense, but he must be in a subdued morbid state, he has been blighted or he is no vaccinate; it is his diseased condition that protects him from smallpox.

Some may, perhaps, say that vaccinosis is the same as vaccinia; this is. however, not so; vaccinosis is vaccinia and something more, for if a person is vaccinated unsuccessfully he has *not* had vaccinia, whereas some of the worst cases of (my) vaccinosis which I have met with were just those in whom the vaccination did not "take," as the saying goes. Hence I must call attention to what I believe is a fact, *viz.* : that it often *does* take deep hold of the constitution without calling forth any local phenomena, and, not only so, but such cases may be even very severe in their *internal* developments, manifested by the supervention of various morbid symptoms after vaccination. Let us dwell a little on this novel assertion, I was going to say *fact*, yet probably very few will admit that it is a fact at all, but only a fad of mine, since everybody holds that if the vaccination does not "take" the individual has remained uninfluenced by the process of putting vaccine under the cuticle. In other words, when a person is vaccinated and does not take; is, in fact, unsuccessfully vaccinated, it is held that said person is proof against vaccination, and we certify accordingly. Everyone believes that the unsuccessfully vaccinated individual has not in any way been affected or altered by the vaccination.

CLOSE AND MINUTE OBSERVATION, HOWEVER, TEACHES ME THAT SUCH IS BY NO MEANS NECESSARILY THE CASE, FOR NOT A FEW PERSONS DATE THEIR ILL HEALTH FROM A SO-CALLED UNSUCCESSFUL VACCINATION. My own conception of the thing is just this : The vaccinated person is poisoned by the vaccine virus; what is called the "taking" is, in point of fact, the constitutional re-action whereby the organism frees itself more or less from the inserted virus. If the person does not "take", AND

THE VIRUS HAS BEEN ABSORBED, the "taking" becomes a chronic process — paresis, neuralgiae, cephalalgiae, pimples, acne, &c. The less a person "takes," therefore (in such a case), the MORE is he likely to suffer from chronic vaccinosis, *i.e.*, from the genuine vaccination disease in its chronic form, very frequently a neuralgia or paresis.

Most practitioners will agree that neuralgia is more prevalent now than ever before within the present age, and experience has forced me to ascribe many such cases to vaccinosis.

If my colleagues object to my aetiopathology of such neuralgiae, perhaps they will favour all with a more satisfactory one. The word neuralgia" covers such a multitude of sins in the world of nosology and pathology that my hypothesis is an exact science compared therewith!

**— Manifold Disease**

I have treated a certain number of other cases, with varied disease symptoms, on the hypothesis that I was dealing with vaccinosis, and often with results little short of startling, but I hardly think it would serve any useful purpose to multiply examples. The foregoing observations embody and exemplify all that is essential of what I have observed and thought on the subject; if other physicians will follow on the same lines, the reward will be theirs and mine; and if they will not, then the reward still is mine in this, that I have cured very obstinate cases of disease by reckoning with vaccinosis as a clinical fact, and as a man I could not do less than, say, what I believe I know on the subject before the world. It remains for others to judge whether the work was worth doing. (XIX 76)

## Vaginal Douche

I hold very strong opinions on the question of intro-vaginal injections : they are altogether damnable and pernicious, shallow in conception, wrong in theory, and harmful in practice. (XXIII 84)

## Varicose Veins

One sees the oddest things in the way of varicose veins in the lower half of the body, but not very often in the upper, as gravitation is enough to empty them when they are higher up. (XVII 113)

I reasoned thus : Veins that dilate in that manner, steadily, slowly, increasingly, must do so from an obstruction in their progression heartwards, just as the little rivulets higher up the stream must fill up when the stream is dammed up lower down. (XVII 113)

**— Treatment**

When a man comes forward with a proposition not generally received by his fellows in his own walk of life, it behoves him to proceed inductively and independently. If he does this he is proceeding scientifically, and trained minds, not being overladen with prejudice, soon know where they are in dealing with his proposition. Experience proves that a proposition may be demonstrably true, and that it may yet meet with only a very limited acceptance; especially is this the case with new truths, and truths that involve unpleasant consequences. And when a person has once committed himself, once taken sides, he is very apt to go on thenceforth for ever — for *his* ever — from the standpoint of a *parti pris*.

May not venous subjects fairly say to the *physicians* — What have *you* all been doing the past two thousand years; have you not, with all your learning, vivisections and mortisections, poisonings and drugprovings, and your never-ending ransacking of all creation for new remedies; have you not herewithal been able to hit upon some gentle innocuous means of bringing back a few dilated veins to their normal calibre? (VI 19)

Oddly enough, the *art of healing*, pure and simple, is not in great repute nowadays; indeed, it is almost a reproach to fling one's self body and soul into the business of healing, and herein try to do better than one's father did. Nay, it is even dangerous for a man of good repute to strike out a new path in therapeutics, and *try* to cure what the solid phalanx of and ancient trades union has ever held to be incurable; if he do, he will infallibly be looked at askance, and no one will thank him, while many will seek to deride and vilify him. The reason of this lies largely in the history of medicine and of mankind; bad ware has been so often brought forward as good that no one may be much blamed for looking with some suspicion on all new notions.

Now, I am coming forward with the thesis that atonic dilated veins may, in many instances, be made to shrink to their original size by the proper use of medicines, administered internally and aided by certain auxiliaries, — in other words, varicosis, haemorrhoids, varicocele and varices are amenable to drug-treatment, and therefore surgery, in this department of diseases of the veins, is to be superseded by medicines. Surgeons will no doubt object to being thus ousted, and will probably not fail to vent their wrath upon me. Good, my ireful brethren, you have done that before in another subject (*Curability of Cataract with Medicines*), and yet truth is gaining thereby, and a certain step in advance has been made.

Of course you will perceive that neither there, nor here, am I originating anything; I have merely been sitting at the feet of Hahnemann, and have come out to do battle for this great truth.

In the sincere hope that some truth-loving and truth-seeking brother may read this, and be desirous of seeking the path I have wandered, I will give it step by step, just as I have come. It is an honourable path, wherein walk many good men and true, who are striving to make the physicians business one of *healing the sick, cito, tuto, et jucunde*; the path is not easy to travel, neither is it always daylight therein, but it has just one safe and sure hand-railing running along it from end to end, and that is ... the LAW OF SIMILARS. There are other guides, but they do not go all the way; they are only here and there, so we will, in the following pages, just hold on to ... LIKE CURES LIKE. We are the more constrained to do so as we know no other safe guide in therapeutics. (VI 23)

## Varicosis

**How to understand Varicosis from Obstruction.** If we dam up a given river at a certain place, all the little streams and rivulets that debouch into it *above the dam* will fill up and swell in volume, and very likely overflow their banks and flood the environs. Now, if we want to get rid of this overflow of the banks, we may certainly raise the banks and so hem in the water, but in this way we increase the volume of the rivulets, and the heightened banks need much and constant attention; but if we go down to the dam and remove it, we have no further difficulty with the streams and rivulets, for they will run on and empty themselves into the river, just as the latter will run on into the sea.

Now so it is with varicose veins from obstruction; the obstruction is the dam that prevents the smaller veins from duly emptying themselves into the larger ones. We may, to continue our simile, heighten the banks by putting on elastic stockings, but the better plan is to go down to the obstructive dam and remove it, for just as the rivulets with the higher banks increase in volume, so do varicose veins that are merely held in by

mechanical support. (VI 3)
Above the level of the heart we do not often meet with varicose veins, because gravitation is sufficient to overcome any moderate obstruction. Below the diaphragm, on the other hand, varicose veins are very common, because here gravitation tends to increase any tendency to varicosis.
A swelled or enlarged liver is a frequent cause of varicose veins of the right leg; a swelled spleen has a similar effect on the venous circulation of the left lower extremity. Constipation has a like effect on either lower extremity, according to where the accumulated faeces lie. In ladies, uterine enlargement and displacement act similarly. One-sided varicosis is often caused by ovarian enlargements. (VI 8)

## Venous Congestions

For it must obviously be much the same thing whether all the cases of haemorrhoids come together or not, — and a dilated vein is essentially the same pathological entity whether it be portal and miscalled liver disorder, or on the legs and termed varices, or at the anus and designated piles, or round the spermatic cord and known as varicocele. (VI 137)

**General Constitutional Venosity.** There are certain subjects whose venous systems are exceedingly prone to ail; if they have anything wrong with their hearts, it is pretty sure to be the venous side of it; if they get dyspepsia, it arises from congestion of the portal system of veins; if they suffer from headaches, it is from venous stasis; if they get constipated, piles develop at once; if they stand much, or wear a tight garter, they get varices of the legs; if the *uro-genetic* system gets irritated or injured, and fails to get tone-giving natural relief, they have varicocele, or menstrual troubles from dilated veins of the ovaries and broad ligaments, as the case may be. They are *constitutionally venous,* and suffer from passive congestions at all turns. (VI 46)

## Women and Operations

It is astonishing with what lightheartedness the belongings of a patient — particularly a number of the women — discuss such operations on *women other than themselves*! (XX 249)

## Part II

# Materia Medica Notes & Therapeutics

### Acne Remedies

There is also a kind of acne that is distinctly of arthritic nature, and this yields well to *Urea 6*; in this variety pustulation is much less pronounced than in vaccinal acne or phthisic acne. Broadly put, vaccinial acne yields to *Thuja occidentalis, Sabina* and *Cupressus*, also to *Silicea* and *Maland* : acne from masturbation, to *Bellis perennis*; phthisic acne, to *Bacillinum*; when the acne is very pronouncedly pustular and scarring, to *Vaccinin.* and *Variolinum*; and arthritic acne calls for *hippuric acid, hippurate of Sodium* and *Urea*. The study of the varieties of acne is highly interesting and instructive, as almost all the great constitutional ancestral diseases show themselves in young persons in the form of acne. Not frequently cases of acne are of mixed pathological qualities, and these need *all* their pathologic *simillima* : Remedies only morphologically homoeopathic to the acne-form only palliate; to really and radically cure they must be *pathologically* similar. What a vast vista! (IX 171)

### Aconite

*Aconitum napellus* is, probably, the most frequently indicated remedy in the scientific treatment of neuralgia. This is as well known in homoeopathic practice as the fact that woollen socks tend to keep one's feet warm. But some people who wear woollen socks have nevertheless cold feet, and in like manner a good many persons with neuralgia have taken *Aconite* and still kept their neuralgia. There is no such a thing as a panacea or specific for all sorts of neuralgia, a sure proof that there is neuralgia and neuralgia, or, in other words, every neuralgia has a pathology of its own. (XIV 3)

Had the homoeopaths done nothing in practical medicine but fix and precisionize the use of *Aconitum* in inflammations and fevers of the inflammatory kind, they would have well merited the undying gratitude of the whole human race. That the use of *Aconite* is thus by them fixed with scientific precision is a matter of common knowledge, and needs no further insisting upon, for "we do not drink our *Aconite* out of a Wilksian mug". (XII 7)

## Acorn Water

With a few people, particularly with those who have suffered from old spleen engorgements, diarrhoea sets in after using it for two or three weeks that makes them feel better. It seldom lasts more than a day, and it is not weakening, but moderate. Hence it is not needful either to stop the acorn-water, or to lessen the dose. (X 49)

## Aurum

In reference to the subject of this little volume Hahnemann says, "*Das Gold hat grosse, unersetzliche Arzneikraefte*" ("Gold has great remedial virtues, the place of which no other drug can supply"); and having myself used it in practice for several years, I have come to regard it in the same light : *I cannot do without it*. To my mind there are varieties of disease that *Gold* and *Gold only*, will *cure*, and others that Gold, and Gold only, will alleviate *to the full extent of the possible*; and not a few of these varieties of disease are of the gravest nature. As a heart-remedy alone it claims the most earnest attention of every medical man.

In homoeopathic practice it is neglected, and in allopathic practice it is practically unknown.

I claim for the following pages only that they constitute a rough Introduction to the Study of Gold as a Remedy in Disease. (II Preface (V))

Beginning with the sensorium, we note how some became *depressed in spirits, plaintive, tearful, melancholy, desirous of death, suicidal, restless, anxious,* and some *timid, irritable, disagreeble, getting into quite a rage at the least contradiction, and wanting to quarrel and going into violent passions.* In some the opposite state of *great hilarity* is noted : and in others *the two states alternate.*

One *sits moping in a corner,* desirous of being left alone, another is *all vivacity,* and has a lively word for everybody.

In some *the memory* is rendered very *acute,* while in *others it becomes almost annihilated.*

Not only does Gold thus affect the brain, but it is a great disturber of the cranial circulation; there are *rushes of blood to the head and brain, headache, giddiness* and *hammering,* and *rustling noises in the head.*

And not only are the contents of the skull thus so materially disturbed in their states and functions, but the bony shell itself is profoundly affected in its life and being, as witness the *pains in the bones of the head,with tenderness on pressure, and the bony lumps to be felt under the hairy scalp.*

The *eyes,* too, are *powerfully* and *painfully* affected, and in one observer the *pupils* were at *first contracted* and *then dilated,* while the vision of another is interfered with; *"he sees indistinctly"*, and there is even *total loss of vision for a moment*; and finally Dr. Hermann is so affected that he sees *only with the lower half of his eyes, as if they were covered superiorly with something black* (see the eye cases later on), and then again he *cannot see anything distinctly, as everything seems double,* and thus objects get jumbled together.

There is a pustular *eruption on the face, neck, and chest,* the *parotid* and *submaxillary glands swell* and *are painful*; the *bones* of the *face* and *nose* are *tender* and *painful,* while the *wings of the nose* are *sore* and *inflamed,* and there is a *sore within them that scabs over.*

The *teeth pain* and are loose, the *gums are sore,* and *so is the throat*; there is an *offensive smell from the mouth* (one of the earliest uses of Gold was to correct foul *breath*), with *a good deal of saliva in the mouth* (the muriate produces inodorous (?) salivation).

The digestive tract is irritated and disturbed throughout; *uneasiness in the stomach,* amounting at times to a *sense of weight, pain or swelling; stitches in the sides; nausea; retching; griping; colic; flatulence; flatulent colic; weight in the abdomen, with icy cold hands and feet; pressing in the right inguinal ring as if a hernia would protrude, an inguinal hernia protrudes with great pain; distention of the bowels with rumbling within; constipation, flatus, diarrhoea; stitches, burning and swelling of anal end of rectum*; in fact, the whole of the intestinal tube is irritated and fretted till it writhes and wriggles, protruding at the inguinal ring, and voiding its contents.

Nor are the kidneys exempt; there *is constant desire to micturate, the urine is like butter-milk, and more fluid is passed than is drunk* (its use in dropsy is very ancient).

The genital sphere is powerfully moved (in these experiments all adult males); a *long dormant appetite is roused in one*, and *generally great orgasm of the parts*, with *all* the known phenomena that *result therefrom*. Their various anatomical parts are fretted; stitches in the urethra and glans, with escape of prostatic secretion; the scrotum itches, the *right testis pains* as if bruised in one observer, and in *another observer the same organ becomes a tumid mass with pressive pain when touched or rubbed against from 6 to 11 p.m.*

Going back now to the respiratory sphere, we note *all the symptoms of a running cold in the head*, and then *congestion and catarrh* of the *entire bronchial lining with the dry and humid stages and cough with dyspnoea and constriction of the thorax, or just the opposite* - viz., unusual freedom of breathing.

The symptoms of cardiac asthma are thus and in the following well depicted : *extreme tightness of the chest with difficult breathing at varying times, great weight on the chest, especially a heavy weight in the sternum*. This latter symptom points to *angina pectoris*, in which I have used it with marked success.

In view of its ancient reputation as a cordial, the cardiac symptoms have a great interest. We read further : *In walking, the heart seems to shake about as if it were loose; at times a single thump of the heart; palpitation of the heart; violent palpitation of the heart; a kind of restless anxiety, arising in the region of the heart, and driving him from one place to another, so that he cannot stay anywhere.*

There are various *tearing stitch-like pains about the body*, and the *spine pained* a prover so much one morning that he *could not move hand or foot*.

There are *tearing pains in nearly all the joints*, and the *muscular system is considerably affected*, so also the *bones*.

There are *wheals in the skin of the lower extremities like nettle-rash that itch, are made worse by rubbing, and are worse out of doors.*

*There is a weary, tired pain in the head and in all the joints in the morning in bed that motion ameliorates.*

*The arms and legs are numb and asleep in the morning on awaking*. (I have cured this symptom, occuring in a middle-aged man, with Gold.)

There is *great liability to catch cold and great sensitiveness of the whole body to all kinds of pain, so that the very thought of pain is almost the pain itself.*

There is a good deal of *wakefulness by day and restlessness by night with bad dreams; "he often awakes in the night in a fright"; "he moans in his sleep"*.

*Chilliness and rigors are very prominent symptoms : "cold hands and feet", "cold down the back", "cold in the whole body", "shivers with cold", shudders with cold in bed", "cannot get warm all night", "in the evening feverish chilliness over the whole body with a bad cold in the head, but not followed by fever or thirst".*

Symptom 440 in Hahnemann is "morning perspiration all over".

This gives a rough outline of the effect of Gold on the healthy human economy. (II 33)

Hahnemann's own idea would seem to be that the pure metal is to be preferred on account of its noble simplicity and superior merits. At first he used the muriate because of its solubility, being influenced by the current literature of the time on the subject, and by those authors who affirm that metallic Gold is totally useless as a medicine because of its insolubility; but then finding that a whole series of Arabian physicians had successively used *finely-powdered Gold*, beginning as far back as the eighth century, and since when *Geber* (*de Alchimia traditio*, 1698) praised powdered Gold as a *"Materia laetificans et in juventute corpus conservans,* : and probably being acquainted with M. Chrestien's works, he set about powdering some for himself, and then proved it on the healthy as we have seen. Hereafter he tells us he only made use of the pure powdered metal, therein following the example of the Arabian physicians. Legrand arrives at the same conclusion — viz., that the powdered metal is the best form of administration.

But the salts of Gold are Gold and something else, still their chief effects justify us in considering them, for practical purposes, as Gold; moreover, they seem to give us a deeper insight into the action of the metal on the economy, though possibly only because they have been experimented with, to the neglect or exclusion of the triturated metal. (II 44)

## Proving of Aurum Foliatum

To get a really concrete conception of what a given drug can do, there is nothing equal to *trying it on your body*. As I, in this, practise what I preach, I made the following short proving on myself.

**Jan. 27th, 1879.** In my usual health and spirits. 12.15 p.m. Take four grains of *Aurum foliatum,* first decimal trituration, dry on the tongue. This sample was most carefully triturated for a long time. My object in making use of the 1x tritutration was to see if our *lowest* trituration had any power. **3 p.m.** While returning from St. Martin's-le-Grand I felt *intolerable itching in the right groin in its inner third,* and here was realised the old proverb, *Ubi dolor, ibi digitus,* the street and the public notwithstanding. **4 p.m.** Having returned, an inspection shows a wheal, now become tender from the violent rubbing that has been carried on every few minutes for the past hour. **5 p.m.** The wheal is gone, but the part remains tender.

**28th.** Sensations in joints and muscles, like one has after unwonted exercise. Feel very strong, with plenty of go in me. Going upstairs I involuntarily take two steps at a time, and run in and out of patients' houses instead of walking. Clearly this is the *primary* action of the Gold; its *first action* as an *excitant and as an exhilarant*. When will the reaction come, and how great will be the recoil?

**29th**. Evening. Proctostasis these twenty-four hours, which is most unusual with me and clearly drug-effect. Renal secretion much less in quantity; feel well.

**30th**. Normal. 11.30 a.m. Take four grains of *Aurum foliatum*, 1x trituration, dry on the tongue. Evening. Very wakeful; well up to work; great mental activity; testes a little swelled and hard.

**31st**. Last night erotic dreams; early in the morning in bed weary pain in right torsal bones, shooting up towards the knee. Pains in the bones of skull soon passing off. Astringent metallic taste in mouth; tongue slightly coated with brownish fur.

**Feb. 4th**. In the groove between nose and cheek a cutaneous lump of the size of a split pea; it irritates, gets picked, scabs over and persists. Feel *not* upto the mark; very depressed and low-spirited; nothing seems worthwhile. After proving *Cundurango* several years since, a small wart on my chest increased in size, and it has continued to grow ever since and is now about the size of a split horse-bean, with irregular hill-and-dale surface; it is beginning to lap over and to catch things. Since commencing the *Aurum* it seems a little flatter. The last two nights I have dreamed a great deal of death. 2 p.m. Take four grains of *Aurum foliatum*, 1x trituration, dry on the tongue. Evening. Am unusually wakeful; am told that I look pale.

**5th**. Dreamy towards morning; am repeatedly told that I look pale and worn; have a dazed feeling in the head.

**6th**. Feel ill; look pale; have pain at the lower part of spine; have had bad nights, dreaming of the dead and of corpses. Take four grains of *Aur. fol.* 1x as before. Evening. Feel fagged, but yet not able to sleep. Feel quite out of sorts. For many days great morbid activity of uro-poetic system; sleep does not refresh; dreams of the dead and of dead bodies. Uncomfortable feeling in forehead; pain at the bottom of spine.

**7th.** Look and feel ill, and although weary, no inclination for either rest or sleep. Having thus taken one grain and six-tenths of metallic Gold. I am thoroughly satisfied that it can make *me* ill. My allopathic brethren maintain that the metal Gold is *inert*! *Sure proof* they have never tried it, properly triturated, on their own bodies. *Fiat experimentum in corporibus vilibus homoeopathicorum*, say they, perhaps. I desist from taking any more of the Aurum as I feel so out of sorts, and my memory is so sharp that I fear the secondary effect in this direction might be serious.

**March 25th**. Still have some pain at the bottom of the spine; the last week or two my memory has been very bad indeed, and I am low-spirited. The before-mentioned wart is flatter and certainly much smaller.

**April 16th**. Memory a little less clouded; still a little pain at the bottom of back occasionally; the wart is nearly gone.

**30th.** Memory getting good again; the wart seems again slightly on the increase. (II 61)

The implantation of the syphilitic virus upon a scrofulous constitution is one of the most intractable of all morbid manifestations, and but few medicines will touch it at all. Gold does. This condition I would term *Psoro-Syphilis*, or *Scrofulo-syphilis*, if I may be allowed to coin an expression to serve the purpose of this paper — viz., to elucidate the curative range of this remedy in this unhappy marriage of two vile constitutional taints. (II 98)

It may be objected that as the use of Gold in dropsy is almost as old as the hills, it cannot be claimed for Homoeopathy. To this I would reply, Gold will only really cure it if homoeopathically indicated; that having a proving of the drug from the hands of that wondrous worker Hahnemann, we have means by which we can *differentiate*, and thus we are enabled to prescribe scientifically. (II 104)

For Gold is no mere function disturber, but a producer of organic change, and hence its brilliant effects in organic mishcief. The vascular turgescence of *Belladonna* and that of *Aurum* are very different affairs. (II 127)

Gold will not make an old organism young, but it will do an old organism good, and, *pro tanto*, it rejuvenates. (II 131)

Now the "other facts" show that *Aurum* affects the brain much more than it does the liver, and quite as much as it does the testes. Hypochondriasis lodged of old in the liver free of rent; it has been many times ejected, and formally located for some time in the testes; latterly it has been a homeless waif. It is satisfactory to learn that its ancient vested rights of domicile are respected. That comes of our living under the reign of law.

***Query*** : Does hypochondriasis ever sit in the ovaries? or in the Ligamenta lata? (II 136)

**Gold in the Treatment of Pining Boys.** Not infrequently one is consulted about the non-thriving, pining condition of boys; they are low-spirited, lifeless; their memories are bad; they are not up to the mark, and are lacking altogether in boyish go; the tongue is commonly coated at the back, and the appetite for plain food is bad. They are the despised ones at cricket and football, and at school they are not wanting in taste for books, but still they take no position in their forms. "I do not know what it is, but he does not seem to get on". These boys are not necessarily vicious or given to naughty habits, but they are maudlin and unmanly fellows.

Examine the testes, and you will find them mere pendent shreds; just on the verge of atrophy.

A short course of *Aurum foliatum*, 3rd trituration, four or five grains three times a day, seems to act like magic on them; they brighten up, eat, work, play, and sleep like boys should; and their comrades begin to take some account of them in the playground and cricket-field. They become altogether more manly, and spend less time over their books, and yet take better places in their classes. Now look again at the before-mentioned glands, and you will find them larger, firm, and well suspended. (II 137)

## Aurum and Mercury

All authorities agree that Gold is chemically cousin-german to mercury; a comparison of their pathogeneses reveals the fact that they are no less so physiologically. (II 140)

## Bacae Juniperi

These berries are a good spleen medicine which I have often ordered for the poor, and sometimes with good effect. The berries must be crushed, and a handful left a long time to draw in four cupfuls of boiling water if you want to see any effect from them. I do not think it is the aethereal oil, but a non-volatile principle of the berries, that acts as a splenic. (X 51)

## Bacillinum

Now I maintain that, taken early, we have in *Bacillinum* a real remedy for phthisis pulmonalis, and for a considerable number of otherwise incurable forms of tuberculosis; and eight years ' experience backs up this affirmation, and Father Time will confirm it. (XVI A PREFACE IV)
Homoeopathy is the winning horse at the Medical Derby of the world, and will presently be hurried past the winning post by Orthodoxy itself as her rider.
And what effect has the past year's experience had upon my own views as to the therapeutic efficacy of Bacillinum? Simply to confirm them : my *"Five Years'* Experience in the New Cure of Consumption" has simply become six; and having enlarged my clinical borders by this additional year's experience, I have only to add that I have nothing to take from my first edition — the further year's observation having fully confirmed the views therein set forth. (XVI A Preface VIII)
In regard to the accumulation of tartar on the teeth, already in my own first proving of *Bacillin.*, I thereafter noticed the falling-off of two or three cakes of tartar from my lower incisors (never before or since); and in many of

my published cases this curious influence of *Bacillin.* has been noticed. (XXII 36)

The best way to get some really good *Bacillinum* (if any one wishes to prepare it) is to take a portion of the lung of an individual who had died of genuine bacillary tuberculosis pulmonum, choosing a good-sized portion from the parietes of a cavity and its circumjacent tissue as herein will be found *everything* pertaining to the tuberculous process — bacilli, debris, ptomanes and tubercles in all stages (such was practically the origin of the matrix of my *Bacillinum*) and prepared by trituration in spirit. In this way nothing is lost. There is, moreover, nothing disgusting in this, which can hardly be said of sputal tuberculinum — one instinctively shrinks from it. Finally, this mode of obtaining our *Bacillinum* will result in our having a fairly constant preparation, and one which will meet all paractical requirements in the present imperfect state of our knowledge. No doubt in the future we shall have elaborate and scientifically-accurate investigations into the characters and qualities of the various bodies that our *Bacillinum* no doubt contains; but we who live now must use the means at our disposal, we cannot let our patients die because we have not now the hypothetically perfect pathologico-pharmaceutical preparations which it is permissible to believe our more favoured aftercomers will possesss; we must work with such tools as we have, and our *Bacillinum* is beyond any question the grandest anti-consumptive remedy the world now knows, and is likely to be for long years to come. (XVI A 139)

## Bacillinum and Clarke

As this little treatise was going to press, I wrote to my friend, Dr. John H.Clarke, the able Editor of the *Homoeopathic World*, to ask him to give my readers the benefit of his experience with the remedy herein recommended, and he replies as follows :

*"30 Claridges Street,*
*London, W."*

"I began to use Bacillin, and the same time I proved it on myself, taking (on December 20, 1890) just the thirtieth, and afterwards the one-hundredth potency. The chief symptoms I experienced were the following :

1. Pain in glands of neck, worse on turning the head or stretching the neck. Right side more affected.
2. Pain deep in head, worse on shaking the head.

3. Aching in teeth, especially lower incisors (all sound). This was felt at the roots, especially on raising the lower lip; the symptoms persisted many months, and I occasionally feel it now. Teeth very sensitive to cold air.
4. Sharp pains of short duration in chest and various parts of body.
5. Pain in left knee whilst walking one evening; passed off after perservering in walking for a short distance.
6. Nasal Catarrh. Pricking in throat (larynx), with sudden cough. Single cough on rising from bed in the morning. Cough waking me in the night. Easy expectoration. Sharp pain in precordial region, arresting breathing. Very sharp pain in left scapula, worse lying down in bed at night, relieved by warmth.
7. An indolent angry pimple on left cheek. This persisted many weeks, and I began to fear it was something worse. After it had once healed it broke out several times at long intervals and even still a slight indentation can be felt at the spot. (XVI A 277)

"I will only add to the above record that I have not found anything to antidote the effects of *Bacillin*, and that I have often given remedies to patients under the influence of it without, apparently, any interference in the acton of either, and further, I have not been able to discover any difference in the action of *Bacillin* made by Dr. Heath and Koch's *Tuberculin* in homoeopathic attenuation; and I should judge that the pathogenesis of Koch's *Tuberculin* collected by me in the '*Homoeopathic World*', vol. xxvi., 1891 would be applicable as indications for the use of either.

*Yours ever,*

*John H. Clarke*

(XVI A 312)

## Bacillinum and Constitutions

Of course, it is not suggested that Bacillinum is a specific for all cases of phthisis, of every kind, and necessarily it will do no good in those cases of phthisis to which it is not homoeopathic; something that will cure every case of any malady bearing a given name is, of course, non-existent.

Still, bacillary phthisis taken early, and complicated with nothing else, is curable by *Bacillinum*, and this I say after eight year's experience at the bedside and in the consulting-room. anything even approaching to it in therapeutic efficacy is thus far absolutely unknown.

Where, for instance, vaccinosis is also present, the vaccinosis must be first cured or the phthisis remains uncured, do what you will.
When there is a primary spleen affection that led up to the phthisis, such a case must be approached from the spleen as starting-point, or the treatment fails. When a liver disease underlies the whole maladive state, and phthisis only coexists with it, the liver malady must be first cured.
When this state arises from an hereditary syphilitic *taint* (I say *taint*, not the disease proper), the specific nosode may be required first.
When the phthisis arises from a cancerous parentage, *Bacillinum* alone will not always suffice, until other remedies have prepared the way.
When the constitution has been damaged by typhoid, by malarialism, by alchololism, by cinchonism, and so on, all these must be therapeutically reckoned with, or success will not reward our efforts. Wherever, in fact, phthisis coexists with other diseases, or taints of diseases, the *Bacillinum touches the bacillary part of the case ONLY.*
When phthisis supervenes upon overcrowding, conventicular or monastic life, excesses of the various kinds, bad food, foul air, chronic sewage poisonings, wounded pride, unrequited love, bad drinking water, active oft-renewed infection from marital or other domestic ties, or from the air, walls, beddings, etc., it wil be in vain to expect the simple administration of a remedy of any kind to cure unaidedly if the active cause still remains present and operative. (XVI A 199)

## Bacillinum and Consumption

But consumption is the ever-present enemy, and I presently formulated to my mind the proposition that there must be some means of finding out whether the virus of consumption could cure consumption or not. I determined to try some of it upon myself, — I not being in consumption. I took it in varying doses at various times, the 30, C., C.C., in the form of pilules. (XVI A 16)

**Effects of the Poison of Consumption upon Myself.** One effect was constant, viz., a severe headache, worse the day after taking the poison, and lasting on till the third day. This headache I felt every time I took it; I fancied the headache from the thirtieth was much worse than from the hundreth. The kind of headache I could only describe as far in, and complelling quiet fixedness. The Headaches recurred from time to time for many weeks.
The next constant effect upon me was expectoration of non-viscid, very easily detached, thick phlegm from the air-passages, followed after a day

or two by a very clear ring of the voice. The third effect was not quite constant, viz., windy dyspepsia and pinching pains under the ribs of the right side in the mammary line. And, finally, disturbed sleep — distressful. There was a little cough on three occasions, but only very slight, and only just enough to raise the phlegm, which came so easily that one might almost say it came of itself. (XVI A 16)

The idea that the remedy of a disease may lie in itself reaches back to the youth of the world. Moses' lifting up the serpent in the wilderness is a symbolic similitude; "take a hair of the dog that bit you" almost formulates a doctrine. The homoeopathic conception can hardly be separated from the idea of curing the disease by a bit of itself, for the simple reason, that if you alter somewhat two things that are identically the same you reduce identity to similarity.

When I speak of consumption or phthisis, I mean the real tubercular disease, the genuine more or less infectious consumption, whether it is of the lungs, brain or whatsoever other part. (XVI A 20)

## Bacillinum and Ringworm

In the first edition I communicated the important fact — many smaller things are called great discoveries — that ringworm yields readily to *Bacillinum*, and that I therefore regard this cutaneous eruption as a tubercular manifestation. (XVI A 161)

## Bacillinum and Thuja

I am here and there struck with the fact that, for instance, *Bacillinum*. will not act till *Thuja* has been given and then it will act beautifully : the vaccinosis evidently barring the way, much as Hahnemann teaches in regard to psora and the use of *Sulphur* intercurrently. (XX 281)

## Bacillinum and Tuberculinum

The difference between our old friend *Tuberculinum* or *Bacillinum* and that of Koch lies in the way it is obtained; ours is the virus of the natural disease itself, while Koch's is the same virus artificially obtained in an incubator from colonies of bacilli thriving in beef jelly; ours is the chick hatched under the hen, Koch's is the chick hatched in an incubator. The artificial hatching is Koch's discovery, not the remedy itself or its use as a cure for consumption.

I think very highly of Koch's remedy, as the world will no doubt call it, and I know that he is on the right track. I am more sure than Koch can be himself, because I used it five years before he knew it, and he has yet to prove that his results are satisfactory. There is one other difference, i.e., the mode of administering it to the patient; I use the remedy in high potency, which is not fraught with the palpable dangers of Koch's method of injecting material quantities under the skin, or, in other words, straight into the blood. Of course, if Dr. Koch's dosage and mode of administration should give better results than we have obtained, then Koch's method will have to be adopted. But my present opinion tends to the opposite conclusion. Still we will leave that till Koch's method has been properly tried. Meanwhile, here is my own. (XVI A Preface XIII)

Who first used the word *Tuberculinum* I do not know; I believe it was Dr. Swan of New York; I had it from Dr. Skinner of London some sixteen or seventeen years ago; but the mode of obtaining it I felt to be altogether too nasty, though the *two hundredth* dilution of any thing whatsoever — even of original sin — is at least — clean ! I believe Dr. Swan is under the impression that he was the first to use and recommend the use of phthisical sputum — his tuberculinum. But in this he is in error; the thing has been done time and again, and records of the practice exist. This, however, does not lessen Dr. Swan's credit; though I presume Dr. Swan had his first ideas from Lux through Constantine Hering. Paracelsus is full of both Homoeopathy and isopathy as I long ago pointed out, and the fact that Hahnemann never quoted from Paracelsus is not to his credit, for he must have read him (XVI A 132)

## Bacillinum — Its Sphere

As to the use of the other remedies, I would specially insist upon the fact that the phthisic virus only acts *within its own sphere*, and that this sphere is very *sharply defined* as to time, and what it does not do soon and promptly it does not do at all. Its action is, if I may so express myself, *acute* : its chronic equivalent is *Psorinum*.

*Second Edition* : When I say *soon* I mean its action *begins* at once — only, of course, as phthisic process are generally chronic, the treatment thereof must also be the same, i.e. chronic. (XVI A 40)

This is quite in accordance with my other experience, when the consumptive process is in full blaze the virus is unavailing. (XVI A 79)

## Bacillinum — Parenteral and Low Dilutions

Phthisis and the tubercular diseases generally have definitely entered the list of medicable diseases. But finally, and for the last time, the remedy must *not* be administered by injection; it must be given in high, higher and highest potencies and the doses must be FAR APART.

To those who can use only low dilutions, I solemnly say . . . Hands off! (XVI A 195)

## Badiaga

What struck me was the enormous number of freckles on his face, and as I had a few times succeeded in ameliorating that condition with *Badiaga*, I put the patient on that remedy for two months. (XXII 59)

## Bellis Perennis

The effects of *Bellis* (common daisy) in this state, that I think of as *autotraumatism*, is often little short of marvellous. (VI 129)

The peculiarity of his insomnia was that he awoke in the very early morning and could not get off again. I have before explained that this symptom is characteristic of *Bellis perennis*. (XVI A 181)

***Bellis perennis* in the Inconveniences of Pregnancy.** It happens to some ladies when they are *enceintes* that they find it very inconvenient to get about, walking being very irksome and almost impossible. In such cases the Daisy soon sets matters right.

Why did I give *Bellis* in such a case? Merely because the inconvenience complained of was due to mecahnical pressure : the tissues were pressed upon, and therefore in a condition precisely like that of a bruise — hence I gave my old friend the Daisy — bruisewort; i.e., it acts upon the muscular fibres of the blood-vessels and upon the tissues, and thus clears the line of these mechanical obstructions. (XXIII 100)

*Bellis per.* is our common daisy; it acts very much like *Arnica*, even to the contingent production of erysipelas; it causes pain in the spleen, and generally symptoms of coryza, and of feeling very tired, person (the writer) wanting to lie down, it acts on exudates, swellings and stasis, and hence in a fagged womb its action is very satisfactory; indeed, in the discomforts of pregnancy and of varicose veins patients are commonly loud in its praise. In the *giddiness* of elderly people (cerebral stasis) it acts well and does permanent good; likewise and particularly in fag from masturbation, in old workmen, labourers, and the overworked and fagged, it is a princely remedy. In the head-sufferings of elderly working gardeners its action is very pretty. Its action in the ill-effects from taking cold drinks when one is hot is now well-known. It is a grand friend to commercial travellers, and in railway spine of moderate severity it has not any equal so far as my knowledge reaches. I think *stasis* lies at the bottom of all these ailings.

When given at night *Bellis* is very apt to cause the patient to wake up very early in the morning, hence I order it by preference to be taken not too late in the day. I have often cured with it the symptom "wakes up too early in the morning and cannot get off again," and here the higher dilutions act much more decidedly and lastingly as a rule and without any side-effects, for here the action is purely homoeopathic and not simply deobstruent. (XXIV 49)

I regard this peculiar property of the Daisy (i.e. for ill-effects of sudden wet chill to heated stomach or body surface) as eminently important, and ask all who may read this to make it known, so that it may be available for such as travellers, tourists, harvesters, soldiers on the march, when they, being heated, have had a cold ducking, or have drunk cold liquids.

I would recommend it also in the acute and chronic dyspepsia from eating cold ices, as the conditions here are indentical, for I have, in such cases, found it an eminent curative agent. (IX 115)

**Traumatic Swelling of Right Breast Cured by *Bellis* Alone.** I adduce the following case (Case 211, Part III) of a swelling in a young lady's breast, rather to exemplify in a neat way the curative range of the DAISY in the treatment of tumours.

No experienced practitioner will deny the important part played by bruises, blows, and falls, in the genesis of tumours and cancer; and hence our anti-traumatics ought to figure much more largely in our therapeutics of growths from blows. Before giving my case I will quote a very instructive note on this very question that appeared as leader in the first volume of the *Homoeopathic Recorder* (Philadelphia), No. 4, 1886.

**Malignant Growths.** "In the preceding number of *The Recorder* there appeared three items concerning malignant growths, which deserve more than passing notice. One is the history of the development of a malignant formation as the result of the frequent mechanical irritation of a simple mole on the face, another recounted the cure of an extensive sarcomatous growth by an intercurrent attack of erysipelas, and the third contained the analysis of a series of cases of carcinoma in all of which there was antecedent injury by mechanical or chemical means; in the latter selection the writer asks in all seriousness : Is cancer, whatever its form, ever primary — i.e.,does it ever originate without previous injury ?

A negative reply to this inquiry is of the highest importance to those who believe in the curative effects of drugs. It deprives the disease-action of part of the mysterious, fateful quality so constantly associated in our minds with these affections, and which terrorizes to some degree the powers of the medical attendant. For we hold that the great majority of physicians, on discovering the existence of a suspicious growth, are strongly impelled to advise the use of the knife as the only sure treatment, nowtithstanding that in cases of undoubted malignancy the value of surgical interference is greatly lessened by the relatively poor results as measured by the added years given to the patient.

Moreover, if the occurrence of an infectious inflammation of the skin has destroyed malignant disease-process in that issue, there is a fairly good basis for the view, reasoning by analogy, that a drug-disease — i.e. a disease produced by the action of a medicine — can, if affecting a part involved in the malignant process, cause similarly efficacious results.

A thorough study of the symptoms of each individual case, with the view of finding the exact simillimum, the exhibition of the latter in different attenuations, if necessary, changing the remedy only when a change of symptoms demands it, and extreme watchfulness of involvement of the neighbouring glandular structures, make up, it appears to us, the duty of the physician.

Whether he would be justified in holding out any hope of cure by internal medication after evidences of systemic infection exist, must be decided by his own experience; but, as there are always cases in which operation is inadmissible, or in which it will not be allowed, opportunities will not be wanting to continue treatment with the properly chosen remedy. (XI 60)

## Brassica Murialis

I have found the *Brassica murialis*, which Dr. Heath tells me should be called *Diplotaxis tenuifolia*, of good service in the lazy livers of relaxing climates, when patients feel as if they could scarcely crawl about from sheer goneness. It is homoeopathic to such, as I know from a fragmentary proving made by myself in 1874 (XVII 93)

## Bursa Pastoris

In my judgement, as I have elsewhere stated, the Shepherd's Purse is pronouncedly a uterine medicine. It is a very notable remedy in uterine sterility — pregnancy frequently occurring during its use. A gentlemen was under my professional care for frequent nocturnal micturition of a gouty character, and I ordered him *Bursa pastoris* Q, ten drops in water at bedtime. On April 8th he wrote me that he could not take such a large dose, as it caused him '"aching and fulness in the head, worse in the morning. " At my request he resumed the medicine (Bursa) in four-drop doses.

June 10th — On this day he brought the medicine back himself to me in the original halfounce bottle, still two-thirds full of the tincture, complaining very much of its "nasty rotten drains smell," and saying he could not take any more of it, for, says he, "it *flushes* my face so much that I cannot take it; I only took three drops this morning, and just see how it has flushed my face."

This symptom being pathogenetic, we thus get another remedy for the flushes, and it would be additionallly indicated in gouty individuals, for *Bursa pastoris* often produces a notable output of gravel. (XXIV 32)

## Calendula

The two symptoms, "chilly hands" and "easily frightened," taken together and in conjunction with liver troubles, would seem to call for Calendula. (XVII 227)

## Carduus

The kind of liver enlargement which *Carduus* cures is in the transverse measurement (XVII 58)

Rademacher first learned its use and never ceased to prize it, notably in blood spitting from liver and spleen engorgements. No remedy, he declares, in our whole drug store can compare to *Carduus* when there are stitches in the side with bloody expectoration. He recommends his readers to note well where the last trace of pain is felt as it dies away, as that is likely to be the primary seat of the real disease. (XVII 74)

Nevertheless, when people's skins are in unhealthy state they commonly treat the skin, or go to a skin doctor who is pretty sure to regard his speciality as the first, and treats the skin, generally *d'en face*, with washes and ointments and the like.(XVII 109)

Riel's proving of *Carduus* shews it to produce pathogenetically : "nausea, uneasiness, pain, vomiting, with inflation of the abdomen etc." (XVII 57)

## Ceanothus

During last summer and this winter I made several provings of *Ceanothus*. To my surprise the first symptoms noticed was a sticking pain in the spleen, and after the continued use of the remedy, there was quite an enlargement of that organ, worse by motion, but at the same time unable to lie on the left side; following this there was pain in the liver, a congestion and enlargement, with sticking pains worse by motion or touch.

"Pain in lumbar region, with a desire to urinate.

"The prover for several days and nights was unable to get any rest, owing to these aggravating pains in the sides; when lying on left side the pain in the spleen was so great I could not lie still, and upon turning over I experienced the same difficulty on opposite side. At this time the urine had a green color, bile being found in the urine, urine frothy, traces of sugar with an alkaline reaction, sp. gr. 1030.

"Pain and weak sensation in umbilical region. A generally weak sensation. Pain and soreness in muscles on exterior part of thighs noticed in every prover.

"Tongue coated in the centre with a dirty white coating. Loss of appetite. Loss of flesh was noted in one prover, with general weakness, and paleness of face.

"Stools become clay-colored, showing an action on the liver.

"One prover who had malaria several years ago developed a beautiful case after a somewhat prolonged use of the drug.

Every physician using *Ceanothus* in splenitis following malarial fever knows full well its wonderful action. Where the spleen is affected from any cause, with enlargement, deep sticking pains, worse by motion, but at the same time unable to lie on leftside, the case will generally yield quickly to *Ceanothus*.

"I have at the present time a case of pernicious anaemia, accompanied by spleen pains, rapidly improving from the use of *Ceanothus*.

"I would suggest the remedy in question for leukaemia, pseudo-leukaemia, splenic anaemia, and Hodgkin's disease. Also, for the so-called bilious attacks, the patient having a dirty white coating on tongue, pain in liver and spleen, with or without clay-coloured stools, possibly with pains in umbilical region, and with it all a general tired feeling.

"When this drug becomes thoroughly known it no doubt will be a great remedy for malaria and its effects" — *Medical Century*. (X 68)

**Ceanothus in Consentaneous Heart Disease.** Where the heart is perturbed consentaneously with a spleen affection, the relief obtained from the use of *Ceanothus* (and other splenics) is often very noteworthy.

The number of cases of spleen affections commonly reported as cardiac is considerable. And even in cases where the heart is really at fault, the easing of the spleen region by splenics is often a great help to the comfort of the heart. (X 71)

## Cedron

To *Cedron* I was led because patient complained very much of coldness in the abdomen : "Oh, my stomach is so cold." (XXIII 19)

## Chelidonium, Myrica Cerifera and Hydrastis

I would, however, just dwell upon the fact that *Chelidonium* will very frequently cure engorgements of the right lung even when it is a concomitant of true phthsis, but it has no influence over the general phthisical state, other than what pertains to, and results from, the lower half of the right lung and liver. As an intercurrent remedy in the hepatic complication of phthisis it is capable of rendering important service.

Likewise as an intercurrent remedy in gall-stones it is useful, as is also *Myrica cerifera*, but both stand far behind *Hydrastis* in this affection. (XVII 48)

## Cholesterine

Ameke claimed to have derived much advantage from its use in *cancer of the liver*. This is a weighty statement, and is *true*. I believe I have twice cured cancer of the liver with it; and in obstinate hepatic engorgements that, by reason of their obstinacy, make one think interrogatively of cancer, the effects of *Cholesterine* are very satisfactory; at times even striking.

I commonly use the 3x trit. in six-grain doses three times a day, but this will here and there act very violently, and when this happened I have found the third centesimal trituration effective. (XVII 119)

*Cholesterine* is my sheet-anchor in organic liver disease in which the commoner hepatics — *Chelid.,Carduus,Myrica,Kalibich., Merc.,* and *Diplotaxis tenuifolia* have failed. (XVII 122)

## Chelone Glabra

*Chelone glabra* — I should like to say that its seat of action is the left lobe of the liver and it *line of action* is in the direction of the navel, bladder, and uterus, while the "line of action" of *Carduus* is horizontal from liver to spleen, or conversely. At the first blush this looks fanciful, but the competent can readily verify it clinically. (VI 11)

From this (treatment of enormous vortex in the right groin, just on Ponpart's ligament) and similar observations I have laid it down for my own future guidance that the *seat of action* of *Chelone glabra* is the left lobe of the liver and its line of action is in the direction of the navel, bladder and uterus. (XVII 215)

## Colchicum

"Rely upon *Colchicum* in gout and you will get plenty of Ponglet's disease," was the advice to me given by a most clean-headed physician. (XXI 28)

My own suspicions are to the effect that *Colchicum* homoeopathic to some of these external manifestations which it effectively gets rid of, but leaves the uric deposits in the blood and tissues. The outside symptoms are gone, the inside disease remains. (XXI 29)

## Colocynth

Personally, I have an idea that *Colocynth* is an ovary-medicine in the Rademacherian sense. But both Gilchrist and Dunham cured their cases simply by considering the totality of the symptoms, and as these distinguished men cannot do the impossible, it must follow that tumours can be cured symptomatically. Dunham, the gentle scholar, the humble-minded Christian physician, is now in heaven, smiling down encouragement upon us who labour on; may his earth-ward smiles strengthen us in our heavenward strivings. (XX 177)

## Conium Maculatum

The late Professor Gunther, of Duisberg, used to give for chronic cough a powder composed of one grain of *Conium* and ten grains or a scruple of oak mistletoe. He had once cured an old gentleman with it. A colleague of mine, an out-and-out sceptic, who had in vain patched away at the old gentleman, did not deny the cure, but ascribed it to chance, to the particular faith the patient had in Gunther, and not to the action of the powder. But I could in no wise agree with his opinion, for although I had at the time but very little experience of *Conium*, still I knew Gunther was a sensible physician, who wrote simple prescriptions, and so must have understood the curative action of his medicines. I once met Gunther over a patient, about whom there was little to say, as he was evidently dying. In the course of our conversation, I begged him to tell me what he thought about *Conium*. He was willing, but, being interrupted by the anxious friends of the patient, only gathered that he set great store by it. I had several times easily cured patients of his of liver coughs, and to whom he had in vain given *Conium*, as I saw from the prescriptions of his that they brought with them; from which I concluded that it was not a sure liver remedy. I had before fruitlessly used *Conium* in painful spleen infections, and hence too hastily concluded, because I was still stupid, that it was not a spleen remedy. Now that I had become wiser, and understood that nature could produce different sorts of spleen affections, I began also to see that while *Conium* might be quite useless in one kind of spleen infections, it might nevertheless be remarkably curative in another kind of spleen disease. Thus I once used it in a case of consensual cough arising from a primary spleen disease. This is hard to cure; all the lung medicines do no good. Of the belly medicines, the only one that would occasionally be of any service was the *Semina cardui*. I now put *Conium* to a very severe test, that is to say, I gave it in cases in which the *Cardui Maria Seminu* failed me, and lo and behold I saw the most beautiful and most astonishing curative action from it. Since then I have never given it up, and as I make no unreasonable demands upon it, it has never disappointed me. I stated earlier on that Gunther gave it in combination with oak mistletoe, but there is nothing in that; I have found it just as active with sugar of milk or sweetwood, as when triturated with oak misletoe. (X 52)

## Cundurango

At this period I was myself still suffering from my proving of Cundurango (see British Journal of Homoeopathy, July 1875), and I had repeatedly proved that the crack in the angles of the mouth was a very characteristic symptom of the drug. The pustules and other cutaneous manifestations of this drug are torpid (see the proving in the British Journal of Homoeopathy and the "Symptomatology" in Allen's Encyclopaedia of Pure Materia Medica, Vol. iv.,p.1 et seq.)

1. *Cundurango* produces cracks in the angles of the mouth, and also cures such.
2. *Cundurango* is in my opinion, an antipsoric, and case appeared to be a psoric manifestation from injury.
3. *Cundurango* has beyond any doubt cured cases of cancer, and this seemed such a case.
4. It seemed to me that the ulcer in the angle of the mouth that started as a mere crack — just supplied the phothogenetic differentiation requisite for knowing whether to give *Hydrastis, Conium*, or what not.

Thus *Cundurango* has undoubtedly cured a number of cases of cancer; but we may say the same of *Sulphur, Thuja, Arsenicum, Conium, Hydrastis, Carbo animalis, Bryonia, Bufo*, or *Galium Aparine*, and hence the point to find out is what characterize or species. The greatest characteristic yet observed of our *Cundurango* is the crack in the angle of the mouth, and hence on theoretical grounds we may say that a case of cancer with a manifestation in the angles of the mouth calls for *Cundurango*. (XIII 11)

## Cupressus Lawsoniana

As, however, I am, so far as I am aware, the first and still the only practitioner to use *Cupressus Lawsoniana*, I may be permitted just to state that I base my use of it upon a fragmentary proving made by myself with the berries and leaves, and from which I conclude that it acts very like *Thuja*; I could not go on with my proving because of the terrible pains it caused in the stomach. I shall refer to it again. Finally, it might be asked : Why did you not stick to the *Thuja* rather than folow it up with *Sabina*, and then with *Cupressus*? Because I have found *from practical experience that ringing the changes on like-acting remedies conduces more quickly to a cure than going on with the same*. (XX 125)

## Dental Neuralgias

Many cases of toothache are neuralgic, and require one or more of the already-named remedies, and such others as *Silicea, Nitric acid, Mercurius, Kreosotum, Hecla lava*. Perhaps three-fourths of the cases of toothache are not due either to caries, necrosis, or abscess, primarily, but to the general state of the constitution; more particularly is toothache, in my opinion, very frequently due to the Stomach, and I have sometimes wondered whether decaying teeth are at times anything more than *constitutional issues*, for I have several times noticed that profoundly dyscratic complaints have taken on increased morbid action soon after the dentist had extracted a bad tooth. Particularly in cases of tumours have I noticed this, and for some time I have been in the habit of forbidding any extractrion of bad teeth until the graver malady had been quite cured, when, oddly enough, the teeth commonly *cease from troubling*. I am well aware that the local inflammatory processes of dental, anal, aural, and vaginal pains-neuralgias, as I understand the term — do indeed give rise to the pain, but I hold that the only real cure of the neuralgia — the pain arising from the local morbid process — is the extinguishment of the morbid condition itself that lies at the bottom of the inflammatory, carious, necrotic, or neoplastic process. In neuralgia how true it is that "things are not what they seem." (XIV 81)

## Ferrum Phosphoricum

*Ferrum* is a most likely medicine indeed on theoretical grounds and from analogy; the sixth trituration of the phosphate is very potent in controlling the vascular system, and it simultaneously affects the blood mass. (VI 143)
*Ferrum Phosphoricum* is a most powerful vein medicine, although its action on the arteries is its prime sphere; it has cured a small aneurism in my hands (the sixth centesimal trituration), and a great indication for it is *throbbing*. It is also a beautiful hypnotic, but those who usually sleep well are often kept awake by it. *Kali chloricum* is indicated in congestions, and specially in swarthy subjects. (VI 148)

## Ferrum Phos and Acidum Fluoricum

That *Ferrum phosphoricum* acts brilliantly in the old, and *Acidum fluoricum* in the young, I can vouch for from my own experience. (VI 151)

## Glinicum

*Glinicum* is none other than *Medorrhinum;* then why multiply names? Only because I obtained the matrix of this myself from a typical case, and macerated it myself in spirit of wine, and so I know what it is and how prepared, and any one else can do the same at anytime and anywhere in the whole wide world. Furthermore, we can use the name *Glinicum* just as we use *Met. alb., Verb. sap.*

In simple georgic and bucolic times our weeds no doubt amply suffice for our ailings; but in these polyandrous days, when late marriages are the rule, and gonococcic fluxes are all over the place, we must need go to the source of the disease for its remedy — for *ubi morbus, ibirremedium* is a blessed fact. *Cinchona* does not grow in cold wet places, that's where we find the willow.

My indications for *Glinicum* are : roused in the small hours of the morning by the pain, acidity, coated tongue, filthy taste and breath, uncleanably dirty tongue, weakness, pallor, chilliness, worse from cold wet; and moreover *Glinicum* is largely a left-sided remedy. *Glin.* wipes out half the cases of sciatica that pass my way. What a record ! (XXIV 47)

## Gout Remedies

A very frequently indicated remedy is gold — *Aurum*, either the *Aurum metallicum*, the *Aurum muriaticum*, or the *Aurum muriaticum natronatum*. And this remedy is all the more frequently called for on account of the past history of some of the worst cases of post-arthritic heart affections.

*Strophanthus* — I generally use the first centesimal dilution — helps much, notably where the mischief lies as between and concerning the liver and the right side of the heart.

Where fatty decay is a prominent feature *Phosphrous* does good, but *Vanadium* is here my sheet-anchor — it meets the atheroma of the arteries of brain and liver to a nicety, and thus fills a unique place as being a real remedy of this organic change, and, as an alternate remedy, *Bellis perennis* is a princely medicine. *Vanadium* 5 and *Bellis* Q *month apart* (with an intercurrent hepatic or two) have in my hands, time and again, restored veritable physical wrecks to health.

*Digitaline* 2x (Keith's) ever holds its own as a cardiac tonic. *Convalaria majalis*, too, is a sure friend in the gouty heart, and the same may be affirmed of *Cactus grandifloris*. The liver, pancreas, and spleen lie physically between the heart and kidneys, and must be con-comitantly considered in some cases. The gouty dyspepsia having had its hearing, the kidney troubles proper loom large in the graver cases, and need the very greatest attention, as in them lie the ground causes of so many constitutional upbreakings. Above all things in this regard we must take into account the state of the arteries as leading up to the shedding of the epithelial cells and the exudation of albumen.

Where there is grit and gravel present, I have had cause to be satisfied with *Urticus urens* Q and *Coccus cacti* Q in alternation at the beginning of the treatment, but their action is not very deep-going. Where the urine is muddy, peasoupy, the ancient *Solidago virga aurea* Q soothes the kidneys gently — I had almost said sweetly-5 drops in a tablespoonful of water is my usual dose. But *Solidago* is also a not very deep -going remedy. *Coccinella septempunctata* acts very like it, but goes down a little deeper and stands midway between it and *Cantharis*, which fits the hot congestive quality of nephritis, but the dose must be infinitesimal. Where there is a renal bleeding, *Terebinth* (not lower than the 3x) has classic claims on our attention. *Phosphoric acid* — about No. 1 is very soothing to the kidneys when the urine is notably phosphatic. In Bright's disease a past grand master in therapeutics has all his work cut out, and he will need all his knowledge, however great, of climate, diet, raiment, and therapeutics. The remedy which, taken by itself, has done most in my hands in chronic Bright's disease is *Mercurius*, about the third trituration. A tincture of cloves, in the same strength, will bring down the quantity of albumen excreted very frequently, and concomitantly there-with there is a rise in patient's feeling of well being. Considering that cloves cause albuminuria, their use as a condiment should be condemned and forbidden. But the more gentle renal remedies, such as *Solidago*, *Coccinella*, and *Coccus cacti*, are very soothing and helpful in alternation with these deeper-going remedies capable of including, and curing, organic change. It is often very helpful in chronic gouty kidney to consider the patient in his or her entirety, and not forget the patients while studying their kidneys. We shall often find that the kidneys are spokesmen for themselves first certainly, but for the liver, heart and arteries, *and skin*, and, indeed, I would affirm of the organ which we call the kidney and of the organism, that the organ speaks for the organism and the organism speaks for the organ, each one "for self and partner." (XXI 150)

**Have we a Remedy or Remedies Essentially Homoeopathic to the Gouty Attack?**

To this I think an afirmative answer can now be given. I propose to show that *Urtica urens*, the common stinging nettle, is such a one, and I think *Natrum muriaticum* has strong claims to be so considered also. But *Nat. mur.* is a classic remedy in homoeopathy; it is well known and much used by such as have gripped the true inwardness of homoeopathic drug-action. As I will presently relate, I have used *Urtica urens* a good deal for some years in ague and spleen affections, and thus it comes to pass that I have had ample opportunities of becoming intimately acquainted with its powers. Patients under the influence of small material doses of *Urtica* will often pass quantities of gravel. (XXI 32)

I have no faith in gout cures unless they thicken the urine. If the heart is weak or atheromatous I commonly rely on *Gold*: and it is a veritable friend in need and indeed. If the skin is fairly normal I use the *Aurum muriaticum natronatum* 3x. In the same dose as the simple muriate, and am generally not disappointed with the results. I have also used *Jaborandi* and its alkaloid *Pilocarpine* with good results. In the treatment of acute gout it is sound practice to keep an eye on the stomach first, the heart next, and collaterally on the reciprocal relations, topographic and pathologic, of the heart and liver and spleen respectively; and this because the heart, with liver, spleen, stomach, and kidneys, are really the "interested parties" in acute gout. When I speak of stomach I really mean the epigastrium and more precisely speaking, the solar plexus - to which *aether*, *zincum*, and *hydrocyanic acid* will bring prompt and efficient help. (XXI 30)

**Urate of sodium in the Treatment of Gout.**

I have used *Urea*, *Uric acid*, and *Urate of Sodium* in gout, and they are of distinct value; they have helped me most and best where the deposits persist: they stir up the lazy deposits, so to speak, and help to eliminate them.

*Daphne*, *Mezerenum* and *Physalis alkekengi* have been used by me in gout off and on with a certain amount of benefit. So have *Bryonia*, *Rhus*, *Pulsatilla* and *Bacillinum*, and many others, each in its own sphere, in accordance with the indications and data of homoeopathic pharmacology, as well as with my own clinical experience. And *Aconite* has helped me up to a certain point many times: notably in the stiffnesses that remain after gout, have I found *Aconite* 3x or 3, given night and morning, of positive avail.

*Bellis perennis* does distinct good in the after-gout debility of the limbs; and *Cypripedium pubescens* (and also the powder *Cypripedinum* 3x) is its equivalent in the sphere of the nerves in the after gout adynamia and neurasthenia. Where there are actual calculi that require solution before they can be passed, *Piperazinum purum* bulks up very imposingly. (XXI 51, 52 & 53)

## Gouty Eczema remedies

The first principle in the treatment of gouty eczema is negative: use no external applications whatever, for the affection is not only constitutional, but it is also mostly compound and complex in its nature : and, I declare most emphatically, that the external treatment of gouty eczema is most dangerous-nay, I would say that it is positively idiotic. Surely, if we have a disease it is better outside than inside, and it, in the end, does not help us to lay the flattering unction to our souls that our family blood is faultlessly pure when it is not. "There is no disease in our family," one often hears; but is it so? Certain breeds are stronger than others, and given families in their blood-lives are relatively less impure than certain others, but people of absolutely clean, pure blood **I have never known.** Our family taints are printed in our skins in very bold type indeed, - only, happily, not every one can read the record.

Where the gouty eczema has become the cutaneous outlet for the constitution, its uric nature has to be borne in mind, and, in such cases, *Acidum uricum* 6, *Urea* 6, and *Acidum lacticum* 6, render notable service.

Where there is much irritation I have used *Persicaria urens* 6, 12, 30, with much benefit. Where the whites of the eyes are dirty-looking and lustreless, *Euonymus taropurp.*, *Diplotaxis* Q, and other hepatics are great favourites of mine in gouty eczema. Where there is a demonstrable sycotic taint, I use all the antisycotics — such as *Thuja, Sabina, Acid. nit., Cupressus, Medorrh.* — with a free hand, but mostly in high and higher potencies at infrequent intervals. And every organ disease must be put right by its appropriate organ remedies.

*Mercurius, Hepar,* and *Rhus ven.* are also very frequently indicated. Occasionally, when the wetting ooze dries up in layers, *Castor equi* has helped me. When the skin is brown, or has brown patches, *Sepia, Iodium,* and *Bacillin* and *Cholesterin* are friends in need and indeed. The ultimate court of appeal is the *Materia Medica Pura*; and the *Repertory* shows the way to discover the right remedies. As a very needful check on aimless wanderings in this field, however, we find an accurate knowledge of the pathology — the morbid biology — of the case in point, and if to this we add the fundamental principle, that in scientific therapeutics the curative range of a given remedy is fixed by its pathogenetic powers and possibilities, we are pretty sure to reach the goal. You cannot, however, hit the target a mile off with a gun that only carries fifty yards-no remedy is therapeutically greater than is the drug pathogenetically. (XXI 159)

## Haemorrhoid Remedies

*Aconitum Napellus* — When a febrile movement accompanies the piles, with dry skin and cephalic-congestion. It is not often called for in practice in this affection, but in plethoric subjects in whom there is determination of blood to the head, a prompt use of this remedy may avert apoplexy. When this is done, see to your patient's diet.

*Acidum Aceticum* — Profuse haemorrhoidal bleeding ; haemorrhage from bowels after checked metrorrhagia; constipation ; malignant disease of rectum.

*Aesculus Glabra* — The greater pathogenic power of this remedy should lead us to think of it especially when there is a paretic state of the legs, and the *cauda equina* is disordered. Carrying the nut on the person is said to cure piles, but I will not vouch for it.

*Aesculus Hippocastanum* — Dr. Hale is of opinion that the *central point of action* of this drug lies in the *liver and portal system*. It is decidedly one of our most powerful remedies for piles *and constipation*. My own notion of its applicability points to those cases in which there are liver, portal, rectal, and spinal indications for its use. Hale says the *absence of actual constipation* differentiates between this and other pile remedies : to this I cannot assent, my own pretty extensive experience with it leads me to say with Dr. Hughes that it is indicated in constipation, and that very strongly. That it is a great rectal remedy is undoubted. Dr. Hart's special indication for it is *throbbing in the abdominal and pelvic cavities*. Lilienthal puts the following symptoms thus : DULL BACK-ACHE, PURPLE HAEMORRHOIDS. Sensation as if sticks, splinters, gravel were in the rectum are said to be characteristic of it.

*Aloes* — Protruding piles, with constant bearing down sensation and prolapse of the bowel; paralysis of the sphincter ani. Aloes stood of old in *evil* repute in haemorrhoidal affections; thus in Nathanael Sforzia's NEUES ARTZNEYBUCH (Basel, 1684) we read, p.34, — *Alle purgierende Sachen, sonderlich von ALOE, alle gesalzenen und gewurtzten Sachen seynd schadlich* (in Piles). So that with our law to lead we know how to use *Aloes*. How is it Sforzia was so enlightened? He was in his day *heterodox*!

*Alumina* — Haemorrhoids worse in the evening; better after night's rest; clots of blood pass from anus; stools hard and knotty like sheep's dung.

*Ambra Grisea* — Itching, smarting, and stinging at the anus; increased secretion of urine, much more than the fluid drunk. Worse in the evening ; also when lying in a warm place, and on awakening. *Better* from slow motion in the open air, and when lying or pressing upon the painful part. Presence of cholesterine in the faeces.

*Ammonium Carb* — Haemorrhoids, Protude, Independent of Stool.

*Ammonium Mur* — Haemorrhoids sore and smarting after suppressed whites; hard, crumbling stools, requiring great effort to expel them ; bleeding from the rectum, with lancinating pains in perinaeum, especially evenings; stinging and itching in rectum before and during a stool; the piles surrounded by inflamed pustules.

*Anacardium* — Lilienthal says : Internal piles, especially if fissured; painful haemorrhoidal tumours; frequent profuse haemorrhage when at stool; great and urgent desire for stool, but the rectum seems powerless, with sensation as if plugged up; great hypochondriasis.

*Antimonium Crudum* — Copious haemorrhoidal haemorrhage accompanying a stool of solid faecal matter;
Mucous Piles : pricking burning; continuous mucous discharge, staining yellow; sometimes oozing away of an ichorous discharge; feeling of soreness in the rectum as if an ulcer had been torn open.
*Apis* — When there is much burning and excesive oedema of the parts.
*Arnica Montana* — Blind haemorrhoids, with painful pressure in rectum, constipation and tenesmus; worse when standing and from cold things. In prolapse from over straining at stool and from violent riding.
*Arsenicum Album* — Haemorrhoids with stitching pain when walking or standing, not when at stool, with burning pain; burning and soreness in rectum and anus; rectum is pushed out spasmodically with great pain, and remains protruded after haemorhage from rectum; BURNING IN ALL THE VEINS, restlessness and great debility, worse at night and from cold, better from warmth; HAEMORRHOIDS OF DRUNKARDS.
*Aurum* — My own use of this polychrest in piles has been confined to syphilitic subjects aggravated by mercurial symptoms. I should consider it especially called for in the *aged* and *in pining* youthful subjects.
*Badiaga* — I have put down the river-sponge as an anti-haemorrhoidal remedy, because Hering says it is useful in the complaints of adults who had manifestations of scrofula in their youth, and because it has a reputation in Russia for the cure of piles. Now there is a class of persons who are strumous and heaemorrhoidal, and hence it may be worth remembering especially when the lung or heart symptoms of Badiaga are present.
*Belladonna* — Bleeding piles; spasmodic constriction of sphincter ani; violent pains in small of back as if it would break; piles so sensitive that the patient has to lie with the nates separated ; scanty red urine; congestion of blood to head; red, hot face; thirst and restlesness.
*Berberis Vulgaris* — Haemorrhoids with itching and burning, particularly after stool, which is often hard and covered with blood; soreness in the anus, with burning pain when touched, and great sensitiveness when sitting; hard stool like sheep's dung, passed only after much straining; constant pulsating stitches in sacrum; fretful and weary of life.
*Bryonia Alba* — Hard, tough stool, with protrusion of the rectum; long-lasting burning in the rectum after hard stool; sharp burning pain in the rectum with soft stool; white and turbid urine; sensation of constriction in the urethra when urinating. *Worse* in the morning, also from motion and from heat. *Better* while lying down, or on getting warm in bed.
*Cactus Grand* — Constipation as from haemorrhoidal congestion; swollen varices outside the anus, causing great pain; itching of anus, pricking in the anus, as from sharp pins, ceasing from slight friction; copious haemorrhage from anus, which soon ceases.

*Calcarea Carbonica* — Haemorrhoids protruding, painful when walking, better when sitting, causing pain during stool ; great irritability of the anus, even a loose stool is painful; frequent and copious bleeding of the piles, or for suppression of habitual bleeding (after sulphur). Perspires a good deal in the head, especially at night. The Calcarea subject is light haired.

*Capsicum* — Piles having swollen ; itching, throbbing, with sore feeling in anus; the tumours are very large, with discharge of blood or bloody mucus from the rectum; blind piles with mucous discharge; suppressed haemorrhoidal flow, causing melancholy; lack of reactive force, especially with fat people who are easily exhausted.

*Carbo Veg.* — Discharge of an acrid, corrosive, viscid humor from the anus, causing much itching and some smarting; oozing of moisture from the perinaeum, with soreness and much itching; protruding large bluish varices, suppurating and offensive, with burning pains in the anus, stitching pains in the small of the back, burning and tearing in the limbs; constipation, with burning stools and discharge of blood to the head, flatulence, slow action of the bowels; epistaxis; dysuria; especially called for in debauched, used-up subjects and in profound adynaemia.

*Chamomilla* — Bleeding piles with compressive pain in the abdomen, frequent urging to stool; occasional burning and corrosive diarrhoeic stools; tearing pain in the small of the back, especially at night; painful and ulcerated rhagades of the anus.

*Collinsonia Canadensis* — Dr. Hale believes that this remedy has the power of contracting the branches of the portal vein — indeed, he inclines to believe that it has this action on all the bloodvessels and even on the heart. It is in common use in America as a vulnerary. It claims a careful study and comes into very frequent use in general varicosis, and any of its varieties, such as haemorrhoids, varices, or varicocele. And if Hale's view of its action is right, those cases of dilated *right* heart, passive portal congestion, with haemorrhoids, would be its triune sphere, and hereby there is always constipation and the cases are chronic and obstinate.

*Dioscorea Villosa* — Dr. Burt got haemorrhoids and yellow, thin, bilious stools with prolapse of the rectum, when he was proving the colic root. In another a haemorrhoidal tumour of nearly four years' standing disappeared while proving it. Its reputation in enteralgia is now well established. Acute painful varicocele from excess in venery, or long-lasting unsatisfied desire, will make us think of *Dioscorea* or Dioscorein. *Dioscorea* is a powerful cardiac, and has cured a case of *angina pectoris* in the hands of Dr. Skinner.

*Ferrum* — Piles, copious bleeding or ichorous oozing tearing pains with itching and gnawing, costiveness, stool hard and difficult, followed by back-ache. We heartily endorse Schussler's recommendation of the *Phosphate*, and that in the sixth centesimal trituration, but very irritable subjects must not take it at night, as it is very apt to keep such awake. It comes in specially after other rectal remedies have done their work, to consolidate the cure by reason of its profound action on the whole systemic cirulatory apparatus.

*Graphites* — Piles with pain on sitting down or on taking a wide step, as if split with a knife, also violent itching and very sore to the touch; burning rhagades at the anus; large haemorrhoidal tumour, protrusion of the rectum, without urging to stool, as if the anus was lame; fissure of the anus, sharp cutting pain during stool, followed by constriction and aching for several hours, worse at night; chronic constipation, with hardness in hepatic region ; moist humid eruption on scalp and behind ears; watery leucorrhoea at the times of menstruation ; piles, accompanied by dizziness.

*Hamamelis Virginica* — The use of this remedy is somewhat empirical, but its power over haemorrhoids and other venous sticlis is such that it stands *facile princeps* at the head of them all. The stasis, its introduction into our practice is thus given : Mr. Pond brought out his Extract of Hamamelis as a remedy for piles. Dr. Constatine Hering was Mr. Pond's family physician, and was induced by the latter to try its efficacy in some diseases, particularly in painful bleeding piles. But its virtues as a pile medicine were well known to the aborigines of North America, and the earlier settlers got their knowledge of it from them. Speaking of it in a letter to Hering, in 1853, Dr. Okie says : "I next made use of Hamamelis in a number of cases of painful and bleeding piles. Those cases in which it has proved most beneficial in my hands are characterized by running soreness, fulness, and at times rawness of the anus; in the back a weakness or weariness, or as the patients graphically express it "Doctor, my back feels as if it would break off."

It is our best topic in all forms of dilated veins. Almost all Americans *en voyage* seems to carry Extract of Hamamelis with them.

*Hydrastis* — This plant has a reputation for many things. Undoubtedly it is a great polychrest. I should think of it for haemorrhoids with jaundice and constipation, some other *Hydrastis symptoms* being present. I have known it *cause* balanitis and yellow balanorrhoea, with such a strong-smelling discharge that the unintentional prover had to keep away from society for several days, and so profuse that he fastened a piece of linen inside of his shirt to help to absorb the discharge, and nevertheless his trousers were spoiled by the flux. The discharge was very yellow, and after it had lasted three days there was phimosis, and on my forcing the prepuce back it cracked in three places and bled. There had previously been nothing whatever wrong with the parts, and from my knowledge of the gentleman and a very careful ocular examination of the parts, I can say that there was no urethritis or urethral flux, and no chancre or chancroid, and there had been no coition of any kind at this time. At the height of the affection one of the inguinal glands became painful and swelled; it all passed off in a week with no treatment but cleanliness. He had taken it about a week, some six or eight very yellow pilules a day, evidently Q or 1x, and "for a stitch in the liver and dirty tongue." To the best of my knowledge and belief the whole series of phenomena were pathogenetic.

*Ignatia Amara* — Sudden sharp stitches in rectum, shooting upwards into the body; vacuation of faeces difficult, because of seeming inactivity of rectum, every violent effort to expel them may produce prolapsus ani; after stool frequent spasmodic constriction of the anus, recurring pains in the anus, compounded of soreness, spasmodic constriction, and pressure; moderate effort at stool causes prolapsus ani; bleeding during and after stool; fissures of anus; haemorrhage and pain are worse when the stools are loose.

*Kali Carbonicum* — Passage of faeces difficult owing to their bulk; sensation as if the anus would be fissured; stinging, burning, tearing, itching, screwing pain, followed even a natural stool, setting the patient nearly crazy and depriving him of sleep; the tumours swell and bleed much; riding on horseback ameliorates the pain for the time being; haemorrhoids complicating *fistula in ano*, especially in the *poitrinaires*.

*Kali Sulphuricum* — Haemorrhoids with catarrh of stomach, and tongue coated with yellow mucus; sensation of faintness in the stomach, and dull feeiing in the head, fearing to lose her senses.

*Lachesis* — Piles protruding and strangulated, or with stitches upward at each cough or sneeze; sensation as of a plug in the anus; rectum prolapsed or tumefied; hammering, beating in the rectum; worse at the climaxis, or with drunkards.

*Lycopodium Clavatum* — Varices protrude, painful when sitting,; discharge of blood, even with soft stool; itching eruption at the anus, painful to touch; itching and tension at the anus in the evening in bed continued burning or stitching pain in the rectum; constipation; ineffectual urging from the contraction of the sphincter ani; flatulence; haematuria; pain in the sacral region, extending to the thighs, worse rising from a seat. *Lycopodium* has undoubtedly cured aneurisms of small calibre; it lessened one in my hands while I was House-Surgeon at the Hardman St. Homoeopathic Dispensary, in Liverpool. Hence its power over *blood-vessels* must be admitted.

*Mercurius* — Large bleeding varices which suppurate; haemorrhage after micturition; haematuria; with violent frequent urging to urinate; prolapsus recti after stool; rectum black and bleeding; pain in the sacrum, as after lying on a hard couch, great weakness, with ebullition and trembling from the least exertion.

*Cyanuret of Mercury* — I have used this remedy in diphtheria with very satisfactory results, and hence it constitutes a part of my usual drug of choice. The enormous activity of all the combinations of the metals with hydrocyanic acid leads us naturally to expect great things from the Cyanide of Mercury. It causes phlebitis and varicosis; it has a grand future. The sixth centesimal dilution is the lowest I ever use of this deadly drug — in this strength it may be given to the tenderest babies.

German homoeopathic practitioners speak highly of *Acidum hydrocyanicum* in varicose ulcers.

*Muriatic Acid* — Piles, suddenly, IN CHILDREN ; the haemorrhoidal tumours are inflamed, swollen, bluish, with swelling of anal region, sore pains, violent stitches, and great sensitiveness to contact, even of the sheets; prolapsus recti while urinating.

*Nitric Acid* — Long lasting cutting pain in rectum after loose stool, with haemorrhoidal troubles; old pendulous haemorrhoids, that cease to bleed, but become painful to the touch, especially in warm weather, haemorrhage bright red not clotted, faint from least motion, bleed after every stool ; spasmodic tearing during stool from fissures in rectum; haematuria, shuddering along the spine during micturition, and urging afterwards.

*Nux Vomica* — Blind, or bleeding piles, irregular piles; stitching, burning or itching of the anus; stitches and shocks in the small of the back, with bruised pains so that the patient is unable to raise himself; constipation, with frequent ineffecutal urging to stool, and with sensation as if the anus were closed and constricted; frequent rush of blood to the head or abdomen, with distension of the epigastrium and hypochondria; haematuria from suppressed haemorrhoidal flow, or menses; ischuria, suppression of urine; backache, must sit up in bed.

*Petroleum* — Piles and fissures at the anus, great itching; scurf on borders of anus; stool insufficient, difficult, hard, in lumps.

*Phosphorus* — Constipation, small-shaped, hard stool, and expelled with great difficulty; discharges of blood from the rectum, also during stool; spasm in the rectum; paralysis of the lower intestines and of the sphincter ani; discharge of mucus out of the gaping anus; stinging or itching at the anus; the piles bleed easily; increased secretion of pale, watery urine; involuntary discharge of urine. *Worse* in the evening and at night, also when lying on the back or left side. *Better* when lying on the right side, from rubbing and after sleeping.

*Podophyllum* — This is a remedy that I, myself, have used but very little, for the very good reason, that of late years a veritable podophyllomania has raged in this country, and almost all patients with anything wrong between liver and rectum have taken it on their own account. This regrettable abuse of a potent remedy must not deter us from bearing it in mind in suitable cases. Hale says : "*Haemorrhoidal affections* are admirably under the control of *Podophyllum*. The specific affinity which this drug has for the liver, portal system, and rectum, as shown in the pathogenesis, enables it to cause haemorrhoids from portal congestion, chronic hepatic affections, and primary irritation, congestion and even inflammation of the veins, and mucous membrane of the rectum. It will be found useful in external piles, for those which bleed and those which do not. The *sensations* it causes in the rectum, anus and haemorrhoidal tumours are similar to the effects of *Aloes*, of which it is a congener."

*Morning aggravation* is characteristic of *Podophyllum*.

*Pulsatilla Nigricans* — Painful protruding piles, with itching and sticking pains and soreness.

*Rhus Tox* — Fissures of the anus, with periodical profuse bleeding from the anus; sore piles, protruding after stool, drawing in the back from the above downwards, pains in the small of the back as if bruised, when keeping quiet; frequent urging to urinate day and night with increased secretion; sore blind haemorrhoids, protruding after stool, with pressing in the rectum, as if everything would come out. Worse at night, from cold, pressure, or rest.

*Silicea* — Haemorrhoids intensely painful, boring cramping sensation from the anus up the rectum and towards the testicles; protrude during stool; become incarcerated. and suppurate; piles protrude with the stool, and discharge bloody mucus; can only be returned with difficulty; fistula at anus, with chest symptoms, aching, beating, throbbing, in lumbo-sacral region : anus is constantly damp.

*Sulphur* — Haemorrhoids blind or bleeding, blood dark, with violent bearing-down from small of back towards the anus : lancinating pain from anus upwards, especially after stool; suppressed harmorrhoids, with colic, palpitation, congestion of lungs; back feels stiff as if bruised; anal region swollen, with sore, stitching pains; considerable qaantity of blood passed with soft easy stool; PAINLESS PILES ; bleeding, burning, and frequent protrusion of the haemorrhoidal tumours : weak digestion, dysuria.

*Valerianate of Zinc* — Dr. Dradwick noticed the fact that in a considerable number of patients troubled with piles, and who were taking *Valerianate of Zinc* for other troubles, the haemorrhoids have, with few exceptions, been relieved. In cases of neuralgia, prosopalgia, spinal neuralgia, and proctalgia, together with haemorrhoids, we may be glad to remember this happy union of *valerian* and *zinc*.

*Veratrum Album* — Haemorrhoids, with disease of lungs, or pleura : painless discharge of masses of blood in clots, with sinking feeling; bruised feeling in sacral region. (Lilienthal.)

*Zincum* — Constipation, stool hard and dry, inefficient, only expelled by hard pressing; sensation of soreness, and violent itching at the anus, as if from ascarides; violent desire to urinate; retention of urine when beginning to urinate. *Worse* in the afternoon and in the evening, also when in a warm room. *Better* in the open air.(VI 155)

## Heart

Then it may be remembered that *Rhus* causes, — palpitation of the heart that is so violent that the body becomes moved thereby; tremor of the heart ; pain in the chest as if the sternum were pressed in ; dyspnoea and oppression of the chest. So we know that it affects the heart very powerfully. (VI 142)

## Helonias

**Helonias in Enlargements of the Uterus, with urinary Trouble.** In all cases of simple organ diseases one of our greatest difficulties is to know which organ remedy is really indicated. How is one to find out? From the provings, no doubt, but with most of our remedies the provings do not tell us enough. Rademacher, following Paracelsus used to maintain that it was impossible to know without organ testing, partly because the *spiritus epidemicus morborum* so often plays a part in diseases. Many of the cases of urinary troubles that come before us are primarily from the womb being enlarged and too heavy — and hence dislocated, and producing irritation at the neck of the bladder, with frequent desire to micturate.

Frequently in dysuria from an inflamed state of the urethra I find *Triticum repens* Q, 10 drops in a little water, frequently repeated, of prompt effect, often giving complete relief in a few hours, and if the ailment is primary to the urethra the relief is an abiding cure; if from a tugging of the heavy womb, the ailment returns again and again, — it is only relief and not a cure. This is true always in the use of organ-remedies for organ-diseases : unless the ailment is primary to the organ acted upon by the organ-remedy, we only attain transitory relief. This I have often before pointed out, and here we need not go any wider afield into higher homoeopathy. *Helonin* fits well cases of urinary trouble arising primarily from a too heavy womb. (XXIII 112)

## Hepatics

**Rademacher's Hepatic.** Rademacher's liver medicines are *Quassia, Chelidonium, Liquorcalc. mur., Nux vom., Crocus,* and *Carduus,* though he does not reckon the last-named as solely an hepatic. (XVII 156)

## Herpes Remedies

Mr. Hutchinson says that *Quinine and Aconite* are the most useful remedies, but that he has had no triumphs. Now, what I would point out to Mr. Hutchinson is this : If he has had no triumphs, how does he know which are the most useful remedies? It is not correct to say that *Quinine and Aconite* are the most useful remedies in the treatment of the after-pains of shingles. As a matter of fact, it is only a common occurrence for either *Quinine or Aconite* to be called for in this affection. How two remedies that only occasionally cure, because only occasionally indicated, can be the best remedies, is a little beyond my simple understanding.

*Rhus tox.* is a much more frequently efficacious remedy for the shingles after-pain than either *Quinine or Aconite;* and of ordinary everyday remedies, *Phosphorus* is, in my experience, the *best,* and by *best* I mean the most frequently curative. Of course the best must ever be that remedy which is pathogenetically most similar to the case in point. And why best? Because it cures.

I think rather too much is made of "age" in referring to shingles. No doubt the after-pains are most troublesome in the old, but the bulk of the cases which have come under my observation have been in the middle-aged, and not in the aged, and I believe shingles is most common in the middle-aged. In the quite young I believe shingles to be relatively infrequent.

Now the homoeopathic treatment of the shingles after-pains is one of the prettiest bits of therapeutic sharp-shooting imaginable, and we can honestly claim to have had very many triumphs without, as rule, either *Quinine or Aconite.* I have myself had the greatest number of cures with *Phosphorus,* but *Rhus tox., Thuja occid., Vaccinin.,* and *Variolin.* constitute a very reliable rearguard, — the last-named being far and away the most certain, prompt and radical. I use it always in high or very high dilutions, and do not readily repeat. If Mr. Hutchinson will follow these lines he will be able to claim many triumphs. (XIV 136)

## Hydrastis

I have before pointed out my fondness for *Hydrastis* in small material doses as an aftercure to the bacillinic treatment. Here (in pelvic consumptiveness) I gave it for a month, but at times I give it for two, and I sometimes use it intercurrently between two courses of *Bacillinum* with much advantage, not that it has any relationship to tuberculosis as such, but it increases the appetite, and patients under its influence put on flesh of good quality. (XVI A 186)

And here I will allow myself to interpose the remark, that *Hydrastis* given as just named fattens up patients after the cure with the bacillic virus in an often truly wonderful manner. The bacillic virus has a well-defined and limited sphere of action, and very frequently needs to be followed by other remedies, as so few cases are quite simple.(XVI A 64)

## Hydrastis & Opium

It is odd that people who have been taking *Hydrastis*, not infrequently think they have been taking-opium. (XVII 85)

## Jaborandi

I have used *Jaborandi* for many years — in fact I wrote a paper on it already in my allopathic days; but though I have used it long, I have not used it often; of late years I have generally used *Pilocarpinum muriaticum* 3x. It is my big shot in mumps. It is well known that *Jaborandi* causes profuse perspiration, ending in a very dry skin. I regard it merely as an organ remedy of the sweat glands, affecting also the parotid and the pancreas. I have known it long, but do not know it well. (XXIV 41)

## Juglans Cinerea

In relation to the use of *Juglans cinerea in angina pectoris*, I was much pleased lately to see that my original observation of the pathogeneric anginal symptoms of this vegetable arsenic has been clinically verified by another observer, viz., Dr. Ussher, of Wandsworth. (XIV 70)

## Leucocythaemia — Splenic remedies

I hav found *Oleum Succini non rectificatum, Spiritus glandium Quercus, Thuja* 30, *Mangan. acet.* 1, and *Natrum sul.* of positively curative effect in leucocythaemia splenica. (X 63)

## Levico

The waters of *Levico* are a very favourite remedy of mine in many skin affections where I need a little tonic, and where it seems of great advantage to give the organism a rest from the effects of high dilutions of the more specifically acting remedies. (IX 216)

I will add that *Levico*, in 5 to 10 drop doses, is a valuable intercurrent help in grave cases where there is much debility, notably after the searching remedies such as *Bacillinum*. (XXII 34)

## Lyssinum

The sufferings of the celibate state, notably in women, are at times amenable to its benign influence, and to this I was partly led by a consideration of the prime cause of rabies, viz., pent-up sexual longings. We will not dwell too much on the subject, but I feel bound to name this, my valuable clinical friend. I use 30 and C. and higher only. And when we reflect on the truly awful sufferings of this lyssic state in the human subject, we must gratefully accept the help which *Lyssinum* can give. Of course, like all homoeopathically used remedies, it fits only certain cases, not by means all, for *Med*. and *Luet*. (both high) also play a great part in such loveless states.

"I am roused in the night with such fearfully horrible, sinful feelings" calls for *Med*.

"No sooner does night come on than I am a prey to such dreadfully sinful desires that drive me mad" calls for *Luet*. Now are all these sin? I cannot think so; to my mind they are no more sinful than colic or neuralgia; they are just the sufferings of our common humanity, and what sufferings too! Much worse than mere pain. (XXIV 13)

## Medorrhinum

**In Angina Pectoris.** Were I asked which is the most frequently - indicated remedy in angina pectoris, and the one that helps radically and really, I should say *Medorrh*. C., CC., and M. I have used it mostly in men, and only in a high dilution. I will not dwell upon the cases I have cured or relieved by it, but its indication with me has been purely historic, and on the principle of taking a hair of the dog that bit you. There is very commonly flatulent dyspepsia present where it is indicated, and often catarrh more or less inveterate : true medorrhoea being the first mother — *Urmutter* — of catarrhs. (XIV 165)

The late Dr. Swan, of New York, once wrote me that he had found *Med.* (high) a good antiodte to the ill effect of influenza, which statement I have very frequently verified. (X 76)

— **Morning Sickness.** *Med.* 1000 for this ailing is a grand friend in need and indeed; many a time ladies have written for "those powders that cure morning sickness," and this is the remedy. The dose is not to be lightly repeated; in this case the first dose aggravated, the third was followed by a cure. (XXII 96)

## Mercurialism & Aurum

What I mean is that if a given individual shows chronic symptoms of mercurialism pure and simple, or mercurial symptoms with symptoms of any given disease, the chronic mercurialism may be successfully combated with refracted doses of Gold. The utter childishness of asserting that Homoeopathy consists in treating acute cases of poisoning with homoeopathic remedies is only equalled by that other pretty assertion that Homoeopathy means to grow giants on infinitesimal portions of a bread crumb. An Australian worthy has lately rediscovered this old mare's nest. And he even accuses a well-known homoeopathic author with inconsistency for teaching the same treatment of cases of poisoning as is recognised by the authorities in toxicology.
Such nonsense is believed by the simple and is hence noticed in passing. Nevertheless, even in acute cases of poisoning, *after the ingested poison has been eliminated, or chemically antidoted, or rendered chemically inert,* the remaining symptoms can truly be successfully ameliorated by homoeopathically cholera remedies. (II 142)

## Mercury

A French writer of fifty years ago says : "In England they use mercury as much as we use chocolate in France". (II 60)

## Mercury & Aurum

Neither do I propose to join in the insane cry of the so-called antimercurialists; on the contrary, if I were reduced to one remedy in the treatment of protean manifestations of this disease, I should certainly choose *Mercury*. *Mercury* is, *facile princeps*, the anitisyphilitic remedy. But the dose? Ay, there's the rub! To do the good without risking the harm is the true test.

Moreover, I do not propose to vaunt the use of Gold in this special disease, but rather to point out that it deserves a very much higher place in the *Armamentarium* of the physician than is accorded to it in general. For centuries Gold has been used with excellent effect in scrofula, heart-disease, skin diseases, dropsy, tedium vitae, melancholia, and the Morbus Gallicus, or syphilis.

In the treatment of some heart diseases, some bone diseases, and of sarcocele, to know the medicinal value of Gold or to ignore it is, just the important difference between curing and failing. But, of course, the metal must be first triturated, so that it may become remedial. (II 18)

## Natrum Muriaticum

There are certain generalizations that have arisen in the evolutionary expansion of homoeopathy that must be rightly and duly appraised if we are to do the *greatest possible* amount of good in practical drug therapeutics.

Thus the general statement that *Natrum muriaticum* antidotes the effects of quinine deserves a certain amount of attention, though of course it is not every case of cinchonism that dynamized chloride of sodium will cure. In this sense I understand the value of the statement that Gold follows Mercurius so well in the syphilitically broken down. (XX 269)

## Nettles

It seems to me that if any honest enquirer is really desirous of putting the truth of homoeopathy roughly, yet readily, to the test, he need only handle a few nice nettles with gloveless hands, when he will find that nettles really do produce nettle-rash; and then if he will treat a few cases of nettle-rash, occurrring as a disease, with some nettle-tea or tincture, he will find that the nettle really does cure the disease nettlerash ! . . . . and, if that is not homoeopathy, pray what *is* it? (XXI 145)

## Bellis Perennis

This (Coccygodynia) is a neuralgia at the very bottom of the spine, where our caudal appendage would be placed were we caudate. Not unfrequently it is of traumatic origin, and I have cured a case of this kind with *Bellis perennis*, and another with antisycotics. I think it is most common in women. (XIV 79)

## Neuralgia, Hypochondria & Enteralgia — Remedies

*Phosphorus*, in allopathic doses, is a very dangerous, and that a very sneakingly dangerous drug, and no one should use *Phosphorus* internally unless they possess the requisite knowledge as to how much will harm and how little will cure. As a tonic for the nerves it is simply murderous. For the neuralgias of the right side under the ribs (hypochondrium) the hepatics must be studied, and the principal ones here are *Hydrastis canadensis, Chelidonium majus, Myrica cerifera, Diplotaxis tenuifolia, Cholestearin, Bryonia alba*, and *Kali bichromicum*. The neuralgias of the left hypochondrium are more or less connected with the spleen, and the remedies here needed will be found in the little work on *"Diseases of the Spleen and their Remedies Clinically Illustrated"*, by the writer. Of course, the neuralgias all down the sides in their walls will require such remedies as *Bryonia alba, Ranunculus, Colocynth, Rhus tox., Cimicifuga racemosa*, and the like. Some very obstinate ones I have cured with *Variolinum* C.

The enteralgias are met with *Plumbum, Dioscoreo villosa, Colocynth*, and their allies. (XIV 75)

## Neuralgia Remedies

*Ferrum* — iron — besides being unquestionably a great blood medicine, is also useful in neuralgia, and in those cases of great debility *where the urine is alkaline* (Rademacher), the acetate in small material doses is *facile princeps*.

Probably few practitioners of experience will deny that we are living in an age of neurosis, where neuralgia is becoming more and more prevalent, and I am strongly of opinion that tea, coffee, tobacco, alcohol, wear and tear and worry, are essential causal factors. Some have advanced good grounds for believing that migraine, or hemicranial neuralgia, is mainly due to coffee.

Enteralgia, I know, is very frequently due to tea and I have some grounds for believing that pig-meat (notably roast pork), shell-fish, and potatoes also contingently cause neuralgia.

In neuralgia of the walls of the chest, *Ranunculus sceleratus* renders good service, and in neuralgia of the heart, made worse by walking, *Arsenicum, Juglans cinerea, Arnica, Bellis perennis,* and *Aurum* are to be thought of. (XIV 31)

## Neuralgia of the Stomach — Remedies

I have often cured this with *Acidum hydrocyanicum* in one-drop doses of the first homoeopathic centesimal dilution. Only physicians may use it, as it requires careful dosing. Of the same nature, and quite safe to use, is the *Prunus virginiana* in five-drop doses of the mother tincture. I learned its use myself of an old lady, nearly ninety years of age, many years ago.

*Zincum* — either the cyanide or the acetate — is a very notable remedy in gastralgia. Many cases of dyspepsia are of a neuralgic character, and the most common and most commonly distressing in this cold wet climate is curable by *Silver* — either the nitrate (Arg-n) or the oxide (Arg-o). A noted physician of the last generation made quite a reputation by his great cures of neuralgia and dyspepsia of the stomach; and his remedy was the oxide of silver. The good man was an active hater of homoeopathy, little weening that his own reputation and success depended entirely upon the homoeopathicity of his remedy to the complaint he cured with its aid. Mankind is apt to hate and despise its best and truest friends. The various neuralgias arising from urethral pyorrhoea — from the gonococci — are usually amenable to *Argentum*. This remedy has a well-earned reputation in *tabes dorsalis,* and is homoeopathic to its pains in some varieties, and *Sabina, Thuja,* and *Cupresus* come close upon it in sycosic neuralgias generally. (XIV 77)

## Nitric Acid

This use of *Nitric acid* in fistula is ancient history with the homoeopaths. Hughes' *"Manual of Pharmacodynamics,"* third edition, well sums it up by pointing out that *nitric acid* manifests great power over the mucocutaneous outlets, — "those parts where mucous membrane is exposed to the external air, and where skin is so shielded and moistened that it approximates to mucous membrane" Hughes, writing still of *nitric acid,* continues, "It exhibits a singular power over the rectum and anus : it has cured prolapsus fistula, and even fissure." (XVI 18)

## Nosoda

I am very sure if Hahnemann were now alive he would have been ahead of us all in the use of the viruses of diseases in high potencies. He, at any rate, would have realized that the greater the virus the greater the remedy; and that not merely as a learning-tinged motto, but as a real guide in practical clinical work. (XVI A (PREFACE IV)

## Nux Vomica

The duskiness of the skin, and the big brown patches on the forehead, led me to give *Nux*. It did much good, and under its influence patient's skin became lighter and cleaner. (XVII 154)

## Nux Vomica & Chelidonium

Where the gall ducts are alone implicated he considers *Nux vomica the right remedy*. Hence *Chelidonium* would be indicated in alcoholia as well as in jaundice when the affection is primary to the "inner liver." (XVII 38)

## Oleum Succini

*Oleum Succini Non Rectificatum*. This is a good spleen remedy. It must be given in small doses, and as people often make a mess of the dropping, it is best to give it in some other fluid. I order it in acorn-water and formerly in acorn-spirit. To six ounces of acorn-water I add half a scruple or a whole scruple of the oil. They do not mix chemically, but if the mixture be well shaken our object is attained; the patient does not get more into his stomach than we intend. The giving them together contains no virtue; at least I have no reason to think so. The *Oleum Succini* does good service in painful spleen affections where with there are convulsive attacks, such as the hysterical and hypochondriacal often have. Only once did I observe its smell cause hysterical convulsions in a woman, but that is a very rare exception to the rule.

Oswald Crollius lays great stress of the importance of rectifying the oil of amber, but what he says therein is not true. The rectified oil is nothing like so serviceable as the unrectified. In general, Crollius is the most honorable and the most straight-forward of all the iatro-chemists, but a man of but small understanding. (X 51)

## Onions, Hypericum

He was a great smoker, and as he stooped one day to light his pipe with a scrap of a French newspaper, he read what was on it, viz., an account of a case of neuralgia of the stumps which had been, cured by eating onions. Of course, onions do make most people sleepy. I have myself cured a case of neuralgia of the stamp with *Hypericum per.* 3x. (XIV 104)

## Ophthalmic Diseases — Important Remedies

*Ammon Mur.* — Hoarseness. Cough at night, when lying on the back. Frequent hawking, with expectoration of mucus. Coldness in the back, especially between the shoulders. *Capsular cataract, dimness of sight, as if obscured by a fog. Flying spots and points before the eyes.* Constipation; stools hard, crumbling. Head feels full and too heavy. Irritability and bad humour.

*Arsenicum Alb.* —Cannot rest in any place; changing his position continually. Vomiting of the ingesta after each meal. Violent, unquenchable, burning thirst, with frequent drinking, but little at a time. Tongue dry, brown, black, cracked. Burning sensation all over the body. *Everything appears green. Sees as through a white gauze. Pulsative throbbing in the eyes, worse after midnight. Periodical headache. Ulceration of the cornea. Burning in the margins of the eyelids. Corrosive lachrymation making the lids and cheeks sore.* Pains are relieved by warm application.

*Aurum Metallicum* — Is especially called for persons with syphilitic mercurial dyscrasia. The least contradiction excites his wrath. *Fiery sparks before the eyes. Vertical half sight. Eyes look protruded. Objects seem smaller and more distant. Fog or smoke before his eyes. Bones around the eyes feel bruised.* Putrid smells from the mouth. Constipation. Stools very hard and knotty. Discharge of fetid pus from the nose. Passes more urine than what corresponds to the quantity he drinks. (V 106)

*Baryta Carb.* — Weakness of memory. Inflammation of the throat with swollen inflamed tonsils. Cracking in the ears when swallowing. Great liability to take cold. Cough worse in the evening till midnight. *Sensation of dryness in the eyes. Scrofulous inflammation, with phlyctenula and ulcers on the cornea. Photophobia. Flying webs and black spots before the eyes.* Paralysis and palsy of the aged persons. Fetid perspiration on the feet. Tearing in the limbs, with chilliness. Dry or humid scurf on the head.

*Calcarea Carb.* — Great liability to take cold and great sensitiveness to moist, cold air. Acidity of the whole digestive tract with sour taste, sour vomiting and sour smelling stools. Profuse and easy perspiration. Intense thirst and great hankering for milk or half-boiled eggs. Catamenia too early and too profuse in fat women. *Pressure, itching, burning and stinging in the eyes. Watering of the eyes in the morning, or in the open air. Dimness of sight. Mist before the eyes when looking sharp. Cutting in the eyes and eyelids.* Vertigo, when ascending a height, walking in the open air, or turning the head quickly. Anguish, with palpitation of the heart. Perspiration on the feet.

*Calcarea Fluorica* — Indurated glands. Syphilitic ozaena, with offensive discharge. Constipation, with inability to expel the faeces . Blind or bleeding piles. *Cataract. Blurred vision. Spots on the cornea. Flickering and sparks before the eyes.* Enamel of the teeth rough & deficient. Mal-nutrition or cavities of teeth. Sore throat, better from warm drinks.

*Calcarea Phos.* — Forgetfulness; can remember things only for a short time. Difficulty in performing intellectual operations. Staggering when rising from a seat. *Aching pain in the eye-balls as if beaten. Ulcers and spots on the cornea. Cataract. Eyes water with yawning. Sensation as of veils before the eyes.* Gums painful and inflamed. Loss of appetite. At every attempt to eat, the belly aches. Belching, followed by burning in the epigastrium. Offensive, hot and noisy stools. Protruding piles; oozing of a yellow fluid. Anal fistula.

*Cannabis Sativa* — Asthmatic attacks; he can only breathe when standing up. Difficult respiration when lying down. Violent palpitation of the heart. Feeling of weariness. *Injection of the vessels of the conjunctiva, great photophobia and lachrymation. Cornea, opaque and vascular. Dimness of vision. Cataract.* Sensation as if intoxicated. Congestive headache. Sensation as of a heavy weight on the vertex. Constipation, Strangury. Burning and smarting pain in the urethra while urinating.

*Carb. Animalis* — Panting and rattling breathing. Sensation of coldness in the chest. Hoarseness. Painful swelling and induration of the glands of the neck, etc. *Sensation as if the eyes were lying loose in their sockets. Senile cataract. Vision of a net swimming before the eyes. Eyes feel weak.* Hardness of hearing. The tip of the nose is red, chapped and burning. Repugnance to greasy food. Weak digestion; almost all food causes distress. Hard and knotty stool.

*Causticum* — Rheumatic affections with contraction of the flexors and stiffness of the joints. Involuntary urination when coughing, sneezing or blowing the nose. Frequent ineffectual desire to defaecate. *Feeling of sand in the eyes. Heaviness of the upper eyelids or ptosis. Burning and itching sensation in the eyes. Flashes of light before the eyes. The sight is bedimmed as though he were looking through a fog. Incipient cataract, with perpendicular half-sight. Cataract reticularis. Warts on the upper eyelids.* Aversion to sweet things. Greasy taste in the mouth. Violent thirst, with desire for cold drinks. Asthma, especially when sitting, or lying down. Rattling noises in the chest. Cough with pain in the hips, and relief by a swallow of cold-water.

*Chelidonium* — Low-spirited and desponding, with inclination to weep. Gnawing sensation in the stomach, relieved by eating. Constipation. *Misty appearance before the eyes. Weak sight. Cannot distinguish letters. Lachrymation. Pain in the eyes, as if pierced by knives. Lamp light aggravates pain in the eyes.* Longing for warm milk. Oppression of the chest. Great debility and lassitude after awaking in the morning. Stiffness in the joints.

*Cinararia Maritima Succus.* — This is the only homoeopathic medicine that has been used externally as a specific for the cataractous affections of the eyes. It is prepared from the juice of the plant and dropped in the eye. *The juice does not appear to produce any inflammation : a slight burning sensation, which lasts for about two minutes, follows its application. There is also more or less lachrymal discharge tinged with the colouring matter of the liquid used. Probably the action of this remedy consists of stimulation of the absorbents, and so far our present experience goes, the improvement produced is progressive and enduring.* The general dosage should be two drops instilled in the eyes three times daily. One should contiune this medicine with some patience for several weeks before any material change will be observed.

*Conium* — *Cataract especially from contusion. Short-sightedness. Things look red. Aversion to light, with out inflammation of the eyes. Sensation of coldness or burning of the eyes in the open air. Ulcers on the cornea.* Vision weak with vertigo, and general debility. *Lids open only with great difficulty.* Frequent micturition, during the night; the urine cannot be retained. Strangury. Constipation, with ineffectual desire for stool. Violent, spasmodic, nightly cough. Chilliness, with desire for heat, especially the sunshine.

*Euphrasia* — Cough only during the day. Oppression of breathing. *Profuse, fluent coryza, with smarting lachrymation and photophobia. Increased secretion of mucus and agglutination of the eyes in the night time. Stitching pain in the eyeballs. Swelling of the eyelids.* Pulsating pain in the head. Frequent emission of clear urine. Stitches in the hips and knee-joints when walking.

*Graphites* — Repugnance to salty food. The abdomen becomes inflated after eating. Stools hard, knotty. The urine smells sour or offensive. *Intolerance to light. Muco-purulent discharge from the eyes. Letters run together when writing. Flickering before the eyes. Everything turns black on stooping. Profuse lachrymation. Eczema of the eyelids.* Moisture and sore places behind the ears. Hardness of hearing. The nails are thick and crippled. Menses too late, too scanty and too pale. Profuse, thin, leucorrhoea with weakness in the back.

*Kali Carb.* — *Cataract, especially of the right eye. Sharp stitches in the eyes. Weakness of vision. Lachrymation. Bright sparks, blue or green spots before the eyes. Puffiness; swelling between the eyebrows and eyelids like a sac.* Especially useful for those who take cold easily and suffer from frequent attacks of tonsillitis. Perspiration easily excited. Great stiffness of the back, unable to stoop. Spasmodic cough, with retching and vomiting. Cough worse from 3 to 4 A.M.

*Kali Iod.* — Principally called for the syphilitic subjects. Darting pain in the region of the heart. Cough with oppression of breathing and salty and greenish expectoration. Pain in the back as if bruised. Ptyalism. Ulceration of the tongue and mouth. *Dim and foggy vision. Sees objects indistinctly. Dull discoloured state of the iris. Burning in the eyes and lachrymation. Syphilitic choroiditis. Iritis after abuse of Mercury. Chemosis.* Chilliness all night, with shaking and frequent waking. At times chilly and at other times profuse perspiration. From least cold repeated attacks of violent and acrid coryza.

*Lycopodium* — Has arrested the growths of cataracts. Weak vision, unable to distinguish small objects even at a short distance. Seems as though one were looking through a fine lattice. Night-blindness. Veil and flickering before the eyes. Black-spots before the eyes. Hemiopia, sees only the left half of objects. Mucus in the eyes, must wipe them to see more clearly. *Cough with copious purulent expectoration. Every exertion causes shortness of breathing. Red, sandy sediment in the urine. Immediately after the meal, the abdomen is bloated. Has a great appetite, but a small quantity of food fills him up to the throat.*

*Magnesia Carb.* — Hardness and stitching pain in the region of the liver. Constipation. Ineffectual urging to evacuate, with small stools, or only discharge of flatus. *Black spots or moles before the eyes. Dimness of vision. Lenticular cataract. Obscuration of the cornea. Dryness of the eyes or profuse lachrymation. Chronic blepharitis. Agglutination of the eyelids especially in the morning.* A short walk tires much. Rheumatic pains in the limbs. Sleepiness during the day. Sour taste in the mouth. Vertigo when kneeling or standing. Pressing headache.

*Mercurius Sol.* — Spongy, easily bleeding gums. Fetid smell from the mouth. Ptyalism. Tongue broad, flabby and ingested. Sorethroat. Violent burning thirst, day and night. Discharge of mucus from the rectum. *Stitches in the eyes. Periodical vanishing of sight : Aversion to light and to look into the fire. Mistinesss before the eyes. Black spots, flies or sparks before the eyes. Ulceration of the margin of the eyelids. Lachrymation. Ciliary infection.* Offensive and oily or sour-smelling sweat. Perspiration gives no relief, and accompanies almost all complaints. Rheumatic pains, worse at night.

*Natrum Mur.* — Chronic coryza, with loss of smell and taste. Ptyalism. Longing for bitter food and drink. Continuous thirst. Evacuations difficult, with stitches in the rectum. Passes blood with the stools. *Unsteadiness of vision; objects become confused. Dim sight, as if looking through gauze or feathers; objects seem covered with a thin veil. Sees only one-half of an object. Fiery zigzag appear around all objects. Eyes give out in reading or writing. Pain in and above the eyes, coming on and going off with the sun. Lachrymation in the open air.* Throbbing, as if little hammers in the temples. Palpitation worse from the slightest exertion or noise.

*Nitric Acid* — Mercurial and syphilitic ulcers in the mouth and fauces with pricking pains. Gums swollen and easily bleeding. Foetor oris. Violent thirst. *Cataract of the right eye. Regions of the eyes sore and painful to touch. Burning pain in the eyes. Vision obscured when reading. Black spots before the eyes. Objects appear dark. Corneal ulcers. Lachrymation.* Varices of the anus swollen, burning and bleeding after every evacuation. Frequent desire to urinate, with scanty discharge of dark-brown, bad smelling urine. Sycotic condylomata.

*Phosphorus* — Especially suitable for lean and slender persons. Great liability to take cold. Painfulness of the larynx, preventing talking. Difficult inspiration. Cough worse in the evening and at night. Burning sensation" over the body. *Mistiness of sight.Gauze before the eyes. Sees halo around the candle. Cataracta viridis. Black moles floating before the eyes. Aversion to light.* Hunger soon after eating. Great thirst, with longing for something refreshing. Vomiting of what has been drunk, as soon as it becomes warm in the stomach. Haemorrhoidal tumour easily bleeding.

*Plumbum* — Obstinate constipation. Stools hard, lumpy, difficult to expel. Violent colic. Painful pressure in the stomach. Intense thirst, especially for cold water. *Cloudiness before the eyes inducing one to rub them. Dimness of vision, especially on right side. Nightly tearing pains in the eyes and forehead. Could hardly distinguish day from night. Eyeballs feel too large.* Vertigo, especially on stooping and on turning the eyes upwards. Strangury. Anxiety about the heart and palpitation. Heavy and difficult breathing. Paralysis of the lower limbs and feet.

*Pulsatilla* — Is especially suitable for the females, who are quiet, mild and yielding in their nature. Cannot describe her ailments without weeping. Feeling of chilliness with pains and thirstlessness with most of the complaints. Vertigo when rising from a seat. *Amblyopia from supperession of menstrual discharge. Dimness of sight, with lachrymation in the open air. Flashing of fire before the eyes. Dryness of eyes and eyelids, feeling better from cold application or bathing. Discharge of muco-purulent matter from the eyes.* Agglutination of the eyelids in the morning. Frequent attacks of diarrhoea, with painless and changeable evacuations. Desire for cold food and drinks.

*Rhus Tox.* — *Is useful in suppuration of the cornea after extraction of the lens; also in pan-ophthalmitis after operation. Eyelids red, swollen, oedematous, especially the upper, and spasmodically closed. Profuse gushing of tears on opening the eyelids. Orbital cellulitis. Cheek under eye dotted with red pimples.*

*Lids agglutinated in the morning, with purulent mucus. Obscurity of vision. Extreme confusion of sight*. Triangular redness at the tip of the tongue.
*Senega*. — Light sleep at night, the least noise wakens him. Very profuse perspiration, especially on the chest, arm-pits and genitals. Perspiration from the least exertion. *Cataract, especially after an operation. Obscuration of sight, with glistening before the eyes, worse from rubbing them. Swelling of the eyelids. Eyes pain as if they were pressed out, as if the eyeballs were being expanded, especially in the evening at candle light*. Cough with copious expectoration of tough mucus. Chronic bronchitis or bronchial asthma. Oppressed breathing, as if the chest were not wide enough. Violent palpitation of the heart. Dyspnoea, as from stagnation in the lungs.
*Sepia — Chiefly called for cataract in women, and who suffer from uterine complaints. Particularly useful in the incipient stage. Sparks before the eyes. Green halo around the candle light. Black spots hovering and swimming before the eyes. Burning pain and pressure in the eyeballs*. Falling off of the hair. Loss of smell or fetid odour from the nose. Ozaena; blowing of large lumps of yellowish-green mucus and blood from the nose. Continuous, debilitating sweats. During menstruation, depression, toothache, headache, bleeding of the nose, and soreness in the limbs. Stools insufficient, retarded, like sheep-dung.
*Silicea — Cataract, especially of the right eye, after suppressed foot-sweat. Spots and cicatrices on the cornea. When reading the letters run together or look pale. Obscuration of sight, as from a gray cover. Black spots and fiery sparks before the eyes. Aversion to light. Ulcers on the cornea. Lachrymation in the open air*. Profuse, sour-smelling sweat, on the head only. Tendency to take cold in the head, which cannot possibly be left uncovered. Obstinate constipation. Stools after being partly expelled, slip back again. Aversion to warm, cooked food. Desires only cold things.
*Sulphur* — Is especially called for dirty and filthy people, prone to skin affections. Aversion to being washed; always worse after a bath. *Burning and smarting sensation in the eyes — dimness of vision, — acrid tears. Feeling as of a splinter of glass in the eyes. Cortical cataract especially of the left eye*. Intense thirst. Desire for sweets and highly seasoned food. Burning sensation in the soles, compelling him to put them out of bed-cover. (XV Chapter VIII)

## Phosphorus

I have used phosphorus in pneumonia and phthisis scores and scores of times with strikingly curative results, so have thousands more. Those who deny this power of phosphorus — I, of course, mean *free* phosphorus —

must bring me more than mere words before I can admit their denial as having any value. (XX 25)

If a normal individual gets chilled and a pneumonia follows as a consequence, the disease that we have to deal with has a no longer existing cause : the chill, which is over and past. What remains is effect, and has located itself in the lungs; the distressed breathing, the cough, the bloody sputum, etc. These are now the disease from alpha to omega.

*Phosphorus* administered as a remedy will cure this *chill-pneumonia*, and there is an end of it; patient gets quite well, little the worse for it.

If a foreign body — say a little nail — gets into the lung substance, and there sets up a pneumonia with distress of breathing, cough bloody expectoration, etc.;; here we have a still existing cause — the nail. *Phosphorus* administered as a remedy will at first, perhaps, seem to cure his nail-pneumonia, just as it did the chill-pneumonia, but then the affair hibs, retrogrades, exacerbates.

The phosphorus is homoeopathic to the pneumonia *per se* but *not* to the nail. The nail is here typical of any material still persisting cause such as weak heart, valvular disease, microbes, &c.

Supposing the pneumonia to be caused by still active and multiplying microbes, the phosphorus would play the same part here as in nail-pneumonia; it could not get rid of the nail; it cannot get rid of the microbes. (XX 26)

## Picric Acid

In the debility from jaundice. I have found *Picric acid* very helpful. I have commonly used it in the third dilution. (XVII 83)

## Post-Influenzal Remedies

*Cypripedium pubescens, Cypripedin, and Scutellaria laterifolia,* and *Scutellarin,* have long been my sheet anchors in post-influenzal neuroses. (XXII 34)

## Pyrogen

I have found that *Pyrogenium* is indeed "the *Aconite* of the typhous or typhoid quality of pyrexia," as Drysdale so tersely puts it.

To what form, then, should we expect *Pyrexin or Pyrogen* to be applicable? The true clue to this is given, I think, by the state of the blood, for that is the most marked and important of the signs of septicaemia; the local congestions and extravasations not being so constant or so grave as respects the issue. If we contrast the characteristic hyperisoton state of the blood in inflammatory fever, displaying its bright colour, buffy coat, firm coagulum, and the adherence of the red corpuscles in rolls, with the septicaemic state of blood already described, showing its dark and dissolved state, loose coagulum, the red corpuscles adhering in clumps, and the increase of white corpuscles, we shall see well-marked grounds of distinction. This latter state of the blood is very similar to, if not identical with, that which belongs to typhous or adynamic fevers, and, indeed, in describing fatal cases of septicaemia after wounds the analogy of the symptoms is so great with these fevers that the word 'typhous' is generally used in describing them.

We shall find it convenient to go back to the terms of Cullen, viz., synocha for inflammatory fever, the typhous or typhoid condition for the low adynamic or asthenic character or quality of fever,and synochus for the mixed kind, which is inflammatory at the beginning and typhous at the end. I do not know that the more accurate discrimination of the typhous, enteric, and relapsing fevers into distinct specific diseases gives any ground for denying the existence of the above distinctions of the character in the pyrexial state in general, and, therefore, we should still keep up the words inflammatory and typhous or typhoid, as expressive of different qualities or characters of fever, and not of distinct febrile diseases.

"As *Aconite* is well known to be the most important of the remedies for the synochal or inflammatory pyrexia, so the most summary indication for *Pyrogen* would be to term it the *Aconite* of the typhous or typhoid quality of pyrexia. This being a condition and not a distinct disease, it is to be looked for as occurring in a variety of disease such as the typhous and enteric fevers themselves always, and more or less it may occur in intermittents, so-called bilious remittents, in certain varieties or stages of the exanthemata, especially scarlatina, measles and smallpox, of dysentery, and of epidemic pneumonias, diphtheria, etc. From the gastroenteric symptoms *Pyrogen* may possibly also apply to some stage of cholera and to yellow fever. It is, of course, to be distinctly understood that this substance is only recommended, at certain stages and phases of these diseases, and entirely as a remedy of a secondary or subordinate character, and not in any sense as a *specific* for the whole disease.

At all events, we easily see from the above considerations that reasonableness of the expectation that any remedy which could moderate and control the concomitant non-specific pyrexia in the specific fevers would thereby palpably diminish the average mortality, even though it could not cut short the specific disease itself. Whether *Pyrogen* be such a remedy remains to be seen; at present we have only to show that a place is open for a possible agent of this kind. (XII 25)

## Quercus

**On a Remedy Homoeopathically Antidotal to the Effects of Alcohol.** For some years past I have been acquainted with a remedy that antidotes the effects of alcohol very prettily, as I will now proceed to show (Case 460, Part III). I enter upon the subject in this place, because it deserves to be made widely known, and also because, in the treatment of gout, the alcoholism not infrequently bars the way. The remedy I refer to is the distilled spirit of acorns — *Spiritus glandium quercus.* (XXI 77)

I might add that the *Quercus* will *cause* giddiness, and it is, moreover, a mild, yet powerful spleen medicine. (XX 205)

**Does the action of the *Spiritus Glandium Quercus* Extend to the Liquor Habit?** I think I must answer this very largely, though not entirely, in the negative. Its action antidotes the alcoholic state promptly and effectively, and the craving is at times greatly lessened, and in here and there a case cured altogether; but speaking broadly, it stops short of the liquor habit. Just as *Urtica urens* will not cure the gouty disposition, except in a small degree, only helping the organism to cast out the gouty product itself, and so leaving it strengthened, so the *Glandium quercus* will not cure the liquor habit beyond a very limited degree. (XXI 97)

## Ring worm and Bacillinum

The metamorphosis wrought in the bad or poor constitutions of ringworm patients subjected to the influence of Bacillinum (high, and mark well. in very infrequent doses) is simply beautiful, and a delight to the heart of the physician who loves his work for its own sake, and the more so if he has a fair share of the milk of human kindness in him. (XVIII 18)

## Ringworm — Sepia & Tellurium

Hughes, in his *Manual of Therapeutics*, says that Herpes circinnatus (ringworm of the surface) is usually treated, and with fair success, by *Sepia*, but that when the proving of *Tellurium* produced so similar an eruption, he (Dr. Hughes) followed Dr. Metcalf in prescribing it instead of *Sepia* for this disorder, and has never failed to cure it speedily thereby. (XVIII 10)

## Rubia Tinctorum

By the way, *Rubia tinctorum* is an excellent remedy in splenic anaemia. I usually give 10 drops of the strong tincture three times a day. (XXII 56)

## Sanguinaria

Dr. Hering says : "This is the best remedy in most cases of migraine or sick headache. Still, it must prove most useful when the attacks occur paroxysmally, namely, every week, or at longer intervals; or when the pains begin in the morning, increase during the day, and last till evening; when the head seems to feel that it must burst, or as if the eyes must be pressed out, or when the pains are digging, attended with sudden piercing, throbbing lancinations through the brain, involving the forehead and top of the head in particular, and being more severe on the right side, followed by chills, nausea, vomiting of food or bile, forcing the patient to lie down and preserve the greatest quiet, as every motion aggravates the sufferings, which are only relieved by sleep." (XIV 106)

Dr. Mills regards what he calls "sun headaches" that is, those increasing in violence with the sun's ascent, decreasing as it declines, when preceded by *scanty urine* and pass off attended by *profuse flow of clear urine*, as indicating *Sanguinaria*, and the *urine symptom as its keynote*. (XIV 109)

## Sanguisuga

I have used *Sanguisuga off.* — the good old leech of glorious memory — for a number of years in some cases of haemorrhage, and at times with striking effect; at times it has failed me. I was first led to use it from perusing a short notice (the reference to which I have unfortunately mislaid) of some physiological experiments performed with it on the continent, from which it appeared the leech decomposes the blood in some way and causes haemorrhage, and hence I conclude that it is homoeopathic to haemorrhage whereof the cause lies in the blood itself rather than in the tissues through which the blood passes.

And this would seem to explain why the bleeding from leech *bites* is often out of all proportion to the actual lesion in the continuity produced by the mechanical *bite*.

I once saw a case of very nearly fatal bleeding from a few leech-bites in the inflamed neck of a young man, and yet the lesions were quite insignificant. Whether the leech has ever been used as an internal remedy by anyone but myself I am not aware. (XX 326)

## Sciatica — Remedies

This common complaint has yielded in my hands most frequently to antisycotics, and that quickly, often too when spas and very violent measures had entirely failed. And *Aconite and Rhus* have at times helped, perhaps, when the pain was due to chronic neurilemmatitis. Indeed, the symptom *pain* might very well be chosen as a test of medical systems were it not for the incapacity of the bulk of mankind, professional, and lay, to see clearly and to distinguish the essential and fundamental difference between curing a pain from the ground and gagging the pain-telling nerve. (XIV 79)

## Scilla

Although I may be in some doubt as to whether *Carbo veg.* really acts healingly upon a diseased spleen, I am, on the contrary, very sure about *Scilla.* I have found it quickly and surely helpful in such painful spleen diseases-affections painful and beyond any doubt in and of the spleen. (X 44)

## Spigelia

**The Neuralgia of Spigelia (Hart).** Periodical headache, generally confined to the right temple, or to the left eye and left temple, pulsating, darting or boring, commencing every morning with the rising of the sun, reaching its height at midday, and gradually declining till the sun sets, and accompanied with pale face, nausea, and vomiting. Aggravated by motion, stooping, noise, thinking, or mental emotion. (XIV 111)

## Splenic Flexure Remedies

But not every case of asthma, due to the spleen, will yield to *Carbo.* Those stomach pains that, as they pass off, lose themselves in the left hypochondrium, and which I put down to the spleen, I have at times cured with *Carbo*; more frequently, however, with other spleen remedies.

Kidney affections, with dropsy, due to primary spleen disease, I have never tried to cure with *Carbo,* because I thus far have managed to cure them with other remedies, and I do not hold it to be right to try experiments from mere curiosity. (X 43)

## Spleen Remedies

Those I have tried are — *Galiopsis grandiflora,* a celebrated spleen remedy of the old time, and not to be depised; and *Rubia tinctoria,* which is also undoubtedly justly credited with being a splenic, but I have not used it often enough myself to be able to say anything satisfactory about it. (X 50)

My first and only literary acquaitance with *Ceanothus Americanus* is the very short empirical account of it in Hale's *New Remedies,* which I read some five or six years ago. Previously I had frequently felt a difficulty in treating a pain in the left side, having its seat, apparently, in the spleen. *Myrtus communis* has a pain in the left side, but that is high up under the clavicle; the pain that is a little lower is the property of *Sumbul;* still lower of *Acidum fluoricum;* a little further to the left of *Acidum oxalicum;* more to the right of *Aurum;* right under the left breast of *Cimicifuga rac.*

These remedies promptly do their work when these left-sided pains are a part of the disease-picture, but they will not touch the pain that is deep in behind the ribs of the left side; more superficially *Bryonia* has it; a little deeper than *Bryonia, Pulsatilla nutal,* will touch it; and so will *Juglans regia,* which poor Clothar Muller proved as a student. But the real splenic stitch requires *China, Chelidonium, Berberis, Chininum sulphuricum* or *Conium,* or *Ceanothus Americanus.* (X 14)

## Thuja

In chronic disease, when the right remedies seem barred in their action, Hahnemann, on the off-chance that it might be due to psora, recommended his disciples to interpose *Sulphur* as the great, most likely, antipsoric. Most of us have found this a very valuable clinical suggestion. Similarly, I have found that vaccinosis frequently bars the way, and then *Thuja* comes in with simply the beautiful effect of a genuine *simillimum.* Spider naevi generally disappear under *Thuja* 30, long used and infrequently repeated. (XXII 52)

## — and Vaccinosis

**On Vaccinosis and its Cure by Thuja Occidentalis, with remarks on Homoeoprophylaxis.** FEAR not, critical reader, this is not an anti-vaccination treatise, for the writer is himself in the habit of vaccinating his patients, *au besoin,* and he believes that vaccination does protect, to a certain large extent, from the small-pox, though the protection must necessarily cease as soon as the vaccinated person has slowly returned to his pristine state of pure health.

The writer starts with this declaration just to clear the ground, and to explain that the following pages are neither pro-vaccinational nor anti-vaccinational in the ordinary sense, inasmuch as their scope is essentially one of aetiopathology and cure, and of Homoeoprophylaxis. — That is to say : the writer's aim is to shew *firstly* that there exists a diseased state of the constitution which is engendered by the vaccinial virus ( the so-called lymph), which state he proposes to call VACCINOSIS, or the *Vaccinial State*; and *secondly*, that there exists also in nature a notable remedy for said Vaccinosis, *viz* : the *Thuja Occidentalis* : and *thirdly*, that *Thuja* is a remedy of Vaccinosis by reason of its homeopathicity thereto; *fourthly*, that the law of similars also applies to the prevention of disease.

*Vaccinosis* does not express merely the same thing as *Vaccinia*, for the latter means the febrile reaction which occurs in an organism after vaccination, with special reference to the local phenomena at the point where the vaccinial pus, or lymph, is inserted. Sometimes, also, the term vaccinia is applied to a general varioloid eruption following vaccination; but here, vaccinia is commonly held to end.

Now all this is included by me in the term vaccinosis, but still *I do not mean merely this, but also that profound and often long-lasting morbid constitutional state* engendered by the vaccine virus, which virus we usually euphemistically term "lymph." Lymph, of course, it is not, but pus-matter — and why a specific virulent pus should be persistently called "lymph" seems somewhat *peculiar*, and is eminently unscientific. As I am a lover of purity, and incidentally also of philological purity, I call this "lymph" pus, because it is pus and not "lymph". The diseased state, then, engendered by this vaccinial pus, by vaccination, is *Vaccinosis* : and in it are not included any other diseases whose causes may be accidentally or incidentally contained in the vaccine pus, — such as scrofulosis, syphilis or tuberculosis. (XIX 1)

## Tonsil Remedies

Many years ago *Baryta carb.* 30 or 12 was in very high repute for the cure of enlarged tonsils. Its reputation was well founded, as I can testify. Taken by itself, it is the biggest tonsil medicine we have. Where the tonsils have enlarged from vaccinosis, *Baryta* will not do much until the vaccinosic quality has been got rid of by *Thuja*, or *Silicea*, or what not. Similarly, where the tuberculosic quality lies behind, *Bacill.* is needed first, and then the *Baryta*, and so on. (XXV 50)

As a rule before these have done all their work there is evidence of amelioration in the child's health, and the enlargement has somewhat lessened.

*Calcarea phosphorica* — say 3x — two or three doses a day follows well; indeed I have often been almost startled at the sudden improvement that will set in under its use : the whole child brightens up, coughs disappear, the intelligence awakens, the ribs stiffen, and the surroundings are well aware that something is being done for the enlarged tonsils.

The third trituration of the *Iodide of Mercury* will often rapidly and radically change the aspect of the enlarged tonsils.

*Calcarea iod*. 3x is often useful in the abjectly strumous.

In puny boys whose testicular development is very backward — in fact can scarcely be said to exist at all — *Aurum met*. 3 trit. is, with me, an old and well-tried remedy; it may often be noticed that, as the testicles take on life and increase in size, the tonsils diminish in bulk.

Where the tonsils are very hard and there is evidently much sclerosed connective tissue in them, the Iodide of *Barium* will help.

In stubborn cases, it will often be necessary to recur again and again to the same remedies, notably to such remedies as *Sulphur* 30, *Calc. carb*, C., *Thuja* 30, *Sabina* 30, *Bacillinum* 30 and C., before all the bars to cure are organically removed.

Sometimes *Baryta carb*. 30 alone will rapidly reduce enlarged tonsils, but alone it does not often suffice.

*Hepar sulphuris* is a classic remedy in enlarged tonsils, and in some cases *Silicea* is the remedy. (XXV 70)

## Triticum Repens

This is our common couch grass that is such a plague to the farmer, and yet if such a farmer has an irritable bladder he will walk over his couch grass, and travel a distance to see a doctor, often getting no help, for school-learning too often engenders contempt for the simple weeds, under our feet. (XXII 115)

## Tuberculinum Kochii

Being more than satisfied with *Bacillinum* I have not needed to have recourse to Koch's Tuberculinum, but in order to be sure that my high opinion of his preparation was warranted I have used *Tuberculinum Kochii* 6 in the form of tincture prepared from Koch's matrix fluid obtained from his Berlin agent, but here I will only say that I have satisfied myself that his fluid is a good anti-tubercular remedy administered internally as a homoeopathic dilution. It seemed to me, however, nothing like so good as *Bacillinum* in its therapeutic effects, and also not equal to the *Tuberculinum Swanii*; but as I have had a good deal of experience with Swan's remedy and much more with *Bacillinum*, and very little with Koch's, I would not prjudice the question, as in the meantime I must consider myself relatively unqualified to give an opinion on Koch's remedy further than to say that it certainly has power over tubercular processes. (XVI A 142)

## Tumour Remedies

Some of the little tumours of the eyelids that one commonly meets with are from a wrong condition of the stomach, the state of the pancreas seems distinctly answerable for a certain number of them, some are apparently a sequel of vaccinia, and odd articles of food are known to cause them in certain people, e.g., roast pork. Often such swellings will rapidly disappear, but not in-frequently they become hard, insensitive, and chronic. A few months of proper constitutional treatment will cure them. The remedies most commonly indicated are *Thuja occid., Argentum nitricum, Natrum sulphuricum, Pulsatilla nig., Hepar sul., Calc., Hydrastis canadensis.* (XIII 4)

## — of Breast, — Remedies

*Acidum aceticum* has a certain reputation for cancerous and benign tumours. Dr. J. C. Peters maintains that it will dissolve the "cancer cell." I have used it with advantage in cancer, but principally as an external irritant, notably in hepatic and pyloric indurations.

*Aconitum napellus* The use of *Aconite* in tumours of the breast is by no means to be despised, as it commands congestion to some extent, which is a great help. Of course it has no direct or specific action.

*Apis mel.* Of this remedy Dr. Gilchrist (a very high authority) says : "I have frequently benefited, if not cured, various malignant and semi-malignant growths with the following symptoms :

Small ulcers with a gray slough, deep, and running into one another; pain, burning; itching or stinging; sharp stinging pain in the ulcer or tumour; pus is of a light yellow colour, and scanty; erysipelatous inflammation of the surrounding skin; dark purple colour of old scars; thirst is either absent or increased for small quantities.

*Worse* in the morning; also from warmth?

"*Better* from cold water and pressure. Left side."

"Has been used in many varieties of tumour, perhaps with special adaptability to cystic formations. I have used it in case of cancerous ulceration with good results a number of times; you will find a case of *ovarian tumour* reported cured by this agent in the *North American Jour. of Hom.*, Vol. xxi., p 553, by Dr. Piersons; also one by Dr. P. H. Hale, in Raue's *An. Rec.*, 1872, p. 173. In the latter case the 1st dilution was used, in the other the high, Dr. Garnsey, of Batavia, 111., reports a case cured, in which he used *Apis* and *Apocyn. can.* in alternation (Am. Hom. Obs., Vol. iv., p. 251). In Helmuth's *Surgery*, p. 1181, a case is reported cured with some remedy in attennuation with *Arsenic*, reported by Dr. Craig. These two last cases are not as valuable as they might be, on account of the alternation of the remedies."

*Apocynum Cannabinum* — It is a solvent unquestionably. I have thus cured a case of adenoma with it, used in the form of an ointment. Its action seems, in such cases, to be powerfully solvent.

*Arnica montana* — The great sphere of *Arnica* is trauma and haematoma. Dr. Lee cured a case of "movable" tumour of the orbit with it.

*Argentum nitrum* — It is sometimes useful in cutaneous cysts, and notably in the hydraemic.

*Arsenicum* — It is a classic remedy for bleeding cancer and many cases cured or ameliorated by it have been published. It has an equally great reputation for the cure of lupus.

*Arsenicum iodatum* — It has cured cancer of the breast, and also of the womb.

*Aurum metallicum* — It is useful in mammary indurations, particularly after *Mercury* has been used.

*Aurum muriaticum natronatum*, taken by itself, is probably the best remedy for uterine tumours that we have.

*Barium* — It has a reputation for lipomata; the carbonate is used, and also the iodide and the muriate.

*Belladonna* — It is used by myself merely for its congestive effects, and of course, in refracted dose it helps and relieves.

*Bellis perennis* — A very grand remedy, but, being only a common weed, is unknown or condemned and despised. It was ever thus. I have already illustrated its use in tumours of the breast. (Case 234, etc., Part III)

*Bryonia alba* — It cured a case of fibroid tumour in the hands of Dr. C. Wesselhoeft. In my judgment, it is an important tumour medicine by reason of its demonstrated effects in arthritic states, and in circum-oophoritic peritonitis; and where the pertoneum is probably involved in the ovarian tumours, it will greatly relieve. The following note on lime is from Gilchrist :

*Calcarea carb.* — Tumours occuring in the characteristic calcarea individual. Tendency to boils; to take cold easily; deficient animal heat; cold feet; perspiration of the feet and head particularly; pus is copious, putrid, yellowish, or white like milk; similar to *Baryt. carb.*, excepting that the subjects are younger. Stapf (*Archives*, vol. iii) reports a case of encephaloma of the eye, which was cured after commencing the process with *Calc.* There is much doubt existing as to the correctness of the diagnosis. Dr. Sumner (N.Y. State Hom. Mad. Soc. Trans., Vol. ix) reports a case of ovarian tumour cured by this remedy (World's Conversion, 1876) reports a case from Helmuth of Sebaecous cyst cured; Dr Alvarez (Med. on rest. Vol. iv. p. 89) a case of lipoma; Prof. Beebe (Loc.cit. a case of fibrous tumour, in alternation with Coni. however, taken from Helmuth. I can report one case of uterine fibroid cured. A number of polypi existed : the large ones were expelled, and the smaller disappeared by absorption. Nasal and uterine polypi have been cured so frequently that no citation of cases is necessary.

*Calcarea phos.* — The indications are similar to those under the carbonate. Perhaps there is a greater tendency to deficient ossification in the case of this remedy. I have thought that the Carbonica is of special value in cases of pedunculated fibroids : the Phosphate when sessile.

*Cundurango* — Indications for this powerful drug have been already given.

*Colocynthis* — Gilchrist and Caroll Dunham have each recorded a case of ovarian cyst cured by this remedy. Sharp abdominal pains lead to its choice.

*Conium maculatum* — I have cured one case of tumour with this old favourite of Stoerk's, and it also has done me very good service in cancer of the tongue.

*Ferrum* — In the cachexia I have found *Ferrum aceticum* in small material dose of great benefit; in fact, I have often interrupted the more constitutional treatment for a little intercurrent course of iron, and with much advantage. Where there is plethora, of course a higher dilution must be used. I like Schussler's phosphate of iron (Ferr. ph.). And the picrate (Ferr. pic.), by reason of its cephalic, hepatic, haemic, and local actions, is a grand remedy.

*Galium ap.* — Drs Bailey and Clifton have had brilliant results with this remedy in cancer of the tongue, particularly the latter, who has probably cured as many tumours by medicines as any living man.

*Galium* was used in combination with glycerine, the indication was evidently "Old Herball."

*Graphites* has a well merited reputation for wens and herpes and tumours in the herpetic.

*Hydrastis canadensis* — The late Dr Bayes, had quite a reputation for tumours, and he set great store by its use.
I too, have used it a good deal and fully endorse Dr Bayes views. Dr Blake cured a case of epithelioma and also one of scirrhus with *Hydrastis*.
*Iodine* — It is not favourite of mine indeed, I hardly know how to use it, as nearly as one I see with a tumour has already had it in some form or other. However, I have used it in tumours of the pancreas with striking effect. (See Rademacher on this remedy in regard to this organ.)
*Kali chloratum* — It is a good remedy for mammary tumour that is little more than a mastitis.
*Lappa major* — I once knew a "Lady Bountiful" who used to cure poor people of swellings with a tea made of the roots of this plant. Her indication was — *the blood.*
*Kali brom.* cured a case of ovarian tumour in the hands of the late Dr. Black.
*Kali iod.* has been used with advantage in cases of supposed epithelioma. So has *Kreosote.*
*Lapis alb.* — The late Dr von Grauvogl introduced this *Urkalk gneiss* for occult cancer, glandular tumours and bronchocele. He was led t use it by having observed the tumourifacient effect of the water containing it. Von Grauvogl sent me a portion to try some years before his death, with a very kind letter which I have preserved and still cherish.
*Phosphorus* — has helped me in mammary tumours when given for menorrhagia, but I have generally used in the bleeding stage in alternation with *Carbo animalis*.
*Phytolacca dec.* — is of undoubted value in mammary tumours, but requires to be given in material doses. In refracted dose I have found benefit from it in mammary *Atrophy*; in one case, the increase in the size of the breasts was notable.
*Platina and Pulsatilla* are remedies to be remembered in mammary tumours, and also *Silicea, Acidum fluoricum, Mercurius,* and many others.
I have myself obtained the greatest help from *theories* of drug action, diatheses, and specificity of seat as well as of action; and medicines that are known as mere organ-remedies will often cure its organ of the disease that caused the tumour, and then the tumour atrophies. (XIII 64)

## Urea & Hecla

Urea (6-12) and Hecla both of which have more than once done me good service in stubborn cases of tumours. The former particularly in gouty persons. (XX 165)

## Urticarial Remedies

*Chloral hydrate* and *Urtica urens* and also *Persicaria urens* are very useful in such cases, and so is also *Bacillinum*. But where the nocturnally appearing wheals are, as it were, echoes from the paternal past, nothing equals the remedy here named as curative. The thing is cured root and branch, recurring occasionally when a new tooth sprouts, when the dose has to be repeated once, or perhaps twice, till the cure is definitely completed. (IX 163)

## Urtica Urens

I subsequently became aware that *Urtica urens* is contingently capable of producing *fever*, as some subsequent experience will show. The fever of the gouty attack is not great but still feverishness is a part of such attacks, and I should not feel sure of the homoeopathicity of a remedy thereto, did it not possess the symptom "fever" in its pathogenesis. (XXI 35)

I call the discovery, of this gravel-expelling power of *Urtica*, *great*; well, it has been *great* to me in my clinical work, and my patients are generally of the same opinion as myself, — so much so that one or two of the commercially minded among them have over and over again urged me to bring it out as my gout medicine; but I have no respect for nostrums or nostrum-mongers, and am quite content to make it known as a most valuable remedy in the treatment of acute gout, as it cuts short the attack *in a safe manner*, *viz*., by ridding the economy of the essence of the disease product, its actual suffering-producing material. (XXI 36)

The nettle is a very curious plant, that appears to follow man the world over. I have read that its original *habitat* is somewhere in Asia, whence supposedly started the wanderings of the peoples. As we all know, it dies down in the winter and shoots out again in the spring. Certain it is that it follows man wherever he goes. I lately inquired of a gentleman resident in Western Australia whether there was any nettle indigenous to that region, and received a reply to the effect that he knew of no Australian nettle, but that the English nettle sprang up everywhere near human habitations. Last year, when in the country for my holidays, I searched about to find out where the nettles best throve, and found that the plant was most flourishing in and at the sides of ditches which carried off the fluid sewage from the cottages, and thus possibly living to some extent on urinous food. This point is somewhat interesting and suggestive.

We must not only take the symptoms and cover them; we must also take the whole pathology, both of the disease and of the drug, and juxtapose the two processes, and then get in behind the symptoms and see whether in addition to the symptomatic similarity there is also coincidence of the drug pathology with the disease pathology, both running from start to goal. The reason why *Urtica* cannot cure the gout disease, but can only cure the gouty attack, is because its pathology goes only up to the product, and stops short of the production. (XXI 101)

By the way, *Urtica urens* is a splendid splenic, whose clinical history I propose to relate another time. (XX 220)

*Urtica* had in old times quite a reputation for gout and sand, and I have repeatedly noticed that patients, while taking *Urtica ur.* Q in the manner just described, have passed large quantities of sand, and in several instances such patients have been alarmed, never having passed any before in their lives.

*Urtica urens* is a very notable splenic (Case 118, Part III), and with its aid I have often cured ague. And for the common manifestations of pure gout, it is my sheet-anchor for years past. I could fill a little book with cases in proof of this statement. (IX 149)

## Urtica urens and Natrum Mur.

It is distinctly curious to note the remarkable effects of *Natrum muriaticum* and *Urtica urens* in gout, as well as in ague and malarialism. (XXI 51)

## Varicocele Remedies

The remedies called for in varicose conditions of the spermatic veins will be frequently the following: *Acidum fluoricum, Pulsatilla, Silicea, Osmium, Acidum Phosphoricum, Hamamelis,* and *Aesculus* according to the symptoms.

*Acidum fluoricum* will be indicated when there are moist palms, pain in the left side, or a history of syphilis.

*Aurum* when the testicles are very small and weak, and in those suffering from mercurialism.

*Silicea* when there are sweaty feet, or when there is a history of a suppression of pedal perspirations, and when there are chilblains.

*Osmium* when it had been produced or aggravated by a deep, hollow, low cough, seemingly coming from low down in the body.

*Acidum phosphoricum* when associated with phosphaturia and pain in the testicle.

*Pulsatilla* will suit many cases and be specially called for in the obese and those of lax fibre and tearful mood.
*Hamamelis* is the prince of vein medicines, especially topically applied. (VI 145)

## Viscum album

*Viscum album* is notable remedy, and has its place in the treatment of angina pectoris. There are certain cases of angina that are synalgiae, starting from given points in the abdomen, sometimes from one ovary, at times from both ovaries, and at others from *beneath* the spleen, rather than from the organ itself. In several of such cases *Viscum album* 1x has helped me. (XIV 164)

## Zincum Aceticum

By the way, for a fagged brain *Zincum aceticum* 1x, five drops in water night and morning, is indeed mighty for good. (see Rademacher's experiment in "Erfahrungsheillehre") (XVI 49)

Part III

# Case Reports

## NATRUM MURIATICUM

### 1. NEURALGIA — FACIAL

*Observation* — Mrs. B., æt. 24, came under my treatment in 1876, in the early months of pregnancy, with very severe neuralgia of the face. The case proved itself very obstinate, and many drugs were fruitlessly tried, but eventually it yielded to *China* given in the form of pilules saturated with the matrix tincture, which drug was chosen because of *perspiration breaking out* when the pain became very bad. The neuralgia constantly re-appeared, and finally *China* ceased to have any effect. Then *Populus tremuloides* was given simply because of its being a congener of *China* and did good, in fact quite cured for the time.

This pregnancy passed and my patient consulted me again, being again enceinte early in 1877, for the same kind of neuralgia, and this time its obstinacy nearly reduced her and her physician to despair.

The case was treated in the old Hahnemannian fashion according to the totality of the symptoms which were very few and apathognomonic, and neuralgia being always bad, and always worse, and apparently not ameliorated by anything.

After many weeks of fruitless endeavours to cure this neuralgia with medicines chosen from the repertory, I turned to Guernsey's *Obstetrics* (2nd edition) and found I had already tried all those given in his list at p. 372, 373, 374, except two; these two I then fairly tried and again failed. So my patient had received *Aconite, Belladonna, Bryonia, Calc-c., Cocculus, Cimicifuga, Coffea, Gels., Glon., Ignat., Mag-c., Nux-v., Puls., Sepia, Spig., Sulph., Verat-a., China, Populus,* and some others. Besides which she had applied, often in almost frantic despair, nearly every known anodyne, so that the soft parts of the face seemed almost macerated.

Here I suggested change of air (what should we poor practical physicians do without this *ultimum refugium*), but circumstances prevented her from leaving Birkenhead for more than a day or two, so her husband took her for little outings to New Brighton and Southport, and Chester, when it was observed that *the neuralgia was worse at the seaside* and better inland.

A happy thought struck me that this might be due to the *salt* in the air at the seaside, and, being moreover absolutely at the end of my tether, I acted on it and gave *Nat. mur.* 30, one pilule very frequently : the neuralgia at once began to get better and in a day or two was quite well. It subsequently returned at intervals, much less severely, but promptly yielded to the same remedy in the same dose. The 30th dilution was chosen simply because some pilules of this strength were in the patient's chest.

The patient was quite satisfied that *Nat. mur.* 30 effected the cure. (I 11)

## 2. SYNOVITIS RIGHT KNEE

***Observation*** — A young gentleman of about 21 years of age came under treatment for Synovitis of right knee with considerable effusion. Patient had a dirty looking skin, was constipated and had many *Nat. mur.* pains in the lower extremities.

$R_x$ *Natrum muriaticum 6.*

Fiat. pul. gr. vj.

Dose — One in water every three hours. Rest in the recumbent position.

I did not see the patient again, but he was observed by my colleague, Dr. Reginald Jones, who kindly gave me the following report : "The medicine purged the patient so severely that it had eventually to be left off; it also produced a great discharge of the urates, the urine becoming very thick therewith.

No other medicine was given and patient was quite well in a fortnight. (I 13)

## 3. RHEUMATIC FEVER

***Observation*** — Mrs. M., æt. 50, or thereabout, had a most severe attack of rheumatic fever, the joints being much swollen, red and distressingly painful. The usual homoeopathic treatment was adopted but with no great success. It was her fifth attack of rheumatic fever. Between the third and fourth week Dr. Jones and I saw her together and found this condition : Ill-coloured skin; obstinate constipation; foul tongue; *urine very pale and limpid*; great depression of spirits; fever, joints red, swelled and painful; great restlessness; low and desponding of the future; sour perspirations; insomnia; bedsores, and great weakness.

We agreed in the opinion that the emunctories had almost left off work and required to be brought back to their duty. A sharp cathartic combined with a diuretic seemed to be indicated by the general condition, but contra indicated by the profound adynamia, and hence the blessing of a *refractissima dosis*. My consultant's observation in Case 2 caused him to suggest the same remedy. So we put patient on *Nat. mur.* 6 trit., as much as would lie on a shilling every two hours in water.

No other medicine was given, and no auxiliaries used.

Next day her urine became a little cloudy; the second day the bowels were moved and the urine had a red deposit; then diarrhoea with loaded urine set in; the swelling, redness and pain in the joints went away; the skin became cleaner looking; the tongue cleaned gradually, the perspirations ceased, her spirits became brighter, and in ten days from beginning the medicine she was in full convalescence, though still very weak.

Patient suffers from chronic asthma with slight emphysema, and is always obliged to sleep in the semi-recumbent position, but for six weeks after this critical evacuation she was able to lie down in bed like anyone else without any dyspnoea.

Many months have elapsed and she is now about in her house and drives out, still asthmatic and has *chronic* rheumatic pains here and there. Her tongue was cleaner for two months than I had known it for the previous three years.

This patient lives ten miles away and was not seen often, but the husband brought daily reports, and when doing so pleaded hard day after day that the *Natrum muriaticum* might be discontinued because of its purging so severely, he fearing lest it might weaken her too much. On that account it was then given interruptedly, but with no other medicine, and the alvine and renal functions fluctuated accordingly.

Hahnemann says (*Chronische Krankheiten*, 2nd edition, vol. iv., p. 348) : "Pure salt (just the same as any other homoeopathic somatic force dynamized) is one of the most powerful antipsoric remedies."

And higher up he speaks of it as an heroic and violent remedy that, when dynamized, must be cautiously administered to patients.

Then he exclaims : "*Welche unglaubliche und doch thatsaechliche Umwandlung! — eine anscheinend neue Schoepfung!*"

Still it goes against all common sense and all one's notions of things, and no man may be blamed for declining to accept such a preposterous proposition, merely on trust; it is scarcely possible to accumulate sufficient facts to get anyone to listen to it, much less to believe it. (XI 14)

### 4.. DEEP CRACK IN LOWER LIP

***Observation*** — At this stage of things I felt curious to know what the sixth centesimal trituration of *Natrum muriaticum* might do to my humble self pathogenetically, I being in my usual health. So I took nearly ℨiv. in about ten days in little pinches dry on the tongue at odd intervals. It produced — no, that is too bold a statement. I got gradually during that time a deep crack in the middle of my lower lip, which swelled and became burning and very painful; the *Natrum muriaticum* may have had nothing to do with it, but I gave it up and both crack and swelling went away. I never had the like before, nor since.

The same symptom is noted by Hahnemann, and Dr. Allen in his *Encyclopaedia* — but removed by the latter from the regional division of the "lips," and placed under "skin" which is not only confusing, but also a mistake. (I 16)

### 5. PAIN EPIGASTRIUM

***Observation*** — Mr. H., æt. 45, came under treatment for great pain in the stomach which sent him to bed and kept him there in great agony. The last year or so he has been subject to these attacks of epigastric pain, and I was sent for to relieve this as on previous occasions, and the wife specially requested me to give something not only for this attack but to use whenever the attacks came on. He had, besides the pain, vesicles on the lips drying up into scabs. I gave *Nat. mur.* 6 trit. gr. vj. every two hours in water; next day (observed by Dr. Jones) it was followed with a great discharge of the urates and a regular attack of gout. Has since remained free from these attacks of pain, and this is now many months since.

It is impossible to tell whether the *Natrum muriaticum* had anything to do with the metastasis of the gout from the stomach to the big toe; moreover it is not now medico-scientifically fashionable to believe in metastasis. (I 16)

### 6. HEMICRANIA AND SEDIMENTOUS URINE

***Observation*** — A girl of 15, suffering from Hemicrania dextra and cloudy, thick, red, sedimentous urine. I gave her *Nat. mur.* 6 trit. and received shortly thereafter a written report "urine quite free from sediment or cloud in a way it has not been for long." The megrim was not affected.

The young lady and her mother attributed the changed condition of the urine to the powders; the urine had been in the abnormal condition for a long time and my ordination consisted only in prescribing the powders. Weeks afterwards the urine continued clear.

This case is not adapted to carry conviction to the mind, as we know that many atmospheric changes and accidental circumstances of all kinds alter the state of the water at once. (I 16)

## 7. VOMITING

*Observation* — A baby on the bottle some three months old. I find it has not slept well for some time and is now very *restless* and *fretful*, and *vomits water*. Give *Nat, mur*. 6 trit. It *at once* began to sleep two or three hours at a time and the watery vomiting ceased. Two days afterwards measles broke out.

The mother conceived a very high opinion of the soothing soporific effect of the powders. (I 17)

## 8. BACK PAIN AND THICK URINE

*Observation* — Mr. P., æt. 26, has had very thick urine for months, and for two months very great pain in small of back, worse on bending and very much worse when digging in the garden. Gave *Nat. mur*. 6 trit. The back pain and turbid urine disappeared in four days and did not again appear. (I 17)

## 9. LEUCORRHOEA

*Observation* — A lady, æt. 54, with Stillicidium lachrymarmum and bad chronic yellow excoriating leucorrhoea — *Nat. mur*. 6 trit.

In one week the leucorrhoea had quite disappeared but the Stillicidium was worse.

Chronic leucorrhoeas are not apt to disappear spontaneously in one week, though its possibility cannot be denied. (I 17).

## 10. AMENORRHOEA, CONSTIPATION AND POLYURIA

*Observation* — Unmarried lady, æt. 24, Polyuria; constipation with much flatus; amenorrhoea these two months. First symptoms *worse at the seaside*. She is rather thin with an ill-coloured skin. *Nat, mur.* 6 trit. In a few days the menses appeared, and the renal and alvine functions became normal.

She had passed her second menstrual period.

A causal nexus between the taking of the *Natrum muriaticum*, and disappearance of the symptoms is not easily established here. (I 17)

## 11. DYSPEPSIA

***Observation*** — A clergyman's wife, about 50 years of age consulted me on February 29th, 1878, complaining of severe dyspepsia with other symptoms of *Natrum muriaticum*. My visit was a hurried one so I did not enter very fully into the case. *Nat, mur.* 6 trit. vj grains in water twice a day was the prescription; it cured in three days these symptoms : "*Hiccup* occurring morning, noon, and night, for at least ten years which was brought on by Quinine; it was not a hiccup that made much noise but shook the body to the ground; it used to last about ten minutes and was very distressing."

How do you know that the hiccup was really produced by quinine? I enquired. She answered : "At three separate times in my life I have taken quinine, for tic of the right side of my face, and I got hiccup each time, the first and second time it gradually went off, but the third time it did not; when the late Dr. Hynde prescribed it, I said, do not give me quinine as it always gives me hiccup, but he would give it me; I took it and it gave me hiccup which lasted until I took your powders; it is more than ten years ago since I took the quinine."

The cure of the hiccup has proved permanent.

This patient is a most truthful Christian woman and her statement is beyond question.

She has been a homoeopath for many years and my patient off and on for more than three years, during which time I have had to treat her for chronic sore throat, vertigo, palpitation, and at one time for great depression of spirits.

She had also previously mentioned her hiccup incidentally but I had forgotten all about it, and on this occasion she did not even mention it, so as far as the hiccup goes the cure was ... a pure fluke! But it set me a-thinking about the Hahnemannian doctrine of drug dynamization for the thousandth time and has seriously shaken my *disbelief* in it.

Hiccough is a known effect of *Chininum sulfuricum* : Allen's *Encyclopaedia*, vol. iij., p. 226, symptoms 370 and 379.

We note from this case that :

1. The effects of quinine, given for tic in medicinal doses to a lady, may last for more than ten years,
2. *Natrum muriaticum in the sixth trituration* antidotes this effect of quinine,
3. While the same substance in its ordinary form, viz. common salt, does *not* antidote it even when taken daily in various quantities and in various forms for ten years. Inasmuch, then, as the crude substance fails to do what the triturated substance promptly effects, it follows, therefore,
4. *Trituration does so alter a substance that it thereby acquires a totally new power*, and consequently that —
5. The *Hahnemannian doctrine of drug dynamization* is no myth but *a fact in nature* capable of scientific experimental proof, and, inasmuch as the crude substance was taken daily for many years in almost every conceivable dose, in all kinds of solutions of the most varied strength it results —
6. and lastly. That the *Hahnemannian method* of preparing drugs for remedial purposes *is not* a mere dilution, or attenuation, but *a positively power-evolving or power-producing process*, viz. *a true potentization or dynamization*. (I 18)

## 12. CONSTIPATION AND HEADACHE

***Observation*** — A lad, æt. 12, living at Parkgate. He suffers for some time from constipation, loss of appetite, dirty looking complexion, emaciation, frontal headache going round to the back, sleepiness towards evening and first thing in morning, urine thick with nasty smell. Excepting the "nasty" smell, which the boy could not define, I find all these symptoms in the pathogenesis of *Natrum muriaticum* in Allen's *Encyclopaedia of Pure Materia Medica* and numbered respectively 529, 353, 251, 885, 64, 970, 561.

Therefore *Nat. mur.* 6, and that six grains in water forenoon and afternoon. After taking 24 powders he returned cured of all the symptoms except the odour of the urine and the emaciation, and "feeling very much better". The prescription was repeated and patient did not return. His father subsequently informed me that the cure was complete. (I 20)

## 13. CHLOROSIS AND HYPOGASTRIC PAIN

***Observation*** — Young lady about 28 years of age : emaciation, chlorosis, for eighteen months, slight bearing down in the hypogastrium, gradually getting worse, and the last week increasing to very severe cramp beginning in the back and coming round to the pubic arch, and, when walking felt severely in the knees, had frequently to sit down to get relief from the hypogastric pain, urine muddy for a long time, obstinate chronic constipation, the mouth is dry but there is no thirst, taste disagreeable, bitter.

Nearly all these symptoms are in the pathogenesis of *Natrum muriaticum*. Hence *Nat. Mur.* 6, twenty-four six-grain powders taken in a fortnight resulted in the *permanent disappearance of all the symptoms* excepting the emaciation and the chlorotic conditions, for which she was put on *Phosphorus*.

As to the emaciation she gained six pounds in ten weeks, but this gain in weight was partly made which under *Ferrum* 6, for haemoptysis, chronic cough and large moist rales in the left lung, and these symptoms having disappeared under *Ferrum* 6, she went into the country "For three weeks and returned with the above symptoms. (I 20)

## 14. CHILLINESS

***Observation*** — Gentleman, æt. 34 or thereabouts, has suffered from a *general feeling of chilliness* (attributed by himself to a poor circulation), for *more than two years, sleepiness and drowsiness* after dinner for two months, compelling him to go and lie down; black spots before the eyes; disagreeable taste in the mouth, sour; watery eyes; urine clear; bowels moved twice a day; looks very pale.

Ordered him *Nat. mur. 6* trit. six grains in water twice a day.

Having taken twenty-four of such powders he paused a few days and returned stating that the *chilliness had quite disappeared* and *also the postprandial drowsiness*, the black spots had quite disappeared but were returning again a little, the sour taste was gone, the watery state of the eyes as bad as ever, *the urine had become cloudy*.

In this case the medicine was evidently quite homoeopathic to the condition of the patient, and it is manifest that the *Nat. mur.* 6 profoundly affected his organism, as the chilliness of more than two years duration quite disappeared, as also the after-dinner drowsiness. (I 21)

## 15. PHLYCTENULAR OPHTHALMIA

***Observation*** — Lad of 12 came under observation on March 30th, 1878, suffering from a group of symptoms that collectively are conveniently called Phlyctenular ophthalmia. The left eye was spasmodically closed from the photophobia. A month before he had caught a cold in this eye, and it had remained closed, inflamed and painful ever since, and was not getting any better. On everting the lids an ulcer in the cornea is observed, resulting evidently from a burst phlyctenula of about the size of a split pea. The dimness of vision from this ulcer determined the parents to seek advice, they fearing the "eye" was being affected. To leave an ophthalmia for month without seeking advice is a phenomenon that will greatly surprise many, but *not* medical men.

The prominent symptom in the case was the great lachrymation, and this is very characteristic of *Natrum muriaticum*. So six grains of *Nat. mur.* 6 trituration was given in water three times a day.

April 6th. Opens his eye wide and sees quite clearly; the photophobia, pain, inflammation and lachrymation gone; the ulcer nearly so.

Continue the medicine.

Excepting some very faint leucomatic streaks the cure was complete in a few more days.

Patient had formerly been long under my treatment for caries of the petrous portion of left temporal bone, and had got quite well of it.

*Sodium chloride* has an ancient reputation as ar antiscrofulosum, as we all know. (I 22)

## 16. GANGLION

***Observation*** — Boy of 9, with ganglion on leg of the size of a small hen's egg. Has been under my treatment for many months with no good result except very slight amelioration from *Sticta pulmonaria*. *Silicea* did no good. On Dr. Schussler's recommendation (*Abgekurzte Therapie, Vierte Auflage*, p. 46, Oldenburg, 1878), I gave *Nat. mur.* 6, six grains in water night and morning.

Three months later I received by letter the following report : "The swelling on the little boy's leg, I am glad to say is much better — *a good deal* smaller, now about the size of a small nut, and rather more in its original position — not so much under the knee joint as it was."

Continue the medicine. (I 23)

## 17. GOUT

***Observation*** — Lady, æt. 63. Regular gout in left big toe and foot. Patient is fond of beer.

$R_x$ *Nat. mur.* 6 trit. Six grains every two hours.

In four days all symptoms had disappeared. Here I *did* order her to leave off her beer, but was ... not obeyed.

Patient since this keeps a stock of these powders on hand, and calls them her "gout powders"; they have since promptly relieved two or three similar attacks, as I learn from her daughter.

Since treating this case I have used *Nat. mur.* 6 trit. frequently repeated, in several other cases of gout, with *very* great satisfaction indeed.

Query : Does the remedy cause an increased elimination of the urate of sodium? I think it probable. (I 23)

## 18. PYREXIA — RECURRENT

***Observation*** — April 21st, 1878. John H., æt. 29, seaman, had fever and ague two or three times a day, with watery vomiting, in Calcutta, in September, 1877. Was in the Calcutta Hospital three weeks for it, and took emetics, quinine and tonics. Left at the end of the three weeks cured; but before he was out of port the ague returned, or he got another, and he had a five months voyage home to the port of Liverpool. During the first three months of this homeward voyage he had two, three, four, five attacks a week, and took a great deal of a powder from the captain, which, from his description, was probably Cinchona bark, then the fever left him, and the following condition supervened, viz., "Pain in right side under the ribs, cannot lie on right side; both left calves very painful to touch, they are hard and stiff; left leg semiflexed, he cannot stretch it." In this condition he was two months at sea, and two weeks ashore; and in this condition he comes to me hobbling with the aid of a stick, and in great pain from the moving.

Urine muddy and red; bowels regular; skin tawny; conjunctiva yellow. Drinks about three pints of beer daily. I recommend him not to alter his mode of life till he is cured, and then to drink less beer. The former part of the recommendation he followed, as I learned from his brother; of the latter part I have no information.

Observation XI. bears directly on this one, we having evidently to do with an ague suppressed with *Cinchona*. Therefore ordered *Nat. mur.* 6 trit. Six grains in water every four hours.

April 27th — Pain in side and leg went away entirely in three days, and the water cleared at once; but the pain returned on the fourth day in the left calf only, which to-day is red, painful, swelled and pits. He walks without a stick.

Continue medicine.

May 4th — Almost well; feels only a very little pain in left calf when walking. Looks and feels quite well, and walked into room with perfect ease without any stick.

He thinks he had a cold shake a few nights ago. He continues to perspire every night; ever since he got the ague the sheets have to be changed every night.

Continue medicine.
May 11th — Quite well. No medicine.
July 20th — Continues well.
The last two reports were obtained by me from his relations, he, being well, not thinking it worth while (notwithstanding his promise to report himself) to come again after the third visit on May 4th.
Considering that patient had been a fortnight here on shore before coming to me, it is not probable that his rapid cure after taking the *Nat. mur.* was due to the climate. Still this is the weak point in the case, if it have any.
Patient and doctor both think the medicine wrought the cure; others may think differently.
It is to be noted that the salt provisions and sea air during a voyage did not cure it. (I 24)

## 19. CHILLINESS AND SLEEPLESSNESS

***Observation*** — Mrs. B., æt. 53. For four or five weeks *cold shakes* many times a day and night, beginning in the shoulders like cold creeps, and going down the back and then all over; cold creeps in legs in bed at night; head cold and sweaty; nauseous taste in mouth; great sleeplessness these four or five weeks, viz. wakes at 2 a.m., and is unable to get off to sleep again.
She is very tearful; merely describing her symptoms brings tears into her eyes.
$R_x$ *Nat. mur.* 6 trit. Six grains in water every four hours.
On my calling a few days later to see how she was progressing, I got the following report : — "The cold creeps and shakes left off after the first powder" (She speaks of the powders subsequently as "those powders that made me warm".). Feels altogether warmer now, not like the same, and sleeps well. She never had ague.
Two months after this I had occasion to see her daughter, when patient (the mother) said, "Those powders did me so much good that I have been better than I had been for years."
Subsequent to the cure I thought I should like to know whether patient was in the habit of partaking of salt with her food; and on enquiring was much astonished to hear the following statement from her :
"About a year ago I was recommended by a friend to take a good deal of salt, as she thought it would be good for me, and since then I have taken about one-and-a-half teaspoonfuls a day often spread on bread."
Query : Was this a case of chronic salt poisoning antidoted by its own

dynamide?

This is a most interesting observation indeed. Here we have a lady who in addition to partaking of salt in the ordinary way with her food, and in her food, had actually partaken of one-and-a-half teaspoonfuls of salt daily for twelve months, and was even still doing so during the cure, and *yet the very first powder of triturated salt* wrought such a marked change. The difference in the look of the patient was also remarkable : at my first visit she came to me in her drawing room with a shawl over her shoulders, and looking evidently cold; at my second visit only a few days later she wore no shawl, and was quite free from any chilly feeling. This lady suffered for years from *Angina pectoris* (true breast pang), and had been given up by members of both schools to the brandy bottle; but under my treatment (extending over two years) she made a complete recovery, having been now quite well of it these 18 months. (I 25)

## 20. COLDNESS IN LEGS

***Observation*** — Mrs. W., æt. 60. Came under treatment for coldness of the legs from the knees to the feet, for three months; she cannot keep them warm in any manner; at night she wraps them up in flannel, and encases them also by day, but still they are cold; the coldness is subjective but not objective; she suffers also very much from sleeplessness and great nervous irritability.

$R_x$ *Nat. mur.* 6 trit.

At the next visit a few weeks afterwards she reported that she had been promptly cured of her old insomnia, and also of the coldness of the legs, but the legs were not as she would like, the coldness having given place to a burning feeling, especially in the veins of the part, which now swell. She no longer wraps up or encases her legs, but on the contrary they are almost too warm.

To continue the medicine.

The cure was permanent. The medicine so improved her nervous state that she still speaks of it as the "powders that soothed her nerves." (I 26)

## 21. CONSTIPATION

***Observation*** — Constipation, of long standing, in a pale anaemic young lady of 23; only one motion in two or three days.

$R_x$ *Nat. mur.* 6 trit. Twenty-four six-grain powders, one in water forenoon and afternoon.

This one set of powders quite cured it; there is now daily stool. Also the menses came on a week late (*very* unusual), and the usual painfulness was absent; they were also not so excessive as usual. (I 26)

## 22. OEDEMA PRAEPUTIUM AND INTERTRIGO

*Observation* — A gentleman, æt. 60, with oedema of the praeputinum (prepuce) for some weeks; severe intertrigo between thighs and scrotum, with a good deal of acrid discharge, and considerable excoriation; this condition has existed for many months, notwithstanding daily ablutions often several times repeated. Patient is arthritic and very melancholy and despondent.
His skin is very dusky and unhealthy looking.
$R_x$ *Nat. mur.* 6 trit. Six grains four times a day.
In a week the oedema and intertrigo were nearly well, and he was in very much better spirits, and at the end of the second week he was well. He continues well, and the skin of his face is lighter in colour, but the colour of that of the trunk remains as before. The change in his mood was quite remarkable. (I 27)

## 23. PAIN JAW (NEURALGIA)

*Observation* — Gentleman of 35. Pain in left side of lower jaw extending to the end tooth of left upper jaw, and up to the left eye, always after food, throbbing wrenching pain, *making the tears come into his eyes*; the pain he describes as terrible, and it lasts about an hour.
He has been in this condition for three months, which coincides with his leaving Liverpool and coming to reside in Tranmere.
Urine high coloured and thick.
The pain evidently proceeds from a decayed tooth.
He sleeps well after the after-supper pain has gone.
$R_x$ *Nat. mur.* 6 trit. Six grains in water three times a day.
In a week he reported : Pain much better, it comes on and lasts only five or six months, *and no tears come into his eyes.*
To continue the medicine.
The next report was that just as he thought he was cured he caught a slight cold, and the pain came on in all its original violence, when a dentist relieved him of both tooth and pain.
Goes under treatment for haemorrhoids. The fact that the pain returned in all its original violence is only what we should expect under the circumstances, and it militates against the case as one of *permanent* cure, but does not invalidate the evidence of the potent drug *action.* (I 27)

## 24. CHILLINESS FROM SCANTY PERSPIRATION

*Observation* — A gouty gentleman of 70. Until three years ago he was in the habit of perspiring freely, but latterly he perspires less, and for *three years* he has always felt *chilly and cold*.

Urine bloody and thick; he urinates with great difficulty, and uses the catheter at night these two years.

He takes *Nat. mur.* 6 trit. for three weeks, and reports that after the first day or two he ceased using the catheter altogether, having sufficient power over the bladder; the urine is free from blood and slime, but still thick, but not so red or brick-dusty; he is more costive than usual, and feels considerably warmer.

He begs to go on with the medicine, to which I agree.

He did not consult me again, but when he came to pay his little bill he informed me that he had gradually got quite well of his chilliness, that his urine had become normal, and that he no longer needed to pass the catheter at all.

The urine may *possibly* have come right of itself, and passing the catheter those two years *may* have been a mere habit and unnecessary; but *how* are we to account for the disappearance of the cold, chilly sensation that had lasted three years? (I 28)

## 25. CHILLINESS AND PROFUSE URINATION

***Observation*** — Gentleman of 50, usually enjoying good health, and of splendid physique. Symptoms : For the last six weeks coldness of the abdomen, from the navel downwards, including the genitals, swelling of the abdomen after late dinner, with flatulence; passes a very large quantity of water with a strong odour; it does not contain any sugar; he is cold about the legs, and is restless at night, with cold creeps from navel down the legs; as he sits on the sofa before me, I notice that he holds both his hands tight over the pubes; and to the enquiry why he does so, he replies that he is so cold about those parts that he holds his hands there to warm them. The sensation is as if his shirt were wet and cold; when he urinates it seems as if he would never leave off for the dribbling. Fearful thirst of mouth, not of the stomach; bowels regular; tongue coated, breath foul. Very despondent of himself.

Takes vapour baths regularly. Here the chilliness, profuse urination and thirst seem the prominent symptoms and, as we all know, they are those of *Natrum muriaticum*.

$R_x$ *Nat. mur.* 6 trit. gr. vj. Fiat pulv. Tales xxiv.

One in water four times a day.

Eight days later : The coldness a great deal better; does not pass quite so much water, and its smell is less bad, the coldness of legs better a great deal, as also that of the pubic parts; the thirst is also much better, so also the tongue; breath sweet; feels better all over; warmer.

Is anxious to continue the medicine, which is done.
He did not come again, so I wrote to him to enquire how he was doing, and received a reply to the effect that the second lot of powders had finished the cure, except a little thirst, for which he intended coming to see me again, but he never did.
From a mutual acquaintance I learn he continues well.
In this case the amelioration commenced immediately after the powders were taken, and as far as I can see the cure can be attributed to them only. (I 28)

## GOLD AS A REMEDY IN DISEASE

### 26. DROPSY LOWER LIMBS WITH DEPRESSION

The following is a case of dropsy of the lower extremities, which came under my observation some two years ago. I was fetched, I think it was one Sunday, to see a lady in Cheshire; it was feared she was beyond recovery. I found my patient, a lady of about fifty, in bed; her lower extremities were swollen, painful, they pitted on pressure, and were worse at night, better in the morning. This oedema had been coming on for a week or two, but it had usually on for a week or two, but it had usually quite disappeared by the morning, and thus caused but very little anxiety, but now it had greatly increased even in bed, and very naturally was causing great alarm. Dropsy is almost always a grave symptom, though not always. In this case I think it was. There was a history of many illnesses, and altogether this drug-picture presented itself :

1. There was dropsy, and patient had
2. Great depression of spirits, amounting to
3. Profound melancholia
4. Then there was great difficulty of breathing, and
5. Weak pulse and feeble heart
6. She was psoric, and had a good deal of
7. Discharge from the nose, that at times contained some blood.

I gave her the *Muriate of Gold* in the third decimal dilution, but I do not remember the exact number of drops or the repetition of the dose, but the dose was not less than one drop (it may have been two or three), and as often as every two or three hours, and given in water.
The case got rapidly well, all the oedema having permanently disappeared in less than a week. Eighteen months after this she informed me she had never since had any return of the dropsy, though her health was

anything but good. This was only a recent case, and, though grave, was yet not severe as to the dropsy, but the despondency was almost a substantive malady.

In this case Gold acted as veritable pick-me-up, and I submit that the remedy was homoeopathically indicated, and the cure a homoeopathic one; about the dose I will not quibble; with me the best dose is the one that cures. (II 102)

## 27. SQUAMOUS SKIN DISEASE

*Case of Squamous Skin Disease* (M. Golfin in Chrestiens Mémoire). — A gentleman, thirty-two years of age, of healthy parentage, and of lymphatic temperament. He has a humid squamous eruption on the left arm and hand. A year previously he had successively gonorrhoea, the itch, and syphilis, which latter was badly treated. Then ophthalmia, eruptions on the skin of an ill-defined character, and finally *dartre* (tetter). Depurative treatment for three months, but in vain.

Short course of treatment with sulphur ointment and another with one of the acetate of lead. Then a repercussion from sulphurous baths : hereafter violent cough, causing great distress with copious expectoration and with pains in the chest. A large blister on the arm, tepid baths and sudorifics, reproduce the exanthem, and the pulmonary irritation yields somewhat to soothing and anodyne treatment. Then treatment with perchloride of Gold rubbed into the tongue and pills of oxide of Gold prepared with potash, and many other remedies supposed to be auxiliary to the treatment with *Aur-m.*

Patient quite recovered, his recovery being preceded by long-lasting perspirations. Is since married and has healthy offspring. (II 110)

## 28. SKIN DISEASE

*Case of Severe Skin Disease; Noli me tangere,* by M. Souchier. Alexandrine D ___, eldest daughter of an inhabitant of Drome, enjoyed good health until she was eleven years of age (she is now, December, 1826, nineteen). At this period her father and mother, who state that they have always had good health, were surprised to see her two cheeks become the seat of a peculiar eruption that the physicians, whom they consulted for her, called *dartre vive rongeante,* and which soon made destructive progress at the end of the nose and around its base, notwithstanding the most appropriate and energetic treatment that could be devised for her at Lyons, to which place they had taken her and placed her under the care of the best physicians. Nevertheless the menses set in between thirteen and fourteen; but this brought no amelioration in her condition, as had been expected. At the age of fifteen all the soft parts of the nose had been eaten away, both cheeks were excavated by the ulcerous inflammation, to the extent of two inches in diameter; she was very thin, glands of neck much enlarged, so also the submaxillary glands, and those in all the bends of the joints. To this horrible state was soon added all the early symptoms of a tuberculous affection of the chest. Alexandrine continued in this wretched condition till the month of May, 1824, without getting either better or worse. At this period the ulcers of the nose and of the cheeks became covered with pretty large excrescences; those situated on the cartilages of the nose, being transverse, closed up the orifices of the nasal fossae, and the nasal fossae were horribly enlarged by the destruction of the wings of the nose. Such rapid progress was all the more inconceivable, as nothing was neglected to thwart and counteract it. Portal's syrup, all kinds of tonics, the most vaunted depuratives, had, as it were, been showered upon her; the most bland diet, and at the same time analeptic, with a view to the state of marasm into which she had sunk, was also adopted. Presently she ceased menstruating and then her parents lost all hope. In November, 1824, a fungous tubercle came in the region of the right eyelid; its progress was very rapid; all the other symptoms of this horrible disease were getting daily worse, when, on the 21st of November, 1824, M. Souchier was consulted, who at once declared the affection to be venereal. The coppery look of the wounds and surrounding parts was the point on which he based his diagnosis, and directed him in the choice of his remedial treatment.

Four grains of the *perchloride of Gold* and of *Sodium,* divided into thirty, twenty-nine, twenty-eight, and twenty-six fractions, were administered to her successively by being rubbed into the tongue night and morning. After the administration of the fourth grain a change for the better was observed in the state of Alexandrine : her cheeks and all the ulcerated parts of the face, which were dabbed with an ointment of Gold (five grains of powdered Gold to the ounce of lard, and altogether fifteen grains were thus used), were two-thirds healed. The excrescences, that at first had become paler, grew less, and entirely disappeared at the beginning of the sixth grain, divided into twenty fractions; the fifth had been divided into twenty-four. The fungous growth of the middle part of the right eyelid had also disappeared at this period. At the end of the seventh grain, divided into sixteen fractions, the cicatrisation of the ulcers was complete and her menses reappeared. The stubborn cough, to which the young patient had been subject from her fourteenth year, and which had sensibly diminished from the fourth grain, ceased entirely at the end of the ninth and last grain of the muriate. She got quite strong, and her physiognomy had, very nearly, resumed its former appearance. The end of the nose, although it had been eaten away down to the cartilages, was covered with a very even scar. The cheeks had again taken on almost their natural rotundity, but they have the peculiar appearance of cicatrised parts, and this face, formerly so horrible, is now not even absolutely ugly. It is now December, 1828, three years since this cure was completed, and it still holds good. The girl whom I see pretty often, *no longer gets the severe colds she was formerly subject to* in the winter months : she had also frequently spit blood. (II 29)

## 29. VIOLENT PALPITATION, FEAR OF DEATH

A young married lady used to be seized in the street with indescribable anguish, great oppression of the chest, and fear of death, and violent palpitation. I do *not* affirm that this was a case of true breast-pang with degenerative change. I tried various remedies, hit off from memory, but did no great good. Then I went to work *a la* Hahnemann (of course, I ought to have done so at first; you need not tell me that), and ascertained the *previous history* of my patient. She had, as a young girl, *an eruption in the bend of her left arm, with rhagades* (Manganese). A truly eminent dermatologist was consulted, because the young lady was going to make her social *debut*, and, of course, required to appear with bare arms. But there was that horrid eruption in the bend of the left arm, and so the *debut* had to be postponed. An ointment was applied; the eruption was — well, sent to the rightabout. She made a brilliant *debut*, soon got married, and began to have a family (once a dead foetus). She was never well — and her children? Scrofulous. I gave her *Sulphur* 30, and before the twenty-four one-drop powders were used there the identical old eruption was again in the fold of the arm. "Just as it was when I went to Dr. — ;" and patient was at once free from all other symptoms. Patient was so satisfied that there was a causal *nexus* between the exanthem in the arm and her distressing trouble, that she refused absolutely any further treatment for fear it might be *cured* (*!*) again. "I do not mind the arm; I can wear long sleeves now."

But this has carried me away from the use of Gold as a heart medicine. (II 119)

## 30. ENDOCARDITIS RHEUMATICA

"A stout young man who had already had several severe rheumatic attacks, was down with violent rheumatic fever accompanied by painful swelling of the joints. On the second day the rheumatism left the joints and attacked the heart, *causing violent irregular palpitation, with great oppression of the heart*. Five venesections, with the usual antiphlogistic arrangements, got rid of the immediate danger to life; but the subsequent treatment did not relieve patient of his *cardiac anguish,* and *hydrocyanic acid* would not afford even transitory relief of this anguish (*Beaengstigungen*)".

Then this prescription : *Aur.-Mur. gr.j. Solv. in Aq. Meliss. zj. Add Syrup. Chamom*; Zij. D.S. Every two hours a teaspoonful. Already the first night (after a few doses) was calm — the first good night since the commencement of the illness. The next day there were only slight indications of oppression and irregular heart-beat. Patient went on several days continually improving, when there appeared a painful swelling of right hand. The patient felt such benefit from it that he became quite sad when his physician, Dr. Spiritus, discontinued it in order to give other remedies to complete the cure. The symptoms I have *italicised* show that Gold was homoeopathically indicated, though it may be questioned whether Dr. Spiritus knew it. (II 121)

## 31. METASTASIS FROM FEET TO HEART

I call to mind a very similar case of metastasis from the feet to the heart, in a lad who had rheumatic fever, brought on by the nurse putting his feet into hot water. Said nurse exultingly informed me at the morning visit that *she* had cured the feet! The next night there was frightful oppression of the heart, somewhat relieved by *Aconite,* but it persisted off and on for days, and the poor lad's heart is damaged to this day.

I confess in all humility that I think Gold was *the* medicine because homoeopathic to the state, but unhappily I did not know it then.

Would that we homoeopaths kept closer to our study of the Materia Medica Pura, and spent less of our valuable time and talents in internecine squabbles about the precious dose and the eternal name of the school. (II 123)

## 32. PALPITATION AFTER LOSS OF BLOOD

I think enough has been said to show that Gold has an important place in the treatment of heart affections of the gravest kinds. But considering the great importance of it in this connection, I will just add very short notes of two other heart cases treated with Gold. They may both be read in Frank's *Magazin*, vol. i., pp. 25, 26. The first of these is that of a lady who, after severe bleeding from the womb, consequent on the expulsion of a molar mass, had *violent palpitation, anxiety,* and *congestion of blood to the head.* Usual remedies did no good. Then *Aur praecipitat* (per fer. sul.) in doses of one-sixth of a grain brought relief after a very few doses, accompanied by this remarkable phenomenon : *"From evening till midnight violent itching beginning in the soles of the feet and then extending to the whole of the body."* The use of the Gold was continued, and the same phenomenon recurred for several days, dininishing in intensity. After the use of two grains of the Gold the heart symptoms were quite cured. We have already noted that Gold is an antipsoric with Hahnemann, and in connection with this case the question suggests itself to my mind whether this fore-midnightly itching was a pure pathogenetic symptom or a psoric crisis? *Itching* is a very prominent symptom of Aurum we know. (II 124)

## 33. PALPITATION, ANXIETY AFTER BLEEDING

Now this one more case and then I have done with the cardiac virtues of Aurum. Four weeks after a normal confinement a lady greatly exerted herself and brought on exhausting bleeding; then a few days afterwards there were *rushes of blood, violent palpitation of the heart, great anxiety, and faintings. Digitalis* and acids brought no change; then half a grain of Gold was given twice daily with rapid good result.

Dr. Becker, who is the author of these cases, mentions a third and similar case in which Gold was given with the same satisfactory result. My obstetric friends, how many such cases do you remember in your practices in which you did *not* remember this cardiac action of Gold? I remember one. *Cactus* relieved it; Gold would have cured it by virtue of the firm grip it gets of the living tissue of the vascular system, and physiologically producing symptoms similar to these.

For Gold is no mere function disturber, but a producer of organic change, and hence its brilliant effects in organic mischief. The vascular turgescence of *Belladonna* and that of *Aurum* are very different affairs. (II 126)

## 34. RHEUMATIC ENDOCARDITIS

While this was at the printer's, the following interesting and instructive case occurred in my practice, viz. :

*Rheumatic Endocarditis* in the course of rheumatic fever. I was fetched one day in February (17th), 1879, by a gentleman in the city to see his wife, a lady of about fifty-five or sixty, who was lying very dangerously ill at the end of the third week of rheumatic fever. This gentleman, who is an old homoeopath of thirty years' standing, and whose knowledge of drugs and disease is really remarkable for a layman, had treated patient himself, and with no inconsiderable success considering the severity of the case, but suddenly the patient's condition became very alarming on account of the rheumatism having apparently seized upon the heart. I found this condition : Patient was propped up in bed and breathing very hurriedly; the lips bluish; tongue dry and coated; anxious expression of face; puffy under eyes; moist rales all over chest, with cough; pulse rapid, compressible, and intermittent; action of heart floundering; loud endocardial bruits; slight dropsy of feet; no appetite at all, could just suck a grape or sip tea; profuse perspirations; limbs swelled and painful, the joints almost as firmly locked as if anchylosed, cannot move hand or foot for pain and from this swelled inflamed state of the joints; flesh of hands puffy; bones of hands swelled, almost immovable, and tender.

I ordered *Aurum foliatum*, 2nd trituration, very frequently. Alone and no auxiliaries.

Why did I order Aurum? Because it affects the heart and respiration very much *like* they were affected in this patient, and because it moreover produces profuse perspiration, profound weakness, anorexia, and great anxiety. Then the bones were greatly affected.

Feb. 18. A little easier. Rep.

19th. Better in all respects. Rep.

20th. Considerable improvement in the action of the heart; breathing comfortable; is out of danger. Rep.

22nd. Continued improvement. Rep.

24th. Quite comfortable. Continue the *Aurum* and take *Nat-sul.* 6 tril. in alternation with it. My reason for alternating was that I thought it imprudent to leave off the Gold, and yet *Nat-sul.* was now indicated.

March 2nd. Is up sitting by fire. Appetite good.

6th. Heart, joints, bones, and hands free from rheumatism; is sitting by fire quite comfortably; appetite good; tongue moist, but slightly furred; feet swell a little towards evening.

This is going to press, and hence I cannot give the sequel; but this case so well illustrates the action of Gold on the organic tissue of the heart that I here insert it.

When I saw patient first I gave a bad prognosis, and had it not been for the Gold I fear it would have been realised. Auxiliaries did not do it, for I used none; faith in the doctor did not cure her, for patient had never seen me before. (II 127)

## 35. DIFFICULT BREATHING, DEPRESSION AND BROWNISH PATCHES

Last week I saw a lady of some seventy odd summers. She had *great oppression at the heart, cardiac difficulty of breathing, weak pulse, and great depression of spirits.* Her skin showed *large patches of a brown* hue, and again patches like albugo. She was unable to rise. I gave her the third centesimal trituration of *Aurum foliatum* in four-grain doses every three hours. Yesterday I found she had left her bed for a few hours; her spirits were bright, appetite better, her breathing easy, and the oppression at the heart much relieved. "I am quite cheered, mamma is so much better, : said the daughter. Six weeks later : She is downstairs, still weak, but very much improved.

The elective affinity shown by Gold for the blood-vessels might make one think of it in incipient atheroma of the arteries in middle and advanced life. I am much impressed with the *visible beating of the carotids and of the temporal arteries in its provings.* In many heart affections, especially in the aged, one sees this. (II 131)

## 36. CASE OF OPPRESSION, PALPITATION AND GREAT DEBILITY

Before leaving the question of Gold in the conditions of the aged, I will note that I lately prescribed it in a low trituration for an old gentleman of eighty-five who had severe *attacks of oppression at the heart at night with palpitation and with great debility.* I sent him twenty-four powders, but before they were finished I received the report that "My father is so much better that he is now only taking one powder a day."

I may seem fanciful to some to talk about remedies for old age, but it is not so in reality, for old age may fairly be treated as a disease, inasmuch as it has peculiar symptoms, the like of which are in the pathogeneses of our drugs. (II 132)

## 37. LOSS OF SIGHT (PARTIAL)

"Mr. I., æt. 24, lawyer, while reading, was suddenly affected with partial loss of sight. Seeking medical advice, he was told that he was suffering from congestion of the retina, and was put under the use of *Mercury.* After a few weeks of treatment (being twice salivated) he lost his sight completely, January 14, 1873. Received *Aconite* 12, first three times, then twice per day. January 30. Could distinguish light from darkness; improved slowly to March 26, complaining of fulness over the eyes and floating specks in vision. He received *Apis* 2c and *Merc-viv.* 30M. March 31. His state was as follows : Feeling of severe pressure from within outward, and from above downward, in both eyeballs, accompanied by dull, heavy aching deep in both globes. On pressure, the eyeballs were more tense and firm than usual. He saw yellow, crescent-shaped bodies floating obliquely upward in the field of vision; sees a little better on looking intently and steadily at an object, *though he sees no trace of the upper half of an object.* In the *upper dark section of the field* of vision, occasional showers of bright, starlike bodies; the lower half looks lighter, and he can distinguish colour, light or dark. By gaslight a number of bright, floating specks and dots are seen. Eyes better by moonlight, and after active muscular exercise. Pupils irregularly dilated; cornea dull, with loss of usual lustre; anterior chamber contracted, colour of the optic nerve entrances of a greenish hue, except round the periphery, which was yellowish white, with a slight trace of pigmentary deposit on lower outer edge of optic disc in left eye, the retinal vessels bent abruptly on their exit from the disc, and closely hugging the floor of the excavation, bent sharply upon the periphery of the papilla; central portion of retinal vessels strongly pulsating; large letters cannot be distinguished, he seeing only something black upon a white ground. *Aurum* was given in the 200th. After three weeks, patient was much improved, could get about the streets alone, being able to follow the cracks in a board sidewalk; the dark half vision had disappeared, seeing as well the upper as the lower half of an object. Five weeks from commencing with *Aurum*, everything looked blue, and objects generally much lighter. May 5. He received *Aurum* M., but was shortly after lost sight of by removing to the West." (II 148)

## 38. HEMIOPIA

A man, æt. 52, accustomed to drink whisky everyday, *Lach* improved, could get about the streets alone, being able to follow the cracks in a board sidewalk; the dark half before his eyes; to this, at a later period, black spots were added, and for the last few weeks he can only see the upper half of objects; their lower half seems to be covered by a black veil. Appetite poor; sleep restless and full of anxious dreams; is sad and would cry all the time. Ophthalmoscopic examination gives no clue. Thinking that it was due to the whisky it was strictly forbidden. *Aurum* cured in four weeks, notwithstanding the patient did not abstain from his accustomed dram. — *Baumann in A.H.Z.* (II 151)

## 39. CHORIO RETINITIS

Some years ago, a gentleman who had taken large quantities of Iodide of Potash complained that the vision of the left eye had been failing for a year and a half. He could not see the upper half of a room or any large object though the lower half was clear. No pains in the eye; objects seem smaller and more distant; has some black spots before vision, is always worse as day progresses, and better in the morning; twitching in the upper lid. On inquiry, it was found that he had syphilis ten years ago, but had not been recently troubled with any secondary symptoms, except that a large bursa-like swelling on the wrist had persisted a long time. Vision was 5/200. Upon ophthalmoscopic examination there was found *chorio-retinitis* (chronic), with an accumulation of fluid beneath the retina, which settled to the lower portion of the eye and caused a large detachment of the retina. Vitreous hazy from infiltration. Right eye normal; refraction normal. Knowledge of the pathological condition here gave no clue to the remedy, and we were obliged, this time at least, to rely upon the symptomatology (as one should be always ready to do). The remarkable symptom of not seeing anything in the upper half of the field of vision is, of course, the most prominent. In addition to the Aurum symptom, we may find under *Digitalis*, "as if the upper half of the field of vision were covered by a dark cloud in the evenings on walking." *Digitalis*, moreover, covers the pathological point, having been found curative in fluid exudations of various kinds. It is also worse in the evening, while *Aurum* is usually worse in the morning. Still taking the history of the case into account, and previous dosing with *Iodide of Potash, Aurum* 200th was given, under which he steadily improved. The haziness of the vitreous almost entirely disappeared, the inflammation of the retina subsided, and in one year the vision rose to and remained at 15/100, beyond which it will not go, for the retina was partly disorganised, and cannot be repaired with retinal tissue. Since then, several cases of the same disease have been treated with Aurum with almost unvarying success, though in some cases no improvement followed, and the remedy only served to arrest further progress of the malady. Many of these cases will be found to follow overdosing by *Potash* or *Mercury*, and perfect vision can never be expected from the nature of the tissue changes. (II 152)

## 40. SUB-CHOROIDAL TUMOUR

One singular case of a man, forty years old, was sent for advice. A large black, sub-choroidal tumour was found behind the lens in the fundus, growing from the inner side. He suffered no pain, but the symptoms of vision were those of *Aurum* (the whole disease had only lasted about six weeks); vision, 5/200. After taking *Aurum* 200th a week, vision rose to 5/80; and in eight weeks more to 5/60, since which time he has not been seen. It was probably an exudation tumour, and may have been absorbed.

Thus we see that Gold is also no mean medicine in diseases of the Eye. We also note that the high dilutions act as well as any other. So Hahnemann said fifty years ago. (II 155)

## PREVENTION OF HARELIP, ETC.

### 41. ACID AND ALKALINE CHILDREN

At the end of the year 1874 I was consulted by a gentleman about his children, the youngest of whom had double harelip. He had some confidence in homoeopathic treatment, and was desirous of knowing whether there were any means of getting the wound to heal well after the operation for harelip that an able surgeon was on the point of undertaking. I recommended the local application of *Calendula officinalis* as an excellent and well-established vulnerary, especially to clean wounds. The operation took place, the gentleman used the *Calendula* as directed, and the surgeon, a man of some experience, declared he had never before seen such a rapid healing process or such a nicely-healed surface in any of the cases of hare-lip on which he had operated.

The reputation of *Calendula* (the common marigold) as a vulnerary is very old, but it survives almost exclusively in the homoeopathic school, in which it is, as you all know, in daily use.

The next older child than the one operated on had, and has, a slight insufficiency of the upper lip, if it were a little worse it would be harelip.

Subsequently the gentleman consulted me in regard to his own health, and after the consultation the conversation fell upon his children, upon the excellent result of the operation, and the rapid healing of the wounded parts. Then regret was expressed, especially as the child was a girl, as of course the neatest scar can never constitute a perfect or pretty lip. At the best it is only passable, and not particularly unsightly.

Finally he said, "In case my wife should have another child, what would you expect the next to be like?"

A answered, "That cannot be determined; but taking all the circumstances into consideration, viz., that your first child is perfect, that your second child has only a slight defect in the upper lip, that your third child has double hare-lip, and that your wife was apparently in good health with these, all equally, I should expect the next to have harelip also, a little worse than the last, and perhaps even cleft-palate."

He further inquired whether anything could be done to prevent it? My answer was, that I knew of no special experience on the subject at all, but as the body fruit could certainly be affected medicinally. I should think hopefully of properly directed medicinal treatment of the mother during pregnancy. I promised to do my best, and he said he would let me know if any further pregnancy should occur, and place the mother under my treatment.

The subject took hold of my mind, and I often animadverted upon it. Many remedies suggested themselves, and many plans of treatment; the one that found most favour with me was to be based upon specificity of seat or local drug affinity. I reasoned that any drug that would specifically affect the upper lip and palate might act as a stimulus to the part if coursing in the mother's blood, and thus bring about complete union of the bilateral parts. But an insuperable difficulty here presented itself — viz., I knew of no such drug with anything like a strongly expressed affinity for the part. Such remedies as *Kali bichromicum, Aurum, Iodine, Mercury, Natrum muriaticum, Mezereum, Phosphorus,* were thought of, but I did not feel the local affinity idea was workable here.

I then thought of tissue affinity or specificity of histological seat, as worked out in its fullest extent of late years by Dr. Schüssler, of Oldenburg, in regard to disease. I thought that a formative element of the tissue might be wanting, and thus condition imperfect development. If we grow wheat, we must supply its elements, as manure, to the soil, and if we grow tissue we must supply its elements in the mother's blood which is the food of the foetus; if the wheat just fails to finish the ear, we concluded formative elements are wanting; if the absolute concrescence of the bilateral parts of the human foetus just fails of completion, we may fairly assume that formative elements are lacking. So I thought. And in order to try to find out *what* was likely to be lacking, I went over embryology a little, and I will ask you to go over exactly the same ground as myself presently, by giving a short *resume* of the development of the involved parts first, and then show how, and what remedy I diagnosed.

The surgeon who had operated on the little girl, and also the family accoucheur who assisted at the operation, were also consulted upon the hoped-for possibility of preventive treatment in the then future; but these gentlemen laughed at the idea, and said the only thing for it was operation, prevention being out of the question.

But we may reflect upon the fact that it is not at all an uncommon thing in our hospitals, and occasionally in general practice, to treat a pregnant person suffering from syphilis very actively with *Mercury*, and the results are on the whole very encouraging indeed; still, as far as I am aware, it is seldom that any physician attempts the intra-uterine treatment of any other complaint, and even here the *idea* has generally been to treat the *mother* only, or principally.

In thinking the matter over, and endeavouring to find some sound reason to guide me in the to-be-attempted preventive treatment of harelip, I was encouraged to hope for a good result from the recorded experience of a few homoeopathic obstetricians who tell us of the successful medicinal treatment of the uterus and of the expectant mother herself; for it seemed no great difficulty, theoretically, to modify the development of the foetus, which grows in the uterus and is fed with the blood of the mother, seeing that both the mother's blood and uterus can, demonstrably, be modified therapeutically.

Now, although I felt the idea of trying to prevent harelip with the help of *specificity of seat* in the ordinary homoeopathic sense unworkable, still this lay in the nature of the case rather than in the nature of the thing generally. Thus in those liable to beget offspring with defects or deformities, or displacements of organs, or parts to which we have approved remedies with specific affinities for such organs or parts, we might, and undoubtedly should, find it of eminent service, and also of the careful application of the homoeopathic law of similars; also of the tripartite pathology of Hahnemann; and of the constitutional states of Grauvogl, and perhaps, even of the *Remedia universalia* of Rademacher.

But to return, let us examine the embryology of the parts involved in harelip and cleft-palate.

Biologists tell us that the face is originally formed of a middle portion proceeding from the forehead, or frontal process, and of a lateral portion on each side, derived from the superior extremity of the first visceral arch. These parts are at first separate.

The lateral and the inferior parts, destined to form the superior and inferior maxillary apparatus, are both derived from the first visceral arch, in which an angular bend appears; the part above this bend being converted into the superior maxillary mass, and that below it into the inferior maxillary apparatus.

The superior maxillary mass, in its growth, approaches the frontal process, and unites with it; a cavity being left between that process and the two superior maxillary masses, which becomes the nasal cavity. By the union of the superior maxillary masses (the superior maxilla and palate bone) of opposite sides beneath this cavity, the separation of the nose from the mouth by the palate is effected.

The mode of development of the face affords an explanation of the abnormal cleft-palate, and the congenital cleft between the upper maxillary and the intermaxillary bones and of those congenital fissures which pass between the intermaxillary and upper jaw, as far upwards as the orbital cavity. Congenital clefts of this kind are thus the *results of an arrest of development occurring during the primitive condition of the parts.* We may, therefore, infer that cleft-palate is due to lack of a due supply of formative material; the superior maxillary masses ossify indeed, but fail to unite in the median lines. If so it will follow that if the requisite amount of formative matter be supplied soon enough to the maternal blood, it will be given off to the foetus, and tissued osseous union will take place, and deformity will be prevented.

But the skeleton may unite in the middle, and yet the soft parts fail to do so; and when this occurs with those the superior maxilla, the deformity known as harelip is the result.

We may regard the basis of the upper lip structure as already differentiated into connective tissue, which is indeed the stroma of the whole body, and all of its organs. When, therefore, the soft parts fail to unite in the median line of the upper lip, and we get the ugly defect known as harelip, we may conclude that the development became arrested from a lack of one of its constituents *in development or functional power*.

All things considered, I concluded it was, in this case, *lack of lime-life*. Then the next point was — which salt of lime? Here the psoric constitution of the mother pointed to *Sulphur*.

My conception was not that there was an actual lack of lime as such, but rather a lack of assimilative or developmental power of the lime-function in the sense of Moleschott and of Schüssler, and that struma or psora (= morbid *x*) was the hindering agent.

I therefore decided on *Calcarea sulphurica*, and believing it was *quality* that was required, and *not quantity*, I determined on the sixth centesimal trituration.

This is how I diagnosed, theoretically, a remedy for this case of presumptive defective formation, and this remedy I made up my mind to give if the lady should come under my care.

A little time elapsed, and the husband appeared to inform me that his wife was believed to be *enciente*. *Calcarea sulphurica*, 6th trituration, one grain night and morning, was prescribed. The lady continued to take it till the end of the seventh month of pregnancy, and during the last two months she took *Lithium carbonicum*, and at full term *she gave birth to a healthy and perfect child.*

In due course a *second* pregnancy took place. The same course of treatment was adopted, and with the same happy result — viz., *a perfect child.*

Since this time I have kept the subject of the intra-uterine medicinal treatment of the human foetus before my mind; but my experience here has since been for the purpose of preventing, respectively eradicating, constitutional taints and hereditary proclivities. Cases other than those two, for the prevention of defect or deformity, have not hitherto come under my observation.

But this further experience of mine I will refer to again, as an interesting paper, published in the *Practitioner* for December, 1878, by Dr. Thomas P. Tuckey, of County Cork, Ireland, here claims attention. Dr. Tuckey is evidently an original thinker. The paper is entitled, "On the Preventive Treatment of Cleft-palate and Hare-lip and some further Remarks on the Relation of the Ovaries to the Sex of the child." (III 107)

## 42. PREVENTION OF CLEFT-PALATE AND HARELIP (1)

Mrs. H., aged thirty-five, mother of six children.

Every one of her children have had hare-lips, two have also had cleft-palate. The disease appeared not to be hereditary, and she could not call to mind any of her family, or of her husband's family, who have had harelips. Is a fine strong woman, but has fearfully crooked eyes; no other deformity. Has always had good health. Her husband, small, but strong and healthy, never has had any diseases while she has been married to him. He and she have both lived all their lives in the country. He is sober, and has always been so. Her first child had simple harelip; no cleft, in palate; does not remember getting any frights when carrying her children.

A pregnancy occurred; Mrs. H. presented herself, and the doctor prescribed the following mixture :

℞ Calcis phos. ʒj. grs. 20.
Calcis carb. ʒj.
Bicarb. magnes.
Chlorid. sodii.
Sodae. phosph. aa ε ss. M.

To be added to an 8 oz. mixture composed of Gelatine, Gum arabic, Syrup of ginger, and Cinnamon water; I drachm three times daily.

As clefts in the palate and lip are said to be due to arrest of development *prior to the end of the third month,* Mrs. H. was at once put on this mixture, which is intended to represent a very rough analysis of the constituents of bone. In any future cases Dr. T. thinks he would grind up the bones of the head of some animal, and give some of the powder instead of the above elaborately constructed mixture.

The essential parts of this mixture are clearly the Lime, Phosphorus, and Magnesia. The little polypharmaceutical performance of adding Gelatine, Gum arabic, Syrup of ginger, and Cinnamon water is not a little amusing.

But to return. The woman took the mixture regularly *until the fourth month;* she went her full time, and was delivered of a girl, without a trace of deformity about her lips or palate; the child was healthy and strong.

[This mixture was a strong alkaline one, and prevented acidity and facilitated child development — T.C.D.] — Quoted by Dr. Thomas P. Tuckey (III 115)

## 43. PREVENTION OF CLEFT PALATE AND HARE-LIP (2)

Hearing of this case, Mrs. L. came to seek Dr. Tuckey's advice. She was the mother of eight children, most of whom had cleft-palate and hare-lips; in four of them the hare-lip was double, and more shocking objects of deformity he had never seen. One boy was perfectly repulsive. The woman believed herself pregnant, and was at once put on the mixture. She went her full time, bore a girl without harelip, indeed, *but who evidently had one in utero,* for the lip, though united, was united *crookedly,* and one side was puckered up, as if by a slight and narrow burn.

This is, truly, a most remarkable and interesting case. (Dr. T.P. Tuckey) (III 117,)

## 44. PIGMENTATION FOREHEAD IN A CHILD DUE TO MOTHER'S LIKING FOR LIVER DURING PREGNANCY

Here I may narrate the following observation : A lady patient of mine was extremely fond of liver, during one of her pregnancies; at least once a week she would partake copiously of it — pregnancy fads are as old as the world. This lady was delivered of a very fine *child that had extensive pigmentation of the forehead,* such as we are wont to see in some ladies during gestation. This brown discolouration gradually disappeared from the baby's forehead in about four weeks. The mother's skin was also in parts very deeply pigmented, but not the forehead. (III 120)

## 45. PREVENTION OF WARTS

Thus, a lady patient of mine has a good many moles and warts on her person, and her husband a great number of warts, some very unsightly, on his. Considering the frequent observations that warts will, at a more advanced period of life, take on increased action, hypertrophy, and become epitheliomatous, their presence in an individual is not only aesthetically undesirable, but may become the source of positive danger to life; at any rate, they are ugly things at the best. Moreover, both of them are rheumatic and constitutionally strumous. This lady has passed through four pregnancies under my observation and professional care, and during each one I subjected her to a course of treatment with the most happy results. The four children were born with unblemished skins — wartless, moleless, and spotlessly pure.

It may be objected that the treatment had nothing to do with this purity of skin, as the interesting babes might have been equally unblemished, without any treatment at all. Of course, I cannot *prove* the contrary, still —

"Like genders like, potatoes tatoes breed,
Uncostly cabbage springs from cabbage seed."

My belief is, and it is based on observation, that those four children would in all probability have all been born with unsightly warts on various parts of their persons had the mother not been treated to prevent it.

The course of treatment followed was in this wise — *a peu pres.*

*Sulphur*, generally in the sixth, twenlfth, or thirtieth dilution (by preference the last-named), was given as the most certain anti-psoric. This was granted time to act, and then followed *Thuja occidentalis* as the anti-sycotic *par excellence*. Lest any specific taint lay in its history, *Mercurius* was given. The lady's teeth are very carious, and hence *Acidum fluoricum* was given for a while; the children have thus far sound toothie-peggies, and teethed normally and without any mediaevally superstitious gum-lancing. (III 122)

## 46. PREVENTION OF SKIN AFFECTION

A lady, mother of several (five) children, was under my treatment for a chronic internal skin affection; her husband had formerly been successfully treated by me, for psoriasis of lower extremities, with *Arsenicum.* The last baby I had treated for eczema while still at the breast, and when it was vaccinated the arm became very seriously inflamed, and the object of anxious care and medicinal treatment. All the five children had had, I was informed, something wrong with the skin, and every scratch with them festered.

The sixth pregnancy occurred, and I treated the lady during the greater portion of it. The principal remedies used were *Psorinum* 30, *Sulphur* 30, *Calc. sulph.* 6, and *Juglans cinerea* I.

The child came in due course; everything was normal, and the little mannikin was the finest of the lot, and remained for two years with a pure skin, and the vaccination caused no inconvenience. All the other children had cutaneous affections before they were a year old, and some of them proved altogether intractable.

The child passed from my observations then, but I have heard that it now has "something on its arm," but what, I do not know. Supposing it to be a cutaneous affection, the result of the preventive treatment would be that it remained free for the first two years of its life; and moreover, it is by far the finest and handsomest of the six children.

Of course, I cannot *prove* that it would have been otherwise if the mother had no treatment at all. (III 123)

## CURABILITY OF CATARACT

### 47. CATARACT CAPSULO-LENTICULAR

A tailor aged sixty, affected with capsulo-lenticular cataract of both eyes, could barely distinguish light from darkness. *Magnes. carb.* 30 was given once a week in alternation with the essence of *Cannabis sativa.* Two months from that time he could read large-sized print. He received several other remedies, but no further improvement was effected. (Dr. Schroen) (V 80)

### 48. WEAK EYESIGHT AFTER TYPHUS

Mrs. B., aged 31, was left after typhus fever with weakness of the eyes and eyesight. Everything appeared as if she were looking through a mist; she could only see outlines of objects, and did not dare to walk out alone. The left eye was most effected; behind the pupil there was an opacity on the lens, the bulb of the eye not affected, the pupil responded to the influence of the light; menses was suppressed. *Pulsatilla, Sepia,* and *Cannabis,* were used without benefit. *Lycopodium* 4 was then given, and six days afterwards the menses reappeared; in two weeks more there was decided improvement of the sight, so that she could discern smaller objects, and in three weeks her sight was entirely restored. — (Dr. Diez in Hyg., 18,457). (V 80)

## 49. EYE SYMPTOMS, DUE TO EFFECT OF SMALL-POX

I have before referred to *Dr. Caspari's case*. It is this : "Mrs. D., aged 36, had small-pox while a child, and her eyes have been affected ever since.
"Her symptoms were : Tears from the right eye, of a corroding, salty nature, which caused constant irritation of the lower lid and cheek; trichiasis of the few remaining eyelashes of the upper lid; conjunctiva pale red; varicose vessels running to the cornea; sometimes a sensation as if sand were in the eye; agglutination of the lids during the night : for six months past she had simple light-gray, lenticular cataract; she could still distinguish very large objects at a distance of four yards.
"After she had taken *Pulsatilla* 9, there was a subsidence of the inflammation and photophobia; her sight was improved; the lens became clearer at its circumference, and the pupil was distinguishable; after a further use of *Pulsatilla* there was observable only a small, grayish speck in the lens; the circum-ference was fully transparent, and the sight only remained slightly obscured.
"The essence of *Cannabis*, and lastly, *Opium* 6, rendered the lens perfectly transparent."
Dr. Caspari examined the eye on several subsequent occasions, but there was no return of any of the former symptoms. (V 81)

## 50. ARTHRITIC OPHTHALMIA AND CORNEAL OPACITY

"Mrs. E., became afflicted with arthritic ophthalmia and leucomatous opacity of the cornea, and after the gradual clearing off of the opacity, the lens was noticed to be of the colour of a beginning cataracta glaucomatosa.
"After receiving *Phosphorus* 3), the lens returned gradually to its former healthy state." (*Arch.*, 8, 3, 156, by Dr. Schuler.) (V 83)

## 51. INFLAMMATION OF EYE AFTER COLD IN FACE

"A gentleman, aged 38, in consequence of a cold in the face, became affected with an inflammation of the left eye, with the following symptoms : Towards the cornea an arterial network was noticed, over which were coursing some larger vessels towards the circumference of the cornea; drawing pain between the shoulder-blades and right upper arm. *Bryonia* and *Puls.* were given without benefit; four days later, however, the inflammation had somewhat diminished, but was followed by nebula of the left eye, in consequence of which the patient could distinguish large letters only; behind the pupil could be noticed an opacity of the capsule of the crystalline lens; the pupil was round, and the iris was also unchanged; there was no photophobia, and no secretion from the eye. The accompanying symptoms were, pressure and distension over the region of the stomach, extending as far as the right breast and lower lumbar regions. Great uneasiness, pressure in the forehead, feeling of heaviness and drawing in the thigh, and sleeplessness.

"*Nux* was given, without benefit; then *Bell.* 3 was used night and morning for two days, with such surprising results that every vestige of disease disappeared." (*All. Homoeopathische Ztg.*, 37. 340). (V 83)

## 52. BLINDNESS FROM ITCH AND FEVER

"M., aged 20, tinsmith by trade, was affected a year-and-a-half ago with the worst kind of itch, and subsequently with fever and ague. Sometimes be had tearing pains in the left eye, and some itching of the skin, to which he paid very little attention; suddenly he noticed, however, that he had become completely blind in the left eye.

"*Symptoms.* — A staring look of the left eye; pupil dilated and immovable; in the centre of the lens there was a slight opacity : his sight was almost extinguished.

*Treatment.* — August 2, *Sulph.* 6; from August 9th to September 23rd, six doses of the same.

"Six days after the first dose, *many pustules appeared on the face and arms*; in the meanwhile his eyesight improved so much that he was enabled to distinguish large letters. From September 13th to September 23rd, *furuncles on the arm made their appearance*; after that the skin became clear again, and the affected eye was as useful as it had ever been before." (*Arch.*, 14, 5, 105, Emmerich.) (V 84)

## 53. FLOCCULENT CATARACT

"A girl, aged 12, had been affected since her earliest recollection with flocculent cataract (probably congenital) of both eyes. She had an operation performed about four months ago, without the least benefit; four doses of *Magnes. Carb.* 200 were also given, without any benefit. Five months later she received *Euphras.* 200, in water; a tablespoonful once a day was followed by some improvement of the left eye. The *Euphrasia* was continued for four months with steady improvement; as soon as the patient ceased to improve *Sulph.* 200 was given, followed by *Magnes. Carb.* 200, one dose every week for five months, at the end of which time the circumferences of the cataracts in both eyes were only just observable. *Euphras.* 200, *Silic.* 200, and *Acid. Nitr.* perfected the cure. The use of spectacles for cataract assisted, however, very much to increase the sight of the child.

"How much the former operation had done towards the cure, referent is not able to say." (*Allg. H. Ztg.*, 35, 205, Rummel.) (V 85)

## 54. IMPAIRED EYESIGHT AFTER SCROFULA

"A farmer, aged 50, of small stature and with light-brown hair, had suffered for the last few weeks with impaired sight; the patient had formerly been troubled with scrofula.

"*Symptoms.* — Patient sees with the right eye only those things which are above him, and with the left eye only those which are at his side; but in all other directions everything appears as dark as night to him.

"Partial opacities of the crystalline lenses were clearly observable; the one in the right eye occupied the larger, and that in the left the smaller half of the pupil.

"*Treatment.* — *Cannab.* 2, three drops daily in water for three weeks, was given without benefit. *Calc.* 3, six doses, at first one dose a day for two days, afterwards one dose every week; before the last dose had been taken, patient had entirely recovered his sight." (*Viertelj. Schr.*, 2, 426. Villers.) (V 86)

## 55. CATARACT FROM MERCURY, ARSENIC ETC.

The following case, I think, although not very successful, is interesting : A lady, æt. 64, widow of a staff officer, has resided many years in India. She has cataract of both eyes these four years, worse of the right. Previously to the discovery of the cataract she had slept for four years in a room lined with arsenical wall paper. In this room she lay with diseased kidneys for nine months. She dreads an operation, and has already received *mercury, iodide of potash, sulphate of zinc,* and *borax* either topically or internally.

The opacity of the right lens has a stellate appearance. There is constant and great photophobia, and much secretion and morning agglutination. The treatment was begun with *Nux. Vomica* 3, and *Sulphur* 30. This was in June, 1876.

July 22. Eyes more confortable. To take *Bell.* 2, and *Lith. Carb.* 3 trituration.

Sept. 12. General health decidedly improved. To bathe the eye-lids with a week infusion of *Calendula* and take *Zinc. Mur.* 3.

Sept. 30, *Calc. Carb.* 3 trit.

Nov. 21. Sight and everything decidedly better. *Arnica* 6, and *Gelseminum* 6.

Dec. 12. *Santon.* 3.

Feb. 12th, 1877. Improvement in sight; can see better to read and write — *Zinc. Cyna.* 3.

March. *Euphrasia Off.* (mother tincture).

April 25. The painfulness after dinner and on first waking is gone. Sight better. On examining with the ophthalmoscope one can see only very slight opacity of left lens; that of the right is whitish and opaque in its upper and outer portion.

*Rep. and Phos.* 30.

June 5. More pricking in the eye and more secretion — *Arnica Montana.*

July 5. Sight better, but pain worse — *Glonoin* and *Euphrasia.*

Aug. 9. The edge of the opacity seems a little less defined — *Acid. Oxal.* 2x.

Sept. 24. Eyes very painful — *Calc. Mur.*, 30.

Jan. 12th, 1878. *Ferrum Phos.* 6 trit.

Feb. 7 *Kali Chlor.* 6 trit.

March 7. *Nat. Mur.* 6 trit.

April 10. Eyelids look much better, not being so inflamed, and the secretion is far less. Rep.

May. 15. Worse — *Kali Chlor.* 6.

June 20. Not better — *Santonine,* 3 trit.

Sept. 25. Slight indications of gout in big toe — *Nat. Mur.* 30.

Dec. 28. No better — *Puls. Nut.* 1.

Feb. 5. 1879. No better — *Aurum Fol.* 1 trit.

March 11. Eyelids dreadfully bad : they smart very much, as if they contained pepper — *Zinc. Sul.* 3 trit.

April 25. Eyelids as sore as ever — *Lith. Carb.* 3.

May 29. *Calc. Mur.* 30.

July 12. Eyelids better — *Elaps. Cor.* 6.

This is the sum of three years' treatment, and is certainly not very encouraging. (V 92)

## 56. CATARACT AND HEART SYMPTOMS

*Observation* — Mrs. __ , æt. 66, came first under observation at the beginning of March, 1877. For eight years previously her sight had been failing, and twelve months before coming from Scotland to consult me, she was examined by Dr. Argyll Robertson, of Edinburgh, who diagnosed double cataract, that of the left eye advanced, and less so that of the right. She has an elder brother with cataract that began at about the same age as did hers.

She has photophobia; great dimness of vision; objects do not seem distinct; cannot see anything at a distance; things at times appear double; her dimness of vision is unquestionably increasing.

I examine the eyes with the ophthalmoscope and note that the opacities are stellate in both eyes, that of the left much larger. Pupils react well to light : very slight *arcus senilis*; is breathless on going upstairs; suffers from flatulence; flushes readily; gets severe spasms at odd times over the stomach; has had erysipelas of the head and face six times, the first time more than forty years ago, and the last time three or four years ago; has haemorrhoids; often gets indigestion.

$R_x$ Tc. *Aurum Muriaticum* 3x. One drop at bed-time.

April 14. Better in *general health,* but the eyes are no better except that work does not strain them so much.

$R_x$ *Glonoin* 2 and *Iodium* 2.

May 16. Still better in general health; *fancies* she sees better.

To continue the medicines.

June 14. "I am thankful to say I do feel a shade of improvement in these bright sunny days. I *used* to feel the sunshine very blinding; *but within the last fortnight I have felt my vision clear for distant objects."*

To continue the medicines.

September 1. "I feel thankful to say I do feel a shade better, can discern objects more clearly.

To continue the medicines.

October 24. "I am *not* sensible of further improvement, but am *better in general health."*

$R_x$ *Hydrastis Canadensis* 1x.

November. "...; about my eyes — I am thankful to say I feel a little improvement, *objects are clearer."*

To continue the medicine.

January 16, 1878. Much the same.

$R_x$ *Ferrum Phosphoricum* 6 trituration. Six grains night and morning.

March 9. Has been reduced by a bad attack of bronchitis.

$R_x$ *Acidum Nitricum* 1. Three drops in water three times a day.

April 26. *I feel my eyes stronger; improvement in my sight is apparent."*

To continue the medicine.

May 22. Much the same. *Natrum Muriaticum* 6 trit.

July 3. No worse.

$R_x$ *Santonine* 3 trit., grana vj.

September 20. Have taken two lots of the powders (=72); no change. But after I had taken some seven of the powders AN ERUPTION CAME OUT ON MY ARMS AND SHOULDERS."

$R_x$ Tc. *Pulsatilla Nuttaliana* 1. Two drops in water forenoon and afternoon.

December 13. "I have continued the drops, which. I procured at Mr. Pottage's in Edinburgh and am glad to say they have done me good; I do feel less of dimness and see things clearer than for some time previous. I do feel hopeful that the cataract is being checked, as I am feeling my sight better than it was six months ago. — P.S. My *general health is very good*. I have scarcely had a headache since I came under your treatment."

To continue the medicine.

February 17, 1879. Is continuing to improve, but reminds me that she is very deaf these many years.

$R_x$ Tc. *Elaps. Cor.* 6.

April 22. "I am glad to say the drops have really done me good; my eyes seem *clearer* and I am *quite sensible of improvement*. Shall be in Edinburgh next week, and can get what you prescribe while there, from Mr. Pottage. We have had a very severe winter, but I have kept well, and the longer experience makes me more convinced that the homoeopathic medicines agree very well with my constitution."

To continue the medicines.

June 27. "i have again exhausted my little bottle I got filled, when in Edinburgh, and feel thankful to be able to say, *my eyes are wonderfully improved*; I am more sensible of this by the last medicine than I have felt by former drops or powders, and my constitution seems in good order considering my years."

To continue the medicine.

September 5. It is two months since I wrote to you; my eyes are wonderfully improved, sometimes I can read a little without the aid of my spectacles : I feel my constitution to be in a very healthy state; I am free of all headaches, and stomach and bowels in good order.

As this lady has been taking medicines now for about two years and a half, and is so well in her general health, and the sight evidently not only vastly improved but *still improving*, I advise abstention from all medication for a time.

I have given the extracts from this lady's letters, and thus my readers can judge for themselves. I have not seen her since the commencement of the treatment. I call attention to the appearance of the eruption, to the lady's age — now nearly 69 — to the fact that her brother has also cataract, and to the vast improvement in her *general health.*

Cataract is a constitutional complaint, and we must treat the person, not the cataract. Thus in this case my first prescription was given for the *heart symptoms,* and it is very evident that the Aurum really benefited the *heart,* and that was the first step up the therapeutical ladder.

As far as I know, an *advanced cataract,* of eight years' growth, does not thus behave between the ages of 66 and 69 when let alone.

November 1879. The report runs : "My breathing is no better, but *my eyes continue well,* my sight is *wonderfully strong.*" (V 93)

## 57. CATARACT (RIGHT EYE) - 1

***Observation*** — Gentleman of high position, 59 years of age, has cataract of right eye, left eye doubtful; his mother had double cataract; 47 years ago an apple hit his *left* eye and permanently injured it; thus more work has been thrown on right eye.

When looking at the moon or a candle, he sees a disk of red.

May 1877. $R_x$ *Arnica Montana,* 1.

June 20. Has an impression that the *left* eye (which was injured) is a *little improved.*

To continue with the *Arnica.*

This gentleman did not consult me again; he seemed vexed because I would not give him any positive prognosis, and announced his intention of going to his eye surgeon again; and, as I know the latter spends his spare time in laughing at homoeopathy, there is no difficulty in guessing the result of the interview.

I never give a positive prognosis as to the curability of any given case of cataract, as I have no sufficient data to go by; I simply say, "Try, and *if we fail* you can *still* have recourse to an operation." (V 97)

## 58. CATARACT

***Observation*** — Maiden lady, æt. 49, came under treatment on January 13, 1878, for cataract. Had taken a great deal of *Platina* 3x. in 5 grain doses, night and morning, for many months! The first day of taking it, it gave her a congestive headache. This I mention, as it *may* have had something to do with the lenticular opacities.

Her symptoms were these : Both upper lids swollen, the left worse; the right eye was the first affected, and is, perhaps the more misty of the two, but in the left eye there is an appearance of white transparent threads, and when inflamed, a crescent-shaped band, like a flame, seems to cross it below the lids, but does not remain; the eyes are often inflamed, especially the left one; there are heat, soreness, and sometimes itching; the eyes are better at the seaside.

$R_x$ *Ferrum Phos.* 6 trit. In 6 grain doses, three times a day.

Feb. 10. "Have felt stronger; the bowels more regular the first week, but less so the week following. The halo I used to see arount a candle-flame has almost disappeared, but seems to have given place to a somewhat greater mistiness; there is also less dread of light, less aching, and less inflammation, so that on the whole the eyes are decidedly stronger."

$R_x$ Trit. 6 *Nat. Mur.*

July 5. "My eyes are much stronger and better in every way."

Pergat.

August 5. "Altogether I am in much better health; the eyes are much stronger; can see distant objects better."

She perspires a good deal in the head.

$R_x$ *Calc. Carb.* 6 trit.

She subsequently informed me by letter, that her vision was very materially improved; she could see distant objects better; from her sitting-room window she could clearly distinguish objects far down an opposite street. She is not desirous of further treatment. (V 98)

## 59. CATARACT AND GOUT

***Observation*** — Case of cataract in an elderly, gouty gentleman, in whom the *Iodide of Potash* A trit. has *decidedly* improved the sight. He is still taking it.

Case of cataract of both eyes in middle-aged gentleman. It began three years ago.

*General Symptoms* — Great liability to catch cold; considerable lachrymation; profound sleepiness after dinner; dry pain in eyes. These symptoms determined me to give him *Natrum Muriaticum*, 6 trit., 6 grains in water twice a day. All those symptoms promptly disappeared, and he continues to take the medicine these many months on his own responsibility; hence it may be presumed that he is getting better. (V 99)

## 60. DOUBLE CATARACT

***Observation*** — Young lady, about 25 years of age, double cataract these three years, perhaps congenital; the right eye has been pricked by Dr. __ .

*General Symptoms* — Perspires in the hands a good deal; menses scanty, slightly painful; renal sphere normal; alvine function tardy; hands and

feet go to sleep, dead, yellow, numb.
$R_x$ *Pulsatilla Nuttal.* 1. Three drops in water, three times a day.
This was in September, 1878.
Oct. 18. Bowels now quite regular; perspires less in hands.
Pergat.
Nov. 28. Hands do not often perspire now; sight *in status quo.*
$R_x$ *Puls.* 3.
Dec. 30. Headaches better; menses more free than formerly.
$R_x$ *Pil. Sul.* 30.
Jan. 30th, 1879. No difference, except that her headache is worse.
$R_x$ *Cina Anth.* 1.
Feb. 26th, 1879. "Stronger and stouter than before treatment : mamma and my sisters think I can see with the affected eye better than I could, but I feel doubtful of it myself."
To continue the medicine.
$R_x$ *Cina Anth.* 1.
April 15. "Can see to read better, but cannot see any better at a distance; the operated eye is not so serviceable as it was."
To continue the remedy.
June 20. "Do not know whether it is the clear sun or the medicine, but I see better; I am afraid it is the sun; my general health is now perfect."
$R_x$ Trit. 6 *Calc. Fluor.*
Aug. 1. No further change.
$R_x$ Pil. *Silicea Terra* 30.
Continues under treatment.
This case looks promising, but time must show. (V 100)

## 61. CATARACT (RIGHT EYE) - 2

***Observation*** — Lady, married, 38 years of age.
*History* — Has lived a number of years in South America, and there suffered from inflamed eyes. Returned to England in May, 1876, after an absence of twelve years. On returning consulted Mr. Shadford Walker, Liverpool for the inflamed eyes; he examined the eyes with the ophthalmoscope and found cataract of right eye. He cured the inflammation and said the cataract must be left alone. Saw Mr. Critcher at the beginning of August, who said it would probably progress very slowly.
Has been under Dr. Drysdale, of Liverpool, with benefit for her general health.
*Present State* — Left pupil larger than the right; has always been weak in the right side of the body; there is opacity of the right lens, though not

very extensive. She cannot see well; has always been myopic; wears glasses; cannot see so well with the right eye as with the left; has always a mist before the right eye.

Has considerable pain in the right side for the past twelve months; before that, suffered for a year from dysentery; pain in the right hip; pain also in an around the right ovary. Menses rather too frequent; is very slightly haemorrhoidal; ankles swell towards night, the right one more than the left.

$R_x$ Tc. *Chelidonium Majus* 3.

Nov. 18, 1876. No change. To go on with the *Chelidonium*.

Nov. 23. The pain in the right side is very much better; it is worse when she breathes; suffers very much from heartburn.

$R_x$ Tc. *Phosphorus* 1.

Dec. 8. Much better in general health; the pains in the right hypochondrium, right hip, and right ovary, very much better; she feels stronger.

$R_x$ Trit. 3 *Natrum Sulphuricum*.

Jan. 9, 1877. Still has pains in the right side, but it is less severe; the right eye very uncomfortable; dreadful heartburn; is very cold; worse in wet weather.

$R_x$ Trit. B *Iridium*.

February. Is now *quite* well in general health, but the mist before the right eye is no better.

$R_x$ Trit. 4 *Acidum Oxalicum*.

April 27. Feeds tolerably well : eye no better. At times gets acute attacks of pain in the right side. Is recommended at such times to take the tincture of *Chelidonium* 1.

$R_x$ Tc. *Euphrasia* 6.

June 20. The eye is worse, it feels uneasy, and is getting more dim; the pain in the side very bad; mouth dry and parched; tongue covered with a thick orange-coloured fur.

$R_x$ Trit. B. *Iridium and Phosph.* 1.

July 24. Eye better; many symptoms of the hydrogenoid constitution.

$R_x$ Trit. 5 *Natrum Sulphuricum*.

Oct. 24. The urine is very turbid; there is very much pain in the uterine sphere.

$R_x$ Tc. *Solidago Virga Aurea* 1x and Tc. *Viburnum Opulus* 1.

May 28, 1878. The eyes water a good deal. *Natrum Muriaticum* 30.

June 15. Pil. *Sanguinaria Canadensis* 6, one before each meal.

*About this period*, but whether before taking the *Sanguinaria* or after, I unfortunately cannot ascertain, AN ERUPTION CAME OUT ALL OVER THE BODY, IN PATCHES, ITCHING VERY MUCH, worse in the inside of the thighs, legs, and arms and chest. It was an erythematous eruption

and lasted only a few days.
August 14. *Natrum Sulphuricum* 4 and Pil. *Calcarea Carbonica* 30.
March 4, 1879. The pain in the right side is now observed only at rare intervals; eyes decidedly better; the lower lid of the right eye twitches a good deal.
To take *Dulcamara* 3. Four drops in water at bedtime for two months.
After writing this prescription, and while engaged in some general conversation, I noticed that my patient's eyes watered a little, and that she used her handkerchief to wipe them. There was no epiphora, the cataract, and as the haziness is gone, it is pretty sure that the cataract has likewise disappeared. With the naked eye, one can detect nothing abnormal. (V 101)

## DISEASES OF VEINS

### 62. VARICOSIS - 1

I was once consulted for a young lady whose left lower extremity was the seat of very severe varicosis : the veins were so badly dilated that the limb had a hideous aspect, — so much so that all idea of marriage had been given up; the well-fitting stocking certainly supported the veins, but otherwise only tended to render the whole limb varicosic. I readily ascertained the location of the dam or obstructive element in the case, viz., there was a considerable enlargement of the left ovary, with severe concomitant leucorrhoea. This ovarian enlargement appeared to me to be due to chronic inflammation of a sycotic nature. I set to work with antisycotics, and in a few months the enlargement lessened, and finally disappeared entirely; and in proportion as the enlargement lessened so the varicosis likewise diminished, and also the leucorrhoea, and finally the varicose veins could no longer be found. The young lady reappeared in society, and she presently married and had her first baby last year. (VI 8)

### 63. VARIX RIGHT GROIN

Less than two years ago a Commander in the Royal Navy, a very healthy, well-preserved man, about forty years of age, consulted me in regard to an enormous varix of the right groin as big as a small orange, and the thing was all the more alarming as the wall of the varix had become thin, and being in the bend of the groin, mechanical support was practically impossible, so of course it appeared that patient would have to quit the service. There being no heart affection, no blood disease, no primary vein disease and no history of any local lesion or disease of any sort, I made a careful examination of the abdominal organs, and could only make out a not very considerable enlargement of the left lobe of the liver. I therefore set about curing the liver, though I did not think the said enlargement sufficient to account for such an enormous varix. However, as soon as the liver had been brought back to the normal, the varix was reduced to a mere nothing, and in a few months the delighted patient hastened off on active service, looking forward to becoming in due course an Admiral.

The remedies which cured this case were *Carduus Marianus* Q, *Chelidonium majus* Q, and *Chelone glabra* Q. For an account of the two former remedies see my "Greater Diseases of the Liver." and my "Diseases of the Spleen and their Remedies" respectively. As to the last-named remedy — *Chelone glabra* — I should like to say that its seat of action is the left lobe of the liver. (VI 9)

## 64. VARICOSIS - 2

Thus several years since a city merchant consulted me for such a state, he being desirous of getting married. Almost all the superficial veins of the extremities were dilated, and also the hypogastric veins; the large varicose veins were about the size of goose quills, the smaller ones about that of crow quills, so the aspect was ugly indeed. After about two years' treatment the veins were reduced about three-fourths, and the marriage has now been fixed for the near future.

I was led to diagnose indurated abdominal glands, from the visible and feelable hypertrophy and induration of his inguinal glands, which were cleary inherited and not acquired. Nosodes were the chief remedies.

The diagnosis of the seat of the dam is of very great importance in these cases. Where one lower extremity is enlarged from perturbed circulation in the deep-lying veins of the limbs, looking like phlegmasia alba dolens, but occurring in the male, and not necessarily with any increase of sensation — the left leg is most commonly involved — the condition would appear to bear some relationship to the spleen, and may, perhaps, be to the spleen, what myxoedema is to the thyroid. (VI 13)

## 65. VARICOSIS AFTER GONORRHOEA

Thus, a gentleman consulted me early in the current year (1894) for a considerable enlargement of the left leg, in aspect very much like the ordinary white leg. He was also suffering from scarring acne, and the skin of his face was very shiny. The spleen was notably enlarged. Patient dated the swelling of the leg to an attack of mountain fever which he had four years ago in Colorado, since when his enlargement had existed. He had gonorrhoea years ago, and had also been twice vaccinated. Vaccination at times perhaps always, causes a certain amount of tumefaction of the spleen, as does also gonorrhoea, and I have over and over again seen varicosis follow common gonorrhoea; examples of this I could cite in numbers.

*Urtica urens* Q in small material doses greatly lessened the enlargement of the leg in a few weeks. I cite this case thus quite shortly, to exemplify the usefulness of diagnosing the dam in cases of obstructive varicosis. (VI 14)

## 66. THE LAMP-LIGHTER'S CASE OF EXCESSIVE VARICOSITY OF THE LEFT INTERNAL SAPHENOUS VEIN

A middle-aged man, by occupation a lamp-lighter, came under observation at the Dispensary for an enormously dilated vein of left thigh. At its highest and largest end, just where it dips down to the femoral vein through the saphenous opening of the *fascia lata*, it was as large as a child's wrist; and near the knee, about the size of a man's little finger, so that there was no inconsiderable danger of its rupturing and causing dangerous haemorrhage. It was not the local expression of general varicosis, but arose from a mechanical obstruction in this wise : Patient had sowed his wild oats lang syne, and as part of the harvest had reaped a big bubo in the left groin. This had sloughed, and been burned with a strong acid, and there resulted as scar, a cicatricial surface of the size of a man's palm, and this scar-tissue in contracting had very much narrowed the entrance of the long saphenous vein, through the opening of the *fascia lata* into the deeperlying crural vein. Then, in those days lamplighters used to do their work with the aid of light ladders, and were in habit of sliding down them scores of times a day, and thus the vein, that had become dilated from the lateral pressure of the venous blood, coursing up the saphena, having such a contracted entrance, became still more disturbed in its function; hence the enormous dilatation.

Patient received *Acidum fluoricum* 6 in pilules, and was directed to take one four times a day, and come and report himself every fortnight till further orders. This he did for several months, with the result that the enormously dilated vein shrank to about one-third of its original size, and this notwithstanding patient's continuance at his usual occupation. No auxiliaries and no local applications or appliances were used, and the diet was not altered. When I saw him last the varicosis had ceased to be of any inconvenience; it was no longer dangerous in anything like the same degree, as the vein felt firm and strong. Considering the irremediable mechanical hindrance at its inlet, the result seemed to me so striking *that I have ever since gone in very strongly for the medicinal treatment of varicosis under all circumstances,* and the satisfaction one has in such medicinal treatment is truly great. (VI 34)

## 67. GENERAL VARICOSIS, VARICOCELE AND VARICOSE VEINS

A gentleman, about thirty years of age, came under my observation on October 17, suffering from chronic prostatitis, varicocele, and varicose ulcers of the legs. At a glance one could see that he was a venous subject; as he was swarthy, pensive, and melancholy, and had long slender limbs. Almost every region of his venous circulation showed signs of dilatation, having an enormous left-sided varicocele, and very pronounced baggy varices of the legs. His internal saphenous veins were like big ropes. Around his left ankle were varicose ulcers, and the whole neighbourhood around was very dark, almost black in places. He stated that this left ankle had been in this state nearly all his life. General health fairly good, except some lack of virility, but bandaging his legs was, of course, burdensome, and the varicocele was very inconvenient, more especially in view of approaching marriage.

$R_x$ *Ferrum Phosphoricum,* 6 trituration ziv. To take four grains in water three times a day.

Nov. 12. The spermatic veins are not any smaller, as far as he can perceive; the veins in his lower extremities are smaller; *and the dark places under the left ankle are turning to a proper flesh colour.*

Repeat the same remedy.

Dec. 8. The varicocele is much smaller — "At one time its existence was very inconvenient; now I hardly notice it," said he. The varicose ulcers have healed up, and the skin around is assuming a healthy hue.

Repeat.

Jan. 8. Has had gatherings in the place where the black patch was. All the varicose veins and varicocele *much* better.

$R_x$ *Kali. Chlor.,* 6 trit., ziv. Four grains in water three times a day.

April 14. The veins are all getting smaller; the foot has *completely* healed (had had it nearly all his life). The varicocele very much better, and also the varices of the lower extremities, the *venae saphenae longae* having notably diminished in size. These few months of treatment have wrought a great change in the patient and in the *man,* and I accordingly gave him permission to get married. he is, of course, not yet *completely* cured of his general varicosis, — the time has been too short for that, — but the improvement is so great that all obvious unsightliness has disappeared, and this is not a small boon to a man contemplating marriage. (VI 47)

## 68. HAEMORRHOIDS - 1

Some six or seven years since, a lady, about 40 years of age, came under my observation. She was suffering from external piles, but otherwise was in perfect health and of magnificent physique. She had taken advice on the subject of her complaint, and an operation had been determined upon, for which purpose she intended to go to her native city Dublin; but a lady friend of hers, having been admitted to her confidence, told her that the homoeopaths were in the habit of treating this affection successfully with medicines. She did not expect to be cured, but thought there could be no harm in trying the homoeopathic method of treatment.

An eight-weeks' course of *Nux vomica* 30, and *Sulphur* 30, resulted in a complete cure. Nothing remained of the tumour whatever. The diet was not altered, and no local application of any kind was used. The case was recent, and not severe, but yet severe enough for her to have been advised an operation.

Thousands of cases of piles may be cured with *Nux* and *Sulphur* alone; almost any dilutions will act, but the thirtieth is more *enduring* in its effects apparently than lower ones. *Sulphur* is a grand polychrest from the crude substance upwards, but. *Sulphur* 30 is a mighty prescription. We get used to its wondrous effects, and cease to marvel thereat, just as we cease to wonder at the electric telegraph or steam locomotion.

I have repeatedly seen *Sulphur* 30 PRODUCE piles, and I once saw Sulphur C. cause a rather severe attack of piles. "I used to suffer from piles. I have cured myself with *Nux* and *Sulphur*, is an oft-told tale. (VI 68)

## 69. VARICOCELE

When practising in Chester I treated a patient at the Chester and North Wales Homoeopathic Dispensary for varicocele. The subject was an Irish workman of herculean stature, and who had syphilis, after getting rid of most of the manifestations of this vile malady, I set to work at the *varicocele*. In this case *Fluoric acid* was indicated, not only on account of the dilated spermatic veins, but because of the *moist palms* and loss of hair. Indeed *Acidum fluoricum* is no mean antisyphilitic remedy in the later manifestations, such as loss of hair, whitlows, and bone disease; so this was given for a number of weeks with very marked benefit, the varicocele having considerably diminished. At this stage the man ceased attending, having gone on a drinking bout, as I subsequently ascertained, (VI 79)

## 70. CHRONIC PILES WITH PROLAPSE OF THE RECTUM

Some three or four years since a gouty gentleman of about 50 consulted me for this distressing malady. For many years he had suffered from haemorrhoids, with prolapse at each stool; he had been treated with various domestic remedies, and by several medical men, both allopathic and homoeopathic, and had obtained temporary relief at various times. Besides this he had a medicine chest of his own, and a Domestic Vade-Mecum, according to whose directions he was in the habit of taking *Nux, Sulphur,* and other such well-known remedies. He was of spare habit, very abstemious in all respects, and a careful liver. His bowels were inclined to be costive, but still they acted most days. All his organs seemed healthy, and there was no evidence of any disturbance in the portal system, but he used, at times, to pass fine sand, like brick-dust. His going to stool was very painful, and the act lasted a considerable period, owing to the state of the rectum; the motion was very hard and usually more or less streaked with blood, and it always brought down the bowel. After carefully washing the part he replaced it with more or less difficulty, and severe pain. On account of this unhappy state, he rarely left his home or family, as it took him nearly three-quarters of an hour to get the matter over, and the bowel washed and replaced. He thought it came originally from lying in the trenches in the Crimea.

In this case there was considerable hypertrophy of the rectal mucous membrane, and also of the subjacent connective tissue, which indeed, is pretty well always present in cases of old standing.

The indications to be fulfilled were :

1. To get this tumid mass dispersed.
2. To get the haemorrhoidal varices to contract.
3. To procure *easy* defecation.

Now, it may be affirmed that many physicians fail to treat such cases successfully with medicines; they look upon them as hopeless. Granted, say they, that simple recent cases yield readily to homoeopathic treatment, but these old-standing cases do not, and they must be either borne or the tumour cut away.

At first sight this seems evident, but a little thought on the subject will shew that it is not *necessarily* so.

Let us remember that we have to deal with venous stasis for the most part hypostatic; and a resultant hyperplasia of circumjacent tissue; this goes on till a tumour is there, and *this tumid mass lies practically without the organism* to a large extent, and hence it is not reasonable to expect to affect it very radically from within, *alone*. At least that is my view of the matter, and I have, therefore, in all very severe cases of piles, made use of remedies externally — usually *Hamamelis*, sometimes *Mikania guaco*.

"Well," some reader will say, "I too have made use of *Hamamelis* externally for years, and yet bad cases for the most part will not yield to it; I have nevertheless to have recourse to the radical operation."

To that I have several things to say. First of all as to the *mode of applying it*. A little reflection will shew that we want the thing applied for a considerable period, and my very successful plan is simply this : — Add to as much water as needful a few drops of *Hamamelis Virginica* Q — I find the ordinary homoeopathic mother tincture acts better than Pond's Extract as a rule, but when the tumour is *very* painful, and active inflammation has been set up, pure Pond's extract of *Hamamelis* may be applied as they use it in America for hurts and sprains. Then take a piece of lint of convenient size, and dip it into the *Hamamelis* solution, and let it become thoroughly saturated therewith; then, on getting into bed the patient is directed to place it on the tumour, or just within the anal orifice, AND LEAVE IT THERE ALL NIGHT. This leaving it there all night is of the greatest importance, and has helped me to cure cases that had baffled some of our very best men, including low dilutionists and the very highest dilutionists. I have noticed that the rock on which the low-dilution men specially are apt to strike is the *recoil* action of their too big doses, while the Hahnemannians, in their laudable consistency, refuse to sanction the local treatment.

The right diet for the haemorrhoidal is a big chapter, and would lead me away from what I am specially pleading for in *bad cases*, viz. : — external treatment, *combined* with the internal. Neither will succeed alone, because external treatment will only aid so long as the mass cannot be thoroughly dealt with from the circulation, and local treatment is only child's play beyond a certain point, and utterly valueless to do more than influence the local mass it entirely fails to *cure* any case of itself, and is to be discontinued as soon as this can be reached well from within; but so long as the mass is, as it were, a something outside of the body, so long must it be dealt with from the outside — a rightly chosen remedy being simultaneously administered internally. The saturated piece of lint, or other suitable material, that has lain all night at the anal orifice, should be burned, and never used a second time; it is important to insist on this, as otherwise the part may get poisoned, as it is difficult to throughly cleanse a *small* piece of linen.

Then, again, all aperients must be *absolutely* forbidden; this is of prime importance, and if a patient (the case being a bad one) will not absolutely give in on this point, I invariably decline the case. There is nothing for it but this. Of course the diet must be modified accordingly. The physician who allows aperients *cannot* CURE bad piles, though he *treats* them with all the skill of Hippocrates, Galen, Sydenham, and Hahnemann combined. Why? Because the peristaltic action set up by the aperient acts from above downwards, and therefore increases the haemorrhoidal mischief mechanically, to begin with, and then by increasing the active congestion, and finally making the hypostasis worse than ever.

Furthermore, it is almost of equal importance *to forbid the patient to go to stool until he positively cannot hold out any longer*; that is of course, in very severe cases. Why? Because haemorrhoidal sufferers have often a knack of *pressing* at stool as if they were parturient; the abdominal press acts upon the whole contents of the belly, and thus the pressure *from above* brought to bear upon the piles will do more harm in a few moments than the best directed efforts of any physician can mend by the time another stool takes place.

It is simply not possible to cure *very severe cases* unless aperients be *totally* abandoned, and unless *all use* of the abdominal press be, for the time, given up.

"But, Doctor, I have taken aperients every day for thirty years, and I *must* have them, and I *must* also have a motion every day, or I am so dreadfully uncomfortable, and have such a fulness in my head; and besides, I dread the suffering of a stool if I put it off, — it is too awful."

Then, patient, go to Mr. Smith and get him to do the necessary operation, for unless you obey in these points, it is simply not possible to cure such a bad case as yours with medicines; with absolute obedience it *is* possible, and very probable.

Be it well understood that the question is now of *very severe* cases where the rectum is prolapsed and perhaps almost strangulated.

In simple cases it is often not needful to bother the patient with any change of diet whatever, but in bad ones it becomes a necessary condition of success.

I have interwoven these remarks with the narration of this case to motive my prescription, which was *Hamamelis Virginica* locally, in the manner above described, and *Aloes Soc.* 6, one pilule four times a day.

This was in August 1876.

Of course it will be objected that as I used *Hamamelis* externally, and *Aloes* internally, I do not know how much of the curative action is due to each respectively. This I grant, and the scientific value of the prescription is thereby lessened, no doubt. The gentleman was away from home at the time at the seaside for his holidays, and this prescription was forwarded to him by post. I had previously seen him through several pretty bad attacks of gout, and he had mentioned his haemorrhoids to me several times, but he never really consulted me about them, because, in truth, he did not believe there was any medicinal cure for them, and he did not intend undergoing any operation for them so long as he could manage to replace them, together with the bowel, after each motion. Now, however, being at the seaside, they suddenly became worse either from the sea air or his long walks, or some other cause through several pretty bad attacks of gout, and he had mentioned his haemorrhoids to me several times, but he never really much worse, that walking had become most painful and barely possible. Hence he applied to me.

He did not write to me again, and remained away about six weeks. Neither did he call upon me on his return, but two or three weeks thereafter I met him accidentally, and then received his warm thanks for having relieved him of his great trouble. He informed me that he was quite well; all the piles had disappeared, and the bowel no longer came down at stool at all; the bowels, too, acted naturally. For fully twenty years this gentleman had almost daily suffered the horrors of a painful stool and prolapsed bowel, followed by the torture of getting it back again. Many months later I attended one of his children for fever, and learned that he continued quite well.

In the face of this experience, is any one at all astonished that I am a strong advocate for the medicinal treatment of piles, and other manifestations of the venous diathesis? In this case I made no alteration whatever in diet, and there was no need to forbid aperients, as he had abandoned them for many years in favour of *Nux*, *Sulphur*, *Belladonna*, and *Opium*, which he knew well how to use. Indeed, alvine constipation was not an important element in this case, it was more a proctostasis. (VI 80)

## 71. HEAMORRHOIDS - 2

In January 1880, a gentleman, about 40 years of age, residing in London, came under my observation. He had suffered for many years from constipation and piles, with prolapse, and he had had a sorry time of it at every movement of the bowels, as the large haemorrhoidal masses came down, together with the rectum, so that the whole resembled a big dahlia in configuration and in colour; moreover, the constriction of the sphincter seemed so great that on my first visit, there seemed no inconsiderable danger of gangrene. His elder brother had suffered similarly, and been operated on very successfully ten or a dozen years ago, but had latterly got as bad as before the operation. My patient's sister, however, a kind-hearted capable maiden lady, who, instead of wasting her precious life nursing poodles, goes into the courts and alleys of this huge city, carrying words of comfort, and healing many with the aid of a Homoeopathic Vade Mecum and a pocket-case of pilules. *From her own experience (!)* she was confident that homoeopathy could cure her brother, and this was the more desirable as he was very nervous and timid, and almost fainted at the very thought of an operation. Moreover, he is by no means a strong man, as indeed no one is at the end of fiteen years of haemorrhoidal miseries and bleeding.

On examination, I found the usual thing : A large purple bleeding mass extending from the anus, causing the patient such terrible anguish that he screamed and cried. He could neither sit, lie, nor stand properly, but found least pain in lying on his side, with knees and chin considerably approximated. The size of the whole tumid mass was about that of a man's fist, and there were small ulcers on the surface, apparently suppurating excoriations.

Besides "having a liver," and being of lax fibre, he was otherwise healthy, though not strong, and of rather small stature.

I set to work in this wise :

1. I propped up the *lower* part of the body, so as to relieve the hypostasis somewhat.
2. I forbade all aperients, and any effort at going to stool : let the bowels absolutely alone.
3. He was ordered to live entirely on slops, rice and other puddings, and stewed fruit for dinner; porridge, with simple syrup (treacle), for breakfast; an ordinary English tea; and gruel for supper. Beef tea occasionally; first every alternate day. No beef or mutton.
4. Pure Pond's Extract of *Hamamelis* constantly applied to the haemorrhoidal tumour, and subsequently the ordinary homoeopathic mother tincture *very much* diluted.
5. Internal medication.

It would be very tedious to give the ups and downs of this case and my reasons for the various remedies employed, but for the advantage of any young practitioner who may chance to read these pages, I will, nevertheless, give the bare skeleton of the treatment. Hahnemann's *Materia Medica Pura* will give him the why and the wherefore.

Jan. 27th.

Tc. *Aloes* 12. At first a dose every half-hour for eight doses, and then every hour.

Those who think the repetition of the dose too frequent, are reminded that the poor fellow lay writhing in agony.

28th. Considerable relief as to pain, especially after each application of the *Hamamelis*. Swelling less tense. No motion, begs for an aperient, and permission to *try* to obtain relief of his bowels. Both absolutely refused, and *reasons given*.

29th. Easier, but otherwise no change.

*Sulphur* 30 every two hours, and continue the Extract.

30th. Same.

31st. Is getting frighteed about his bowels, as they have not acted.

$R_x$ *Kali Carbonicum* 30 every two hours. (He had a cough.)

Feb. 2nd. Easier, but still no *sensible* diminution in the size of the tumour; he is beginning to sleep better, and getting resigned to his fate, though he is afraid of an inflammation of the bowels from retained faeces.

3rd. The *Kali Carb.* 30 is continued, and *Sulphur* 30 given in alternation with it.

Feb. 5th. The tumour is decidedly less tense, and there is now but very little actual pain, and the part has a much healthier hue — not so purple. Bowels still locked, which alarms him; only my threat to throw up the case keeps him from using an aperient.

$R_x$ *Æsculus Hippocastanum* 6 every two hours.

9th. Notable amelioration. No action of the bowels. Continue the *Æsculus.*

12th No action of the bowels; renewed complaints of patient thereat.

$R_x$ *Tc. Æsculus Hippocastanum* 30 four times a day.

13th. Comfortable action of the bowels, with no straining at all. Haemorrhoidal mass withering.

Continue.

15th. The same.

17th. Making very rapid progress; bowels act daily, painlessly and easily, and the patient is able to put on his dressing-gown and lie on sofa. The piles are vastly improved, and the prolapse has disappeared. Continue.

23rd. Continued progress. No change in medication. Drives out, and has

white meat for dinner.
March 2nd. His condition is eminently satisfactory in all respects the bowels act beautifully every day; of the whole anal trouble there is now scarcely anything to be seen beyond a thickening like a ring around the anus, and a large fold of skin in which the tumour had been encased.
$R_x$ *Ferrum Phosphoricum 12x* trit. morning and afternoon.
17th. He is quite well. Nothing remains at the seat beyond a small fold of the skin like a pucker, of the size of a hazel nut, though patient is not conscious of its presence. He has now a daily motion as an act of pleasure — no piles, and no prolapse. Had not been in such a condition since his youth!
Rx *Arsenicum album* 30 twice a day, for its constitutional effect.
April 28th. Continues in all respects well. Beyond the little pucker of skin at anus everything is normal, and this exists unknown to him, and is barely noticeable, being only a shrivelled fold of the skin about the size of a horse bean probably the large tumour had so stretched the skin that it cannot readily contract to its primitive condition.
This case has given me very great satisfaction, and will, I trust, shew those who are faint-hearted, whenever brought face to face with a bad case of haemorrhoids, that even bad cases are perfectly amenable to homoeopathic, postural, and dietetic treatment. (VI 100)

## 72. PILES

At the end of the year 1876, while practising at Birkenhead, I was requested to visit a gentleman residing in the neighbourhood, and on arriving at his house was received by his wife, who told me the following : — For many years this gentleman then about 55 years of age, had been a martyr to piles, difficult defecation and prolapse of the rectum. The bowels acted daily, but it was in the very deed a chirurgical operation in its actual etymological sense, as the faecal mass could not be dislodged without manual aid, often after a syringe, and then the prolapsed gut had to be replaced together with an enormous haemorrhoidal mass. It must be admitted that life at such a price is dear, yet the patient had got used to it, and did not even complain. He thought it inevitable, and naturally shrank from an operation which had been often recommended to him by men of both schools and by his experienced friends. But so long as the daily manual reposition succeeded and the bleeding was not excessive, he bore it; now, however, it had come to the usual pass, the tumour would no longer go back, simply because it was too large and *in erection*, for in severe cases of piles with prolapse the whole mass at times has the physical characters of a tense *corpus cavernosum*.

He has borne it till it could be borne no longer, and had finally decided to send for Mr. B_____ to cut the whole thing off; but his wife was afraid lest he should not get over the operation, and therefore sent for me to learn whether medicinal treatment offered any hope. I explained my views, and, after very much deliberation, the patient decided to try the medicinal treatment to please his wife; he did not, himself, believe that medicines could touch such a severe case; this was also, I was informed, the opinion of Mr. B_____.

Now, it happened that this eminent surgeon, and bitter hater of our blessed homoeopathy, had a very similar case just opposite in the same road, and the two families being friendly, and the cases similar, notes were compared about them. Mr. B_____ operated on his patient, a lady, and I began to treat mine with medicine; he ridiculed me openly, and by name, and I had to wait, for my victory was not yet. Of course I was not sure of succeeding; I merely thought there was hope and promised to do my best, and my best is when I am sitting at the feet of Hahnemann.

Bland soft diet was ordered, and patient put into the right posture, such as I have already explained.

*Hamamelis* was applied locally, and *Aconitum, Belladonna, Nux, Pulsatilla,* and *Sulphur* came into play in succession. The first was on December 9th. At first we did not make much headway, and many were the doubts and fears at this period; I myself did not then sit so firmly in the saddle as I do now.

On December 21st. *Æsçulus Hippocastanum,* third centesimal trituration, every 4 hours. This was continued till recovery, and its action was most brilliant : in six weeks my patient was well enough to go to his business in Liverpool. He was not only cured of his haemorrhoids and prolapse, but his bowels acted naturally and he felt himself stronger. It was now my turn to laugh at my chirurgical *vis-a-vis,* for his patient was *longer* recovering from the operation than mine was from medicinal treatment, and twenty-two months later she was as bad as ever, and then . . . came over to homoeopathy, and was cured.

But to return to the case under consideration : the patient remained under observation and took *Acidum fluoricum* 12 during the months of March and April; in May and June *Natrum Sulphuricum,* 3; and in July *Hydrastis Canadensis* 1.

The *Hamamelis* was used with occasional interruptions for six months, discontinued, as he was as well as if nothing had ever been wrong with his rectum and haemorrhoidal veins. Some of the treatment in this case was directed to the liver. This gentleman has remained well to this day, and that is more than three years since*.

Believe me, my dear allopathic brother, you may deride homoeopathy till the end of your life, but it is true nevertheless.

In the end homoeopathy will have to kiss the cast ... *Magna est veritas criproevaleol.*

**Note to Second Edition** : I heard from this gentleman six years later, viz., January 1886, about his daughter's health, and learn that he himself still continues well, and — strange to say — also grateful! (VI 111)

## 73. CYANOSIS

There will be no harm in giving the following practical case of Blue Disease for what it is worth : —

*Morbus Caeruleus, Cyanosis,* or Blue Disease. Whether this was due to a permanence of the *foramen ovale,* and thus allowing the passage of the venous blood from the right auricle to the left, or to other abnormal apertures in the septum of the auricles and ventricles of the heart, or to any other maldisposition or abnormality, or to patency of the *ductus arteriosus,* I know not, but the subject was a young man of 25 or thereabouts. He had been a labourer in laird's ship building yards for years, but latterly had become unable for work. On my visiting him, I found him sitting propped up in a chair, his face of a deep purple blue colouration, with which we are all familiar as Cyanosis, and considerable oedema of the lower extremities, and hydrothorax; the dyspnoea was very great, and the distal ends of his fingers were clubbed in a most extraordinary degree, worse than I ever saw in the most advanced case of phthisis; a hacking cough; difficulty of speech; racking pains in all his bones and joints, so that he could neither move them nor yet remain quiet. That was just the character of the pain : *made easier by motion*. A more perfect picture of inhuman ugliness in a human being it was never my lot to behold, and this was rendered, worse by the hanging jaw and large oedematous face, and glaring bloodshot eyes. And yet his mother fondled and petted him as only mothers can ! After going over the case and learning that the cyanosis had been from his birth, and that he had only been so bad as at the present for a few weeks, I set about treating the most urgent symptoms, viz., the rheumatic pains. *Rhus toxicodendron* was given at frequent intervals. Now comes the strange part of the story : The *Rhus* not only gradually cured the rheumatism (which I expected) but it cured the oedema, the hydrothorax, the dyspnoea, *and actually lessened the general venosity very considerably,* and in course of time even his clubbed finger ends went a little smaller. As nearly as I remember he took the *Rhus* for about three months, and he then resumed his work as labourer.

That this was a mere *fluke* on my part I need not say, neither do I now comprehend *how* the amelioration came about, — I merely narrate a most interesting clinical fact. During a period of about two years subsequent to this he used to put in an appearance at the Wirral Homoeopathic Dispensary every month or two to be treated for various little colds, and the like, and then I left the neighbourhood, so I do not know what became of him, but so long as I remained at Birkenhead he continued to work in Laird's shipyards.

I do not merely mean that this poor fellow got over his rheumatism, oedema, hydrothorax, and dyspnoea, and was then merely as blue as he had previously been, but his ordinary blueness had very materially diminished — about one-half — as his mother and the neighbours very loudly and unanimously maintained. Here the choice of *Rhus* for the *kind* of pain was strictly scientific; its having brought about a remarkable amelioration in an old-standing case of *morbus coeruleus* is an empirical fact that I do not understand, and of which I therefore can offer no explanation.

This empirical use of *Rhus* I have since remembered with advantage.

## 74. BLUE-FACED BABIES

I have never since met with another case of regular *morbis coeruleus,* but I have had to treat very young babies with cyanotic faces, and have here used *Rhus* 3. with striking benefit. One was an eight-month child, whose circulation was apparently not quite normal, as its face was very pale and bluish. It was not purple by any means, still everybody remarked "how peculiar, bluish, its face was." *Rhus* 3 was given, one pilule three times a day, and the beneficial effect was unmistakable, for within a very few days the face assumed a normal colouration. In several other cases in little infants in whom I had noticed a bluishness of the face, or just of the lower lips only, I have used *Rhus* with undoubted benefit; the bluishness disappeared. Quite lately a little *blonde* of two, with a *blue* lower lip, was ordered *Rhus* by me, and the blueness disappeared in a fortnight, *Quo modo*? (VI 123)

## 75. HAEMORRHOIDS IN CONNECTION WITH ENGORGED SPLEEN

A well-nourished healthy lady of fifty years of age came under observation in April 1880, complaining of the following series of symptoms ... Pain in the left side corresponding to the region of the spleen, so bad that she cannot lie on the left side; with this pain in the side there are two other disturbances, indicating that a kind of vascular turgescence — an *orgasmus humorued* — underlies the whole, viz. : palpitation of the heart, and piles. With these also some indigestion and a feeling as if the visceral contents of the abdomen were being pulled down.

$R_x$ *Tc. Ceanothi Americani* 3x. ziv. Three drops in water three times a day. She came from the country, so I did not see her again; but as I asked for a report in a fortnight, her husband wrote at the end of that period to say that she was well and needed no further attention.

The case of this lady rather interested me, as some six years previously she came under my care for chronic headaches that seemed climacteric; I treated her for these headaches, but could not make any impression upon them, and then on going over the various organs I found that the urine contained a small quantity of albumen. This our ordinary remedies removed in about two months, and the headaches disappeared. About a year later the albuminuria again returned in a very slight degree, and with it some cephalagia; both yielded at once to the same remedies, and she had remained well till she came with the splenalgia and haemorrhoids. I suspect, therefore, that the old albuminuria was not due to any kidney mischief, but to venous congestion of the kidneys. (VI 124)

## 76. VARICOCELE WITH VENOUS ZIG-ZAG

This was a well-nourished, healthy looking gentleman of 29 years of age. He first came under observation on April 16th. He had sinned against his own body formerly, and, being happily enlightened on the subject of bodily chastity, had for years given it up, and ever since been seeking to regain his self-respect and bodily vigour. By the way, when will fathers become sufficiently *manly* to teach lads how to become men?

On carefully examining him, there were four points that came out :

1. There was an endocardial *bruit de souffle* most audible at the xiphoid cartilage.
2. The before-mentioned *venous zig-zag* line on the chest.

3. A left-sided varicocele these seven years; not very large.
4. He had once had a slight attack of piles — none now.

*Diagnosis* : General varicosis expressed especially in the right heart, vena portae, and spermatic veins.

*Treatment* : *Tc. Bell perennis* 1, ziv. Five drops in water three times a day.

June 2. Feels better in himself, the old feeling of *blightedness* left by the miserable habit of youth has gone. The effects of *Bellis* (common daisy) in this state, that I think of as *auto-traumatism*, is often little short of marvellous. But I cannot go into that at present. The varicocele is better; the endocardial *bruit* is less audible, he *feels* his heart comfortable now, the venous zig-zag is slightly better — less distinct, but I am not so very sure about this, having only the eye to go by.

$R_x$ *Tc. Acidi fluorici* 6, m. xxiv. Sac. lac. qs. Div. in p. aeq. xxiv.

To take one powder in a little water at bedtime and report progress in a month.

July 3. The varicocele is smaller; it formerly became very much more distended towards evening, especially after his having been on his feet a good deal all day, and notably *worse in hot weather*; but now he has no inconvenience from the varicocele *even after being on foot all day in this hot weather*. The endocardial bruit can now be heard only with difficulty. I hear very well indeed with both ears, yet the acuity of the right one is greater than that of the left (is it so in everybody — *i.e.*, do the ears differ *normally*?) and this quality of my hearing I make use of for differential diagnosis when using the stethoscope. Now I could formerly easily hear this bellows murmur with either ear, now I can barely hear it with the right aided by the stethoscope. By the way, we want some clinical acoumeter to aid us in coming to an opinion as to the quantitative value of endothoracic sounds for many of these bellows murmurs proceeding from the heart *do* disappear under treatment, may be they are only haemic but anyway we want to gauge them.

Patient is informed that in my opinion he is well, and fully fit for marriage. To this end he had sought advice. Of course, the result requires consolidating with some further medicinal treatment, by taking a drop or two of *Acidum fluoricum* 6 at bedtime does not seriously interfere with any human duties even if they be marital. (VI 127)

## 77. VARICOSIS - 3

A young lady, just over twenty years of age, had very bad varicosis of the left lower extremity, for which she had long worn an elastic appliance with much ease to the pains. Dancing and riding made the leg unbearable; and hence these pleasures, usually considered natural to her age and position, had been given up. The dancing she did not care for, as her views of the serious reality of life led her to think that rhythmic romping was unseemly, but she missed the riding very much. On my telling the Countess, her mother, that the case could, I thought, be cured by medicines. I was not believed. I found the left ovarian region occupied by a swelling of about the size of a baby's fist : it was very tender and there was very distressing leucorrhoea of long standing. I directed my attention to curing the ovarian swelling that appeared to me to be the cause of both varicosis and leucorrhoea. It might be too tedious to detail the two years' treatment, but the result was as I foretold : the ovarian swelling very slowly disappeared, and so did, *pari passu*, the varicosis and the leucorrhoea. The elastic stocking was, of course, abandoned, and riding was resumed. Once or twice I had to treat a threatening return of the ovarian swelling, but eventually the cure proved permanent. The mother received my prognosis gracelessly, and was quite thankless for the cure; but a physician who stands up for new theories and a heterodox practice must put up with antecedent gracelessness and subsequent thanklessness, and if he fail must bear the reproach of impurity of motive. By special grace it may not sour him. (VI 132)

## 78. VARICOSIS OF RIGHT LEG

B., an unmarried lady, of about twenty-two or twenty-three years of age, the daughter of a staff-officer, was brought to me by her mother some time since suffering from varicosis of the right leg, for which she was wearing the usual elastic stocking. Her sister had previously been operated on for ovarian disease, and on percussion and palpation a swelling in the region of the right ovary was readily made out. She complained also of pains in the right ovary and right breast at this period.

The further course of the case was just as in the last, only the amelioration was comparatively very quick.

I might enumerate other cases of unilateral varicosis, but these two exemplify all I have to say on the subject, merely emphasizing the point that unilateralness of effect leads me to seek unilateralness of cause, and both are usually on the same side of the body. (VI 135)

# DISEASES OF THE SKIN

## 79. ANGINA PECTORIS FROM SUPPRESSED SKIN DISEASE

One Sunday morning, some ten years ago, a gentleman ushered his wife into my consulting-room because she had been taken with an attack of *angina pectoris* in the street, on her way to church. Though only a little over thirty years of age, if so much, she had been subject to these attacks of breast-pang for several years : they would take her suddenly in the street, nailing her, as it were, to the spot, and hence she no longer went out of doors alone, lest she should faint away or fall down dead, as was apprehended.

An examination of the heart revealed no organic lesion, or even functional derangement, and I could not quite see why a comparatively young lady should get such anginal attacks. She had been under able men for her *angina*, but it got no better, and no one could apparently understand it. I prescribed for her, and saw her subsequently at her home, to try and elucidate the matter. I let her tell me her whole health-story from her earliest childhood. She said she was getting to the end of her teens, and was preparing to come out, but she had some cracks in the bends of her arms that were very unsightly; these cracks in her skin had troubled her from her earliest childhood. Erasmus Wilson was consulted; he gave her an ointment which very soon cured her skin, and the patient came out socially, made a hit right off, and got married in due course. She had always felt very grateful to Erasmus Wilson for curing her arms, for otherwise, "How could I have appeared in short sleeves."

But there soon followed dyspepsia, flatulence, dyspnoea, and palpitation, and finally the before described attacks of *angina pectoris* threatened to wreck her life. Moreover, she had borne one dead child. As I have already said, there was no discoverable cardiac lesion, and from the lady's health-history I gathered that this cure of her skin (though to me the one important point) was of no casual importance.

I gave my opinion that her skin disease had never been *really* cured, only *driven in* by Wilson's ointment, and that her angina was in reality its internal expression or metastasis. No one believed it, however. I began to treat her antipsorically, and very soon — I think it was less than a month from the Sunday morning visit — the old cracks reappeared in the bends of the elbows, *and from that time on she had no further attacks of angina* at all, and thenceforth she bore living children. (IX 91)

## 80. SPECIFIC ENEXANTHEMATIC ASTHMA

Not long after the before-mentioned experience I was consulted by a Liverpool gentleman for asthma of a very severe type. He was somewhere near forty, and had the appearance of a very old man, partly from the habitual bent position, from his shortness of breath, and partly from loss of sleep and much physicking. About a third of his life was spent in these attacks of asthma. In listening to his life-history, I noticed that he dated his asthma to a cold caught during a child's disease with a cutaneous eruption, and also, judging from his subjective 'symptoms, I concluded that he was suffering from an enexanthema, an internal skin disease of a specific nature. I treated him nearly a year on this hypothesis, and he got a strange coppery condition of the skin, which peeled of almost all over his body, much of his hair falling out at the same time. He was forthwith free of his asthma, and never had it again during the two following years, at the end of which period I lost sight of him. His skin became quite healthy, and his hair grew again. (IX 5)

## 81. ASTHMA, PSORIASIS AND ENLARGED LIVER

A gentleman of thirty came under my care some years since, suffering from asthma, enlargement of the liver, psoriasis, and eczema. When his skin was very bad, his breathing was well; and conversely if his skin got well; he was almost sure to get an attack of asthma, particularly in certain places. I treated his liver and his skin for many months — in fact, for nearly three years. It is now nearly two years since he had any attack of asthma, and he is well of both skin and liver, though sun and wind still affect his skin unduly. (IX 7)

## 82. HYDROCEPHALUS, ECZEMA — LATENT VACCINOSIS

In the early part of the year 1885 I was requested to see the only surviving child of a country clergyman, who had been given up by three medical men, as it had water on the brain. The child's head was of the usual hydrocephalic type; he was alternately wake and delirious at night, and he talked nonsense by day at intervals. Their local doctors had taken a consultant's opinion, and they agreed that the boy was suffering from tuberculosis of the meninges with infusion, of which a little brother had previously died. The child's life-history was told to me, and I underlined the facts that he had had eczema, and had been twice *un*successfully vaccinated. After the *un*successful vaccinations (want of organismic reactionary power) the eczema almost disappeared, and very soon the present disease began. I treated the case thus causally *ex-hypothesi*; a severe pustular eruption, and then patches of lepra and eczema appeared, and at the end of about six months' treatment I was able to discharge the little patient, cured of his water on the brain and of his skin diseases. I saw him the other day, and learned that he continues well and has grown a good deal, (IX 8)

## 83. ECZEMA CAPITIS SUPPRESSED — FATAL ISSUE

About nine years ago the wife of a staff-officer brought her bony little baby to me : it had the milkcursty scalp, so horrible to aesthetic mothers — in fact, it had *crusta lactec, or eczema capitis*. The scalp appeared one solid crust of scabs, but the child seemed perfectly well and jolly. I prescribed for the child *constitutionally*, and forbade all local treatment. The lady's father, however, was a retired physician of repute, and he went to stay at the daughter's house. Seeing the grandchild's eczema, he told the mother to use an ointment to the scalp. She told her father of my warning not to put anything on the bad head, but the old gentleman over-ruled it, and prescribed *unguentum zinci*, which soon healed the eczema. About a fortnight later I was suddenly summoned by telegram to see the child : it had been taken with convulsions from effusion on the brain, and the local doctors were already nonplussed. I did my best to get the eczema back on the surface of the scalp, but totally failed; the child died, and the grandfather sobbingly cried, "Oh ! that zinc ointment." (IX 10)

## 84. DOUBLE CATARACT FROM SUPPRESSED ERUPTION

A middlesex grocer brought his bright little boy of six or seven to me about two years since : the boy had double cataract, and was quite blind. Said the father to me : He used to have an eruption on his head, but that was cured by the doctors at the — Hospital for Diseases of the Skin. And soon *after* he was cured of his eruption we noticed his sight was failing — before that his sight was all right. (IX 11)

## 85. ECZEMA OPHTHALMIA

A lady of fifty came under my care in October 1879. Two years previously she had had eczema of the vulva, with much nocturnal irritation. Dr. W. cured it with bran water and vegetal diet. In August 1879 she got eczema behind the right ear, when her physician gave her *Graphites* 3x and *Merc. sol.* 3x in alternation.

In September of the same year she went to A — , and there met a doctor, who gave her a saline draught, and an ointment containing zinc, lead, and mercury, to be applied at night.

This cured the eczema. She came to me for an inflammation of right eye, that came very soon after the eczema was cured. I explained to her that the ophthalmia and the eczema were really the same thing, and advised constitutional treatment, to which she consented. She *was worse at the sea-side,* she was constipated, her skin was dry, *salt* beef caused constipation and faintness, and she was low-spirited. *Natrum muriaticum* 6, trit., and other remedies, cured her constitutionally, and she had not had any return of skin disease or ophthalmia, when her husband called on me, on June 2nd, 1885, or more than five years thereafter. (IX 12)

## 86. OSSIFIED HEART FROM SUPPRESSED ECZEMA

In the year 1874, I was attending a country squire for eczema of the whole body of a very bad type, — in fact I never saw a worse case. He could not undress without laying a sheet on the carpet, as the quantity of dried scabs that fell off was really considerable : after undressing he was in the habit of using the coal-shovel to shovel them up. I treated him to the best of my ability for a long time, but in vain; he grew rather worse than better. I called in a consultant of very great experience and world-wide reputation, and we treated the case together; but the eczema defied us, and so did the patient too. He sent for me one day, said he was sick of the weary, weary "constitutional treatment" of which I was always telling him. I solemnly warned him against local measures, such as baths and ointments, saying : "Remember this, Mr. __ , I acknowledge that I have quite failed to cure your eczema with my 'constitutional treatment,' at which it pleases you to poke fun, but *you yourself never enjoyed better health in your life,* although your eczema is indeed almost as bad as ever. You are disgusted with your foul disease, and you mean to be rid of its outward expression, come what may. I am sorry for you." He went to an eminent special skin doctor, now deceased, and in a few months was cured of his eczema by means of ointments, washes, and mineral waters.

For four years I did not see him, and then he called to consult me *about difficulty of breathing* that had been slowly creeping on for several years, — in fact was first felt not long after his being cured by Mr. S. of eczema. I should have said that the patient in question told his skin doctor of my warnings anent his eczema, and this gentleman made light of it, declaring that it was my incompetence to cure that deserved attention, and used such language about me professionally that my patient would not allow my name to be mentioned in his house for nearly three years. Then his dyspnoea became a serious matter, and his physicians all failed to cure it, though they all declared that his lungs were sound. At last he found that an extra glass of champagne, a tiny incline, the gentlest game of croquet, all upset his breathing, and the doctors' skill failing, too, he went to the South of France, and to spas, and then to lung specialists, but all to no purpose — his breathing slowly and surely grew worse. Finally he came to me, "to please his wife." He seemed quite well to look at; there was no trace of his former eczema on his skin; his lungs were all right, but his heart was irregular in its action, and there was neither apex-beat nor radial pulse. No medicines did him any real or permanent good, though many well-chosen remedies relieved his various symptoms; in fact, I cured all his symptoms over and over again, and then he died of his disease. We had a *post-mortem* examination of the body, and found ossification of the heart in about two-thirds of its extent, with osseous and quasi-osseous adhesions to the diaphragm and shrinking of the liver.

No doubt, to my mind, about the genesis of the degeneration of the internal organs. When Nature was prevented from speaking as eczema by Mr. S.'s skin-gagging, she used the internal parts wherein to deposit the irritant material which produced inflammation and ossification of the most vital organ — the heart — rendering a continuation of its functions impossible. Such are the facts, and such my reading thereof. (IX 14)

## 87. DISAPPEARANCE OF PSORIASIS AND TRACHOMA AFTER ERYSIPELAS

Striking instances of internal affections being cured by some outward, or other acute manifestation constantly recur in medical literature. A few years since I was reading in the *London Medical Record* (April 15, 186, p. 155, *et seq.*), that —

"Dr. Porfiry G. Bazaroff, of Belyi Klutch, records (*Proceedings of the Caucasian Medical Society*, No. 18, 1885, p. 433) the case of a highly scrofulous soldier, aged 22, who was admitted with general psoriasis vulgaris of two years' duration, severe trachoma of long standing on both sides, and enlargement of the cervical and submaxillary glands. The treatment failing to relieve any of the patient's extremely obstinate and troublesome affections, the regimental surgeons resolved upon placing him on the roll of 'unfit for service.' About that time, however, the patient was suddenly attacked by erysipelas of the face and head. There was nothing peculiar either in the course or in the treatment of the disease. The erysipelas disappeared in seven days, and with it the trachoma, the glandular swellings and psoriasis (first of the face, then — after two hot baths — of the remaining parts) also disappeared, leaving no trace. 'In fact, in a week an "unfit" became quite a healthy man,' the author adds. Dr. Bazaroff mentions, also, a rather obscure case of a young soldier, who had suffered from daily and nightly incontinence of urine, of two months' duration, and who got rid of the symptoms after an attack of erysipelas of the face and head. In another patient, a boy, aged 22 months, with congenital hydrocephalus of the progressive kind, a mild attack of scarlatina was followed by a steady diminution in the bulk of the head (in a month the large circumference lessened a centimetre, the minor 3), an improvement in his general state, &c. Two months later, however, the child died from general convulsions. [Dr. M. Tumpovsky recently published a case of disappearance of ascites from erysipelas (see the *London Medical Record,* May, 1885, p. 19,) Dr. K. Koltchevsky saw a case of trachoma cured by erysipelas (*Ib.,* July, p. 296). Dr. Mishtolt's patient was cured by the same disease from sarcoma (*Ib.,* January, 1884, p. 11). In the *Vratch,* Nos. 38 — 41, 1882, Dr. F. J. Pasternatzky, of Professory J. T. Tchudnovskys clinic, details two cases of the disappearance of hepatic ascites under the influence of typhus fever, and a case of renal dropsy cured by relapsing fever. In the *St. Petersburg Med. Wochensch.,* No. 43, 1883, Dr. Schmidt published a case where erysipelas of the chest had caused a rapid disappearance of an enormous pleuritic exudation — *Rep.*]"

All this surely proves that topic disease is not local, but *organic and organismic.* (IX 20)

## 88. ECZEMA WITH INTERNAL METASTATIC SYMPTOMS

A few years since — May, 1886 — I met with a very striking example of the intimate connection that exists between a skin affliction and internal symptoms. I had seen the lady in town and prescribed for her on April 13th, 1886, and I received the following letter, subsequently. I give it just as I received it, and will let it tell its own simple though instructive tale :

"A few days after I came to see you I was very unwell — at the usual time — which commenced four days too soon, and lasted nine days. On the fourth day, Sunday, April 18th, I was taken at 5 A.M. with fainting, etc., as before; took brandy just in time to prevent going quite off. This was followed by sickness, alternate heat and chill, and I was unable to take any food without causing sickness; I was so ill that my brother became anxious, and sent for the nearest homoeopathic doctor. The sickness continued frequently until he arrived about 1 P.M. I was very weak and in my room for some days.

"During this time the eruption on hands and face disappeared, and the cracks healed, but as soon as I recovered it broke out again and was worse than ever on my face, large patches of spots continually running, with heat and irritation. Both face and hands were much swollen, and eruption extended to wrists and neck — right side of neck below the ear being swollen and tender.

"After a few days the fingers and backs of hand became very badly cracked; for ten days I could scarcely use my hands, and they are still very sore; there is less tendency to heal than usual, and considerable irritation; the joints of fingers are also swollen."

This lady had previously had catalepsy on various occasions, and she consulted me for the neurosis principally. (IX 23)

## 89. ERUPTION ON SCALP — CATARACT

The following case is very instructive, as showing the nature of a skin affection of the head (scalp), and its power of expressing itself in the lens if compelled to retire from the outer integument.

Towards the end of the year 1880, a boy of four was brought to me from the South of England. His sight was good until he was about two years old, when he had incipient cataract in the right eye, then in the left one, and at the age of three he was blind.

I elicited the following noteworthy anamnestic point : He used to have great irritation of the skin ever since he was a few months old; when between eight and nine months old he was treated for it with "Sulphur ointment, a lotion, and medicines."

After the first medicine which I ordered him an eruption came on his skin, and more particularly on the scalp, and he began to see. His mother reported that he altered in his gait, for whereas he formerly looked straight out before him fixedly at the light, now he bends forward. He further astonished his parents by remarking that there was a certain colour in the painted ceiling, pale green. There was also slight but evident change in the opaque lenses themselves.

Now, although I had given to the parents, as my opinion, that the cataract was a direct consequence of the cured (suppressed) skin affection from which the child had suffered, still, no sooner did my medicine begin to bring back the eruption to the scalp than the mother forthwith applied some zinc ointment she had in the house! The zinc ointment did its work very promptly and effectually; the eruption disappeared, and so did the returning vision, — *i.e.*, the boy went quite blind again, and remained so. He also began to talk, laugh, and cry in his sleep again as he had previously done.

The further course of this case showed most conclusively that the opacity of the lenses, and the scalp eruption, stood in causal nexus, — that is to say, they had a common cause. Orthodox medicine *cured* the eruption with ointment, then came the cataract, which is again *cured* by operation. Truly, we live in an age of wisdom and enlightenment. (IX 27)

## 90. PUSTULAR ERUPTIONS - 1

Mr. J — , a hale-looking, middle-aged London merchant, came under my observation on November 3rd, 1881. Said he, "I am not a homoeopath, but twenty years ago I had eczema, and the allopaths could not touch it, so I went to a homoeopathic doctor, and he cured me." And he went on to say that he believed in homoeopathy for skin diseases. On the left leg he had a pustular eruption, due, he believed, to a bruise. He had also eczema of the ear, and he volunteered the information that ever since his second vaccination he had been subject to eczema. The eczema of twenty years ago was soon after the re-vaccination.

$R_x$ *Thuja Occidentalis* 30. Four three-drop powders to the two dozen. To take one, dry on the tongue, three times a day.

He came in a week nearly well; the pustules had at once begun to wither.

The *Thuja* was repeated, but in less frequent doses, and the patient subsequently sent word by his brother to say that, his skin was well, and he himself too busy to show himself as he had promised. (IX 31)

## 91. PUSTULAR ERUPTIONS - 2

Miss __, æt. 18, was re-vaccinated in July, 1881, at her parents' country residence, thirty miles from London, by the local surgeon, with "lymph" direct from the calf. The operation was very successful, and she had a very "fine" arm. But as the "arm" was just at its greatest perfection she got an eruption on her chin, covering its whole extent and involving the lower lip. The thing was very unsightly, and had a singularly ugly, repulsive aspect. The gentleman who had done the re-vaccination was of opinion that Miss — had got some of the vaccine virus on to her finger-nails and inoculated herself by scratching. The sequel, however, showed that the chin manifestation was from within. The surgeon had ordered applications, two of which were vaseline and zinc ointment, but the eruption on the chin was not to be got rid of. The young lady had to wear a dense veil to hide her face when driving out. She was brought to London for my advice, and I gave *Thuja* 30. In a fortnight; she was out and about, and only some diffused redness of the skin remained, but no scar or thickened skin. Now, it might be objected to this case that the *Thuja* had nothing to do with the disappearance of the eruption, because it was just the history of the disease; it ran through its natural course and died, I thought that to myself at the time of prescribing it; but against this was the fact that the arm had healed already, and it had passed the natural course of vaccinia by at least a fortnight when I first prescribed the *Thuja*. But to have a test, I gave her brother, who also had a somewhat similar pustular eruption (and who had been re-vaccinated at the same time), but more spare, and instead of being on the chin, it was around the left nostril, I say, to have a test, I gave this brother of Miss — — *Antimonium tart.*, which is also, as every one knows, apparently homoeopathic to such a pustular eruption.

This is the brother of Miss — — (*Observation iv.*)

The two eruptions were similar, though the boy's was comparatively trivial, and of the same age, and from the same cause, *i.e.*, from the vaccine virus. The patients went into the country, and in two or three weeks' time the mother wrote that the young lady was quite well : "the medicine soon put her right," was her expression, but the boy had "a bad cold in his head; nose-bleed; left side of nose swelled and red; two little spots of matter, the size of a large pin's head, at the edge of the nostril, and below it, having something the look of — -'s chin; his arm is also not well, and he has had four little pocks about the vaccination marks." I sent *Thuja* 30, and he was reported well in ten days.

If any one can account for the cure of these two cases independently of the *Thuja*, his ingenuity is greater than mine. That they were causally connected with the re-vaccination admits of no doubt whatever. (IX 33)

## 92. HAIRLESS PATCHES ON CHIN

Mr. ___, a London merchant, came under my care on July 27th, 1882, to be treated for some roundish hairless patches on either side of his chin, which began four months ago. The larger patch on the right side was about the size of a florin. Had also an old hordeolum on his right lower eyelid.

Has been twice vaccinated; the second time, twelve years ago, did *not* "take."

$R_x$ *Thuja Occidentalis* 30 (4 in 24). To take one, dry on the tongue, at bedtime.

Sept. 7th. — The bald patches are smaller, the one on the left side nearly gone. Has, apparently, a very bad coryza — (?) organismic reaction.

*Rep.*

Oct. 17th. — The bald patches are gone; the old hordeolum also gone. The closely-shaven beard is now uniform, the previously existing white bald patches being completely covered with hair.

I give this as an interesting cure by *Thuja*, but I am not very sure that the disease was really due to vaccinosis, because of other points in his clinical history. Still it might have been so, as the hair is very powerfully influenced by the vaccine poisoning. Thus Kunkel observed both a very weak growth of hair and an excessive growth, especially in wrong places, as effects, he believed, of vaccination. Therefore, let it stand as a doubtful case of vaccinosis for what it may be worth, — but there can hardly be any reasonable doubt as to the cure of the case by *Thuja*.

Here it might not be amiss to observe casually that the presence of sties on the eyelids is often, in my opinion, a symptom of vaccionosis. This case is not without practical importance, inasmuch as hodiernal medicine hands over a sty to the chirurgeon's art; and all the time, poor old dame, weens herself so very much superior to scientific therapeutics usually called homoeopathy. The conceit of the orthodoxly ignorant is truly sickening. (IX 37)

## 93. ACNE OF FACE AND NOSE AND NASAL DERMATITIS

A young lady, about twenty years of age, was brought by her mother to me on October 28th, 1882. Patient had a very red pimply nose, not like the red nose of the elderly bibber, or like that due to dyspepsia or to tight-lacing, but a pimply, scaly nasal dermatitis, which extended from the cutaneous covering of the nose to that of the cheeks, but appearing more as facial acne. The nasal dermatitis was, roughly, in the form of a saddle. Of course, this state of things in an otherwise pretty girl of twenty was painfully and humiliatingly unpleasant to her and to her friends, — in fact, it was likely to mar her future prospects very materially, more especially as it had already existed for six years and was making no signs of departing. She also complained of obstinate constipation. The pimples of the nose and face used to get little white mattery heads. In trying to trace the skin-affection back to its real origin I ascertained that the patient was re-vaccinated six years ago, but she could not remember whether the nose was previously affected or not. This re-vaccination was unsuccessful, *i.e.*, it did *not* "take."

$R_x$ *Thuja Occidentalis* 30.

November 30th. — Pimples of face decidedly better. Nose less red. Constipation no better.

$R_x$ *Thuja Occidentalis* 100.

January 3rd, 1883. — The face is free. Her mother gratefully exclaims, "She is wonderfully better." I ask the young lady which powders did her *most good*, she says, "The *last*." The skin of the nose is normal, but the constipation is no better, and for this she remains under treatment.

That *Thuja* cured this case is incontrovertible; but that it was a case of vaccinosis is not quite so certain, though it is far from improbable. The re-vaccination and inflammation of the skin of the nose were referred both to six years ago when she was in Switzerland at school; but patient could not remember which was first — the bad nose or the vaccination. (IX 41)

## 94. DISEASED FINGER-NAILS

On December 22nd, 1882, a young lady of twenty-six came under my care for an ugly state of the nails of her fingers. Naturally a lady of her age would not be indifferent to the state of her nails. These nails are indented rather deeply, and in addition to these indentations there are black patches on the under surfaces of the nails, reaching into the quick. Very slight leucorrhoea occasionally. She had chicken-pox as a child of eleven. On her shoulders there is an eruption of roundish patches forming mattery heads. Has been vaccinated three different times; the last time two years ago, and the nails have become diseased *since* this last vaccination. The black patches have existed these eighteen months.

Looking upon this — diseased condition of the nails as evidence of chronic vaccinosis, I ordered her *Thuja* 30 (one in 6).

March 19th, 1883. Has continued the *Thuja* 30 for just about three months, with the result that within a fortnight from commencing with it the black patches under the nails began to disappear, and there is now no trace of them. The indentations are notably better. The eruption on the back has not been modified, and for this she remains under treatment; but I thought this much of a case of nail disease would be of some interest, and the more so as it it not easy to demonstrate drug-action on nail growth at all.

The foregoing cases sufficiently exemplify the causal nexus existing, as I believe, between vaccination and diseases of the skin. However, by no means must be attributed all skin affection, following closely or remotely in the wake of vaccination, to the pathogenetic effect of the vaccine virus itself; it *does* cause numerous skin diseases without a doubt, but it also, and frequently, *rouses latent disease* for which anti-vaccinial treatment will, of course, not suffice. (IX 44)

## 95. RINGWORM OF SCALP — CATARACT

At the beginning of 1883 a boy of six was brought to me, from Yorkshire, with opacities of both lenses. The failing of his sight was first noticed in 1881. Had been under an oculist of repute, who had given some drops to be put into the eyes, but these drops could not be used after the first instillation, as they "made the child like a dead'un for days." Has been delicate all his life, and notably worse since the measles in the summer of 1880.

Had ringworm of the scalp in the summer of 1879, which was cured by internal (probably tonic) and external treatment. The father says he is "wick," which he explains means *lively*. After four months of Sulphur 30, and then of the 200th, this report came — "My boy is still improving with his eyes slowly, they have not that large, glaring appearance, look more natural and he has not been excited in his sleep; I think his head is cooler."

A little later I received a letter to say the boy had "ringworm on his scalp again!" That was the last I heard of him.

The connection of cataract and various skin affections has long been noticed and written about by numerous authors, but the doctrine is not accepted by many. On this point I take the liberty of referring to my treatise on Cataract.

## 96. SCABIES — CATARACT — FURUNCLES

Young man, æt. 20, had had the itch one year and a half ago, of which he got rid by internal and external use of medicines. Later, he had an attack of intermittent fever, which he cured with pepper and whisky. A short time since he discovered that he could not see with his left eye. The eye had a dead look; pupil was enlarged and immovable; in the middle of the lens there was an opacity, as if it had been punctured by a needle; the lids and conjunctiva were somewhat reddened. On holding the hand quite near to the eye he could dimly discern the fingers. August 2, *Sulphur* 6; August 9, SEVERAL PIMPLES ON THE FACE AND ARMS. Sight better. *Sulph.* 6, which was repeated on the 19th, 26th, and 29th of August, and on the 3rd and 23rd of September. THERE APPEARED A NUMBER OF FURUNCLES ON THE ARMS; the eye looks natural again, and he sees as well as ever before. — (Fr. Emmerich, "Arch." XIV. iii,p. 105. In Raue.)

And then (pp. 77-78) —

Dr. Bernard gives an epitome of fifteeen cases from Ruckert's *Klinische Erfahrungen.*. (IX 50)

## 97. CRUSTA LACTEA

The fifteenth is this : Crusta Lacta disappears and cataract supervenes which latter is cured with *Spirit Sulph.* (*Autore*, Schoenfeld).
Dr. Bernard also notes that in several of the cases habitual perspiration re-appear, or a custaneous eruption either appears or re-appears.
Need we any further proof that cataract is a *cutaneous* affection? (IX 51)

## 98. TETTERS

Dr. Becker treated a carpenter who had been affected for some time with tetters about the face, which disappeared after a while without his taking any medicine, but his sight became impaired, everything appeared in a place different from its real position, so that he was unable to use his tools properly.
The pupils presented a misty, smoky appearance, as in the forming stage of cataract. He received *Spirit Sulph.*, ten drops three times a day; *the old eruption re-appeared*, and he now saw everything in the right position, but otherwise his sight was not improved.
Then on March 22nd, *Aq. Silic.* was administered in doses of seven drops daily, and this was followed by a great improvement in his sight. He perspired easily, and had much perspiration about the feet. Deposit in urine like lime.
July. — A rheumatic inflammation of the foot set in. (IX 52)

## 99. SUPPRESSED PERSPIRATION OF FEET

The same gentleman treated a lady whose feet generally perspired freely and then became very dry, and thereafter she noticed that her sight became affected in such a manner that everything she looked at appeared to be enveloped in a cloud, she could only read large print.
*Aq. Silic.* was administered in doses of ten drops twice a day. *The accustomed perspiration of the feet returned again* in about a month. Her eyesight became much better. Two months latter, at the time of menstruation, her eyes became worse again, and she then took twenty drops of *Ac. Silic.* three times a day, after which she improved very much, could read better, and continued taking the same remedy. (IX 54)

## 100. SCABIES — AGUE

M., aged 20, tinsmith by trade, was affected a year and a half ago with the worst kind of itch, and subsequently : with fever and ague. Sometimes he had tearing pains in the left eye, and some itching of the skin, to which he paid very little attention; suddenly he noticed, however, that he had become completely blind in the left eye.
*Symptoms* — A staring look of the left eye; pupil dilated and immovable; in the centre of the lens there was slight opacity; his sight was almost extinguished.
*Treatment* — August 2. — *Sulph.* 6, from August 9th to September 23rd, six doses of the same.
Six days after the first dose, *many pustules appeared on the face and arms;* in the meanwhile his eyesight improved so much that he was enabled to distinguish large letters. From September 13th to September 23rd, *furuncles on the arm made their appearance;* after that the skin became clear again, and the affected eye was as useful as it had ever been before, — ("Arch." XIV., v., p. 105. Emmerich.)
Of the connection of the skin and the lens embryologically and pathologically I will say no more, merely referring those interested in the subject for further information to "Curability of Cataract." (IX 55)

## 101. THE STERNAL PATCH - 1

One often meets with liver affections connected with cutaneous manifestations.
I would like particularly to refer to a patch of eruption on the skin covering the lower part of the sternum, which I have several times found co-exist with heart disease and swelling of the left lobe of the liver. In my case-takings I call it in the "sternal patch."
I have four such cases in my mind at this moment. The first I will narrate is that of a mayor of a large town in the north — He had a patch of brownish lichen on the sternal portion of thorax, of the size of a woman's palm; with it were associated an enlarged liver and a cardiac affection, evidenced by palpitation, systolic murmur, and general uneasiness. He came to town to see me at odd intervals for about two years, and was then discharged cured. I treated him antipsorically and organopathically, the most notable benefit being derived from *Carduus Marianus* in five drop doses of the strong tincture given three times a day. (IX 57)

## 102. STERNAL PATCH - 2

The second, I remember, was a Manchester merchant, with the same kind of cutaneous patch on the sternum, and very notable heart trouble, with arcus senilis as a concomitant. Here the case and comfort brought by the *Carduus Marianus* were very striking. Under date of January 31st, 1883, I find in my case-book these words of the enthusiastic patient, — "It had a most marvellous effect; soon made me right; the patch went away in a fortnight; had had it for years."
This gentleman has remained under my care, calling upon me at ood times when in town, and during the past two years has had, besides the strong tincture of *Carduus, Bellis perennis* 1, *Aurum metallicum* 4, *Vanadium* 6, and *Acidum oxalicum* 3x, and some other remedies, and I consider him vastly improved, and his life — speaking commercially — worth 40 per cent. more than previously. (IX 59)

## 103. STERNAL PATCH AND LIVER DISEASE

The third case was that of a New York merchant, who suffered from liver, and had come over to Europe to consult a physician, as he seemed to get no better from the treatment of his New York advisers. I found his liver very much enlarged, and also the before-mentioned sternal patch of skin disease. I gave him *Carduus* in like dose to the foregoing, and he came in a week declaring himself quite well. I advised him to remain awhile under observation, to see if the cure proved permanent, but he hurried out of my room in great glee, and I never saw him again. (IX 60)

## 104. STERNAL PATCH AND ENLARGED LIVER

The fourth case in which I found the sternal patch and enlarged liver, giddiness, and palpitations of the heart, was that of a London lawyer. Here the liver got well, and the heart too, together with the giddiness, but it needed a course of antipsoric treatment to finish the cure of the patch of diseased skin. I might say the same of a fifth case, — an officer in the Royal Navy, where this patch co-exists with hypertrophied liver, and in which the affair has a specific air about it, probably inherited. (IX 61)

## 105. CHIN AND THROAT AFFECTIONS

At the commencement of 1873 a young lady came from a distance to consult me in regard to her throat. She told me she had originally relaxed sore throat, and went to Mr. — -, who cauterized it a good many times, and she used gargles and other local means on his advice. Her throat became better, but she then got a series of quinsies. Then came recommendations of changes of air and tonics. She had thereafter nothing to complain of in her throat, but her chin had become the seat of some nasty spots. For these she returned to the same gentleman, who cured the chin with ointment. After her chin got well her throat again troubled her. Renewed cauterizings; throat again cured. Then the face and chin were covered with spots and pimples afresh. She went on for six years under the most many-sided surgeon of the day, who writes so very philosophically about the pedigree of disease, but who treats his patients generally locally all the same, absolutely unmindful of the twaddling dictum about "gleams of a fruitful suggestion." Well, as this young lady's chin and throat persisted in playing hide and seek, she felt constrained to try something else. I went into the case carefully, and found that the real *seat* of the constitutional disturbances giving rise to the symptoms in the throat and on the chin was neither in the throat nor in the chin, but in the *ovaries*, and so, of course, the silly treating of the throat and chin had led to nothing. (IX 62)

## 106. THE ABSURDITY OF SPECIALISM

Probably it would not be easy to obtain a more striking example of the absurdity and futility of ordinary local treatment usual with most of the so-called specialists than this :

Miss Mora — , twenty-four years of age, was brought to me in June 1885, that I might give my opinion of her case. My treatment was not sought at that time. Twelve years previously she had scarlet fever, and following thereon, measles. Ever since then she has been deaf. She has been subject for varying periods and to various places.

Now, she is actually under two specialists; one treats the ear, and the other is treating her hay fever. In addition to these two learned brethren, her mother is also treating her "nettle-rash" with domestic homoeopathy.

With all this local tinkering and pottering and domestic messing, she is no better. No one has attempted to take a view of her entire economy as a living unity. Is it any wonder that all these fruitless measures have made the poor girl almost bewildered? (IX 65)

## 107. RELATIONSHIP OF SKIN AFFECTIONS TO INTERNAL ORGANS

As illustrating the *general* nature of skin affections, and their intimate relationship with other organs and parts, I will narrate a part of the history of a lady of rank, now forty odd years of age.

Originally, some fifteen or more years ago, she had badly ulcerated legs, and her local surgeon cured them quickly with an ointment. Soon after this cure — of which both patient and doctor were very proud — she had ulcers on the eyes, which a late eminent oculist cauterized, without being able to get rid of them; then a very noted London physician saw her, and said he thought the ulcers on the eyes were due to the too rapid cure of the ulcerated skin of the legs, and ordered her to use vinegar compresses over her shins, with the object of inducing fresh ulcers; but, *at the same time*, he ordered her to use golden ointment to the eye ulcers, — which golden salve forthwith cured them. The vinegar compresses produced an eruption on the legs, as they will on most people.

How this unctuous physician could give an opinion that the eye affection arose from the quasi-cured leg ulcers, and then forthwith order an ointment to cure the eye ulcers on precisely the same lines, might at first sight seem strange, only one knows of him that he mistakes a jumble of second-hand clinical tips for laws of therapeutics.

Presently the poor patient found that getting rid of corneal and conjunctival ulcers with golden ointment was anything but a cure of the disease essentially, for the next step of the progress of the disease was *in* the eye, *not on* it. The *inside* of the eye not lending itself to unctuous handling, it was sought out with the — knife! The operation had to be repeated several times. Well, it's a long, weary, story, and patient is nearly blind, and almost eyeless these several years.

I was listening to this history two days ago, and the poor lady exclaimed, "Ah! if I had but never used that golden ointment." (IX 68)

## 108. ECZEMA — ENLARGED OVARY — CHRONIC OOPHORITIS

It is about two years since a lady of forty came from a distance to see me; she was an invalid, and had not had a month of good health for many years. I found her suffering from chronic oophoritis of the right side, which recrudesced every month at the menstrual time, and which was often accompanied by circumscribed peritonitis. The ovary was enlarged to about the size of an orange, was very tender, and was clearly attached by post-inflammatory adhesions to the peritoneum. The dysmenorrhoea was very terrible, and the periodical peritonitis was quite an illness. She had leucorrhoea, and her visage told the tale of great and repeated sufferings. Treatment has quite cured her, and she now leads an active, useful life; but that is not the point I wish to dwell upon, but rather upon its origin.

I found from her history that she used to suffer from eczema; she went to Erasmus Wilson, who prescribed "zinc ointment and other things," and quickly cured it (the eczema). Patient herself *denied* "ever having had anything the matter with her skin;" it was her relations who told me of the old eczema.

People have certain preconceived ideas of diseases : if they know you are suffering from "liver," they smile; if you have anything wrong with your brain, rendering you insane or vicious, they are afraid of you and lock you up in an asylum; if you have anything wrong with your skin, they shun and despise you, little weening that the same or a like morbid essentiality may be at the bottom of them all. And hence, when questioned about their "skin." people not infrequently stop short of all the truth. (IX 71)

## 109. TUMOURS AND THE SKIN

An eminently instructive case came under my observation on August 13, 1885. A lady, just over 50 years of age, came to consult me with regard to a tumour in her right breast, I having successfully treated a lady friend of hers for a similar affection. But it is not about this tumour, as such, that I wish to speak, — it is the antecedent constitutional condition of the patient that bears on my present thesis, viz., the systemic nature of skin diseases. Well, this lady had suffered from red angry pimples on her face, chin, chest, and back all her menstrual life, with coincident neuralgia of right ovary. She had in vain used washes, ointments, and baths for the skin; only temporary ease and amelioration resulted. But about a year before the date of this visit, she fell with her right breast against a bedstead, and a few months later she noticed a hard lump in her right breast, and her family physician, with a consultant, urged immediate operation, to avoid which she came to me. Just as postscripts are said to contain the real *raison d'etre* of a given epistle, so the parting observation of a patient often throws a strong light on a case. And so here. As she rose from her chair to go, she said. "... It is very funny, doctor, but my skin has been so much clearer since the lump came, — in fact, I have very few pimples now; I dare say that has nothing to do with it, but I thought I'd just mention it." (IX 98)

## 110. HABITUAL PERIODICAL FACIAL DERMATITIS

Miss P., æt. 30, came under my observation on September 24th, 1879, and gave the following history — Ever since she was 12 years old she had been subject to an eruption of great bumps in the face about every three weeks, sometimes less, sometimes more; at one time barely to be seen, at another looking like Phlegmonous Erysipelas. This eruption coincided with the commencement of the menstruation. Going back to its origin, I elicited the following curious fact :

Just before her twelfth year, she was one day out in the fields in sultry weather at hay-making, and while thus greatly heated she fell head foremost into a brook; and some days thereafter she broke out all over head and face with an eruption "just like small-pox." Her whole face and ears were covered, and discharged so much that her mother had to tie a handkerchief round her neck to prevent its dropping on her clothes. She was indoors eight weeks with it. "Since then," she exclaims, "I have had any amount of medicines and greases, and all sorts of things, but they never did me one bit of good!" She had often a terrible sinking at the stomach, as if she had a large hole wanting filling up, together with a pressive headache at the top. Bowels regular, menses very painful — a hot, bad pain across the hypogastrium at the beginning.

*Bellis* was considered a capital remedy for such as had partaken of cold drink when the body was overheated. This is, of course, an extension of this application of its use, but the same idea underlies it. How do we know but cold drink taken into a heated body produces internal erysipelas? If, in the end, this idea be found to bear useful therapeutic fruit, it will doubtless be found in strict conformity with the law of similars. All my observations tend to that conclusion. But considering *Bellis perennis* as analogous in its action to *Arnica* gives a fair reason for its use in this case, as *Arnica* both causes and cures Erysipelas.

Therefore $R_x$ Tc. *Bellis per.* 3x ziv.

S — Three drops in water three times a day.

Oct. 22nd — Face is quite well; has not had a speck for the past fortnight or more. It left gradually. She is actually; menstruating (it began yesterday), and her face is quite free for the first time at the beginning of the flow in her whole menstrual life, which began *eighteen years* ago !! Her bowels have become *confined*, and she has now, but only after food, *a queer shaking, beginning in the pit of the stomach, and going up to the throat*, precisely as if she had been running fast.

To take two drops only once a day, and come again in five weeks.

Nov. 24th — Has continued well of the eruption; last poorly time not a spot!

She came occasionally for two or three months to report herself, and thus I can affirm that it so far remained permanently cured.

The *Bellis* did *not* affect either the sinking at the stomach or the pressive headache on the top of the head at all; so, early in December, I gave her *Sulphur* 30, *one drop* at bedtime for twelve days, when these two symptoms also disappeared. It is to be noted that these two symptoms were of much later date than the facial dermatitis.

Of course, my reasoning in the foregoing case might be faulty, but I think it shows that the Daisy is a notable remedy, and this virtue of a common weed lying everywhere at our feet deserves to be made very widely known. People of any experience do not need to be told that the ill effects of drinking cold drinks when the body is heated are very serious at times, and always inconvenient. Of course, it is not confined to the drinking, as the idea is *sudden wet chill to heated stomach* or *body surface*. This property of the daisy is the more valuable, as we know of no other remedy in our vast Pharmacopoeia that possesses it; and, beyond myself, I believe no one is acquainted with it. Most of what I here write has been lying in a drawer of my writing-desk for years, and this little clinical tip ought long since to have been published, for it may be a good while before another lover of the fair Daisy stumble against old Schroeder's generalization in a humble receptive mood. I regard this peculiar property of the Daisy as eminently important, and ask all who may read this to make it known, so that it may be available for such as travellers, tourists, harvesters, soldiers on the march, when they, being heated, have had a cold ducking, or have drunk cold liquids.

I would recommend it also in the acute and chronic dyspepsia from eating cold ices, as the conditions here are identical, for I have, in such cases, found it an eminent curative agent.

I should like very much to dilate on the remarkable therapeutic virtues of the Daisy, but this is not the place. This much is, however, apposite, for the Facial Dermatitis was one that would certainly be classed as a Disease of the Skin, and internal treatment alone cured it. — Q.E.D.

Quite lately I have information of the cure by *Bellis perennis* of a severe case of Facial Acne, produced originally by patient's rushing about in the cold air while her face was in a very heated condition. (IX 107)

## 111. ICHTHYOSIS

A lady of 73 years of age came to consult me in the month of March 1885 for loss of vision due to double cataract. In dealing with cataract I always go at once to a consideration of the skin, and here the find was instructive; her skin was very thick, dry, hot, and scaly, notably on the extensor surfaces, with long cracks here and there. In her movements patient is exceedingly slow, spending as much as two hours at her very simple morning toilet. Though her skin had never been other than dry and scaly, it is getting much worse of late years. Her lenses were opaque and of a milky colour, and the epidermic scales light-coloured, though not particularly pearl-like, — just a case of chronic diffuse hypertrophic keratosis.

This lady has continued under my observation up to the present time, and so would now be in her 79th or 80th year. She was nearly blind when she came to me, being just able to find a large object; thus with a little groping and feeling with her knees she could find a chair to sit upon. There were temporary improvements in vision here and there, and the lady has still a very small amount of vision. But on the other hand, there has been a very distinct improvement in her skin, which is neither so thick nor so scaly, nor so much cracked. And considering the age of the patient and the very long duration of the affection, I think the improvement in her skin very noteworthy indeed, and her various ailings have been from time to time much relieved as well. During the five and a half years she had from me many remedies, -- *Calcarea fluorica* 6, *Psorinum* 30, *Natrum muriaticum* 30, *Psor. C.*, *Thuja* 30, *Lactuca vir.* 3, *Galium aparine* 1x, *Platanus occidentalis* 1x, *Graphites* 30, *Ichthyol* 30, *Baryta mur.* 3x, and here — August, 1887 — there was very distinct amelioration both in the skin and lenses. *Calcarea hypophosphorosa* 3x, *Aconitum* 3x, *Aurum Muriaticum Natronatum* 3x. *Pulsatilla, Bryonia, Borax, Betula Alba Q, Juglans cinerea.*

The remedies that were of very distinct advantage were *Barium* and *Platanus.* Under *Barium* for several months patient increased in vigour and well-being, and under the *Platanus* for several months also her skin admittedly underwent considerable improvement.

The *Betula alba* patient credited with rendering the skin much more comfortable, but complained that it affected the upper part of the body only.

A friend of this aged lady spoke slightingly of the treatment of this case, inferring that as the case was not cured, the whole thing was a fiasco. But I pointed out that what results from the treatment is strong evidence of beneficial drug action in a very inveterate case at an advanced age; that the lady's discomforts have been greatly alleviated; that at 78 her skin is actually *much better* than it was at 73; while at 73 it was getting worse and worse, her skin at 78 is not getting worse, but better.

The fact that the lady's span of life is dwindling has nothing to do with the clinical evidence of curative results from drug-action, or rather the greater the age of the patient the more remarkable the evidence. We must remember that what we call life is to each individual of us a varying quantity, according to our respective ages, and at 78 life to this lady is *what remains to come after 78*! It may not be much, but it is *life to her* : in other words, alleviating an old patient is, medically speaking, not diminished because the patient benefited may not have long to live by reason of advanced age, —

"At six I well remember when
All folks seemed old at ten."

(IX 129)

## 112. ECZEMA OF SIXTEEN YEAR'S STANDING — ELEPHANTIASIS LABIORUM VULVAE — LIFE-LONG CONSTIPATION

A strong, well-preserved lady, 70 years of age, came under my observation on October 9th, 1890, telling me she had very severe eczema for the last sixteen years, and now for some time past has what has been called dry eczema of the vulvar lips, and there is also a patch of "dry eczema" over her right eye. Both the vulvar lips of the right side were hugely enlarged, and appeared as a big flap of elephantine nature, scaly, shiny, deeply pigmented, reddish in spots, dry and itchy. Patient, though English and long resident in England, is, nevertheless, of West India birth, having left her birthplace and came to this country at the age of 6 years, — *i.e.*, sixty-four years ago. I mention this point because I do not remember ever seeing a case like this before, and hence presume it cannot be common in London, or generally in this country. The irritation was very bad; worse after sitting or walking much, and also at night, when it keeps her awake; it is much worse in the cold weather, diminishing much in the warm weather of summer. Patient enjoyed good health, and has never had anything beyond measles, scarlatina, and pertussis. She complains of being chilly. Nothing seemed to account for so severe an affection in an otherwise strong, healthy lady. There had been in all three vaccinations, the third one having been unsuccessful, and was in 1871. The eczema had first obtruded itself upon patient's attention sixteen years ago, — *i.e.*, subsequent to this third unsuccessful vaccination.

*Thuja* 30.

October 30, 1890 — The little patch of eruption over the eye is well, the labial swelling is less, the mass softer, and patient exclaimed, "I feel quite different."

$R_x$ *Sabina* 30.

November 20. — Not any further improvement.
$R_x$ *Vaccininum* 30.
December 18 — The bowels have acted twice every day, and she had been constive all her life; has been always in the habit of going six or seven days without any motion, and then art and physic had to do it. "Dr. Bell (homoeopath) treated my constipation for long, and finally gave it up as a constituional peculiarity."
Rx *Maland*. CC.
January 8, 1891. — Patient cried out to me on this day : — English, French, German, allopathic and homoeopathic, — all have tried at my costiveness in vain, and now the bowels act so well." The elephantine skin of labia steadily improving.
Feb. 5 — Skin healing well bowels not quite so comfortable.
$R_x$ *Vaccininum* 30.
Feb. 26 — Skin affection improving; bowels act comfortably. "I have never felt so well in my life."
$R_x$ *Nux* 30, under which the bowels went back.
March 19 — *Vaccin.*, 30.
May 21 — Well; bowels act quite regularly and comfortably; and though patient feels not quite comfortable at the vulva, objectively the skin is quite normal.
At the end of November the skin continued quite normal, and hence we may conclude that the cure is a perfect one.
Nine months later — The cure holds good. And this radical cure of an old-standing ailment in a lady of 70 years of age, — the remedies used being all given internally, and not only so, but in dynamic doses (and frequently), — this cure, I say, is noteworthy, and tells well for my thesis that skin diseases are of constitutional nature, and must be so regarded and treated. *Natura [organismus] sanat, madicus curat*. (IX 127)

## 113. ACNE AND SWELLED NECK

On February 10, 1891, an unmarried lady, well on towards 30, came to consult me for roughness of the skin of the face, and acne. She did not mind her cough, it was not so very bad, nor did she make much ado about the rather profuse expectoration of phlegm. She did not even complain of her enlarged tonsils or leucorrhoea, and as for her chilblains, they only came in very cold weather. Said she, "It is my rough skin and this horrid neck." The "horrid neck" was made up of a one-sided enlargement of the neck, consisting of a very much hypertrophied submaxillary gland and tonsil of the same side, with some puffiness of the surrounding areolar tissue, so that the side of the neck appeared "horrid," — *i.e.*, shapeless, and neck and face ran into one another, the jaw-bone line being lost. *Thuja* 30 for a month distinctly lessened the size of the glands (submaxillary and tonsil), but cough and phlegm were not touched.

*Bacillinum* C. was followed by much improvement, the unshapeliness having changed : the jaw had become well defined, and thus neck and face no longer ran into one another, while the left submaxillary gland stood out by itself. The tonsils had gone down, but the quantity of phlegm, though less, was still considerable. I then went up to *Bac.* 1000.

"Those powders did a wonderful thing for my skin : it went quite clear."

July 21, 1891. — Patient is quite well; skin clear; tonsils normal; left submaxillary enlargement gone; neck restored to its pristine shapeliness; and not long after this she was engaged to be married and in the early autumn the marriage came off.

My reading of the whole case was to the effect that I was dealing with vaccinosis and scrofulosis bordering on tuberculosis. May I put pertinent question to any dermatologist or surgeon in this wide world of ours : What would you have done in this case.?

August 1892. — Patient continues quite well, as I learn from her mother, lady X. (IX 132)

## 114. ULCERATIVE ERUPTION OF VULVA

A lady of 50 years of age, for many years married, but childless, came under my care for troubles connected with the climaxis, not the least of which was vaginal and vulvar irritation, as well as a very extensive ulcerative eruption all over the labial and vulvar region extending at times as far as an inch and a half on to the circumvulvar region, but when it came into the common intigument it took more the form of eczema, with a few pustules here and there. The flat ulcers in the labia and nymphae had plagued her years ago, and been cured (silenced) by cauterization. $R_x$ Tc. *Platin. Mur.* 3x, three drops in water twice a day.

In a month the eruption had materially diminished, having lost its pustular and purulent character, and the vaginal discharge had entirely ceased.

Here (May 27, 1887). *Lachesis* was ordered, and with advantage.

July 7, 1887 — The thing has returned.

$R_x$ Tc. *Aurum mur. nat.* 3x, four drops in a tablespoonful of water night and morning.

This completely cured the eruption with its concomitants, the remedy having to be once subsequently repeated; in all, the *Auric salt* was taken during, about thirteen or fourteen weeks. There has been no return, and the lady continues in excellent health and condition. I used no local application whatever. And here I may state, once for all, that I hardly ever order local applications of any sort in cutaneous affections. If in any of my cases herein recited any local applications are used, the fact will be stated; but I believe in no case herein communicated was any local application whatever used, so far as I am aware. Not only so, but I commonly specially warn my patients against all ointments and lotions whatever, as I find that Goulard's lotion, Zinc ointment, Citrine ointment, Golden ointment, and the like, may be found in very many households, and it is very difficult to prevent their being used.

The use of remedies applied as ointments or lotions is absolutely bad; and when I read of the homoeopathic treatment of skin diseases whereby ointments and lotions play a part, my respect for the quality of such treatment is small indeed. It is wonderful how people will cuddle and fondle the ointment pot; and "Regular Medicine" would be indeed badly off without its grease pot and clyster. I often think the use by the homoeopaths of their *Calendula cerate* or ointment comes dangerously near the thin end of the wedge of the vulgarly-conceived putty-and-paint treatment of the medicines of the schools.

It is almost incredible, but the discovery of a new fat for an unguental excipient is an event of the first magnitude in the dermatological world, the vault of whose heaven is still ringing with the echoes of the wonders of veseline and lanoline. And what does it all amount to?

A pat of pig's lard. (IX 135)

## 115. PITYRIASIS RUBRA - 1

Although the Vienna School classifies this rather rare affection with eczema, I cannot see myself whereon the classification is based; but I have only had to treat two typical cases of it, both being of the cutaneous covering of the chest, and two or three cases of symptoms of the rim of the hairy scalp, which were distinctly of the same nature. The patient here referred to came to me on December 22, 1885. A powerful peer of this realm and a great Nimrod, with flesh as hard as nails, he came to be treated for a maddening neuralgia he had picked up on the banks of the Nile; remedies having cured his neuralgia he showed me his chest, which was the seat of a big patch of red pityriasis that he had had for a number of years, — the precise number I do not know. I saw him, off and on, for nearly five years, and gave him a not inconsiderable portion of our Pharmacopoeia (and our Pharmacopoeia is not small — *see*

Allen's "Encyclopaedia of Pura Materia Medica !"), but the pityriasis rubra remained ... Pityriasis rubra. I should say the big patch was composed of a series of smaller patches, all more or less circular or segments of circles.

One day I was reading in an old German book that some sailors — British, I think — many years ago, in some of the Pacific islands, ate of a fish called erythrinus, and came out with a peculiar red rash that became chronic, and which the doctors took for a form of syphilis.

Dr. Alfred Heath, F.L.S., with his wonted devotion and disinterestedness, procured this erythrinus for me, and prepared it homoeopathically, and I, on March 23, 1889, ordered as follows : $R_x$ Tc. *Erythrinus* 1 zj., five drops in water night and morning. I did not see the patient after for about two and a half years — viz., September 1, 1891. When I inquired of him about the "red patch of his chest," "Oh," said he, "you cured that long ago with that big bottle of stuff you sent me," i.e., — the ounce bottle of *Erythrinus* 1. (IX 140)

## 116. PITYRIASIS - 2

The second case of pityriasis which I treated with this *Erythrinus* is greatly improved, but by no means cured. The father of the gentleman who was cured by *Erythrinus* had had syphilis, as I ascertained from an indirect but very reliable source.

The father of the second case died of what seems to have been aneurism of or near the heart. It may therefore be worth while to ascertain whether pityriasis rubra be not a syphilitic manifestation in the second generation. That it is worthy of note that the second patient to whom I here refer, — who is not cured, and is still under my treatment, — came to me originally for heart disease characterized by distress in the heart region, palpitation, irregular heart-beat, and much distress on walking, particularly up hill.

For this cardiac affection (which the regimental surgeon said would be fatal) I prescribed *Aurum muriaticum* 3x, at one time three drops, and at another time two drops, and finally five drops, in a tablespoonful of water three times a day. This cured the heart rather slowly, but the patch of pityriasis *became twice as large*. This vicarious phenomenon between heart and the skin of the thorax I have observed over and over again. So that when an individual has an eruption on his chest, he is not wise to let any skin specialist treat it from the narrow standpoint of the specialist, lest heart disease supervene. See here anent my remarks upon the "Sternal Patch." By the way, the "Sternal Patch" is in the lowest third of the sternum, rather to the right; this thoracic pityriasis patch is rather to the left, and just over the arch of the aorta. The "Sternal Patch" is not a brown, so-called, liver mark, but an eruption; the importance of this eruption lies, I think, not so much in the kind of eruption as in the fact that when it vanishes from the surface, without being really cured from within, symptoms of heart disease, more or less grave, at once supervene. The more one really studies skin diseases the more one is struck with their *habitats*, which are often constant and characteristic. What are the internal pathological conditions corresponding hereto? Without doubt such exist, and have also a definite significance. (IX 143)

## 117. ARTHRITIC URTICARIA — RECURRENT

A lady of position, nearing 70 years of age, of very abstemious habits and a strict dietarian, had been for years subject to violent and severe attacks of gouty nettlerash, taking her suddenly, now in one part, now in another, and compelling her to hasten to her own apartments to apply hot wraps to allay the furious itching. She had been under most of the better-known homoeopathic physicians in England one time and another, and had obtained a little temporary relief sometimes, but not much, so that she had given up all hope for long, and only consented to try again at the earnest solicitation of a friend. When she took my prescription into her hand, she exclaimed, "Oh! that's your tincture of nettles " that's no good. I have tried that under Dr. —, and my dear old friend the late Dr. Hilbers also gave it to me." She persisted in it that *Urtica* would do her no good, but I persuaded her to take it (*Urtica urens* Q), five drops in a wine-glassful of warm water three times a day; and much to her surprise, it did her so much good that she continued to take it for some months, and then discontinued its use, considering herself cured.

In connection with this case it is worth remembering that *Urtica* had in old times quite a reputation for gout and sand, and I have repeatedly noticed that patients, while taking *Urtica ur.* Q in the manner just described, have passed large quantities of sand, and in several instances such patients have been alarmed, never having passed any before in their lives.

*Urtica urens* is a very notable splenic, and with its aid I have often cured ague. And for the common manifestations of pure gout, it is my sheet-anchor for years past. I could fill a little book with cases in proof of this statement. (IX 146)

## 118. DYSPEPSIA — VOMITING — NEURALGIA — NEURASTHENIA — ACUTE ECZEMA

A married lady, childless, 55 years of age, came to me on July 12, 1887, quite broken down in health; it was thought the final break-up of the constitution was at hand. The most prominent and most distressing symptom was perhaps her attacks of faintness and her inveterate and severe dyspepsia, though she felt her nerve symptoms very much. She was afraid of being alone, going about in fear and trembling. Nervous heart-beat; spleen very much enlarged (affirmed that she had had ague every spring until she was nearly thirty years of age); a good deal of neuraligia in the left side of head and face. She is intolerant of cold, and revels in this July heat. This lady is an amateur artist, and paints a good deal these many years, and wonders if her frequent attacks of vomiting have any connection therewith. She formerly had variola and measles, and has also suffered from urticaria. But the fact that she had been twice vaccinated seemed to me the most proximate and least questionable therapeutic indication. Hence I started off with *Thuja* 30.

August 11 — The patient was quite well till two days ago! No vomiting; slight neuralgia only; no fainting attacks; tongue now thickly coated.

The next most obvious point to attack was the greatly enlarged spleen and the chilliness.

$R_x$ *Caenothus Americanus* 1. Six drops in water night and morning.

December 1 — My patient came this day and bitterly complained that the *Ceanothus* had done no good at all, and had, moreover, brought back all the old symptoms, which the *Thuja* powder had so much benefited. The neuralgia is bad again, and the patient very earnestly requests that she have the old powders again.

So *Thuja* 30 was again prescribed in very infrequent doses.

January 17, 1888 — Has a bad attack now on these eight days, and there is a little eruption on the tips of her toes and fingers; no vomiting.

$R_x$ *Ignatia amara* 1.

February 19 — Much better; in fact, feels wonderfully well, *but she has "broken out all over with an eruption of water and matter."* And she now has ceased to be cold, and is, on the contrary hot.

$R_x$ Tc. *Juglans regia* Q. Five drops in water night and morning.

March 27 — The skin has improved a good deal; as the eruption dies away the locus turns brown; the eruption is now worse on the hairy scalp; she feels sick and dizzy. Never had any eruption other than

urticaria till after she took the *Thuja* from me. Much better in all general respects.
$R_x$ *Rep.*
May 8 — Been sick again, three times; many brown marks where the eruption was, otherwise she is well and the skin is quite healthy. The spleen, however, continues pertrophied.
$R_x$ *Urtica urens* Q. Five drops in water night and morning.
October 6 — Bowels costive; feels tired and bilious, and complains very much of feeling shivery and cold *Natrum muriaticum* 6 trituration cured these symptoms, and patient was discharged cured.
July 1893 — The cure holds good. (IX 149)

## 119. STRUMOUS ECZEMA IN BABY, CURED BY *BACILLINUM* CC.

One meets not infrequently with bad cases of eczema in babies that are apt to end in marasmus and death : the eruption in such cases is almost all over the body, wetting, more particularly in certain more or less circumscribed patches, and driving the poor little patients almost mad with irritation, particularly at night. I had such a case this last summer in a baby of only a few months of age, and who was partly on the cursed bottle. Did I say cursed bottle? I will withdraw the wicked word and ask my readers to allow me to substitute for it —, well, I mean the strongest word of condemnation known in our language. In this particular case the mother did her best, so the use of the bottle could not be avoided, and its use was only partial, the mother giving all she had.
Well, I had treated the eczema for some weeks with no benefit, when one afternoon I was suddenly summoned into the country to see this poor bairnie, and a sorry sight it was.
Mother and nurse were at their wit's end to know how to keep the wet patches from sticking to the clothes, fat-besmeared rags only sufficing for a very short time. Hardly any sleep at night from the furious irritation. I then remembered that I once cured an elder baby-brother of this little patient of eczema of the scalp with *Bacillinum*, originally suggested by the ancient scars in their father's neck, now well hidden behind his long beard there-fore ordered for my wee patient *Bucill.* CC. in infrequent doses.
In one week the report ran : "... Baby is much better, and now sleeps and feeds beautifully."
I need only add that the remedy quite cured the case, and the little lassie got quite well, and so remains. Such cases are very apt to end fatally whereof I have been in times past more than once the sorrowful witness;

but then I knew nothing of *Bacillinum* in high potency, or, indeed, in any potency.

The patient in question had not at that period been vaccinated. (IX 154)

## 120. INVETERATE ECZEMA

An American gentleman, 63 years of age, came under my observation on May 14, for a very severe eruption on the skin — inveterate eczema — of many years' duration. Latterly it has been getting much worse and more extensive, and extends now to the penis, prepuce, and eyelids and conjunctivae. There was a specific air about it, but this was strictly denied, a gonorrhoea only being admittedly historic.

I began with *Platanus occidentalis* Q, but in eight days from its commencement patient returned to me, bitterly complaining that there was no improvement.

May 21 — Six grains of *Aurum metallicum* three times a day. This did him some good certainly, but not very much. Then followed *Mercurius solubilis Hahn.* in a low trituration, and it was soon clear that we had hold of the right remedy, but it would not quite finish the cure, though it came very near doing so. A month of *Kali chlor.* 3, and patient considered himself cured, except the redness of the eyes. This ophthalmia was cured by *Jequirity* 3x, six drops in water night and morning. I saw this gentleman a year and a half later, when he declared himself quite well in health and free from eczema. (IX 157)

## 121. GOUTY ECZEMA

In the autumn of 1891 a gentleman of about 60 years of age consulted me in regard to a very severe form of eczema occupying the genital, perineal, anal, and crural regions : the surface was red, raw, shiny, scaly in part, and in part moist. The thing caused him very great distress. The first two prescriptions did him no real good, so on November 27th, 1891, I prescribed the *hippurate of sodium* in the fifth centesimal dilution in ten-drop doses, administered every night and morning, I sending him enough to last a month.

I saw no more of him till the spring of 1892, and then I inquired of the skin trouble. "Oh! that tincture cured me completely." To be quite sure it was so, I carefully examined the parts, and I did the same again four months later, when he called to ask me to suggest a place where he might with advantage spend his holiday. I found no trace of eczema on either occasion, and patient continues in good health. I have seen and treated a good many cases of eczema, and am just beginning to recognise its rather numerous varieties from the aetio-pathological standpoint, and I shall yet have more to say on the subject : here let the simple narrative of the case cured by the *hippurate of sodium* suffice. (IX 159)

## 122. LICHEN URTICARUS

A sixteen-months' old baby was brought to me by its mother on November 27, 1886, to be treated for wheals on its body that became much worse in the warmth of the bed : the distress of the child was great; it got hardly any proper sleep.
R. *Syph* CC.
January 13, 1887 — These little powders quite cured baby in less than a fortnight."
August 30, 1887 — "Baby's skin continues quite well."
Cases of wheals in the skin of young children are very common, and the irritation they cause as the sufferers get warm in bed is often almost maddening. I have known such patients toss and roll about almost every night, and not infrequently roll out of bed in their tormentors. *Chloral hydrate* and *Urtica urens*, and also *Persicaria urens* are very useful in such cases, and so is also *Bacillinum*. But where the nocturnally appearing wheals are, as it were echoes from the paternal past, nothing equals the remedy here named as curative. The thing is cured root and branch, recurring occasionally when a new tooth sprouts, when the dose has to be repeated once, or perhaps twice, till the cure is definitely completed.
Where the primary causation is from the effects of vaccination, *Thuja, Sabina. Cupressus, Vaccininum*, or *Malandrinum* may be used, *Thuja* generally sufficing; and I have required *Acidum nitricum* in some case. (IX 161)

## 123. CROP OF SOFT WARTS ROUND THE ANUS

A middle-aged married gentleman came under my observation in the summer of 1892 complaining of severe indigestion of long standing : a good deal of epigastric distress and pain characterized his dyspeptic state. Incidentally he complained of a most uncomfortable state of his anal region, and on examining this part to ascertain the cause thereof I found a number of small warts arranged almost in a ring round the orifice. A gonorrhoea of many years ago, as also several vaccinations, sufficed to constitute the diagonosis of Hahnemannic sycosis, and, indeed, *Thuja occid.* in the 30th centesimal potency, and of infrequent administration, quite cured the dyspepsia, and also the anus. I carefully examined the anal region, and found that the ring of small soft warts had quite disappeared. "I feel all right there now." (IX 164)

## 124. NASAL ERYTHEMA

A lady, 53 years of age, came under my professional care in the summer of 1890, with erythema of the nose, or as we might call it, dermatic rhinitis. The nose was all red and swelled up, the inflammatory action not in any way extending to the cheeks, but involving the right eye a good deal. In fact, patient, is of opinion that the right-sided conjuctivitis was the starting point of the nasal erythema, and she tells me that she is subject to this ocular inflammation, off and on, for many years.

Anamnetically there is not much to note, except that the lady had been vaccinated seven or eight times, but it had only taken three times.

Under *Thuja* 30 the erythema was half gone in three weeks, and patient had visibly improved in condition. After two months of the *Thuja* the eye was quite well, the erythema still only half well. Finding that the nose scabbed inside, I put patient on *Kali bichromicum* 5, five drops in water night and morning for a month, and then patient was discharged cured. (See the pathogenesis of *Kali bi.*) (IX 165)

## 125. LIFE-LONG ERUPTION ON SCALP

A single gentleman, 35 years of age, came to consult me at the end of August 1887 for a coppery eruption of his scalp that he had had as long as he could remember. Besides this eruption he complained much of chronic insomnia and failing memory. I first gave him the strong tincture of *Fagus cup.*, five drops in water night and morning, but after a month — viz., on September 30 — he complained that he was no better in any respect, — sleepless, forgetful, restless; the eruption bad; his breath very foul; liver slightly enlarged; spleen large and very hard.

*Syp.* CC.

Nov. 11 — "I have slept famously;" and both he and I were of opinion that his hair had gone darker. The eruption distinctly better.

$R_x$ *Spiritus glandium quercus* Q five drops in water night and morning.

Dec. 12 — Eruption nearly gone; the spleen pains a little now; insomnia quite a thing of the past.

$R_x$ Tc. *Carduus Marianus.*

He reported himself quite well of his coppery eruption on January 13, 1888, and two years later it still continued well, and since then I have no further tidings of him. (IX 167)

## 126. CHRONIC CROPS OF BOILS AND ACNE

A young city man, 21 years of age, just entering a very important city firm, came under my observation on March 21st, 1888, complaining that for the past six years he had been suffering from crops of boils. They are worse on his nape and face; at this moments there is one on the nape, and also one on his nose. There are also mattery spots — acne — all over his shoulders. Patient is very rich and rather good-looking, and it is therefore not astonishing that he had been under the professional care of the leading physicians and surgeons and skin specialists of London, to the number of ten. Finding quite a goodly collection of vaccinial scars on both arms, I inquired what number of times he had been vaccinated. Answer : Four times. Urine has a specific gravity of 1020, and the glands of his neck are visibly swelled. I had him about ten weeks under *Thuja occidentalis* 30, very infrequently administered, and the boils and acne pustules all waned and went and came no more, much to patient's amazement, and, indeed, to my own, for I had not expected such a prompt and perfect cure. I subsequently often saw him with his younger brother, and so know that the cure was definite. The case was clearly one of pure and uncomplicated vaccinosis without the dash of consumptiveness that so often lurks behind severe acne.

There is also a kind of acne that is distinctly of arthritic nature, and this yields well to *Urea* 6; in this variety pustulation is much less pronounced than in vaccinial acne or phthisic acne. Broadly put, vaccinial acne yields to *Thuja occidentalis, Sabina* and *Cupressus,* also to *Silicea* and *Maland*; acne from masturbation, to *Bellis perennis*; phthisic acne, to *Bacillinum*; when the acne is very pronouncedly pustular and scarring, to *Vaccinin.* and *Variolinum*; and arthritic acne calls for *hippuric acid, hippurate of sodium,* and *Urea.* The study of the varieties of acne is highly interesting and instructive, as *almost all the great constitutional ancestral diseases show themselves in young persons in the form of acne. Not infrequently cases of acne are of mixed pathological qualities,* and these need *all* their pathologic *simillima.* Remedies only morphologically homoeopathic to the acne-form only palliate; to really and radically cure they must be *pathologically* similar. What a vast vista ! (IX 169)

## 127. ECZEMA OF EXTERNAL EAR AND MEATUS

Miss Ethel S., 14 years of age, was brought to me on September 29, 1891, suffering from a skin affection showing itself as eczema of the outer ear and meatus, the surface of which was wetting, shiny, and in part scaly, and the discharge would at times dry up into scabs. She has very large tonsils; her throat is swelled and irritable, and in the early morning she feels sick. Her father was formerly cured by me of eczema; and hence the young lady was brought to me. She was cured in about six months, the remedies being *Med*. 1000, and *Bacill* 1000 and CC.

This young lady's father's sister has also been cured by me of eczema, and her brother is now under my care for very severe eczema.

There is a tragic circumstance connected with my professional relationship with this socially important family, and it is this : Fifteen years ago I was treating a wee child of another branch of this family also for eczema that extented to the greater part of the poor mite's whole body. I explained to the parents that I regarded the eczema in question as of a very pronouncedly constitutional nature, and that it was this constituional disease that caused the truly terrible eczematous ooze, the skin being merely the medium of relief of the organism. Hence I gave my opinion that it would be dangerous to use local applications to the skin, lest the relatively fair general state of the patient should be impaired; nearly all the glands were enlarged, and primarily so, and not merely from cutaneous irritation, to which conclusion I came from finding such hypertrophied or indurated glands in parts where there was no active eczema.

What I am trying to say just amounts to this : My treatment just amounts to this : My treatment was given up in contempt because I would not give any ointment or wash whatever, and the services of an eminent dermatologist were secured. Things went on very smoothly for a very few weeks, but the patient not long afterwards died "of weakness and exhaustion."

In my judgement she died of the practical application of the dermatologist's gross ignorance of dermatology : bedaubing and besmearing the skin with medicinal substances was the work of this probably well-meaning medical man; but oh! the shallow, shallow work! (IX 198)

## 128. ACUTE UNIVERSAL ERYTHEMA AND CHRONIC RHEUMATOID ARTHRITIS

A maiden lady, 56 years of age, came to consult me on October 16, 1890, for pretty severe rheumatoid arthritis of three years' standing, affecting hands, feet, elbows and knees. Although fifty-six years of age her menses are regular. She has just returned from Buxton, which, she thinks, did her a little good. Her hands are swelled a good deal, so that they are not of much use to her. She has strumous scars in neck. The pains are described as worst when she starts off, and worse in the evening, and worse on the East Coast than in London. Patient had been vaccinated three times. *Bacillinum* C. was given for a month.

November 25, 1890 — The improvement is very great indeed, — in fact, quite startling, for all the pain has gone and the swelling has sensibly diminished; feet better; can stand better; and, moreover, she sleeps so much better.

To continue the same medicine.

December 5 — Patient hurries to me to show me the dreadful state of her skin, which is covered all over with acute erythema, rather papular. She describes the irritation as terrible in the heat ... and ... the rheumatism had gone.

January 1, 1891 — With very great difficulty I prevented this lady from putting something on "to cure" the erythema; in fact, I did not quite succeed, and the case that seemed perfectly cured is not quite cured really, as the hands are stiff again and somewhat swelled.

$R_x$ *Thuja occidentalis* 30.

February 19, 1891 — The hands are not so well.

$R_x$ *Psor* 30, and a month later *Bacill.* C. finished the cure.

The point of greatest interest to me in this narration is the vicarious erythema.

I saw a middle-aged lady yesterday whose hands are swelled and much disfigured by rheumatoid arthritis. The lady's sister tells me that the late Sir Erasmus Wilson once cured the lady of eczema; and we know well what the great Erasmus's "cures" were. (IX 201)

## 129. ECZEMA IN A CHILD OF THREE

On May 10th, 1888, a lady brought her three-year-old little boy to me to be treated for eczema in the bends of the knees; these regions were pretty badly affected, and the little man's cervical glands were considerably enlarged. As the eczema was most trying in the warmth of the bed, I gave *Syph.* CC. in very infrequent doses for a month.

June 7 — Much better, notably of the glands, but the eruption still itches in the warmth. *Acidum uricum* 6, zij., three drops in water night and morning.

August 1 — Nearly well, *Acidum hippuricum,* the same as the previous prescription.

This finished the cure. (IX 205)

## 130. ECZEMA GLANDIS OF SIX YEARS' DURATION

An unmarried rufous gentleman, 32 years of age, came under my observation on May 18, 1887, for left-sided varicocele and eczema of the glans and of the sulcus of the penis; the eruption had been there for six years. Patient was *pucean*. He informed me that he had formerly had eczema on his head. I first gave him *Clematis erecta* 1x five drops in water twice a day, but with no benefit. In June and July, for about five weeks he was under *Malandrinum* 30, with very great amelioration; and thereafter, for about the same length of time, he had from me *Melitagrinum* C.

This cured the eczema, and patient ceased attending. At the end of the year patient said there was a very little of the eczema still in the sulcus, but he did not think it worth while being treated for it. (IX 207)

## 131. ECZEMA

A married lady, 30 years of age, mother of two children, was brought to me by her husband on December 4, 1891, with pretty severe eczema that had been bad during the past eight months, and being specially bad in the bends of arms and on the face, and worst of all around the mouth; most distressing of an evening. Her lips are dry. cracked, "for ever peeling." Pateint's condition was so bad, her general state so debilitated, her appearance so old, worn, and weary, that I felt it to be imperative to better her blood life and pull her together, so to speak, before setting about a scientific cure of the case, so I put her on *Levico* Q for a few weeks, and then upon *Bellis perennis* Q for a month, when patient would not come any more, even to please her husband, remarking, "Oh! I'm getting on nicely now, I do not want the doctor." (IX 208)

## 132. RINGWORM, EÇZEMA, ACNE AND ASTHMA

A powerful, somewhat asthmatic gentleman, 58 years of age, came from the north to consult me on the 12th August 1891, telling me a history of slight winter asthma for many years; this he keeps down with Turkish baths, which he has taken regularly every since he was 21 years of age. His appearance on being undressed was as if he had small-pox of moderate severity, only the pustules are those of acne. He tells me he had "three ringworms across the belly" in the month of February 1881, which he got cured with ointments; and then he got eczema, and got this also cured with ointments; and then came this pustular eruption which ointments will not cure.

$R_x$ *Bacill* 1000.
August 26 — Much better.
*Rep.*
September 8 — "Those powders are too much for me; they cause me bad breathing and sickly feeling; worse in the morning; the skin is rather better; there is no matter in it now."
He is much afraid of the powders, "they act so powerfully."
October 2 — The skin is cleaning.
$R_x$ *Rep.* (CC.)
October 16 — Much better.
*Rep.* (C.)
October 30 — The chronic difficulty of breathing (the asthma) has gone, the breathing beig now normal.
The same remedy was repeated a few times. (IX 209)

## 133. BRAWNY DERMATITIS

An elderly gentleman consulted me on Nov. 12, 1890, for an eruption of the skin, that I can only call brawny dermatitis. It was all over his body, and had been there for years, and itches a great deal. This gentleman was discharged cured in less than a year, and still continues well. The remedies I used were *Persicaria urens* 30 and 3 *Urtica urens* Q, and *Sodium salicylate*.
Patient formerly suffered from chronic rheumatism, but ceased to do so after this rash came out.
Now he has neither skin disease nor rheumatism. (IX 212)

## 134. VERY SEVERE SYCOSIS

On September 26, 1890, a London professional man, 41 years of age, married, and in fair general health, came to me as a *dernier ressort*, and on the earnest solicitation of friend and neighbour. Said he : "I have always ridiculed homoeopathy, and do not believe in it the least little bit, but I am in despair; I have had this beastly skin disease for twelve years (pointing to his chin and face), and I have been under treatment all the time by the most eminent surgeons of London; altogether I have been under eleven different doctors, — of course all allopaths."
Patient's chin and face co-extensive with his beard, was a "mass of corruption," — *i.e.*, dried up, caked together mattery ooze, which he was obliged to get off very frequently with the aid of poultice, when the surface was red and angry and shiny, the sticky stuff at once beginning

to appear again. An ointment he uses keeps it down pretty well in the summer months, but is powerless from autumn to spring. He has also very severe pyorrhoea alveolaris; his gums have receded, and the bulk of his very beautifully formed teeth have already fallen out entirely, or stand out from the gums ready to fall out; his breath is starcoraceous. and his gums and mouth generally he described as "rotten." He has had recurrent opthalmia many times. He tells me he has used scores of ointments, and been very severely handled by the skin specialists, having undergone scarifications and epilations at many different times. Patient has been twice vaccinated. The feeling in the diseased part he describes as stinging. My treatment was continued till June 10, 1892, when I was able to declare him as he declared himself, *well*. Treatment extending over all these months necessarily comprises a number of remedies, the case being so severe and of such long standing. Practially patient had all the leading nosodic and other antisycotics as well as *Zincum acet.* 1, *Jequirity* 3x, *Levico* Q, (the strong water), *Chelidon majus* Q, and *Calc. sulph.* (IX 213)

## 135. OFFENSIVE PERSPIRATIONS — PERIODICAL HEADACHES

An unmarried lady, 38 years of age, came under my care on July 11, 1892, principally for *headaches* and *offensive perspirations*. Patient had lived some years in India, where she had ague badly. The headache was really brow-ague at a spot over the right eye, very bad at 7 P.M., and recurring every eleven dayas. The perspirations were described as *sour, onoiny, nettly*.

$R_x$ *Trit.* 6 *Nat. mur.* Six grains three times a day.

August 9 — The powders brought back the ague, of which patient had long been free. Thereupon she immediately took quinine.

Perspiration less offensive.

$R_x$ *Nat. mur.* 30.

September 12 — Quite free from headaches, and the perspiration has ceased to be offensive. The cure had held good when I last saw patient in February 1893. (IX 217)

## 136. LICHEN URTICARIUS

A bonny boy, 2 years of age, was brought by his mother to me on the 7th of August 1890 for lichen urticarius. But there was an even more distressing feature in this case, for this mite of a boy was already an inveterate masturbator. The urticarious spots were usually at their worst when he got warm in bed, or hot at any time. He had seatworms, picking his nose a good deal. He was about a year under my treatment, and was then discharged quite cured, not only of his cutaneous affection, but also of his nose-picking and of his secret habit of mauling himself about; for it was noteworthy that while he would pick his nose freely enough before folks, and even notwithstanding their forbidding it, he did not masturbate other than in secret.

The remedy that cured the skin affection was very evidently *Bacillinum* C. during one month at the beginning of the cure, and the same remedy in the two-hundredth dilution later on. The remedy that cured his secret habit was very clearly *Platina* 30, under which he was during three separate (not consecutive) months. There were inter-current ailings — cough, cold, anorexia — and *Thuja* 30, *Ipec*. 1, *Ledum* 3x, and *Med*. CC. respectively came into play. The precise parts played by these other four remedies in this case I could not quite determine. More particularly, I do not know which cured the seatworms. But, as before stated, I am very sure the lichen was cured by the *Bacill.*, and the masturbation was cured by the *Platina* 30.

[On the subject of *Platina* in this regard, see Grauvogl's *Lehrbuch*.] (IX 219)

## 137. ECZEMA OF EARS OF SEVEN YEARS' STANDING

On August 20, 1887, a little girl of nine was brought to me for an ill-smelling discharge from the ears, that was said to have started after she had had dysentery seven years previously. In the fold of the left arm a little eczema. Although only nine years old the child had been twice vaccinated, and was clearly quite blighted thereby.

After being under treatment by *Thuja occidentalis* 30 for a month, my note runs, "Vast improvement all round."

After a few weeks respectively of *Sabina* 30 and *Sulphur* 30, patient left cured at the end of the year 1887. (IX 224)

## 138. FLAT PAPILLOMA IN THE ANAL REGION

A childless married lady, a little over 30 years of age, came under my observation on July 19, 1887, for certain very distressing symptoms in the anal region, preventing sleep at night : worse at 2 A.M. On examining the parts I found the anal opening surrounded by haemorrhoidal buttons and on the tip of one of these a flat papilloma about the size of a split horse-bean. By day the whole region was exceedingly uncomfortable only, but by night its soreness prevented sleep.

$R_x$ *Syp*. CC.

August 16 — Very much better indeed; sleeps now quite well. An examination shows that the papilloma has quite disappeared.
Patient remained another couple of weeks under my treatment for the haemorrhoids. These quite disappeared during that period under the influence of, first, *Spiritus glandium quercus* Q, and then of *Euphorbia amygdaloides*. (IX 225)

## 139. PRURITUS ANI

A general staff-officer, no longer young, came under my care on Dec. 11, 1891, complaining bitterly of being roused up at night with fearful itching at the anus. An examination of the part showed only the very slightest degree of eczema. Being of opinion that the pruritus was due to port wine, I ordered *Spiritus glandium quercus*, ten drops in water night and morning. This cured the pruritus. When I next saw the general he said, "That's all right; now I want something for my bronchitis." The complaint was chronic winter catarrh of the bronchial lining. The *Aceticum Lobelioe*, in four-drop doses every four hours, quite cured this in about three weeks. (IX 227)

## 140. BAT'S WING DISEASE — LUPUS

A maiden lady, 48 years of age, from Shropshire, came on August 5th, 1892, to consult me for an eruption on her nose and two cheeks, the figure thus produced being responsible for the designation of bat's wing disease. The eruption is getting very, very slowly worse for the past twelve years. The skin peels off in little flakes, leaving the underlying skin red, and this again dries and in its turn peels off, but very, very slowly and the whole of the skin is not involved, there being healthy skin between. Patient's father is stated to have died of decline at 57 years of age, and her mother, patient tells me, died at 52 of mesenteric atrophy. One of patient's brothers died of phthisis, and her other six brothers all died in infancy. Her three sisters are alive. Patient has had active treatment, principally *Arsenic* and *Mercury*.
$R_x$ *Bacill*. CC.
September 2 — The bat's wing is half gone!
$R_x$ *Rep*.
Sept. 30 — Nose quite free, except in the right side near the eye, where it is *more active*.
Patient informs me that she has been three times vaccinated.
$R_x$ *Thuja* 30.

Nov. 4 — There is just one small spot of the eruption left, near the corner of the eye. A good deal of haemorrhage from the rectum.
$R_x$ *Bacill.* CC.
December 9 — Patient writes me under this date from her home : "I have *no trace of the disease left*, but the piles have bled on four occasions. I was so well while taking the powder."
$R_x$ *Rep.*
January 13, 1893 — The skin remains quite well. "I eat double."
And four months later the lady's sister, in answer to my inquiry, informed me that patient continued perfectly well. (IX 228)

## 141. PAPULAR RASH

An unmarried lady, 23 years of age, was brought to me by her elder sister on Dec. 15, 1890, for a very disagreeable rash on the body. The patient had had measles, whooping-cough, chicken-pox, and jaundice during the course of her little life, and had also been twice vaccinated. Her menses were irregular; she suffered from nose-bleed. The eruption occupied the skin over the chest, stomach, and duodenum, and itched a good deal on going to bed. Patient is very costive, anaemic, and complains pretty eloquently of flatulent dyspepsia. Her spleen is enlarged; she twitches and jumps (starts) a good deal; is better in the evening, worse in the morning.
$R_x$ *Thuja occidentalis* 30, in infrequent doses.
In two months patient had gained five pounds in weight and was quite well, barring an enlarged spleen and little spells of nose-bleed. This was cured in a few weeks by *Urtica urens* Q, ten drops in water at bed time, and the young lady has continued to thrive ever since, so her mother told me quite lately.
I have often maintained the reality of vaccinosis as a orbid entity, and as the years roll round I become more and more certain of my thesis. See my little treatise *"On Vaccinosis"*. (IX 231)

## 142. EPIDEMIC ECZEMA

The only epidemic of eczema, apparently contagious, within my experience was one that broke out in the spring of 1891 at a very large public school near London.
The news came to me thus :
*March 16, 1891.*
"Dear Sir — On or about the 5th of this month a spot appeared over the eybrow of the bearer (my son). Thinking it merely a bruise received the

previous day whilst playing football, a piece of gum paper was put over the place.

"A few days served to show that the thing was more than a simple bruise, so we sent him over to Dr. ____, of ____; he also thought it merely an unhealthy wound, ordered on a bread poultice, and gave some ointment to be applied when 'the wound' was cleaned. At the end of two days I felt sure the diagnosis had been wrong, and so sent the boy over again to the doctor. It was then pronounced to be eczema."

"*Rhus tox.* inwardly, and zinc ointment externally, were prescribed and a fish, fruit, and vegetable diet insisted upon."

"This morning the thing has assumed such alarming proportions that my husband and I felt we must have your advice regarding it."

"Three of the boys playing in his team have broken out with the same kind of eruption."

There were quite a number of cases besides these, patient's brother being one of them.

The eruption itched very much in the evening, and had spread a good deal when the lad called upon me with the just-cited letter of his mother. The *iodide of sulphur* in the third trituration, and six-grain doses frequently repeated, cured the eczema in both lads in about six weeks, and there had not been any return of it. (IX 233)

## 143. ALOPECIA AREATA - 1

A married gentleman, 34 years of age, came under my observation in the month of April 1894; circular baldness in patches here and there, also both ends of moustache are gone; much indigestion and phlegm for many years, and these symptoms led me to prescribe *Thuja* 30; and when he returned after a month of this remedy he complained of the violent action of the *Thuja* 30. "Those powders have so upset me that I have had to keep my bed."

No medicine.

July 17 — Mending very beautifully, but quite lately the hair is falling out again very badly.

No medicine.

Aug. 20 — $R_x$ *Bacill.* 30.

Oct. 23 — Hair growing everywhere very well.

$R_x$ *Rep.*

He called a year later with catarrhal symptoms of chest.

$R_x$ *Rep.*

And twice subsequently the same remedy was repeated. Discharged quite cured in the fall of 1896. (IX 245)

## 144. ALOPECIA AREATA - 2

A married lady, 35 years of age, mother of three children, was brought by her husband to see me in the spring of 1897, for certain nerve symptoms, and . . . "I have a bald patch on my head, about the size of a shilling, also two small wens on the left side of my head in the hair."
April 1 — *Bacill.* 30.
May 4 — Wens gone; urine very thick. *Tub. test* C.
June 1 — "I am much better; the scurf in my hair is very troublesome, but I believe the hair is growing on the little bald patch which I showed you."
June 29 — Not quite so well; very scurfy scalp.
$R_x$ *Tub test.* C.
July 27 — *Bacill.* C.
We had here arrived at a point where further progress seemed barred.
Aug. 26 — $R_x$ *Thuja occid.* 30.
Sept. 23 — "I have been to my hair-dresser's, and he tells me I have not nearly so much scurf on my head, and the bald patch is quite covered with hair." (IX 247)

## 145. LOSS OF MOUSTACHE

A staff-officer, 59 years of age, came under my observation in 1894, first for debility, that remained after influenza. After being under *Urtica ur.* and *Cypripedium pub.* Q for six weeks, he was practically well; "but," said he, "look at the left side of my moustache; the hair is all coming out, and in places the hair of my head. I can't sleep."
April 2 — $R_x$ *Bacill.* 30.
June 11 — Some vomiting; sleepless broken; the hair is visibly thicker, the roundish patch no longer so evidently circular.
$R_x$ *Rep.*
Aug 15 — Nearly well. Moustache much thicker.
$R_x$ *Rep.*
Oct. 24, 1898 — Well; moustache flourishing.
This case is intersting, because only one remedy was used all the time (infrequent doses), and the influence of this upon the hair-growth was quite evident. At the beginning of the treatment the moustache had almost gone on the left side, and at about the centre of this left side it was practically hairless, and even on the right side the rest while well-grown moustache was indeed a sorry thing. It is more than two years since patient was discharged cured, and the cure holds good to date. Said I the other day to his daughter, "How's your father's moustache?"

"Oh! it's all right; as good as ever, but much more grey; poor dear papa, he *was* in a way about his moustache." (IX 249)

## 146. ALOPECIA AREATA - 3

A very tall lad, fifteen years of age, came under my observation in March 1893, to be treated for alopecia areata of moderate severity. "Large bald patches." There were scars in the right side of the neck, where glands had seemingly been excised; some not very large indurated glands in both sides of the neck and in both groins. The young man's skin almost literally covered with severe acne. "A mass of pustules" is the note in my book — the patches had not the dry, clean, ivorylike surface we are accustomed to see in alopecia areata, but they were sticky and shiny, and he scratched them a good deal. This led me to *Mal. C.*, and a seemingly perfect cure resulted in three months. And eighteen months later a lady friend of patient's family said to me, "You made a wonderful cure of General X _____'s son's head."
In April 1895 the young man turned up again, but this time with only one bald patch over his left ear, "Size of a crown piece."
$R_x$ *Mal. C.*
May 2 — Patch smaller, and hair growing on it. — *Rep.*
June 6 — No further progress.
$R_x$ *Bacill.* 30.
July 16 — Hair growing; neck-glands going down. — *Rep.*
Sept. — Well.
Two years later — His cousin informs me that the cure holds good. (IX 251)

## 147. ALOPECIA AREATA - 4

The Countess, X _____, aet. 50, mother of a family, came under my observation for bald circular patches at the back of her head, that have been there only a short time she thinks, and for which she has been under eminent specialists, who say it is a nerve affection. Her ladyship has a marvellous head of hair particularly for one of her age, and hence it would seem almost more strange that she should have perfectly bald circular patches in amongst such a mass of hair, strong and long reaching, a little armful in quantity, down to her hips. But so it was.
Four to five months under *Bacillinum* resulted in a perfect cure; the patches lost their shiny aspect and slowly covered with little hairs, and in about six months it was impossible to find them. The cure holds good to date.

Most of the cases of alopecia areata that have come under my care have been persons naturally blessed with uncommonly fine heads of hair. (IX 253)

### 148. ALOPECIA AREATA — SEVERE CASE - 5

Lady X ____, married, childless, 41 years of age, came under me in April 1896. She wore a wig, and had numerous typical bald areas all over the scalp, and what little of the scalp was not affected by the alopecia, the hair thereon was cropped as stubble. She had tried so many things, and so many physicians, surgeons, and hair professors, that she had quite given up all idea of ever being any better — had indeed become quite callous about it, and did not as a matter of fact consult me about her alopecia at all, but about recurrent cysts; and it was only by accident that I discovered the alopecia one day when the wig was off, because of the great heat.

The case concerns us here only for the alopecia areata, and as very many constitutional remedies were used, I am not able to say what remedies cured, but in less than a year, the alopecia was quite cured, and a year after beginning the treatment the wig could be entirely discarded, but the new hair was not yet long enough for her to dispense with some artificial hair arrangement at the back.

"All my life," she gave as the duration of her alopecia; so a complete cure with remedies within a year is not bad. *Thuja* 30, *Bacill.* 30, *Sul.* 30, *Psor.* C, *Hydrastis* Q, and *Urtica* Q, were amongst the remedies used, and that they, or some them, cured, admits of no doubt whatever, as no local application whatever was ordered by me, and the case had gone on for so many many years, inspite of the best and the worst treatment known in this London. (IX 255)

## DISEASES OF THE SPLEEN

### 149. PLEURO-PNEUMONIA SINISTRA AND SPLEENO-MEGALY

Some years since I treated a lady for "violent vomiting, pain all up the left side, cough with expectoration, profuse perspiration, and fever." She was not a native of the place, but came only for a short visit, and took lodgings in a small house facing a meadow on the banks of the river; the locality was at one time a part of the port, but was many years ago reclaimed. At my first visit she told me she often got inflammations on the chest with cough, and finding considerable fever, cough, pain in left side, and dulness on percussion of the same side, I quickly ticketed it *pleuro-pneumonia sinistra*, and gave *Acidum oxalicum*, which seemed to cover all the symptoms, and to correspond also to the supposed pathological state within. *Oxalic acid* somewhat relieved the vomiting, but nothing more, and I then gave various remedies, such as *Aconite, Bryonia, Phos., Ipec.*, and thus elasped about three weeks, but patient remained as ill as ever. Then I went into the case with very great care, and examined my patient very thoroughly, and, see, there was *inflammation of the spleen*. I gave her *Ceanothus Americanus* in a low dilution, and all the symptoms, subjective and objective, disappeared right off, and my previously ill-treated patient was sitting up in a week, and quite well in a few more days. I had never before met with splenitis in the acute form, and, indeed, it is a very rare disease in this country. (X 14)

## 150. CHRONIC SPLENITIS - 1

*Ceanothus*, one of which I well remember; it is this :
*Chronic Splenitis* — A young lady of about 26 years consulted me for a chronic swelling in the left side under the ribs, with considerable cutting pain in it. She stated that it was worse in cold damp weather, and she always felt chilly; the chilliness was so severe and long lasting that she had spent the greater part of her time during the previous winter sitting at the fireside, and now she was looking forward to the winter with perfect dread. In the summer she had felt nearly well, but the lump and the chilliness and pain nevertheless persisted, but it being warm, she did not heed it much, it being quite bearable.
*Ceanothus Americanus* quite cured her of all her symptoms, and subsequent observation proved its permanency. Often during the following winter she called my attention to the fact that she was not chilly and felt well. (X 16)

## 151. CHRONIC SPLENITIS - 2

Another case which I treated at a later date was that of a young man somewhat similarly suffering.
*Chronic Splenitis* — This young man had been sent to my dispensary, and was occupied in the post-office in some light but ill-paid employment. His whole trouble consisted in *severe pain in the left side in the region of the spleen*, and he had long vainly sought relief of many,

probably at dispensaries. He therefore put in an early appearance at my new dispensary to try the new doctor, probably on the well-known principle of the new broom. He had become quite low-spirited and began to fear he would become totally unfit for work, and naturally that was a very serious matter for a young married man. He told me he had formerly helped his wife in her household matters, doing the heavy rough work, but the pain in his side had now become so bad that he could not carry a bucket of water into the house or even sweep up their little yard, as handling the broom pained him so dreadfully. I was pressed for time, and prescribed *Ceanothus Americanus* in pilules of a low dilution, and promised to go into his case that day week, meaning to percuss the part and ascertain whether the spleen was enlarged. He returned that day week almost well, and the following week was quite well. At my request he again reported himself some time afterwards, and he still continued well. (X 16)

## 152. CHRONIC HYPERTROPHY OF SPLEEN

*Chronic Hypertrophy of the Spleen* — A middleaged lady consulted me, shortly after the above case, for a *severe pain in the left side and a large swelling in the same position*. Remembering the last case, I said I must examine the side. She objected, so I declined to treat her; then she said she would think about it and consult with her husband on the subject. In a fortnight or so she returned (driven by the severe pain in the side), and I examined the side and found an enormous spleen occupying the entire left hypochondrium and reaching inferiorly to about an inch above the crest of the ilium; it bulged towards the median line and ran off to an angle laterally. It was of long standing.

Gave *Ceanothus Americanus* in a low dilution.

This lady being very intelligent I begged she would allow me to examine the side again after I had finished the treatment. She promised to comply.

Fourteen days after this she came full of gratitude, and reported that the swelling was smaller and the pain considerably less.

To continue the medicine. She never consulted me again, but as she was a near neighbour of mine I often saw her, and somewhat six months afterwards she called to pay my fee, and then informed me that she had soon got rid of the pain entirely and the swelling was much smaller, so she had discontinued the medicine altogether, and did not deem it needful to trouble me again.

This is the usual thing. People will not be at the trouble of seeing the doctor as soon as they are better, they seem not to understand any interest one feels in the case. We can only make periodically reliable examinations of patients in a hospital; in private practice it is extremely difficult, as all practitioners know to their chagrin. Still, *faute de mieux*, we must put up with these fragments. This patient has had no children, and had a very fresh complexion. (X 17)

My next case is also one of *Chronic Hypertrophy of the Spleen*, though only about half the size of the one just narrated. Subject : A poor woman of about 30 or 32 years of age, whom I was requested to see by a very kind-hearted benevolent lay minister. She is the mother of several children, very poor, ill-fed, and over-worked, but withal a good, respectable woman, and very clean. She had a considerable and very painful swelling in the left side under the ribs, that had been there for some time, and latterly she could not get up on account of the severe pain. I carefully examined the tumour and satisfied myself that it was a very much swelled spleen, and the pain seemed to me to be due to its pressing against the ribs. I marked its size on the skin with ink, made her engage not to wash off the ink mark, and promised her I would call in a week, having first prescribed *Ceanothus* as in the other cases. But the fates were against my laudable plan, for I received a message, the day before my next visit was due, to the effect that Mrs. ____ felt herself so much better that she was up at her housework, and begged me not to call again, as she thought it unnecessary. (X 19)

## 153. CHRONIC SPLENITIS, CHILLS AND LEUCORRHOEA

Some four years since, perhaps a little more, I treated a lady of about 55 years. She complained of rigors at frequent intervals, and pain in left side, both of long standing.

The leucorrhoea had lasted some twenty years, and was profuse, thick and yellow. She had been for years under the best allopathic physicians of her native city, and finally given up as beyond the reach of medical art, evidently on Moliere's principle that *"Nul n'aura de l'esprit ques nous et nos amis."* Nevertheless, the patient bethought her of homoeopathy, and came under my care. Her last physician had finally suspected cerebro-spinal mischief, and hinted at incipient paralysis.

The pain in the side was the most prominent and distressing symptom, and for this I prescribed *Ceanothus*. In a month the pain was entirely cured, *and also the leucorrhoea*, while the cold feeling was very much diminished, but not quite cured. I have also never succeeded in quite curing it with any subsequent treatment. I watched the case for nearly four years, and am thus enabled to state that the pain in the side and the leucorrhoea never returned, and the chilliness never again became very bad, but still she had it a little when I saw her last. (X 20)

## 154. ENLARGED SPLEEN MISTAKEN FOR HEART DISEASE

A few years ago I was attending some of the members of a family of position in London, and at my various visits I occasionally heard of an invalid daughter of the family suffering from a hopelessly incurable disease of the heart, for which she was said to be under a West-End physician, who was thought to devote himself especially to diseases of the heart. The heart was said to be enormously enlarged, and the patient had had to give up first dancing and then hurrying, and finally she was only allowed to walk very slowly and carefully, lest the hugely enlarged heart should rupture. Several physicians had examined the case, and all were agreed as to its cardiac nature. I had never seen the young lady, and took no particular interest in the frequent narrations of her heart troubles; they are common enough. Time went by, and the mother used to speak of her "poor invalid daughter" with increasing despondency, finishing up one day with the remark that the unfortunate girl was no longer allowed even to walk, as the doctor considered even that now fraught with danger. "Is it not sad?" said she. "Would you like to see her?" I declined, saying, I never cared about seeing other physicians' patients.

More time elasped, and finally I was requested to take the case in hand. I demurred at first, because such hopeless cases are as unsatisfactory as they are painful.

At last I consented to take over the case, and I appointed a time to call and examine the patient.

During all my professional life, I have rarely been more taken aback than I was after I had made my examination of the patient, for I found the heart not only not enlarged, but of the two rather abnormally *small*, although apparently the cardiac dullness extended a foot down the left side. But this dulness on percussion was due to an *enlarged spleen* which pushed up the diaphragm and left lung by its bulk, till the heart and the spleen gave one continuous dull percussion note. Patient had many genuine symptoms of real heart disease — dyspnoea, palpitations, inability to lie on the left side, faintness — but these were due to the mechanical hindrance to the heart's action produced by the spleen bulking upward so much.

That young lady I met three weeks ago looking blooming, and as agile as possible, and she has done her share of dancing, tennis, etc., for some years.

*Ceanothus Americanus* cured the enlargement of the spleen for the most part, though it swelled again two or three times at some months' intervals, and *Ferrum phos.*, *Conium*, *Thuja*, *Berberis*, and other splenics, came into play before patient was really well. Looking at the case now with the advantage of wider experience and more and more matured views of biopathology, and with the patient fully six years under my observation, I regard the affection as primary disease of the leucocytes due to vaccinial infection, the spleen being disturbed secondarily, and then the heart mechanically. I am confirmed in this view by the fact that the spleen would not leave off swelling up at certain times till I had cured the vaccinosis. That prince of splenics, *Ceanothus Americanus*, readily cured the splenic engorgement, but did not touch the blood disease which caused it. This is the inherent defect of organopathy, that it is not sufficiently radical in its inceptive action, but the like remark applies to every other pathy more or less, because the primordial cause is more or less elusive, and generally quite beyond positive science, which only admits of what it knows, and will not seek to encompass the unknown by the processes of thinking and reasoning. Because in former times philosophy made science impossible, the votaries of science now round upon philosophy, and sneer it out of view. *To trace back proximate effects to remote causes is now ridiculed in medicine because mere science is productive of gross-mindedness, incapable of following the fine threads of the higher perception.* (X 21)

## 155. HEART SYMPTOMS DUE TO SPLEENO-MEGALY

It was also about the same time that I was at the house of patient in London, the wife of a general officer and the conversation fell upon the general's heart affection, and also upon that of their *charwoman*. I learned that the lady of the house took a certain interest in her charwoman because she had seen better days and had an invalid husband depending on her labour more or less. This charwoman was, it was said, suffering from an incurable disease of the heart, causing her terrible distress; on rising in the morning she would have to fight for her breath, so that it would take her often three-quarters of an hour to get dressed, having to pause and rest from the dyspnoea and its effects, nevertheless she persisted in thus getting up and dressing, and did as much charing as she could get. Her pride would not allow her to beg of her friends. Such was the story, and I really felt curious to see the charwoman, and promised to do what I could, though from the account given me by the general's wife, I certainly thought it quite a hopeless case.

Calling a few days later, I saw the lady and the charwoman, and having duly examined the latter, I promised to cure her! She was to come to my city rooms, and report herself every fortnight. On returning from the bedroom to the drawing room, the general's wife accused me of cruelty in this raising the poor old woman's hopes "when," exclaimed she, "you *must* know it is impossible." I tried to explain that it was a case of enlarged spleen, and not the heart disease at all, that the charwoman was suffering from, and that the palpitations and fightings for breath were the mechanical sequels of the splenic engorgement, but my patient evidently did not believe it, for she wound up by saying, "As you will treat her for nothing, I hope you may succeed, and it is very kind of you, but you must know that the poor woman has been under various doctors, and all have declared it incurable heart disease, and I merely wanted you to tell me of something to relieve and ease the poor old thing."

This was towards the middle of October. A careful physical examination showed that the heart-sounds were normal, but there was much beating visible in the neck, and the heart's action was laboured. In the left hypochondrium there was a mass corresponding to the position of the spleen, and dull percussion note was elicited not only in the left hypochondrium, but also in the right, and all across the epigastrium, or pit of the stomach, from side to side.

The following notes were put down at the time : "Heart-sounds, normal; apex beat, exaggerated; splenetic dulness extending up to the left mamma; the whole region very tender, so much so that she cannot bear her clothes or any other pressure." The prescription was : *Ceanothus Americanus* 1x zij, five drops in water three times a day.

November 14 — Has been taking the Ceanothus five weeks to-day, and has taken altogether three bottles of it, viz., zvj. It has nearly stopped the pain in the left side, which had lasted for quite twenty-five years. This pain came on suddenly, especially if she drank anything cold. She would get an indescribable pain under the left ribs, and she would have to fight for breath, and the dyspnoea would be so severe that it could be heard in the next room, frightening everybody. She had ague thirty years ago in Northamptonshire. Repeat.

November 29 — Not much pain left; the cold feeling still there, but nothing as it was. Repeat.

December 20 — Has the pain in the left side, but very little; *has not had any of those attacks of fighting for breath*; she can walk better, and the side is much smaller, which she knows from her dress. In her own opinion she is less in the waist by two inches. Before taking the medicine, for very many years she was compelled to pause in the morning when dressing, and lie down on account of the beating of heart, but this has all gone; on examining by palpation and percussion I find the dulness diminished by four inches in the perpendicular, and by about the same from side to side. However, there is still some tenderness on pressure, and the swelled spleen can still be felt towards the median line and inferiorly. She can now do her work (charing) very much better. $R_x$ *Tr. Ceanoth-Am.* 1, four drops in water three times a day.

January 10 — The pain is gone; has now no pain in walking, and she is a great deal stronger and better. The coldness in the pit of the stomach has gone. Repeat.

February 7 — In the left hypochondrium there is now nothing abnormal; the old ague-cake has disappeared, there being no dull percussion note. Her own conception of the size of that portion of the enlarged spleen that used to stretch across the pit of the stomach to the liver is thus expressed by her : "I used to say it was as big as a half-quartern loaf." Not only is the lump gone, but she is much stronger; she now wears stays again, and fastens her clothes with comfort. She again gets some cold feeling in the pit of the stomach, but not much. Her liver seems considerably enlarged, and there is still too much beating of the blood-vessels (veins) in the neck. In my opinion the condition of the blood-vessels calls for *Ferrum* 6, which I now prescribe, and when that has done its duty — as it surely will — the liver will call for attention. But what I wanted to bring out was the specific affinity of *Ceanothus Americanus* for the spleen, and its consequent brilliant effects, as the *simile* only grounded on the homoeopathic specificity of seat, which some say has no existence.

This poor woman thus took *Ceanothus* during about four months in small appreciable doses : at first the 1x and then the 1 centesimal.

The existence of the hypertrophy was ascertained by percussion and palpation, and subsequently I ascertained by the same means that it had ceased to exist. Although patient took the drug for four months I could not find that it affected any other organ — liver, kidney, bowel — save and except the spleen.

The dyspnoea and palpitation were cured certainly but these arose, I submit, from the engorged condition of the spleen itself.

As far as I could ascertain, the secretions and excretions were not affected in the least degree; the remedial action must, therefore, be considered specific. My conception of the cure is simply this, that the specific *Ceanothus* stimulus persistently applied restored the spleen tissue to the normal. This homoeopathic specificity of seat suffices only in simple local disturbances; it is only a *simile*, not a *simillimum*. The latter would, I apprehend, have affected the liver also and the right heart, and I should then not have needed further detail treatment.

This charwoman continued to attend to my rooms for some months, and *Ceanothus Americanus* and other indicated remedies cured her of her "incurable heart disease;" and I saw no more of her for some time, when one day she was ushered into my consulting room. She came up to where I was sitting, told me she was perfectly well, could do any work with ease, and — then occurred one of the sweetest things in my whole professional life — the old lady (and *what a lady*!) put a tiny packet on my desk, tried to say something, burst into tears, and rushed out!

I never saw her again, and have often since wished I had kept that particular sovereign and had it set in diamonds.

## 156. SUPPOSED CONSUMPTION : CHRONICALLY ENLARGED SPLEEN

The case I am about to relate is not without practical interest. The subject is a fine young Anglo-Indian of about 21 or 22 years of age, who a couple of years since, commenced preparing for the study of medicine in London. His father was my patient, and told me, as he left for the East, that one of his boys, whom I had casually seen, was going to remain in London to study medicine as a profession, rather than as a hobby, as said father has done for many years.

Two years elapsed, and then my patient returned from the East, and came to see me on his own account, and I incidentally inquired about the medical student. "Ah! he is better now, but he had to give up the study of medicine, as the professor said he was going into consumption. He had spitting of blood, and they sent him to America. He has returned, and is better; but I am still anxious about him, as his breath is very short. He looks very well."

The young man came in due course, and a very careful percussion and auscultation of the chest revealed nothing but a very large spleen filling up the left hypochondrium, and clearly impeding both lungs and heart in their action.

I ordered *Ceanothus Am.* 1 in five drop doses.

He took the drops for a month or so, and came again on the 16th of February, 1887, telling me he breathed easily and comfortably, and demonstrated to me that he was inches smaller round the body, by showing me his waistcoat and trousers that were previously tight, but now uncomfortably loose, so much so that he laughed at their bagging. Evidently his pulmonary symptoms had never been phthisical at all, but were merely mechanical from the engorgement of the spleen. (X 30)

---

## 157. SPLENALGIA

A lady came to me complaining of the following series of symptoms ... Pain in the left side corresponding to the region of the spleen, so bad that she cannot lie on the left side; with this pain in the side there are two other disturbances, indicating that a kind of vascular turgescence — an *orgasmus humorum* — underlies the whole, viz., palpitation of the heart and piles. With these also some indigestion, and a feeling as if the visceral contents of the abdomen were being pulled down.

$R_x$ *Ceanothus Americanus 3x* ziv. Three drops in water three times a day. She came from the country, so I did not see her again, but as I asked for a report in fortnight, her husband wrote at the end of that period to say that she was well and needed no further attention.

The case of this lady rather interested me, as some six years previously she came under my care for chronic headaches that seemed climacteric; I treated her for these headaches, but could not make any impression upon them, and then, on going over the various organs, I found that the urine contained a small quantity of albumen. This our ordinary remedies removed in about two months, and the headaches disappeared. About a year later the albuminuria again returned in a very slight degree, and with it some cephalalgia; both yielded at once to the same remedies, and she had remained well till she came with the splenalgia and haemorrhoids. I suspect, therefore, that the old albuminuria was not due to any kidney mischief, but to venous congestion of the kidneys. (X 31)

## 158. PAINFUL ENGORGEMENT OF SPLEEN WITH VARICOSIS

Some cases of varicosis will not get well till you cure the spleen of its — perhaps slight — enlargement. Thus, a hale gentleman of 70 odd years consulted me early in 1887 for varicose veins, particularly below the knees. The veins on the surface of all four extremities get knotty and painful. There is a pain under the left ribs, which is worse when he has urinary urging. The splenalgia he has had these ten years.

I perscribed *Ceanothus* 1. It cured the splenalgia and painful vein-knots in a few weeks. He is now comfortable under left ribs for the first time for ten years. He is also not so short of breath. The stricture of the urethra, of which he also suffers, was not affected by the *Ceanothus*, and he remains under my care to see if the stricture will also yield to treatment. (X 32)

## 159. CHRONIC ENLARGEMENT OF SPLEEN WITH HEART SYMPTOMS

An unmarried lady of 49 years came to me in January, 1887, for a supposed affection of the heart. Being rather stout, she was thought to have a fatty heart. She complained of numbness and heaviness down the left arm for a considerable time, also of a pain under her left ribs at times ever since her childhood, and over which part she had had blisters and poultices from most of her many physicians, generally with relief for the time being. An examination showed the heart to be normal, but disclosed an enlargement of the spleen. Patient has suffered from whites all her life.
She took *Ceanothus Americanus* 1, five drops in water night and morning, for two months : I had ordered it for one month only, but she found herself so much better from the medicine that she got a second bottle of it on her own account, and continued taking it for just two months, when she came to inform me that she felt quite well, and percussion showed that the spleen had returned to its normal size. The leucorrhoea was a trifle better, but not much, and for this affection she remained under treatment. The spleen engorgement had been cured by the spleen remedy, but the constitutional state had remained unaltered; but with this I am here not concerned. (X 33)

## 160. VOMITING — CHRONIC AND SEVERE HYPERTROPHY OF SPLEEN

On June 16, 1881, an unmarried lady of 23 years of age, residing on high ground in London, came to me saying she suffered from chronic and severe vomiting, debility and emaciation. The vomiting began about midsummer, 1880, at first once or twice a week, and it has been gradually getting worse, so that she now vomits generally about half an hour after every meal, though occasionally she will miss a meal and not vomit. She has lost 13 lbs. in weight since January last. Menses are getting scant. There is a very considerable area of dulness on percussion in the left hypochondrium, and when she is sick she feels pain under the left ribs. She often gets caught with a pain under left ribs; and besides this left hypochondriac pain, she gets a clawing pain in the pit of the stomach, not seemingly connected with it, and apt to last the whole of the day. Lifting her arms seems to pull her stomach and hurt in the middle. Cannot wear stays, because their pressure hurts; she dons them, but is compelled to put them off every few hours. There is a clear space of about an inch between the area of dulness on percussion of liver and spleen respectively. She flushes at times. She is generally chilly, sitting by the fire when others do not, and she goes to sit by the kitchen fire when there is no fire anywhere else in the house. Cannot walk upstairs other than very slowly, because of dyspnoea. The vomit is sometimes nearly black, as if she had been drinking coffee; at times it is watery, at others just the food.

$R_x$ *Ceanothus Americanus* 1, zv. Five drops in water three times a day. She took no other remedy, and was discharged cured in about seven weeks. The patient had previously been under an able homoeopathic practitioner, who had treated the case purely symptomatically, and thus failed, for the very sufficient reason that the symptoms which he treated were secondary to the engorgement of the spleen, and so his remedies all failed. God forbid that I should say one disparaging word about symptomatic treatment as such, for we but too often have only the subjective symptoms to go by, but where an exhaustive physical diagnosis is possible, it should always be made, and should stand in importance far before merely subjective symptoms, as these may be, and often are, consequently in this sense delusive.

For, in this case, it must be manifest that vomiting due to an enlarged spleen can never be cured by remedies that physiologically produce vomiting, but by such as will bring a large spleen back to the normal. (X 34)

## 161. ENLARGEMENT OF SPLEEN — AGUE CAKE

In November, 1886, a *poitrinaire* lady of 29 came under my observation complaining of indigestion, flatulence, and palpitation, with cough and considerable debility. The flatulence is worse in the evening. The right lung gives a dull percussion note almost all over the front aspect. There is an endocardial bruit, best heard at mid-sternum. The spleen fills the entire left hypochondrium, while in the right side hepatic dulness runs up, seemingly almost to the nipple. There is slight increase of vocal resonance on the right side of thorax. The skin across the epigastrium is very brown. Had a cough ever since she had fever in Malta three years ago; also frontal neuralgia.

*Chelidonium* 1 cured the swelling of the liver, and reduced the spleen a trifle. *Ceanothus Americanus* 1 restored the spleen to the normal, but did not touch the neuralgia. *Thuja occidentalis* 30 cured the neuralgia, and I am now endeavouring to go deeper into the case to find out the etiologic *x* of her constitution, which causes me to state that she is *poitrinaire*, the anatomic basis of which is a sodden phlegmy, bronchial lining; but what is the etiologic moment thereof?

This case also illustrates both *the insufficiency of the organopathic conception and also its practical utility.* (X 36)

## 162. QUASI-HEART DISEASE

A city gentleman between 30 and 40 years came to see me on November 25, 1885, for heart disease, from which he had suffered for fifteen years. He has been under quite a number of eminent physicians, tried changes to spas, and been for climatic benefits east, west, north, and south, at all times and seasons. Cruising about in yacht does him most good. For the past several years he has been under Sir — for his heart.

I find his heart rather small, its action irregular and endocardial bruit most audible below and to the left of the left mammilla. He gets very chilly, and his fingers often go dead in the early morning : the so-called "poor circulation" so frequently accused. He is languid, anaemic, seemingly barely able to rise in the morning. Has been vaccinated three times, but only took very slightly the first time.

The lungs are flat; the spleen notably enlarged.

The most distressing symptom is his nocturnal palpitation.

$R_x$ *Ceanothus Am.* 1. Five drops in water three times a day.

After taking the *Ceanothus* thus for a fortnight, the cardiac and splenic dulness no longer ran into one another, and the palpitation and numbness were much better.

Regarding the case causally as partly from vaccinosis, I gave *Thuja* 30 infrequently, which did him so much good that he stayed away for a month. *But a very ugly patch of eczema had come out in the right axilla! and he subsequently got shingles on left thigh.*

The quasi-heart disease was gone, and has not returned, and the further course of the case presents no relevancy to my present thesis. Strange to say, the endocardial bruit had also quite disappeared.

The foregoing entirely chips from my own workshop, I think it would be well to give an example of what Rademacher's organopathy really is, by reproducing in rough and ready translation the bulk of his chapter on Disease of the Spleen from his great life-work, the *Rechtfertigung,* already referred to. (X 37)

## 163. ASTHMA DUE TO SPLEEN DISEASE

A man who, in his youth, had had a moist eruption all over his body, which eruption was fruitlessly treated with medicines, but went away of itself in adult life, but left behind an ugly fish-skin-like epidermis, began to complain of tension in the left hypochondrium, becoming at times a little painful. He did not, however, consult me for this, but for shortness of breath. I soon ascertained that he had had the tension in the hypochondrium much longer than the asthma, and so thought he was suffering from a disease of the spleen, and which I thought the more likely, as he had never had the least the matter with his lungs. Well, I did not give this man *Carbo,* but another remedy, and the complaint got visibly better. When it had reached a certain stage of improvement, he was hard hit by a then prevailing liver fever, which in his case implicated the chest. This chest affection, however, did not consist in the previous asthmatic attacks, but in pain in the side, with cough and bloody expectoration. He got well, but hardly was he able to be up all day when the old asthma came back worse than ever. Thinking the liver complaint might not be quite cured, I gave him a good hepatic, but the asthma remained. Here I gave him the spleen remedy — the splenic — which had done him so much good before the acute affection came on. The man asked for it himself, but it did no good at all. Asthma and cough remained, and instead of picking up after his acute disease with good night's rest, the asthma drove him every night out of bed. I now gave him *Carb-v,* which soon altered the face of things. Cough and asthma lessened; the latter soon disappeared altogether, so that the man was able to make the hour and half walk home to his friends, who had given him up.

But not every case of asthma, due to the spleen, will yield to *Carb-v.* Those stomach pains that, as they pass off, lose themselves in the left hypochondrium, and which I put down to the spleen, I have at times cured with *Carb-v* more frequently, however, with other spleen remedies.

Kidney affections, with dropsy, due to primary spleen disease, I have never tried to cure with *Carb-v,* because I thus far have managed to cure them with other remedies, and I do not hold it to be right to try experiments from mere curiosity. (X 42)

## 164. CHRONIC ENLARGEMENT OF THE SPLEEN WITH HEMIHYPERAESTHESIA, CEPHALALGIA, DYSPNOEA, ORTHOPNOEA, CONVULSIONS.

A more remarkable case of its kind I never observed. Subject : A young lady towards the end of her teens, of good family, and at a finishing school in London. Had been treated at home for hysteria of a severe type both homoeopathically and hydropathically, the latter consisting of the cold douche when a convulsive attack was on. The cold douche was only once applied, and nearly killed the patient. Many months after it was applied, when the patient was in a state of what seemed to be approaching death from exhaustion with violent delirium, she literally yelled at what she imagined was some one approaching the bed to throw water on her. It would fill a little book to give a complete history of her case, so I will summarize it as briefly as may be.

At first, and for a year or two, I treated her for *attacks*. Said "attacks" I had never seen, but I put them down as a form of epileptoid seizure, though it was distinctly stated that the convulsions were mostly left-sided. Sometimes violent palpitation of the heart was essentially the attack; at other times dyspnoea, orthopnoea; and always a pain in the left side under the ribs, going up and down : and patient, no matter how violent the convulsive attacks, was never quite unconscious. I was not able to see an attack, and could never get a really clear description of them. "Dreadful fighting for breath" coming on in attacks, with pain in the left side, was the essence of all the descriptions given to me. I treated the case, but without doing any real good and finally she was seized with an attack so violent that the parent telegraphed from the country to me to know what to do, and I felt it too serious a case to be treated by me at a distance, and so I wired back that I resigned the case to their family physician, himself an eminent homoeopathic practitioner, who also had formerly tried his hand at the case, but in vain.

Many months elapsed, and I heard only indirectly about the case; and then the friends, in sheer despair and disgust at the obstinancy of the attacks of what their family physician said was a severe form of hysteria that would not go away for good, but ever and anon came like a domestic explosion, creating unrest and tension, brought her to reside near me in the neighbourhood of London, and this was at the beginning of the winter of 1886-87. The attacks soon came, and I had the opportunity of observing them. On entering the room I thought I heard steam coming out in short, sharp "whists" from a kettle-spout, but I found it was patient's expiratory efforts. The dyspnoea was very great, and the convulsions most violent, being always confined to one side — the left — but varying as to position on the trunk, being at times in the nape, then on a level with the nipple, then in the lumbar region, sometimes so bad that the body would be bent like a hoop, and the movements very often sent patient flying either against the bedstead, over on to the next bed, or on to the floor; and hence we had to pad all hard objects. Some of the convulsive contortions were awful to behold, and most of her friends devoutly hoped and prayed that she might die. For some weeks I was the only one who believed recovery possible, so long, so violent, and so exhausting were the convulsive attacks. Myself, I only lost heart once, and that was after a series of attacks of convulsions lasting for hours, and leaving only short intervals. Her friends several times fetched me, in the night, believing patient to be dying.

The thing went on for months, and I was able to get slowly at some constant characteristics.

1. When out of the attacks patient was comparatively well in herself, and looked well, only as time went on, and the attacks lasted for hours with great violence (relays of two, and sometimes three persons being required to hold her down), she became very weak from exhaustion.
2. The appetite was poor, the tongue coated, the bowels obstinately confined.
3. The left side of the body (trunk) was so tender that she could not bear the least pressure. Touching it gently with one finger even made her wince.
4. The spleen was considerably enlarged, and the whole region excessively tender.
5. She had a *constant* fixed pain in the left half of skull, worst about midway between ear and the sagittal suture, and she usually held her head in left palm.
6. Warmth was agreeable, and cold aggravated very distinctly, and particularly frost and snow; violent attacks always came on whenever it froze. "Thunder has always tried me."
7. There was pronounced periodicity, sometimes irregular, but also at times and for weeks together as regular as a clock, there being two, three, or four attacks in twenty-four hours.

I could not agree that the case was one of hysteria, as the family physician thought. In the very early part of the treatment I treated her for epilepsy, but did her no good. Then, in view of the enlarged spleen, I gave *Ceanothus Americanus* and other spleen remedies but in vain.

She was at times feverish, and had *Aconitum*; very flushed in the face, and I ordered at first *Belladonna*, and then *Lachesis*, but in vain.

*Phosphorus, Gelseminum, Zincum, Cuprum, Ignatia, Nux-v, Puls.*, and many such were equally useless. *Aranea diadema, Cicuta,* were no better.

*Sulphur* and *Plumbum* did a little temporary good, and we thought *Cuprum* and *Acid hydrocyanic* eased the convulsions a little, and also *Mikania guaco*. Essentially they did no real good.

The fixed, constant, and often severe pain in the left side of the head at last compelled me to assume the presence of a tumor in the brain, perhaps of a vascular nature. *Silicea* and a number of other remedies were given on this hypothesis, but the patient seemed practically uninfluenced by them.

Heretofore I had treated the case from the particular standpoint, as well as from that of the entire organism, and had failed, so I thought over the case afresh, and came to the conclusion that Rademacher's account of the action of *Oleum succini* made that drug appear a likely remedy. I therefore prescribed the non-rectified oil in five-drop doses three times a day. That was early in March. . . . In forty-eight hours the convulsive attacks ceased, and in three weeks the hemihyperaesthesia. The pain in the head — in fact, the whole series of morbid phenomena — slowly disappeared. So I am now disposed to regard the case as a primary disease of the spleen from the very beginning, the convulsions and head pain being consecutive thereto. This is the *kind of cure* one meets with in Rademacher, and which gave the tone to his life and practice.

When I say kind of cure, I mean an obviously bad case of disease not mending of itself, and cure straight off — generally jugulated.

After taking the *Oleum suc.* for six weeks I very carefully percussed and palpated the left hypochondrium, which was no longer tender, and the enlargement of the spleen had quite disappeared, though patient said the side was at *times* tender still, and the pain in the head still persisted a very little. No convulsion since the second day of taking the *Oleum succini*. (X 55)

## 165. SPLEEN TROUBLE MISTAKEN FOR HEART DISEASE

"Visiting a resident patient one day twelve months ago, I got into conversation with a lady visitor living in Newmarket, who informed me that the previous ten years of her life had been spent mostly in bed or on a couch. Heart disease, her family physician had diagnosed, as well as several professors. I informed her after having made a rapid physiognomical diagnosis that she had a very good heart, and that she could be cured in probably a few months. — Tableau.

"After four months' treatment she was nearly well and stopped treatment for three months. An attack of influenza brought on the old spleen trouble again, but six weeks' treatment brought her round again. There was slight ovarian complication in this case.

"I used *Ceanothus Americanus* with a small dose of *Chel.*, and she like it flavored with *Am. carb.* and *Tinct. capsici*.

"I have usually two spleen cases every week — sometimes more. Sometimes the spleen is very much enlarged and always painful — sometimes complicated with tender left lobe of liver, and also the latter enlarged, and *Ceanothus* has in every instance hitherto removed the spleen trouble, and I have only failed in one case of enlarged and tender left lobe of liver, associated with enlarged and painful spleen. *Ceanothus* has cured the latter, but as yet, this liver baffles me. I put it down to my own ignorance."

Turning over the leaves of the *Homoeopathic Recorder* of May 15, 1900, I saw something about my old friend *Ceanothus*, and which I forthwith proceed to commandeer. (X 66)

## 166. SPLENIC ANAEMIA AFTER INFLUENZA

A couple of years ago I was called upon to treat a case of splenic anaemia after influenza in a young married lady. It would yield to nothing; eminent physicians tried their hands after the family doctor had in vain done his best. I tried, but also in vain. The late Dr. Swan, of New York, once wrote to me that he had found *Med.* (high) a good antidote to the ill effect of influenza, which statement I have very frequently verified. It failed here. When we were all in despair (residence at the seaside had also failed) I bethought me of the fact that pigs fed on modder get their tissues coloured red, and on that idea I gave Mrs. X. 60 drops of *Rubia Tinctoria* Q in water daily. She picked up immediately, the extreme pallor yielded, the dyspnoea lessened, patient and her husband were loud in their praise of the remedy and begged to be allowed to continue it which was done, and a perfect recovery was the result. (X 70)

In several such cases of anaemia I have used the *Rubia Tinctoria* with great advantage. As I have before stated, *Rubia Tinctoria* was one of Rademacher's splenics. I call to mind the case of a maiden lady of 52, who was brought to me in February 16, 1899, for anaemia and debility of a very obscure nature. There had been no period for six months. I prescribed *Rubia Tinctoria* Q, 10 drops in water night and morning. In six weeks she declared herself nearly well. The medicine was continued, and in another two months she was discharged cured. (X 71)

## 167. CONSENTANEOUS HEART DISEASE

Where the heart is perturbed consentaneously with a spleen affection, the relief obtained from the use of *Ceanothus* (and other splenics) is often very noteworthy.

The number of cases of spleen affections commonly reported as cardiac is very considerable. And even in cases where the heart is really at fault, the easing of the spleen region by splenics is often a great help to the comfort of the heart.

Thus a patient of mine who suffers from valvular disease these many years consulted me anew in the spring of 1900. The valvular condition was, of course, unalterable, and the heart distress was pretty bad from supercompensatory hypertrophy; the greatest distress was under the left ribs, and patient was often chilly, and, moreover, in his youth he had had ague.

A few drops of *Ceanothus* two or three times a day brought very great relief, so much so that patient became very loud in its praise, and continued taking it for three months. He told me yesterday that no medicine he had ever taken had ever brought so much comfort to his heart : "The palpitation has almost ceased, I can lie down flat in bed, and can sleep lying on either side, and I pass much more water." Where the congestive distress lies in the liver region, hepatics play a similar part, as this gentleman's remark to me proved, when he said, "I remember you used to give me *Chelidonium*, but that was when the pain used to be in the right side, and that is why I always keep some *Chelidonium* by me in case." (X 71)

## 168. ENLARGED SPLEEN

"A cabman, aged 50 years, living at Boscombe, near Bournemouth, who had been operated on some two years back at the Bromptom Cancer Hospital for what appears to have been enlarged spleen, wrote to me in the beginning of August under the following circumstances :

"It seems that this man and Marrell, whose case of cancer of the pylorus I refer to in my work on *Cancer and Cancer Symptoms*, had occupied adjoining beds in the hospital, and he, having met with Marrell, whose case had been looked upon in the hospital as quite hopeless, immediately started for London to consult me.

"As he arrived too late, he subsequently wrote me a letter which I received when on my holiday, and which I answered on the 13th August by forwarding a prescription of *Ceanothus Americanus* Q gtt. vii; aq. zij, five drops four times a day in water.

"From his letter, as well as from an interview with him on 12th September, I gathered these particulars.

"He had been dragged forward by a bolting horse when driving, and the bar of the phaeton had pressed heavily upon the diaphragmatic region, and this was followed by severe pain, especially in the splenic region, which swelled up and became more and more painful. After suffering in this way for a year, he was admitted to the Cancer Hospital, and after being there for a month, was operated on for enlarged spleen. Before the operation the pain was very great, and certainly the operation relieved this, but after the operation he continued to get weaker and weaker, and his weight went down; in the two years since then he has lost two stones, and is becoming more and more enfeebled. His face is florid, and blood rushes to his face and head, making the face scarlet and the eyes blood-shot and dim and he staggers with weakness. He has to hold on to things when standing, and then the lower part of his body and legs get cold and his hands and fingers numb. A vein running up the right temple enlarges, especially in the morning, to the size of his little finger. The local sensations are thus described in his letter :

"Now as to the place where the operation was, it seems to bubble up, relief coming from pressures, and if it does not work like this, I am worse. Then under my ribs the left side is like a bird fluttering."

"On 12th September he came up from Boscombe to see me, having taken two bottles of medicine. His testimony then was that he was better in every possible way, and that whereas, before taking the medicine, he could not do the lightest yard work for three hours together, he could now keep at work all day. The vein on the right temple had not shown up since he began the *Ceanothus*, and the urine, which before had been thick and scanty, was now clear and free. The bowels were acting naturally, though sleep was poor. On examining the side I found a dull hard mass posteriorly and immediately below diaphragm, and a hard band 2 inches by 2 inches in front, just above the extensive scar of the operation and below the diaphragm.

"The inference from local examination would be either that the entire spleen had not been removed, or that new growth had taken place since the operation. Anyway, the distinct and pronounced relief given by the *Ceanothus* could not be questioned.

"I may mention there was no history of anguish seizures or of chills and perspirations at any time of the disease." (X 72)

## 169. AGUE MEDICINE : URTICA URENS

The stinging nettle is a splenic of very high order. I will content myself with giving one case of ague cured by it.

A young officer, 29 years of age, was invalided home from Burma with malarial fever and a swelled spleen in the spring of 1893. He had had quinine, arsenic, and iron, but was not improving or free of fever.

March 2. — $R_x$ *Urtica urens* Q; ten drops in water night and morning.

March 16. — No fever at all; much sediment in urine (quite normal).

May 20. — No fever.

June 22. — No fever. Discharged cured.
As I have entered so largely into the question of the value of *Uritica urens* in my booklet, entitled *Gout and its Cure*, I will refer my readers for further information here anent to its pages. (X 75)

### 170. PAIN LEFT HYPOCHONDRIUM — DR. CLARKE'S CEANOTHUS CASE

One Sunday morning about a year ago an American lady brought her daughter, aged 14 years, to me, complaining of severe pain in the left side. They had just arrived in London, having landed at Liverpool a day or two before, and the history of the case was this : During the voyage, as the patient lay in her berth, she stretched over to reach something in the cabin, and was immediately seized with a violent stitching pain in the left side. It was thought at the time that the pain would soon go away, but it did not. And after landing, the pain persisted and grew rather worse, so that the plans of the family, which were to proceed to the continent in a few days, were jeopardized.
As it is always well to localize exactly a pain or an ailment whenever possible, I asked the patient to undress, and I found that the pain was not in the chest wall or abdominal muscles, as the history would rather suggest it to be, but was deep in — in the spleen, in fact. Moreover, percussion showed that the spleen was quite considerably enlarged. The pain was > by lying on the painful side.
As it was Sunday and the pharmacies were likely to be closed, I put a powder of *Ceanothus* 30 on the patient's tongue there and then, and gave her a prescription for the same medicine to be made up later on, with instructions to come and report on the Tuesday following. She came in due course, and reported that in two hours from receiving the dose the pain had gone — before the prescription was made up. I again examined the side, and the splenic dulness had gone back to normal.
So we see that my original claim for *Ceanothus Am.*, that it is a homoeopathic remedy in the ordinary sense is substantiated. (X 76)

## FIFTY REASONS FOR BEING A HOMOEOPATH

### 171. PLEURITIS RHEUMATICA

Some years since I was suddenly summoned to the suburban house of a city merchant, who had caught a chill two evenings before on returning from a political meeting. When I arrived, an exquisite case of pleurisy, *pleuritis rheumatica*, presented itself.

The gentleman's wife informed me that she was much exercised in her mind, as many friends had strongly urged her not to have homoeopathy in such a serious case. All very well, said they, perhaps, for women and children, but she surely was not going to risk her dear husband's life in the hands of a homoeopathic practitioner? No, she would have Dr. X., who lived nearby. But though, as a rule, *L'homme propose et la femme dispose*, in this case it was the other way about. The husband flatly refused any other than homoeopathic treatment, and hence my presence. He was in a raging fever and much pain, and merely moaned, "Doctor, give me relief from this pain, and procure me some sleep."

I gave *Aconite* and *Bryonia* — strong.

Next day he was already a little round the corner, and not in much pain, unless he incautiously turned. "Doctor," said he, "my friend Mr. — in — road over yonder, has, I am told, something of the same thing as I have, only more in the shoulder, and he has sent to me to beg me to give you up, and have his medical man, who lives nearby, and who is considered a very clever man — what am I to say?" I replied, "Tell him from me that I shall have you well in your city office in a few days at work, and that on your way home from the city you may call, and you will *still find* him *ill*, and then you can tell him your experience, and compare notes!"

And so it happened, in a few days — I do not remember the exact number — my patient went to his city office, did a small amount of work, and on returning home called on or sent to his said friend, who was still in great pain, and remained so for some time. (XI 12)

## 172. STIFFNESS IN SHOULDER

The gentleman referred to in my last case (No. 171) (my patient's friend), after he got over his acute sufferings went to a specialist for gout, but was still so stiffened in his shoulder and side that he was not able to do his office duty, and after remaining faithfully under his own doctor for a further period and still not getting well, finally — What? Came to me! And what next? *Bryonia alba*, *Chelidonium majus*, and *Sulphur*, cured him in a few weeks.

It seems to me that *Aconite* and *Bryonia* alone, if well studied and rightly used, would convert the whole world to homoeopathy, at least I see no escape for any honest unprejudiced man.

But prejudice is well-nigh almighty. As Bolingbroke says, "It may sound oddly, but it is true, in many cases, that if men had learned less, their way to knowledge would be shorter and easier. It is, indeed, shorter and easier to proceed from ignorance to knowledge than from error. They who are in the last must unlearn before they can learn to any good purpose; and the first part of this double task is not in many respects the least difficult, for which reason it is seldom undertaken."

Did you understand anything about homoeopathy? I would explain to you why I gave the *Bryonia,* why it was followed by *Chelidonium,* and why *Sulphur* had to be interposed; as you are, however, ignorant, you must take it empirically. (XI 13)

## 173. CHLORAL HYDRATE IN LETHARGIC SOMNOLENCY

Those who have watched *old* chloral-eaters may have noticed that they slowly get lethargic, somnolent, and listless. Towards the end of the chapter of chronic chloralism there is a condition of fatty degeneration of a slow, lazy type, and the very mode of death seems peculiar. I have seen a case where the subject of chronic chloralism lay for days a-dying; she was for several days so that it was very difficult to determine whether she was dead or not.

Occasionally one comes across a remarkable case of somnolence, and then the narcotics are to be thought of by the therapeutist.

I will shortly relate two such cases from my own practice.

No. 1. A lady about forty-five years of age, stout, fresh-looking and the mother of a family, was the subject of remark of her friends, on account of her lethargy and sleepiness. Her weakness was such that even crossing the street was almost impossible; the weakness was peculiarly lethargic, a kind of listless heaviness. She was almost constantly asleep; she would get up in the morning after a good night's rest and, even while dressing, she seemed compelled to sit down, and no sooner seated but she would fall asleep. This state of things went on for weeks and months, and her allopathic adviser did his best in vain. After she came under my care I tried first *Arnica* and then *Opium,* with but indifferent success, when all at once I bethought me of the great similarity of the case before me to that of a confirmed old chloral-eater of my clientele. *Chloral* in a low dilution cured my patient, and she again became brisk, active and wide awake. (XI 14)

No 2. An elderly lady came under my care on April 21, 1881, for lethargy, languor, and somnolence.

$R_x$ Trit. 2x *Chloral hydrat.,* 6 grains in water every three hours.

May 7. Under this date I find these notes in my case book : "Feels a different creature; vastly improved; less lethargic, and decidedly less languid."

She then got the third decimal trituration in lieu of the second, and only two doses a day, and then needed no further treatment, as she subsequently informed me when calling with her husband. (XI 14)

## 174. CANCER BREAST AND DEEP CRACK ANGLE OF MOUTH

Subsequently I had to treat a case of cancer of the left breast in a middle-aged woman, but patient had *also a deep crack in the angle of her mouth* on the left side, with thick indurated edges, probably of an epitheliomatous nature. I think you would have agreed with the diagnosis had you seen the case. I therefore reasoned thus : We know empirically that *Cundurango* can cure some cases of cancer; I now know from the direct experiment on myself that it causes the angles of the mouth to crack; the homoeopaths maintain that likes, *ergo, Cundurango* ought to be the curative agent in this case.

The patient took a homoeopathic preparation of the remedy steadily for about three years, with gradual, slow amelioration, and eventual perfect cure. Since then eight years have elapsed, and she is still in excellent health. I think it must be manifest that, had it not been for homoeopathy, this cure could not have been wrought, and patient must long since have died of the dire disease. (XI 15)

## 175. FATTY LIVER, ATHEROMA OF ARTERIES

Ever since the year 1878 I have been in the habit of using *Vanadium* as a remedy in a class of cases that, outside of homoeopathy, you cannot touch — I mean in certain cases or atheroma of the arteries, and fatty degeneration. I had been in the habit of using *Phosphorus, Antimony, Arsenic,* and the like, but was not satisfied with my result in certain cases : nothing satisfies *me* but a *cure*. So I went farther afield, and thought I had found what I wanted in *Vanadium,* whose *physiological* effects I studied in the *Proceedings of the Royal Society*. I got the differential points from an article in the *Journal of Physiology* by Mr. G.F. Dowdeswell entitled "On the Structural Changes which are Produced in the Liver under the Influence of the Salts of Vanadium." In a word, let me say that it consists in true cell destruction, the pigment escaping, the liver being hit hardest. I had a case on hand of fatty liver, atheroma of the arteries, much pain corresponding to the course of the basilar artery, large deeply pigmented patches on forehead, profound adynamia, and so forth.

Well, my patient was then over seventy years, and was very clearly breaking up and going to pass the big bourne whence no man returneth. Thanks to the use of *Vanadium* (I used the soluble ammonium salt) in homoeopathic preparation, chosen according to the homoeopathic law, that lady got quite well, and remains so, being now hard upon eighty years of age, and hale and hearty. (XI 16)

## 176. PAIN IN RIBS AND SPLEEN REGION WITH LEFT EYE AFFECTION

A lady living in Kensington, came to me on June 5, 1882, with a sore, gnawing pain in her left side, the pain being at times sharp and darting, and seated just under the ribs, in the region of the spleen : *worse* at night when she got warm in bed. Concomitantly herewith the left eye is involved : its *puncta lachrymalia* are very red. This is a comparatively simple case of disease, yet withal very painful, and patient came to me *to be cured*. I am sure as a "regular" this case would completely baffle anyone. Without a scientific law to guide you, you would not be able to tackle the case curatively at all. It offered no particular difficulty to me, and I cured it with an essence of the common European walnut! Fancy the walnut tree for such a case! We call it *Juglans regia,* and I gave five drops of the first centesimal dilution in water three times a day. Would you like to know the scientific "why" of this case? Only homoeopathy and the mundane doings of the late Clotar Muller can tell you.

Here again, you see how the law of similars gives executive potentiality to one's knowledge of drug physiology. (XI 17)

## 177. PAIN IN RIGHT HYPOCHONDRIUM

I have given a case of pain in the left hypochondrium cured by *Juglans regia;* not many weeks after that case was cured, as stated, a young lady came to consult me in regard to a very similar pain, but hers was of the *right* side, at the bottom of the right lung. She had had it for three months, and was pulled down by it a good deal, having become weak and anaemic.

*Chelidonium majus* 1, five drops in water night and morning, cured it specifically in just a fortnight.(XI 18)

## 178. HICCOUGH

In the early part of 1883, a young lady was brought to me suffering from a number of morbid symptoms, the most promising of which was

*Singultus* (hiccough). She would get it in attacks lasting about half an hour each, and of these there were generally four a day. In view of the concomitants — emansion of the menses, leucorrhoea, thirst, much saliva in the mouth — I considered that the hiccough was reflected from the uterus. You know something of the views I hold on vaccination and the theory of vaccinosis, which I have elsewhere sought to establish and defend. Well, I proceeded on these lines and gave *Thuja*, but it did no good. I followed with *Sepia*, which is a classic remedy with the homoeopaths for leucorrhoea, but it also did not help. What did I do ? I went to the law of homoeopathy and to the prophet Hahnemann ! Now my patient was *thirsty*; her *tongue was coated*; she had *nausea*; her *mouth filled with fluid*; she had *headache*; she *yawned* a good deal; she had *hiccough*; she complained of great *weakness*, and of *fatigue in all her limbs*; and altogether her symptoms were very much like those of *Cyclamen*, as given in Hahnemann's *Materia Medica Pura*, and THEREFORE if the old seer's notion of similitudes was worth anything, *Cyclamen* ought to cure my patient, and so it did. The third decimal nearly cured her, but not quite; and so I went down to the second decimal when the menses appeared. But the second decimal dilution did not seem to act so well as the previously used third, and hence I harked back to the third. Then, as the hiccough was *not quite* well, I went down to the first decimal, and then for the same reason shot up to the thirtieth centesimal, when no more remedies were needed for the hiccough! (XI 19)

## 179. DYSPEPSIA

A clergyman's wife of about 50 years of age consulted me on February 20, 1878, complaining of severe dyspepsia with other symptoms of *Natrum muriaticum*. My visit was a hurried one, so I did not enter very fully into the case. *Nat. mur.* 6 trit., vj grains in water twice a day was the prescription; it cured in three days these symptoms : "*Hiccough* occurring morning, noon and night *for at least ten years*, which was brought on by quinine; it was not a hiccough that made much noise, but 'shook the body to the ground'; it used to last about ten minutes, and was 'very distressing.'"

"How do you know that the hiccough was really produced by quinine?" I enquired. She answered; "At three separate times in my life I have taken quinine for tic of the right side of my face, and I got hiccough each time; the first and second time it gradually went off, but the third time it did not; when the late Dr. Hynde prescribed it I said, do not give me quinine as it always gives me hiccough, but he would give it to me; I took it, and it gave me the hiccough, which lasted until I took your powders; it is more than ten years ago since I took the quinine."

The cure of the hiccough has proved permanent.

This patient is a most truthful Christian woman, and her statement is beyond question.

She has been a homoeopath for many years, and my patient off and on for more than three years, during which time I have had to treat her for chronic sore throat, vertigo, palpitation, and at one time for great depression of spirits.

She had also previously mentioned her hiccough incidentally, but I had forgotten all about it, and on this occasion she did not even mention it; so far as the hiccough goes the cure was . . . a pure fluke! But it set me a-thinking about the Hahnemannian doctrine of drug dynamization for the thousandth time, and has seriously shaken my *disbelief* in it.

Hiccough is a known effect of *Chininum sulfuricum* : Allen's *Encyclopaedia*, Vol. III, p. 226, symptoms 370 and 379. (XI 19)

## 180. SORE THROAT, HEADACHES AND HICCOUGH

On March 29, 1887, a young lady of 10 years was brought to me, her mother complaining that she suffered from bloodlessness, languor, biliousness, sore throat, nausea, faintness, frontal headaches, matutinal lassitude, poor memory, sour breath, risings in the throat, *hiccough*, white and scant motions, pain in the left side on going up hill. I found an endocardial bruit, best heard at the base, and very notable enlargement of the spleen. Patient could not stand cold, had been only once vaccinated, had had varicella and measles.

I consider vaccination a disease, and I have ventured to call it *vaccinosis*, and have written a small book on the subject; however, I am not concerned with that theme here, but with the greater subject of homoeopathy, which leads to the same prescription as my theory of vaccinosis. *Thuja occidentalis* 30 in infrequent doses *cured the hiccough*, reduced the spleen by about one-half, oddly enough, the endocardial bruit also disappeared. The cure of the hiccough by *Thuja* is, however, the point I desire to call your attention to more particularly. Now note that I have offered you three cases of hiccough, one cured by *Cyclamen europaeum*, the second by *Natrum muriaticum*, and the last one by *Thuja occidentalis* : this diversity of remedial measures for a symptom such as hiccough exemplifies alike the spirit of homoeopathy and the immensity of its mastership over disease. Nevertheless, to an outsider who does not understand homoeopathy, this diversity of remedial measures constitutes a great stumbling block, and has prevented many able, conscientious investigators from understanding it, and yet this is *the strength* of the system, rendering, however, its practice disgustingly difficult. All nature is our pharmacopoeia — that is, for any homoeopath who has grasped the subject, and who has learned to walk without crutches, and who is WILLING TO WORK! And although I have thus narrated three cases of hiccough cured by as many different homoeopathic remedies, still if you were to ask me what remedy I would recommend you to try for hiccough, I should only be able to say, "*that* remedy (not necessarily either of my three) which can be proved to be pathogenetically like the to-be-cured case of hiccough." (XI 21)

## 181. APHONIA

A well-known soprano singer came to me with aphonia : the throat was what is commonly called follicular and congested. You may have heard that the homoeopaths think a good deal of *Arnica* for the ill effect of bruises, hurts, sprains, and the like; in fact, for trauma in general. Well, after using numerous remedies in vain, it slowly became manifest to me that the *aphonia* in question was from an overstrained state of the vocal chords. Moreover, patient had a small pustule on the nape, and mattery pimples on the skin.

*Arnica* cured the case, affording in its physiological action symptoms similar to it.

You will perhaps say that this *aphonia* case is also not a mortal malady. Will you once for all disabuse your mind of the very vulgar professional and popular error, according to which the homoeopaths are said to claim to cure the incurable! Just note, at least for *your own information*, that the homoeopaths make no such claim; what they say is this : Homoeopathy cures what can be cured *much better* than any other system of medicine hitherto made known to the world. The homoeopaths do *not* maintain that other systems are valueless, or that the homoeopathic system is faultless, only that thus far in the art-treatment of disease by remedies. Homoeopathy, by very long odds, beats all the records. Do you see ?

When I say that homoeopathy does not claim to cure the incurable, that leaves the queston of curability an open one; Homoeopathy does *not* accept anything as incurable because certain physicians who are "regular" declare it to be so. *Incapacity to cure does not render the uncured incurable.* Kindly take a mental note of this, because what "regulars" consider incurable may, or may not, be so considered by the homoeopaths. My old pleuritis trouble was declared and proved to be incurable by and for the entire faculty, and yet the *Bryonia alba* of the homoeopaths cured it ! (XI 23)

## 182. ERYSIPELAS

Some years since an eminent member of the Society of Friends wrote to me, stating that he had for a number of years been suffering from erysipelas of the face at odd intervals. I ordered him *Arnica* in a rather high dilution and in infrequent dose, and thereupon his erysipelas faded *and came no more.* Long afterwards he wrote me a very grateful letter, giving me much undue praise for having wit enough to see that the Almighty has His laws in therapeutics for the guidance of His poor, sick children.

I have it from you that *Arnica* causes erysipelas; I will not doubt *your* statement; you may now take it from me that *Arnica* cures erysipelas. *You* know the bad character of *Arnica* in that it is apt to *cause* erysipelas; I tell you of its good fame, viz. that it possesses the power of curing erysipelas, and the intellectual link that completes the little chain is the law of likes that God put into the mind of one Samuel to explain to the world. (XI 24)

## 183. QUINSY

I was summoned by telegraph to a very severe case of quinsy. I hastened to the suffering damsel, and found that various remedies had been used in vain, and the patient was in great distress, having been for twelve hours unable to swallow even a few drops of fluid. Not even the juice of one grape would pass, and some operative interference seemed absolutely imperative. I gave five grains of the third centesimal trituration of a remedy you may not be acquainted with, but which the heterodox homoeopaths quaintly call *Baryta carbonica,* and which is now generally known as the *Carbonate of barium.* In about a dozen hours patient ate a basin of bread and milk. I have often cured quinsies before in the same way and I beg you to believe that the little trick has been done thousands of times by others. (XI 25)

## 184. PAIN IN RIBS AND LEGS AFTER RECURRENT FEVER

John H., aged 29 years, seaman, came to me on April 21, 1878, telling me that he had had fever and ague two or three times a day, *with watery vomiting,* in Calcutta, in September, 1877. Was in the Calcutta Hospital three weeks for it, and took emetics, quinine, and tonic. Left at the end of the three weeks cured; but before he was out of port the ague returned, or he got another, and he had a five-month voyage home to the port of Liverpool. During the first three months of this homeward voyage he had two, three, four and five attacks a week, and took a good deal of a powder from the captain, which, from his description, was probably *Cinchona* bark; then the fever left him, and the following conditions supervened, viz. : "Pain in right side under the ribs; cannot lie on right side; both calves very painful to touch, they are hard and stiff; left leg semiflexed, he cannot stretch it. In this condition he was two months at sea and two weeks ashore and in this condition he comes to me hobbling with the aid of a stick, and in great pain from the moving.

Urine muddy and red; bowels regular; skin tawny; conjunctivae yellow. Drinks about three pints of beer daily. I recommended him not to alter his mode of life till he is cured, and then to drink less beer. The former part of the recommendation he followed, as I learned from his brother; of the latter part I have no information.

The hiccough case bears directly on this one, as we have evidently to do with an ague suppressed with *Cinchona*. Therefore ordered *Nat. mur.*, 6 trit., six grains in water every four hours.

April 27 — Pain in side and leg went away entirely in three days, and the water cleared at once; but the pain returned on the fourth day in the left calf only, which to-day is red, painful, swelled, and pits. He walks without a stick.

Continue medicine.

May 4 — Almost well; feels only a very little pain in left calf when walking. Looks and feels quite well, and walked into room with perfect ease without any stick.

He thinks he had a cold shake a few nights ago. He continues to perspire every night; ever since he got the ague the sheets have to be changed every night.

Continue medicine.

May 11 — Quite well.

I will here urge you to make a profound study of salt in all its bearings; but its being such a grand calorifacient in refracted dose, and during this deadlock of ague and cinchona, will surely entitle it to be considered a very good reason for being a homoeopath, since it cannot be so used on any other than homoeopathic ground. (XI 26)

### 185. FACIAL NEURALGIA

Not many years ago the daughter of a London alderman was suffering from fearful neuralgia of the face; at intervals she had had it for years, and no trouble or expense had been spared in endeavouring to cure it. Their ordinary family adviser was a homoeopath, but he had not managed to cure this neuralgia, notwithstanding several consultations with colleagues; and other men of eminence had been consulted, but to no avail.

I found that the pain was worse in cold weather; worse at the seaside; better away from the sea — inland, i.e., not so frequent or severe, and when the pain came on the eyes watered. A pinch of the sixth trituration of *Natrum muriaticum* in water three times a day cured my young patient in about three weeks. (XI 27)

## 186. COLD SHIVERING FITS

Some years since I was attending one of the children of a widow in the neighbourhood of London, and having made a pretty good therapeutic hit — *homoeopathically,* — she said she should like to consult me on her own account for her nerves; and when we had gone into that matter, she said, "Ah, I suppose it is no use to consult you about my cold shivering fits; no one can do them any good." They were in this wise; on going to bed at night she began to shudder and shiver, and on getting into bed and lying down, she would shiver to such a degree that her teeth chattered, and the movements of her body shook the bed. She had suffered this for years, and had been under a number of physicians for these cold shivers, but no one had ever touched them. She named five well-known homoeopathic practitioners who had in vain tried their hand at it; one of these has since renounced homoeopathy and all its ways, and previously he had tacitly given up the use of dynamized remedies, and loves now to ridicule them. Still for all that, and all that, dynamized *Natrum muriaticum* cured these cold shakes promptly and permanently Long afterwards this lady wrote that she kept a bottle of the medicine on her bedroom mantelpiece *au besoin,* or as we physicians so, neatly put it, *pro re nata,* but never needed it.

I call *Natrum muriaticum* my calorifacient. (XI 28)

## 187. NATRUM MUR. FOR AILMENTS NEAR SEA

A lady, wife of an officer, came over from India, to be under my care. The difficulty in her case lay in this, that she was to stop with her husband's friends, who have a lovely place near the sea, in Sussex, but it usually upset her so much that she could not stay there. "And you know," said she, "it is so very unfortunate for I can stay there for nothing, and have the use of a carriage, and everything is so very nice; and yet I am obliged to decline going there, and have to go to nasty lodgings by myself, which of course I have to pay for." Why can you not live at your husband's place? "Oh ! it is the sea; I am just the same on board ship, dreadfully ill."

Well, the burden of my song is just this — *Natrum muriaticum*, 6 trit., so modified this lady's state that she was not only able to stay at said place, but actually thereat enjoyed being and sitting by the sea. (XI 29)

## 188. HEADACHE

The young wife of a country squire came to me, at the beginning of the summer of 1887, with severe headache at the back, that had made her life sour for a good twelvemonth; she always woke with it; it was throbbing; and during the menses she also had a frontal headache. Left ovary a little swelled and tender. *Thuja occidentalis* in a rather high dilution and in infrequent dose cured her right off. She waited three months to see if the cure was real and then wrote me a grateful letter of thanks. (XI 30)

## 189. MENORRHAGIA OF FIFTEEN YEARS' STANDING

The lady was 51 years old, and so you may call it metrorrhagia if you so prefer, but there had been no break in the menses, which were still regular. She came to me in October, 1882, and told me of her trouble, and that it dated from a miscarriage fifteen years before. She had often flooded at her confinements. *Phosphorus* 200 cured her. She went much smaller in the waist, and told me she "felt like a young girl". She had other intercurrent remedies — *Lachesis*, *Ferrum*, *Thuja* and *Arnica*, but it was the *Phosphorus* that cured the haemorrhage, I having to return to it three separate times, with month between, and the last time I used *Phos.* 100th potency. (XI 31)

## 190. EXOSTOSIS OF RIGHT OS CALCIS

Dr. Carth Wilkinson went once to Iceland for a holiday, and observed that the animals which fed in the pastures where the finer ashes of Mount Hecla fall, suffered from immense maxillary and other exostoses. Being an adherent of the scientific system of medicine founded for us by Samuel Hahnemann, he brought some *Heclae lava* home with him, and it has been already successfully used to cure affections similar to those which it is capable of causing.

On July 3, 1880, a young lady, aged 15 years, came under my observation with an exostosis on her right os calcis, somewhat smaller and a little flatter than half a walnut-shell. It was at times painful. Patient was in other respects in good health and well nourished, but her teeth were not very sound. She goes blue in winter, and suffers also very badly from chilblains both on hands and feet, worse on hands.

$R_x$ Trit. 2 *Heclae Montis lavae,* 5 iv.

S — Six grains three times a day.

17th. The exostosis is decidedly smaller; it never pains now.

*Pergat.*

September 25. The exostosis has entirely disappeared; the two heels being compared, no difference between them can now be discovered. (XI 32)

## 191. CRANIAL EXOSTOSIS

The case was published long ago, and so I will not trouble you with details : suffice it to say, that the man who had the bony growth in his skull was completely and permanently cured by me with Metallic Gold in homoeopathic preparation. Nor is this a isolated case of the kind; the thing has been done oft before, any time during the last fifty years, and even before that. (XI 33)

## 192. COUGH (FOUR CASES)

**Case I.** I happened to read Jones's proving in Hale's *New Remedies* some six or seven years ago, and I was much struck with the character of the cough. I fancy the thing that helped to impress it upon my mind was the fact that I had had just at that period a lady under my care who was suffering from a cough that came on after lying down at night. I had been tinkering away at this cough, and could not cure it; so I blamed the damp house in which the lady resided, and its proximity to a brook prettily hidden among the willows close by. *Hyoscyamus, Digitalis,* and a number of other remedies came into play, but the cough would not budge a bit. Need I tell the heart-rending tale that the patient lost faith in her doctor (the writer) and in his much-vaunted pathy, and set about healing herself with quack medicines and orthodox sedative cough mixtures? Of course, I felt humiliated, and I therefore made up my mind to read my *Materia Medica* a little more diligently. It was quite evident that the cough was a curable one, for the most careful physical examination failed to detect anything besides a few moist rales that tallied with the moderate amount of expectoration.

Failures are very instructive at times.

Just after having received my congé from this lady, I was reading Hale's *New Remedies*, and came across Dr. S. A. Jones's proving of *Aralia racemosa*, where he says : "At 3 p.m. I took ten drops of the mother tincture in two ounces of water. An interesting book caused me to forget my 'dose'. The events of the night jogged my memory very effectually." He goes on to say that he retired to rest at midnight, feeling as well as ever, but he, "had no sooner lain down than he was seized with a fit of asthma".

I put down the book — Hale's *New Remedies* was not quite so thick then as it is now — and said to myself, "That's Mrs. N.'s cough, that is just how she goes. She lies down and forthwith begins to cough, to get laboured breathing, and to make her poor hard-toiling husband wish he were a bachelor" : at least he might have wished it, for ought I know to the contrary.

A little time elapsed, and the writer was sent for to see one of this coughing lady's children with eczema. The bairn's common integument having been prescribed for, I timidly inquired about the cough. "Oh," said Mrs. N., "it is as bad as ever; I have tried everything, and do not know what to do." I sat down and wrote :

$R_x$ Tc. *Aralia racemosa* 2, and it cured *citò, tutò, et jucunde* and that not because *Aralia* is good for coughs, and has an affinity for the respiratory organs merely, but because *it is capable of causing a cough like the one that was to be cured.*

Case II — *Tussis Araliae* — A lady came under my observation last summer. She resides in the West End of London, and had been under competent homoeopathic treatment for her throat, and had certainly derived benefit, but still her cough did not leave her, so that she was on the point of removing from London and going to the South, whereof she is a native, she and her friends having become apprehensive lest her chest should become affected. Her cough was not identical with Mrs. N.'s, but the only difference was that it *did not come on till after a first sleep* of not long duration. Patient would go to bed quite well (so did Mrs. N., and so did Dr. S. A. Jones) and lie down and go to sleep, and *after a short sleep,* would wake up with a severe fit of coughing that would last an hour or more.

*Aralia* 3 cured it entirely in a few days, and she gave up all idea of returning to the South.

Case III — *Tussis Araliae* — A child of not quite six gets croupy coughs in damp weather that usually yield to *Dulcamara*. Occasionally, however, there remains the kind of nocturnal cough described in Case II, viz. she will go to bed, lie down, fall off to sleep, and presently awake with a violent bout of coughing. Originally, before thinking of *Aralia,* I had in vain given *Hyoscyamus, Gelsemium, Aconitum, Spongia, Hepar, Dulcamara, Phosphorus,* and *Bryonia.* Then the early nocturnal character of the cough determined me to try *Aralia,* and with prompt effect. (XI 34)

Case IV — *Tussis Araliae* — An asthmatic gentleman of 50 years of age, with moderate **emphysema** of the lungs, has long been under my care. At first he was almost always short of breath on exertion, and had bad nocturnal attacks of dyspnoea and cough. A prolonged course of constitutional treatment has at last partially cured him, but when he catches a cold he gets an attack of bronchial catarrh with *early nocturnal cough.*

It would be tedious to give the treatment of his whole case, but it will suffice to say it consisted principally of antipsorics and hepatics.

One day this gentleman said he wished I could give him a medicine *for his cough,* to have by his bedside at night, because otherwise when he caught cold (as at this time) he would go to bed quite well, fall asleep, and presently awake with a violent fit of asthma that would last from one to two hours, more or less; then he would get up a little phlegm and go to sleep again.

I prescribed one-drop powders of *Aralia* 3x, *pro re nata.* The next time I had occasion to see this gentleman he exclaimed, "I thought those powders would have killed me. I took one as you directed, when my cough became much more violent than I had ever known it, but it soon ceased, and has never returned."

He keeps some of these powders by his bedside ever since, and on various occasions they have helped him, thus far unfailingiy. He has not had an aggravation since the first time of using them.

These cases are samples only, but they teach a useful lesson : to give more than these would be irksome.

It will be seen that *Aralia,* although a new remedy, is a comparatively old friend of mine, and I can confidently commend it for *early nocturnal cough* that *occurs either immediately on lying down,* or MORE COMMONLY *after a first fore-midnightly sleep.* (XI 35)

## 193. ANEURYSM

It may be about three years ago, or thereabouts, that it was my duty to give an opinion on the state of a gentleman of middle age, resident in London, and who was considered in a dying state. He had not much faith in any medical man, or in any pathy, and had for years wandered from one physician to another for his serious heart disease and frightful dyspepsia. The allopaths did him most good, he thought, on the whole, with their remedies, but the good effects did not last. The prescriptions showed that his state had been correctly diagnosed, and not badly treated from their standpoint. He received in turn cordials, iodides, antacids and tonics, but his disease — aneurysm of the aorta — got worse.

The homoeopaths had treated him symptomatically — and he had plenty of symptoms — and once or twice he really thought he was cured for a day or two, but then he became suddenly as bad as ever — his aneurysm evidently got larger.

When I first saw him he seemed almost moribund, and had received the last rites of the Church.

After going over his case well, and taking into account the state of his tissues and organs and the size of his aneurysm, so far as that could be determined, I gave as my opinion that he might slowly get better, and be eventually cured of his disease.

That gentleman has since married, and the aneurysm, though not yet quite gone, is slowly yielding to homoeopathic treatment, freely applied under diagnostic common sense.

The principal remedies were *Aurum met.*, *Chelidonium majus*, *Carduus*, *Ceanothus*, *Glandium quercus*, *Aconitum*, *Ferrrum*, *Cactus grand.*, and *Baryta muriatica*, the first-named and the four last being direcctly — specifically — curative. My knowledge of the use of *Barium* is due to Dr. Flint, and this is not the first or second time that Homoeopathy has cured aneurysm.

I saw my patient walking along the street a few days since with his wife, and I was quite struck with his healthy, ruddy appearance. The power of Homoeopathy over aneurysm gives my twenty-fifth reason for being a homoeopath — and that lands me just half-way with my fifty reasons. Have you thus far conceived any greater respect for Homoeopathy, or can you explain *all* my reasons away ? At least you are beginning to see that my statement at your uncle's house was not boastfulness, but a mere statement of fact. Pray understand that I am not in the least desirous of making you, or anybody else, a homoeopath; it makes no difference whatever to me. Nor does it make any difference to truth : truth will get on very well without any of you.

Nor do I anticipate any particular good from all this scribbling of my fifty reasons to you; I do it just to substantiate my own position, and slap the jeering ignorance of orthodoxy in the face. (XI 36)

## 194. DISEASE OF KIDNEY

It may be half a dozen years ago that an unusually beautiful, sweet girl, a good way in her twenties, residing in an important provincial town, was noticed to fade and get weak, with peculiar ill-defined throat symptoms, weakness in her back, rectal and uterine irritation, weakness and emaciation. People could not think what had come over her. She is one of those human highbreds who will not cave in, but, if duty calls, will go on till they drop : till then, existing on their "go" rather than on their physique.

In life they are commonly misunderstood, and because they can put on a spurt or clear a very high-fenced difficulty *au besoin*, the unknowing and non-observant think they are really strong, but are lazy or sham.

"Oh! she nursed her nieces for weeks and never had her clothes off, but did not seem to mind a bit, and now she would have you believe she is so delicate; she shams, it's all put on." But it is not put on at all : if you examine their heads you will find the animal sphere almost entirely absent.

Dr. R.M. Tuttle, speaking on this point, says :

"Some men can do with ease as much physical labour as would kill other men. The same is true of mental labour. A man like Gladstone can take on himself a course of work the mere attempting of which would effectually silence any one else. He is a man with a large, highly organized brain, but he possesses, besides, the well-balanced organs of animal life which are required to generate the energy that such brains can transmute into intellectual force. *To be able to do the full measure of work of a man, it is necessary to be a good animal.*"

The lady in question has the most exquisitely intellectual development, a wonderful arch of cerebrum, but no occipital power worth while.

Well, the patient had been through a domestic trial and had *bent*; some thought she had *broken*.

A good, kind, gentle allopathic physician, who was wont to attend the family, also attended her, and diagnosed Bright's disease of the kidneys. Said she to her mother : "I am truly sorry to have to tell you that Miss — has a disease of the kidneys that cannot be cured; you must take care of her; she must wear flannel all over, and avoid cold and damp; she may last with care a very long time, but you must not expect her to get well."

Much family council was held together, and the outlook being dark and hopeless, the young lady was brought to me.

Homoeopathy cured her in about eight months, and the young lady thereupon got married, and has now several bouncing children, and she herself continues in good health. Not a vestige of albumen has been in the urine for nearly five years. What cured her? *Mercurius vivus.* She took two doses a day for many months. I did not hit it right off, but tried two or three remedies at first without avail.

This is my twenty-sixth reason for being a homoeopath, and it alone were amply sufficient; and whether it be God's will that I die to-night, or live for another fifty years, I feel that while I do live I am in duty bound to fight the good fight of Homoeopathy with all the power I possess : were I to do less I should be afraid to die.

Young man, the responsibility of *not* being a homoeopath is very terrible. (XI 37)

## 195. POST-ORBITAL NEURALGIA OF TWENTY YEARS' STANDING

This case (which came under observation on January 9, 1882), is one of considerable interest on various accounts. Its subject, a lady of rank, over fifty years of age, had been in turns, and for many years, under almost all the leading oculists of London for this neuralgia of the eyes — i.e. terrible pain at the back of the eyes, coming on in paroxysms, and confining her to her room for many days together; some attacks would last for six weeks. Some of the neuralgic pain, however, remained at all times. Her eyes had been examined by almost every notable oculist in London, and no one could find anything wrong with them structurally, so it was unanimously agreed and declared to be *neuralgia of the fifth nerve.* Of course no end of tonics, anodynes, and alteratives had been used. The oculists sent her to the physicians, and these back again to the oculists. The late Dr. Quin and other leading homoeopaths had been tried, but "no one had ever touched it".

Latterly, and for years, she had tried nothing; whenever an attack came on, she would remain in her darkened bedroom, with her head tied up, bewailing her fate. To me she exclaimed, "My existence is one life-long crucifixion!"

I should have stated that the neuralgia was preceded and accompanied by influenza. In the aggregate these attacks of influenza and post-orbital neuralgia confined her to her room nearly half the year. In appearance she was healthy, well-nourished, rather too much *embonpoint,* and fairly vigorous. A friend of hers had been benefited by Homoeopathy in my hands, and she therefore came of me "in utter despair".

There are the simple facts of the case, though they look very like piling up the agony! Now for the remedy. The resources of allopathy had been exhausted, and, moreover, I have no confidence in them anyway : Homoeopathy — and good Homoeopathy, too, for the men tried knew their work — had also failed. Do-nothing, now much in vogue, had fared no better. I reasoned thus : This lady tells me she has been vaccinated five or six times, and being thus very much vaccinated, she may be just suffering from chronic vaccinosis, one chief symptom of which is a cephalalgia like hers, so I forthwith prescribed *Thuja* 30. It cured, and the cure has lasted till now. The neuralgia disappeared slowly; in about six weeks (February 14, 1882) I wrote in my case-book, "The eyes are well!"

As I have not heard from the patient for some time, I am just writing a note to her to know whether the neuralgia has thus far (December 30, 1882) returned. The reply I will add.

Of course, it does *not* follow that because *Thuja* cured this case of neuralgia of some twenty years' standing, that *therefore* the lady was suffering from *vaccinosis*; that *Thuja* DID CURE it is incontrovertible, and my vaccinosis hypothesis led me to prescribe it. More cannot be maintained. At least, the case must stand as a clinical triumph for *Thuja* 30 — this much is absolute.

In reply to my enquiry, I received the following :

"January 1st, 1883.

". . . I have been in very much stronger health ever since I crossed your threshold, and excepting one or two *attempts* at a return from the enemy, I have been quite free from suffering . . ."

This lady continues well of her post-orbital neuralgia at the time of going to press. After the disappearance of the neuralgia she had several other remedies from me for dyspeptic symptoms. (XI 39)

## 196. CHRONIC HEADACHE OF NINE YEARS' DURATION

Miss G — , aet. 19, came under my care on March 12, 1881, complaining of bad attacks of headache for the past nine years. She said it was as if the back of her head were in a vice, and then it would be frontal, and throbbing as if her head would burst. She was very pale, and her forehead looked shiny, and in places brown.

These "head attacks" occurred once or twice a week.

Tendency to constipation; menses regular; an old sty visible on left eyelid; poor appetite; dislikes flesh-meat; liver enlarged a little; had a series of boils in the fall of 1880.

Feet cold; used to have chilblains. For years cannot ride on an omnibus or in a cab, because of getting pale and sick, skin becomes rough in the wind; lips crack; gets fainty at times.

To have *Graphites* 30.

April 13 — Appetite and spirits better, but otherwise no change. Questioned as to the duration of the head attacks, she tells me the last but one continued for three weeks — the last, three days. Over the right eye there is a red, tender patch; *has two or three white-headed pustules* on her face.

Was vaccinated at three months, re-vaccinated at seven years, and again at fourteen. Had *small-pox about ten years ago.*

Thus here was a case that had had small-pox ten years ago, or thereabouts, for she could not quite fix the date, and had been vaccinated three times besides, once subsequent to the small-pox!

$R_x$ Tc. *Thuja occidentalis*, Ziv. 3x.

To take five drops in water twice a day.

May 13 — Much better; has only had one very slight headache lasting an hour or two; the frontal tender patch is no longer tender; no further faintness at all. Lips crack. The pustules on the face gone, and skin quite clear.

To have *Thuja* 12, one drop at bedtime.

June 17 — Was taken ill yesterday fortnight with soreness of stomach; fever; nausea and perspiration. Subsequently spots broke out like pimples — eight on the face, one each on the thumb and wrist, one on the foot, and two on the back; they filled with matter, were out five days, became yellow, and then died away. Her mother says the symptoms were just the same as when patient had the small-pox. Her headaches were well just before this bout came on.

July 1 — Continues well.

July 27 — The headaches have not returned.

February 24, 1882 — The cure holds good, for she has had no headache, and is otherwise well. She had subsequently some other remedies for the little tumour on her eyelid, and for a small exostosis on lower jaw, but she had received nothing but *Thuja* when the cephalalgia disappeared, and it was two or three weeks before the next medicine followed.

Some months after this date this young lady was brought by her mother merely to show me how well she was, and to take final leave of me; two years later I learned from her mother that she continued well, so the cure is permanent.

An interesting feature in this case is the curious attack which came on at the beginning of June. My reading of it is that it was really a proving of *Thuja*, or a general organismic reaction called forth by it; and this sent me often up to the thirtieth dilution in my subsequent use of *Thuja*, though I have occasionally found the third decimal dilution answer better than the thirtieth.

But this is not the point of my thesis, for this case was cured by the low dilution, and when the low dilutions cure, and cure promptly, even though not very agreeably, but well, it cannot be necessary to go up any higher, especially as one's faith is sufficiently on the stretch without it. (XI 41)

## 197. ENLARGED GLANDS. APEX-CATARRH

Master C —, aet. 11, came under my care on August 18th, 1881, complaining of a cough, worse at 7.30 p.m.; he also coughed by day and through the night, but it did not wake him. He perspired fearfully, worst on the head, and worse during the night. Over upper half of left lung one heard moist cracking *râles*. The cervical lymphatic glands at the top of the apex of left lung were indurated, and distinctly "feelable". He weighed 5 stone 4 lbs. The vaccination scars were on the left arm, and the glands over the apex of the right lung were not indurated. Induration of the lymphatics on the left side of the neck (the vaccination, being performed on that side) is the rule after vaccination, as anyone may observe for himself if he will take the trouble to examine a *healthy* child just before vaccination and any time thereafter. I say, *any time thereafter*, for the thing generally persists for a very long time, unless cured by medical art.

$R_x$ *Thuja* 30, *m. ii.* Sac. lac. q.s. Fiat pulv. Tales xxiv. One, three times a day.

August 27 — Is well of cough, but the sweats continue. To take no medicine.

September 6 — The most careful examination of chest reveals no *râle*; there is no cough; the sweats have quite ceased; the said cervical lymphatics cannot be found. The boy now weighs 5 stone 8 lbs., so that he has gained 4 lbs. in weight since he got the *Thuja*.

Discharged cured.

The boy had been at school, and was sent home to his parents by the school physician on account of his obstinate cough, and because his general symptoms excited alarm. To me it appeared to be the first stage of phthisis. That the boy should increase in weight at home just after returning from school is, of course, not necessarily due to the medicine; home life, too, would improve his nutrition generally, and would perhaps also account for the disappearance of the apex-catarrh, cough, and perspirations. But what is to account for the disappearance of the induration of the cervical glands? (XI 42)

## 198. ACNE OF FACE AND NOSE, AND NASAL DERMATITIS

A young lady, about twenty years of age, was brought by her mother to me on October 28, 1882. Patient had a very red, pimply nose, not like the red nose of the elderly bibber, or like that due to dyspepsia or to tight lacing, but the pimply, scaly, nasal dermatitis, which extended from the cutaneous covering of the nose to that of the cheeks, but appearing here more as facial acne. The nasal dermatitis was, roughly, in the form of a saddle. Of course, this state of things in an otherwise pretty girl of twenty was painfully and humiliatingly unpleasant to her and to her friends; in fact, it was likely to mar her future prospects very materially, more especially as it had already existed for six years, and was making no signs of departing. She also complained of obstinate constipation. The pimples of the nose and face used to get little white mattery heads.
$R_x$ *Thuja occidentalis* 30.
November 30 — Pimples of face decidedly better. Nose less red. Constipation no better.
$R_x$ *Thuja occidentalis* 100.
January 3, 1883 — The face is free! Her mother gratefully exclaims, "She is wonderfully better." I ask the young lady which powders did her *most good*; she says, *"The last"*. The skin of the nose is normal, but the constipation is no better, and for this she remains under treatment.
That *Thuja* cured this case is incontrovertible. (XI 43)

## 199. NEURALGIA OF RIGHT EYE

Mr. ____, a gentleman of position and means, about fifty years of age, came to consult me on June 28, 1882, for a neuralgia of the right eye. He complained of almost constant pain in right eye ever since Christmas 1881, i.e. just about six months. Had had neuralgia in head and shoulders in 1866, and so much morphia had been injected in his shoulders by a doctor in Scotland that it almost killed him : for seven or eight hours it was doubtful if he would recover.
Has a brown, eczematous, itchy (at night), eruption on both shins and between the toes. The neuralgia of right eye, and for which he comes to me, is bad both day and night, but rather worse at night. Mr. (now Sir William) Bowman had examined the eye and declared it to be neuralgia, the eye being normal. Mr. White Cooper had done the same.
On my enquiring when he was last vaccinated, he seemed completely frightened, and stammered out rapidly, "I should not like to be vaccinated again."
"Why?"

"I was very seedy the last time I was vaccinated; in fact, I felt awfully ill for about a month," and he again hurriedly protested that he would not like to be vaccinated again. The vaccination that had made him so ill was either in 1852 or 1853.

This seemed to me to be a case of vaccinal neuralgia, and therefore I ordered *Thuja* 30, in infrequent dose. This was on June 28th, 1882.

July 8th. — But very little pain after the first powder. To have the same medicine again.

The cure proved permanent, and is interesting as proof of the rapidity with which the *most like* remedy can cure a neuralgia. (XI 44)

## 200. DISEASED FINGER-NAILS

On December 22nd, 1882, a young lady of twenty-six came under my care for an ugly state of the nails of her fingers. Naturally, a lady of her age would not be indifferent to the state of her nails. These nails are indented rather deeply, and in addition to these indentations there are black patches on the under surface of the nails, reaching into the quick. Very slight leucorrhoea occasionally. She had chicken-pox as a child of eleven. On her shoulders there is an eruption of roundish patches, forming mattery heads. The black patches have existed these eighteen months.

I ordered *Thuja* 30 (one in six).

March 19, 1833 — Has continued the *Thuja* 30 for just about three months, with the result that within a fortnight from commencing with it the black patches under the nails began to disappear, and there is now no trace of them. (XI 44)

## 201. ACUTE OPHTHALMIA

On May 28, 1875. I was sent for to see a lady suffering from acute ophthalmia. She informed me that her friend Dr. Mahony, of Liverpool, had recommended her to try Homoeopathy when she should again require medical aid, and had also mentioned my name to her. She seemed rather ashamed of calling in the aid of a disciple of Hahnemann, and was very careful to lay all the blame upon Dr. Mahony : for, said she, I know nothing about it. My patient was in a darkened room, and hence I could not well see what manner of woman she was; but I soon learned she was the widow of an Indian officer, had spent many years in India, where she had had ophthalmia a great many times, and that she was in the habit of getting ophthalmia once or twice a year, or even oftener, ever since. It generally lasted several weeks, and then got better; no kind of treatment seemed to be of any avail. Did I think Homoeopathy would do her any good ? I replied that we would try it.

I made an attempt at examining the eye, by lifting up one of the laths of the Venetian blind to let in the light, and then everting the lid; but the photophobia and consequent blepharospasm were so great that I barely succeeded in recognizing that the right eye was a red, swelled mass, while the left one was only comparatively slightly affected; in fact, a case of ophthalmitis. A more minute examination was impossible, as the pain was so great that the patient screamed whenever any light was let into the eye. I took a mental note of the chief symptoms, notably of the fact that the inflammation was chiefly confined to the right eye, and went home and worked out the homoeopathic equation; I was specially anxious to make a hit, and so I spent about half an hour at the differential drug-diagnosis. The drug I decided upon was *Phosphorus*. Thus —

$R_x$ Tc. *Phos.* I*m*. xij. Sac. lac. q.s. Div. in p. aeq. xij.

S. — One in a little water every hour.

That would be *about* the one-hundredth part of a grain of *Phosphorus* at a dose, or rather less.

I called the next day, about eighteen hours therafter, and my patient opened the door herself, slightly screening her eyes with her hand, and quite able to bear a moderate amount of light. The inflammation was nearly gone; the next day it was quite gone.

Patient's amazement was great indeed; in all the twenty years of these ophthalmic attacks she had suffered much, and had had a number of doctors, including London oculists, to treat her, but to no purpose. And yet she had been treated *actively*, and there had been no lack of physic and leeches, and also no lack of medical skill; but there was lacking in their therapeutics the one thing needful . . . THE LAW OF SIMILARS.

How was it that I, with no very *special* knowledge of the eye or its diseases, and with only usual practical experience, could thus beat skilled specialists and men of thrice my experience ?

Was it, perhaps, greater skill, deeper insight into the disease, more careful investigation of the case ? By no means. . . . It was just the law of similars, patiently carried out in practice.

My dear allopathic *confrére*, WHY are you so very simple that you leave us homoeopaths with this enormous advantage over the *best* of you ? Any little homoeopathic David can overcome the greatest allopathic giant if he will only keep to his Materia Medica, *and the directions of Hahnemann*. And the good thing lies so near, and is so constantly thrown at you. If we homoeopaths were only to make a secret of our art, you would petition the Government to purchase it of us!

But *revenons à nos moutons*. My patient was naturally very grateful, and said, "If that is Homoeopathy, I wonder if it could cure my cataract?" On examining the eyes now with some care one could readily perceive that there were opacities behind the pupils, that of the right being the much more extensive. She then informed me that she had had cataract for some years, and was waiting for it to get ripe so as to undergo an operation. She had been to two London oculists about it, and they agreed both as to diagnosis and prognosis, and eventual operative treatment. She had waited a year and gone again to one of these eye surgeons, and been told that all was satisfactorily progressing, although but slowly; it was thought it might take another two years before an operation could be performed. Her vision was also getting gradually worse, and she could not see the parting in her hair at the looking-glass, or the names over the shops, or on the omnibuses in the street; could see better in the dusk than in broad daylight.

In answer to her question as to the curability of cataract with medicines, I said I had no personal experience whatever on the subject beyond one case, and I thought that from the nature of the complaint, one could hardly expect medicines to cure it, or even effect it at all. Still, some few homoeopaths had published such cases, and others had asserted that they sometimes did really succeed in curing cataract with homoeopathic treatment. I added that, inconceivable as it was to me, yet I had no right to question the veracity of these gentlemen, simply because they claimed to do what *seemed* impossible.

In fine, I agreed, at patient's special request, *to try to cure her cataract with medicines* given on homoeopathic lines !

I must confess that I smiled a little at my own temerity. But I consoled myself thus : What *harm* could it do to treat her while she was waiting to get blind. At the worst I should *not* prevent it !

So it was agreed she should report herself every month or so, and I would each time prescribe for her a course of treatment.

All this was there and then agreed to.

She took from May 29th to June 19th, 1875, *Calcarea carbonica* 30, and *Chelidonium* I, one pilule in alternation three times a day. Thus she had two doses of the *Calcarea* one day, and one the next, and conversely of *Chelidonium*.

There were indications for both remedies, though I cannot defend the alternation : I hope I alternate less frequently now.

Then followed *Asafaetida* 6, and *Digitalis purp.* 3.

Then *Phosphorus* 1, and subsequently *Sulphur* 30, and then *Calcarea* and *Chelidonium*.

Thus I continued ringing the changes on *Phosphorus, Sulphur, Chelidonium, Calcarea carbonica, Asafoetida,* and *Digitalis,* till the beginning of 1876. On February 17th, 1876, I prescribed *Gelseminum* 30 in pilules, one three times a day. This was continued for a month.

Then I gave the following course of drug treatment : *Silica* 30 for fourteen days; *Belladonna* 3 for fourteen days; *Sulphur* 30 three times a day for a week; and then *Phosphorus* 1 for a fortnight.

A month or so after this date — March 20, 1876 — I one morning heard some very loud talking in the hall, and my patient came rushing in and crying in quite an excited manner that she could almost see as well as ever. She explained that latterly she *seemed* able to discern objects and persons in the street much better than formerly, but she thought it must be fancy, but that morning she suddenly discovered that she could see the parting in her hair and she at once started to inform me of the face and, *en route*, she further tested her vision by reading the names over the shops which she previously could not see at all.

I ordered the same course of treatment again, and in another two months the lenticular (*or* capsular) opacities completely disappeared, and her vision became and remained excellent.

She had never any recurrence of the ophthalmia, and she remained about a year and a half in my neighbourhood in good health. She then went abroad again, and in her letters to her friends since, she makes no mention of her eyes or sight, and hence I fairly conclude that she continues well.

The patient's age is now about fifty or fifty-one.

I have detailed this case somewhat circumstantially, so that my conversion to a belief in the medicinal curability of cataract may appear to others as it does to me.

This case made a considerable stir in a small circle, and a certain number of cases of cataract have since come under my care in consequence, and the curative results I have obtained in their treatment are extremely encouraging.

And I may add that I published this in the year 1880, and since then I have partially or completely cured a number of cases of cataract with remedies, and this power I possess because I am priviledged to be a homoeopath. (XI 45)

## 202. CATARACT - 1

Mrs. V. — , aet. 66, came under my observation on May 20, 1884. She came through a friend whose cataract had been cured by me with medicines.

Mrs. V.'s history is this : In November, 1882, and in April, 1883, she had been operated upon for cataract of the right eye. Inflammation set in, and eye was lost. Now her left eye has cataract, the lens having a grey look, and her vision is much impaired; she wears spectacles, but can no longer sew or thread a needle with their aid. her father and his sister had cataract. patient's skin is scaly and pimply, more particularly that of the face.

$R_x$ Tc. *Sulph.* 30. ziv.

S — Five drops in water night and morning.

August 30 — Since last date I sent her a medicine, but omitted to note it. She thinks her sight clearer.

*Calc. carb.* 30.

October 29 — "I am thankful to say my sight keeps better, only I am nervous, and everything falling makes me jump."

*Thuja* 30.

December 2 — "I feel my sight improving."

*Causticum* 100.

January 1, 1885 — "I am thankful to tell you my sight is much better; I can now see wonderfully well to read and write with my spectacles on, and I can see very well to go about or do anything in the house without the spectacles."

Rep.

March 25 — "Cannot bear the light so well; the eye which is blinded waters very much."

*Psor.* 100.

April 28 — Bad cold.

*Puls.* Ix.

May 2 — On this day the patient paid me her second visit, and the note in my case-book runs, "The left lens is decidedly less milky; can see to thread a needle."

Rep.

July 2 — "My eye is not quite so clear."

*Silicea* 30.

August 27 — No change.

*Causticum* C.

October 3 — Better of self, and sees better.

4 Rep. (XI 49)

## 203. CATARACT WITH STIFF TONGUE

Mrs. — , aet. 81, came under observation at the end of the year 1880, suffering from cataract of both eyes, diagnosed by various physicians and specialists. Her vision was much impaired; reading had become impossible, and she could barely recognize a person in the street, or the pictures on the walls of my consulting room. Thinking the case hopeless, principally on account of her advanced age, I did not enter with my wonted minuteness into her case, but gave *Chelidonium* 1x, five drops in water night and morning, on pathological grounds.

February 2nd, 1881 — She came and said she felt more comfortable in her *mouth*, her tongue being less hard and stiff; vision the same. Thinking there might be yet a glimmer of hope for the venerable lady — at least that absolute blindness might possibly be averted — I went into her case with greater care. I found she had occasional diplopia, and things seemed farther off than they really were. But the thing that had long distressed her was this : *On awaking in the morning her tongue was as hard and stiff as a board*. That this should have any connection with the cataractous lenses was not apparent; still it was the *most constant*, *peculiar*, and *characteristic symptom*, and, moreover, a very distressing one. I turned up a Repertory, and finally decided on *Sulphur iodatum* (see Symptom 40 in Allen's *Encyclopaedia*). Considering the general character of the remedy, and the pathology of the disease, I did not hesitate, but gave six grains of the fourth centesimal trituration every night at bedtime.

March 21 — My report for this day in my case-book reads thus : — "Hardness and stiffness of tongue *gone*, and she had it two years; it was quite distressing; sees *decidedly* better at a distance."

She came by rail to town to see me, and a married daughter was in the habit of meeting her at the station. When she first came to me she was not able to recognize her daughter on the platform, but this morning she recognized her already at quite a distance, and that readily, and can as readily discern my pictures.

Rep.

July. — Vision much improved; can now read an article in the newspaper.

$R_x$ *Iodium* 30.

August — Receive word from the daughter that patient now sees so well that she does not propose continuing treatment any longer. She reads books with large print comfortably.

September 15 — A lady friend of the patient called abour her own condition, and remarked, "Mrs. — now reads the paper from an hour and a half to two hours every day."

She is now eighty-two years of age.

London, September, 1881. (XI 51)

## 204. CATARACT - 2

The lady came first to me in June 1884, being then fifty-eight years of age, and as clear-thinking, hard-headed a sceptic as ever you saw. The diagnosis was made by an eminent specialist, whose opinion you would not dream of doubting. You see he is so sweetly orthodox ! If he were to turn homoeopath, however, he would not (thereafter) know a lens from a broom-handle !

I looked humbly at the lenses — both of them — and found them uniformly milky-opaque; but as I am not an oculist, and besides, am so sorely heterodox, you will not care to know how the lady's lenses appeared to my optics; so just take it parenthetically as it were, that *to me* they were "kinder darkish like"; cataract our orthodox specialist calls it ! Well, I discharged her cured in July, 1887, and able to read *No.* I.

In case you should care to know what remedies this lady took, I subjoin a list, viz. *Urea* 6 and then 12, *Psorinum* C, *Calc. carb.* C, *Sulphur* Q, *Silicea* 30, *Thuja* C, *Calc. carb.* 30, *Causticum* C, *Silicea* C, *Caust.* 30, *Lapis alb.* 30, *Sulphur* 30, *Conium* 1, *Calc. fluor.* 30, *Graphites* 30, *Chelidonium* Q, *Hepar* 3, etc. etc. The reason for giving them I cannot explain here, but the patient's lenses are now so clear that she sees to thread needles. (XI 52)

## 205. ACUTE MANIA

It is more than a dozen years ago that I, in the North, attended a very wealthy lady, about seventy years of age, for acute mania. The friends had, under the advice of the local practitioner, decided to send her to an asylum, but I objected to that course, being very sure she would never come out again. I have had charge of an asylum myself, and *know well* that, therapeutically, anyone that goes to an asylum is lost. They are treated with great kindness, and kept from harm amd mischief, but as to curing them — well, the "mad doctors" never even try ! and, indeed, it is useless to treat the demented allopathically. But good genuine Homoeopathy would cure half the inmates of our asylums. You will question my statement, I dare say, but it is the bare simple truth all the same. It has been well and learnedly argued in theory and often proved in practice, as you may find for yourself if you will refer to our heretorelative literature.

Homoeopathic (and other!) practitioners are often hoodwinked by the personal surroundings of a patient, and to be pitchforked into a nest of unbelievers to cure a desperate case is verily no pleasant position to be in, as any physician of the homoeopathic ilk knows but too well.

Now, my patient had a lady companion who casts a withering glance at my humble self, and I knew instantly that *she* would baulk me in my efforts to cure, unless I prevented it. So I informed her that either she or I must go, or she must solemnly promise to obey all my orders with regard to the patient, "for," said I, "you do not believe in Homoeopathy, do you ?" "No indeed, I do not !" And that young lady's look of scorn and contempt !

Thanks to *Baptisia* and other common homoeopathic remedies my patient made a complete recovery, and never had a relapse. (XI 54)

## 206. WINDY DYSPEPSIA

The weather is bad to-day, so I am not busy in my chambers; sick people cannot get out in this dreadful weather, and that gives consulting physicians a little time to ruminate. However, a gentleman of seventy-five whom I have just converted to Homoeopathy, was here just now. He came to me last August, and what fixed my attention was his striking resemblance to the late Lord Cairns, who, by the way, was a homoeopath, as was also Archbishop Whately, *the logic Man*. Fancy the great logician a homoeopath !

Well, my patient had been to many eminent physicians in this London of ours for what he called "windy dyspepsia". He is in great and almost constant pain, full of foul flatus, constant diarrhoea, often involuntary, which is a terrible distress to him.

He was greatly improved in a few months, and the remedies which did it were *Arsenicum* 5, *Nux vomica* 5, *Sulphur* 5, *Lycopodium* 12, and *Colocynthis* 3x.

Said the old gentleman, somewhat sententiously, "These medicines seem to suit me." (XI 56)

## 207. WARTY GROWTH IN MOUTH

An officer in the army brought his twelve-year old daughter to me on November 13, 1886, telling me that she had something growing in her mouth. A similar growth had come a year ago, when his family surgeon excised it; in six months from the time of the operation it had grown again, making it difficult for the child to eat her food, as it caught the tongue and teeth, and then bled. This time the doctor ligatured if off thoroughly, leaving a hole, and informed the father that this time he hoped its roots were got rid of. Now it has grown again at the side of the

said hole. On examining the mouth I find in its left side, just to the left of the fraenulum linguae, a warty fleshy excrescence, of the shape of a cock's comb, about a quarter or an inch broad at its base, and nearly a quarter of an inch high. Patient has normal teeth; the tongue is coated and she is very pale. I ordered *Thuja occidentalis* 30 internally, in infrequent dose, and a mouth wash of *Thuja* Q, two drops in a dessertspoonful of water night and morning; to keep it bathing the growth as long as possible, and then expectorate.
As this brought the growth down to the size of a pea, treatment was discontinued, but she then bit it on three successive occasions, whereupon it again took to growing, and on January 1887, when I saw it, it was about as big as a horse-bean. This time I ordered *Sabina*, just as I had previously ordered *Thuja*. Under the *Sabina* patient took on a healthy look, but a small piece of the growth still persisted, when I ordered *Cupressus lawsoniana* in like manner as the *Thuja* and *Sabina* had been used. That was in March 1887, and I did not see her again. But I met her father in October on another matter, when I enquired about the case, and he replied, "Oh, she is quite well; the lump has been gone a long time, but the hole is still there." (XI 56)

## 208. NEURALGIA

A lady of sixty, of the *Vielle noblesse catholique anglaise*, came to me in December, 1886, sent by her daughter, whom I had cured of neuralgia. The daughter had neuralgia of right side of head very badly, that she thought originally came from a *coup de vent*. She spent the winter of 1885-86 in Nice, and one day sat next to a gentleman at the *table d'hote*; they compared notes about their state of being, when it transpired that the gentleman had previously suffered from the very same sort of neuralgia, and in the identical spot, and that for many years until he came to me, when I (thanks to Homoeopathy) cured him.
The lady was forty years of age, and came to me in April 1886; the pain was in the right side of brow, face, ear and neck, and had been on ever since the preceding November.
*Thuja occidentalis* in a rather high dilution and infrequent doses cured the neuralgia in a few weeks, and the lady in question has thought this brilliant cure of her neuralgia of itself sufficient for becoming a homoeopath. (XI 57)

## 209. DEAFNESS

Having begun in my last communication to give you a case of deafness, I fell back on a case of neuralgia that had been suggested by it, and so that leaves the deaf lady to do duty now. Well, she came in December, 1886, because I had cured said neuralgia.

"You cured my daughter's neuralgia, so perhaps you can cure my deafness."

It was a case of long standing that had been under the best aurists, and they had syringed it and done their poor little best, giving temporary ease, but not touching the essence of the complaint, which was due to chronic inflammation and swelling of the walls of the external meatus on both sides.

In five months the lady was quite cured, and the remedies were *Thuja*, *Psorinum*, *Sabina*, and *Ceanothus*, and one other.

This lady has also become a homoeopath, and now employs for her family the homoeopathic practitioner living near her house. (XI 58)

## 210. ENCHONDROMA INDICIS CURED BY CALCAREA FLUORICA ALONE

A maiden lady of sixty came to consult me on October 13, 1883, telling me she had a shiny swelling on her left index finger, which had been there for about eighteen months. The lump was hard and painful, and of about the size of a small split walnut, but rather flatter. Patient was very nervous and depressed.

$R_x$ trit. 3x *Calcarea fluorica*. Six grains four times a day, dry on the tongue.

October 27 — Very great improvement.

$R_x$ Rep.

November 3 — The cartilaginous nature is now clearly to be felt.

$R_x$ Rep.

10 — The swelling continues to get softer.

$R_x$ Rep. (dry on the tongue).

17 — Still progressing; softer and smaller; on its middle finger side it has taken on inflammatory action, as if it were going to gather, being hot, red, and more swelled.

$R_x$ Rep.

24 — The tumour is softer and smaller, and patient is beginning to bend her finger, which had previously become quite impossible.

$R_x$ Rep.

December 1 — Still improving.

$R_x$ Rep.

15 — Finger is much more normal in colour, and still progressing. Patient went on with the same remedy until a short way into the new year. I saw her the last time on December 29th, when she was nearly well.

If I remember rightly Grauvogl was the first to use and to recommend the fluoride of lime for enchondroma.

The interest of this case lies not so much in the importance of the tumour (it was only the size of half a walnut, or thereabouts), but rather in the fact that only one remedy was used, and no other, and no change was made either in diet or place of abode. The lady had a hard lump on her finger for eighteen months; she took a course of *Calc. fl.*, to the choice of which Homoeopathy led me, and the lump went away. — Q.E.D. (XI 59)

## 211. PAIN IN BREAST AFTER TRAUMA CURED BY BELLIS

Miss L.C., aged thirteen years, came under my observation at the end of July, 1879. About eight weeks previously a miserable lad in the street hit her on the right breast with considerable violence; from that time on, this breast became swollen and very painful, until at length she was quite unable to lie on her right side. Patient's mother was *poitrinaire,* as was also her brother, and my experience teaches me that the members of *poitrinaire* families are particularly liable to suffer from blows

At first no notice was taken of the young lady's complaints, but week after week went by, and she persisted in referring to the pain, in her breast. Whether any domestic means had been employed I do not now remember, but eventually I was sent for, as vague notions of tumour and cancer rendered the parents uneasy. On comparing the breasts, the right one was found to be by much the larger, being swollen and very tender.

I thought this a very proper case for testing the antitraumatic virtue of the old English bruisewort, and hence prescribed thus :

$R_x$ Tc. *Bellis perennis* 3x. ziv.

S — Three drops to be taken in water four times a day. The result was a very rapid disappearance of pain and swelling, and in a fortnight patient could lie again on the right side. And a few days later an examination showed that the swelling had entirely disappeared.

Nothing whatever was applied to the part, no change was made in diet, mode of life, or place of abode, and as the thing had already existed for eight weeks, the positively curative effect of the *Bellis* can hardly be denied, which is the one point this case is meant to exemplify and to teach, and that because it is so very difficult to demonstrate positively the effect of any *one* remedy when the tumefaction has become a genuine neoplasia, or hyperplasia. In this case, there was, of course, no hyperplasia. Too many of my cases prove this. (XI 62)

## 212. TUMOUR IN THE THROAT

A married lady of fifty-four came on August 8, 1883, to consult me about a lump in her throat. In the left side of the top of the neck there was a hard body about the size of a hen's egg, but flatter. The tumour had been there for a very long time, and with it she had had much throat irritation. it was situated to the left and behind the larynx, but whether actually connected with the oesophagus or larynx, I could never quite satisfy myself. It moved up and down with the act of deglutition.

$R_x$ Trit. 3x. *Sul. iod.*, ziv., gr. vj. ter die.

August 22 — No change.

$R_x$ *Psor.* 30.

October 5 — The throat — i.e., the fullness, uneasiness, pain and distress in the throat — is very much better, and the tumour has sensibly diminished in size.

$R_x$ *Thuja occid.* 30.

November 1 — The tumour is about half gone.

$R_x$ *Psor.* 30.

29 — The tumour about two-thirds gone : general health good.

$R_x$ *Thuja* 30.

December 21 — There is some tickling in the throat. The tumour is larger again, and the patient feels choky.

$R_x$ *Psor.* 30.

January 14, 1884 — The tumour has again sensibly diminished in size.

$R_x$ *Psor.* C.

February 8 — Tumour still swollen.

$R_x$ *Merc.* viv. 5.

March 3 — "I feel the lump very much less, about half its original size," said the lady. She has much rheumatism in ankles and knees.

$R_x$ *Silicea,* 6 trit., in frequently repeated doses.

31 — Has been visiting a friend suffering from consumption, and since then has spit a little blood-streaked phlegm; has a good deal of tickling in the throat.

$R_x$ *Psor.* 30.

April 16 — No coloured expectoration for a week, and then very trifling; the tickling in the throat is better, but the throat feels very rough. The tumour is rather smaller.

$R_x$ *Sul. iod.* 3x. Six grains three times a day.

30 — No coloured expectoration for the past week; the tickling in the throat is very much better, but talking brings it on. The tumour has lately not altered sensibly in size, but it is more self-contained,

and one can now demonstrate that it is not connected with the larynx, being in the areolar tissue behind and to its left. Has a good deal of rheumatism.

$R_x$ Tc. *Condurango* 1, ziv. Five drops in water three times a day.

May 21 — Thinks it is not so well; tickling sensation in the throat is worse. Feels the spring. The throat is worse in the morning and when tired.

$R_x$ *Thuja* 30.

June 10 — Throat rather better; has only had the coloured expectoration once, but the voice is hoarse, and she feels her throat weak. Has rheumatism in ankles and knees, worse after motion. The tumour is a trifle smaller.

$R_x$ *Urea* 6.

June 11 — More blood-coloured expectoration. Has had all the symptoms of a cold; aching all over with tingling, and feeling giddy and ill; aphonia; much tenderness in the neck; rheumatism better; urine thick (unusual); violent tickling in the throat with scraping and dryness; *the tumour is nearly gone.*

The throat symptoms are worse night and morning, and when she is tired.

$R_x$ Tc. *Phytolacca decandra* I, ziv., gtt. v., n. m.

August 6 — Better in every way; the tumour is barely to be found.

$R_x$ Rep.

September 3 — Feels practically well. I can find the small remains of the tumour only with great difficulty.

$R_x$ Rep. (at night only).

November 13 — Still a little uneasiness in the throat.

$R_x$ Trit. 2x *Sul. iod.*

28 — Nearly well.

R Rep.

December 31 — The tumour cannot be found, but she still complains of a husky voice.

$R_x$ *Tril.* 4 *Kali brom.*

I did not see the patient again for some months, as the tumour had quite disappeared, and she herself felt quite well, but she came to me again on.

April 10, 1885 — Complaining of tickling and irritation at the old spot.

$R_x$ *Psor.* C.

May 11 — She feels easier in the throat, but the tumour is returning.

$R_x$ Trit. 3x *Sul. iod.*

November 25 — The lump is still increasing.

$R_x$ *Psor.* C.

This lady came again on February 15, 1886, and for the last time on April 30, 1886, when I discharged her cured. I see her son occasionally on his own account, and thus know that she continues quite well, and has a very healthy general appearance.*

Confess candidly, do you not wish Homoeopathy were socially *tres comme il faut*, and to be had for the asking ? A lady of high rank said to me three years ago. "If you were *not* a homoeopath, Dr. Burnett, I could make your fortune." Said I, "Well, my lady, I am very sorry not to enlist you in the laudable undertaking of making my fortune, which would be at least very nice for those dependent upon me; but I *am* a homoeopath, and fortune or no fortune, I thank God for this much of His truth."

It is late and I am tired, but I trust you will be able to read my cacography. (XI 63)

* 1896 — No return of the tumour, and patient continues quite well of herself.

## 213. TUMOUR OF RIGHT BREAST IN A MAN*

Although tumours of the breast are much more common in women than in men, still they do also occur in the breasts of males, more particularly in later life. Such a one is the following :

On April 23, 1881, there came to me a rather tall, spare, cachetic-looking gentleman, a London professional man, of about seventy years of age, telling me that ever since the previous February he had been greatly worried, and this was followed by a sensitiveness in his left nipple, which soon passed off and went to the right nipple, wherein it still was. On examining the part I found it the seat of a hard, tumid mass of the size of a pigeon's egg. Patient first noticed it was swelled a month previously. It is not actually painful, but there is a sensation of fullness and uneasiness, and he cannot lie on it, hence it arrests his attention.

$R_x$ *Psor.* 30, m. vi., s. I. q. s., ft. pulv., tales xij., j nocte.

May 7 — There is still a sensation of fullness in it; patient thinks it is softer, in which opinion I share. It is a little smaller. Since taking the powders he has had some bilious attacks.

$R_x$ Rep.

May 21 — It is much smaller; there is much less sensitiveness, and patient can now sleep lying on his right side, which was previously not possible.

$R_x$ Rep.

May 28 — The sensitiveness is now confined to the nipple alone, still he can sleep lying on it. He is constipated, and his tongue is thickly furred.

$R_x$ *Hydrastis canadensis* 3x, ℥iv.
S — Gtt. v., nocte maneque.
June 14 — The sensitiveness still continues, but it has very much decreased.
Rep.
July 2 — Less sensitiveness; tumour still decreasing in size; on the sternum, on a level with the nipple, there is a scabby eruption of the size of a three penny piece, having a red ground, the rest being yellowish. He is still constipated.
$R_x$ Tc. *Hydrastis canad.* 6, ℥iv., gtt. v., n. m.
July 23 — He has scabs on the scalp; a yellow scab at the middle of the sternum; also on his hands. The nipple is no longer sensitive at all.
$R_x$ Tc. *Thuja occid.* 30, in infrequent doses.
August 13 — The tumour has disappeared, with the exception of one of the size of a hazel nut. There is still some scaly eruption on the sternum.
*Psor.* 30 (two to a month).
September 16 — No trace of the tumour to be found. There is still a patch of reddish scaly eruption on the skin of the chest.
$R_x$ Tc. *Chelidon. maj.* 3x. gtt. iij., nocte.
October 13 — No trace of tumour; still a circular patch at mid-sternum. Bowels a little relaxed.
$R_x$ Trit. 6, *Nat. sul.*
October 27 — Well; and has a healthy complexion, whereas it was, at the beginning of the treatment, quite earthy.
Six years have elapsed since then, during all which time the patient has remained well of the tumour — i.e. it has never returned. Two or three times or more in every year the gentleman is in the habit of coming to see me, "To be kept in repair." Before I began the treatment I was importuned by his friends as to whether I was *quite* sure it was safe to forgo an operation, "which you know, Sir J. — says is the only *chance* !"
(XI 66)

* So rare are such cases that I have never seen but three such.

## 214. ANGINA, DEPRESSION

One can hardly have to deal with a more formidable affection than *Angina pectoris*, and in its treatment Homoeopathy can do great things. It is, however, a mighty mistake to treat the cases all alike, as quite a number of different diseases give rise to the usual anginal symptoms; the cases must be diagnostically and therapeutically differentiated if they are to be really *cured*.

A short time since it was my duty to see a lady in Belgravia with *Angina pectoris*; unwonted domestic drudgery, loss of loved ones, fright, loss of fortune, had led up to it.

Apart from the anginal attacks there was a chronic, constant pain across the praecordia, running away under the left breast. For years blisters had been applied at intervals with temporary relief, till they could no longer be borne. Patient was very depressed, sulky, and morose; the menses suppressed. *Aurum metallicum*, 3 trituration, 6 grains every four hours, cured the constant pain in a week, and the anginal attacks have thus far not recurred, and patient smiles now and is bright. The menses have, however, not appeared, and for this she remains under treatment. (XI 68)

## 215. DROPSY LOWER LIMB WITH DEPRESSION

The following is a case of dropsy of the lower extremities which came under my observation two years ago.

I was fetched, I think it was one Sunday, to see a lady; it was feared she was beyond recovery. I found my patient, a lady of about fifty, in bed; her lower extremities were swollen, painful; they pitted on pressure, and were worse at night, better in the morning. This oedema had been coming on for a week or two, but it had usually quite disappeared by the morning, and thus caused but very little anxiety, but now it had greatly increased even in bed, and very naturally was causing great alarm. Dropsy is almost always a grave symptom, though not always. In this case I think it was. There was a history of many illnesses, and altogether this drug-picture presented itself :

1. There was dropsy, and patient had —
2. Great depression of spirits, amounting to —
3. Profound melancholia.
4. Then there was great difficulty of breathing.
5. Weak pulse and feeble heart.
6. She was psoric, and had a good deal of —
7. Discharge from the nose, that at times contained some blood.

I gave her the *Muriate of gold* in the third decimal dilution, but I do not remember the exact number of drops or the repetition of the dose, but the dose was not less than one drop (it may have been two or three); and as often as every two or three hours, and given in water.

The case got rapidly well, all the oedema having permanently disappeared in less than a week. Eighteen months after this she informed me she had never since had any return of the dropsy, though her health was anything but good. This was only a recent case, and though grave, was yet not severe as to the dropsy, but the despondency was almost a substantive malady.

In this case Gold acted as a veritable pick-me-up, and I submit that the remedy was homoeopathically indicated, and the cure a homoeopathic one; about the dose I will not quibble; with me the best dose is the one that cures.

This happened just ten years ago, and the lady is still alive and fairly well. (XI 69)

## 216. RHEUMATIC ENDOCARDITIS IN THE COURSE OF RHEUMATIC FEVER

I was fetched one day in February by a gentleman in the city to see his wife, a lady of about fifty-five or sixty, who was lying very dangerously ill at the end of the third week of rheumatic fever. This gentleman, who is an old homoeopath of thirty years' standing, and whose knowledge of drugs and disease is really remarkable for a layman, had treated the patient himself, and with no inconsiderable success considering the severity of the case, but suddenly patient's condition became very alarming on account of the rheumatism having apparently seized upon the heart. I found this condition : patient was propped up in bed and breathing very hurriedly; the lips bluish; tongue dry and coated; anxious expression of face; puffy under eyes; moist bubbling small rales all over chest, with cough; pulse rapid, compressible, and intermittent; action of heart floundering; loud endocardial bruits; slight dropsy of feet; no appetite at all, could just suck a grape or sip tea; profuse perspirations; limbs swelled and painful, the joints almost as firmly locked as if anchylosed; cannot move hand or foot for pain and from this swelled, inflamed state of the joints; flesh of hands puffy; bones of hand swelled, almost immovable, and tender.

I ordered *Aurum foliatum* (pure gold), 2nd trituration, very frequently. Alone and no auxiliaries.

Why did I order *Aurum* ? Because it affects the heart and respiration very much like they were affected in this patient, and because it, moreover, produces profuse perspiration, profound weakness, anorexia, and great anxiety. Then the bones were greatly affected.

February 18 — A little easier, Rep.

19 — Better in all respects. Rep.

20 — Considerable improvement in the action of the heart; breathing comfortable; is out of danger. Rep.

22 — Continued improvement. Rep.

24 — Quite comfortable. Continue with *Aurum* and take *Nat. sul.* 6th trit., in alternation with it. My reason for alternating was that I thought it imprudent to leave off the Gold, and yet *Nat. sul.* was now indicated.
March 2 — Is up sitting by fire. Appetite good.
6 — Heart, joints, bones, and hands free from rheumatism; is sitting by fire quite comfortably; appetite good; tongue moist but slightly furred; feet swell a little towards evening.
This case so well illustrates the action of Gold on the organic tissue of the heart.
When I saw the patient first I gave a bad prognosis, and had it not been for the Gold I fear it would have been realized. Auxiliaries did not do it, for I used none; faith in the doctor did not cure her, for the patient had never seen me before.
Patient's recovery was complete. (XI 70)

## 217. ANGINA PECTORIS FROM SUPPRESSED SKIN DISEASE

One Sunday morning, some ten years ago, a gentleman ushered his wife into my consulting room because she had been taken with an attack of *Angina pectoris* in the street, on her way to church. Though only a little over thirty years of age, if so much, she had been subject to these attacks of breast-pang for several years; they would take her suddenly in the street nailing her, as it were, to the spot, and hence she no longer went out of doors alone, lest she should faint away or fall down dead, as was apprehended.
An examination of the heart revealed no organic lesion, or even functional derangement, and I could not quite see why a comparatively young lady should get such anginal attacks. She had been under able men for her *angina,* but it got no better, and no one could apparently understand it. I prescribed for her, and saw her subsequently at her home, to try and elucidate the matter. I let her tell me her whole health-history from her earliest childhood. She said she was getting to the end of her "teens, and was preparing to come out, but she had some cracks in the bends of her arms that were very unsightly; these cracks had troubled her from her earliest childhood. Erasmus Wilson was consulted; he gave her an ointment which very soon cured her skin, and the patient came out socially, made a hit right off, and got married in due course. She had always been very grateful to Erasmus Wilson for curing her arms, for otherwise, "How could I have appeared in short sleeves ?"
But there soon followed dyspepsia, flatulence, dyspnoea, and palpitation, and finally the before-described attacks of *angina pectoris* threatened to wreck her life. Moreover, she had borne one dead child. As I

have already said, there was no discoverable cardiac lesion, and from the lady's health-history I gathered that this cure of her skin (though to me the one important point) was to her of no causal importance.

I gave my opinion that her skin disease had never been *really* cured, only *driven* in by Wilson's ointment, and that her angina was in reality its internal expression or metastasis. No one believed it, however. I began to treat her antipsorically, and very soon — I think it was less than a month from the Sunday morning visit — the old cracks reappeared in the bends of the elbows, *and from that time on she had no further attacks of angina at all*, and thenceforth she bore living children. (XI 71)

## FEVERS AND BLOOD-POISONING

### 218. FEVER

**Case I.** Miss C. M. A., aet. twelve years and eleven months, was taken ill in February 1885 at her parents' seat in Sussex — one of the healthiest spots in the country. On the right of *Monday the 16th* she had a headache; felt hot and sick, and could not sleep.

On *Tuesday the 17th* she went to London for the day; felt sick, cold, and hysterical on her homeward journey; was very sick on reaching home; had headache; was restless, and talked a good deal in her sleep. Her mother gave her *Pulsatilla.*

On *Wednesday the 18th* she stayed in bed to breakfast; she was feverish, disinclined for food, and hysterical; complained of pain in her abdomen; all her bones ached; her legs felt as if she could not move them. Her mother gave her *Aconite* and *Chelidonium* in alternation.

On *Thursday the 19th* she was much the same as on the preceding day; she cried a good deal; fancied she saw mice and people about in her bedroom; tongue thickly coated; cannot bear any talking, noise, or light. Her mother continued with the *Aconite,* but substituted *Merc. sol.* for the *Chelidonium.*

On *Friday the 20th* I find this note recorded : Did not sleep last night for more than half an hour at a time; muttered and talked and tossed about in her sleep; complains of headache; pains in her back, arms, and jaws; she dozes for a few minutes and then awakes wandering in her mind; will partake of nothing but water and a little milk.

| *P.M.* | *Temperature* |
|---|---|
| 6 | 103.2 |
| 8.45 | 104 |
| 11 | 103.4 |

With an *Aconite-resisting* temperature of 103° to 104° the child's mother — a clever, capable, and altogether a remarkable woman — knew that danger was ahead. She knew well, from practical life-experience, that when *Aconite* fails to bring down the fever, you must prepare for the enemy of pyrexia properly so-called, or for a more or less sericus something. Accordingly the local allopathic medical man was called in, and he very carefully examined the patient, but found nothing but a spot on the left tonsil. The temperature he found to be 103.4° and the pulse 132. In the absence of pain or distinct feature beyond the pyrexia, he gave as his opinion that it was an attack of herpes, of which he had had some cases in the neighbourhood, and in that *Aconite* and *Baptisia* had done no good, and after a due examination of the patient, it was very clear that we had to do with a case of gastric fever of the gravest kind.

Had Rademacher or Kissel, Guttceit or Rapp been living and practising in the neighbourhood, I think it likely highly probable, that they would have known the right remedy corresponding to the epidemic genius of the disease. But I had no means of knowing what that genius was, or its corresponding remedy; and with a nearly constant temperature rising to almost 105 degrees Fahrenheit, there was no time to be lost, the less so as the temperature had been slowly and steadily rising for days.

Beginning at 9 P.M. on Saturday the 21st, five drops of *Pyrogenium* 6 was given every two hours.

Diet ordered was : beef-tea, chicken-tea, water, juice of apples, and grapes. Also cold water compress to abdomen, to be renewed every four hours.

In view of the very great importance of the question under consideration, viz., the efficacy or non-efficacy of this powerful agent in true typhoid — in the treatment of which all therapeutists to date have had to sing so small — I propose to give the day-book kept at the time in the sick-room verbatim.

***Sunday, 22nd.***

| | |
|---|---|
| 1 A.M. | Medicine (*Pyrogen* 6). |
| 2 A.M. | T. 104° |
| | Slept. |
| 4 A.M. | Medicine. |
| 6 A.M. | Medicine. |
| 8 A.M. | T. 103.6°; beef-tea, 1• oz. |
| 8.40 A.M. | Medicine. |
| 10.40 A.M. | Medicine. |
| 11.10 A.M. | Apple water. |

| | |
|---|---|
| 12 A.M. | T. 104.4°; beef-tea. |
| 12.40 P.M. | Medicine. |
| 1.25 P.M. | T. 104°; sponged; apple water. |
| 1.50 P.M. | Chicken-tea, 1• oz. |
| 2.35 P.M. | Medicine; compress. |
| 3 P.M. | Passed water. |
| | Slept 1/4 hour; delirious. |
| 3.50 P.M. | Beef-tea, 1• oz. |
| 4.35 P.M. | T. 104.4°; medicine. |
| 5.45 P.M. | Chicken-tea. |
| 6.30 P.M. | Medicine. |
| 8.30 P.M. | T. 103.4°. |
| 9.15 P.M. | Chicken-tea; compress. |
| 9.45 P.M. | T. 104° |
| 10 P.M. | Medicine. |
| 11 P.M. | Apple water. |
| | Very restless, wishing to get out of bed. |
| 12 P.M. | Medicine. |
| | Asks to have her mouth wiped out with vinegar and water constantly, "it feels so slimy." Head aching. Has rags constantly on forehead and face sponged with Eau-de-Cologne and water. At her request washed her feet. |

*Monday, 23rd.*

| | |
|---|---|
| 1.30 A.M. | Chicken-tea; passed water. |
| 2 A.M. | Medicine; less restless. Slept 1 hour |
| 4.15 A.M. | Medicine. |
| 4.45 A.M. | Chicken-tea, 2 oz. |
| 6.15 A.M. | Medicine; passed water. |
| 8 A.M. | T. 101°. |
| 8.10 A.M. | Medicine. |
| 9.40 A.M. | Beef-tea and Murdock's food, 2 oz. |
| 10.30 A.M. | Medicine. |
| 12 A.M. | T. 102.4°; chicken-tea,2 oz. |
| 12.40 P.M. | Medicine. |
| 2.15 P.M. | Beef-tea and Murdock, 11/2 oz. |
| 2.35 P.M. | T. 103°. |
| 2.55 P.M. | Medicine; passed water. |
| 4 P.M. | T.103°. |
| 4.20 P.M. | Chicken-tea, 2 oz. |

| | |
|---|---|
| 4.55 P.M. | Medicine. |
| 5.30 P.M. | Passed water. |
| 6.25 P.M. | Beef-tea and Murdock, 3 oz. |
| 7.15 P.M. | Medicine. |
| 8 P.M. | T.101.6°. |
| | Slept 20 minutes. |
| 9.30 P.M. | Medicine. |
| 10 P.M. | Chicken-tea, 2 oz. |
| 11.30 P.M. | Medicine. |
| 12 P.M. | T.100.8°. |
| | Passed a good deal of water; character changed; very high colour but less thick on standing. |

***Tuesday, 24th.***

| | |
|---|---|
| 1.45 A.M. | Medicine; passed water. |
| | Slept 1/2 hour. |
| 2.15 A.M. | Slept 20 minutes. |
| 3.15 A.M. | Chicken-tea; slept 45 minutes. |
| 4 A.M. | Medicine. |
| | Slept 45 minutes. |
| 6 A.M. | Medicine; passed water. |
| 6.30 A.M. | Chicken-tea. |
| 8 A.M. | T.98.2°. |
| 8.10 A.M. | Beef-tea, 2 oz. |
| 9 A.M. | Medicine. |
| 10.15 A.M. | Beef-tea and Murdock, 3 oz. |
| 12 A.M. | T.100°. |
| 12.15 P.M. | Medicine. |
| 1 P.M. | Chicken-tea, 2 oz. |
| 2 P.M. | T.101°. |
| | Slept. |
| 3.30 P.M. | Medicine; passed water. |
| 4 P.M. | T.102.4°. |
| 4.10 P.M. | Beef-tea and Murdock, 3 oz. |
| 6.30 P.M. | T.100.8°. |
| 7 P.M. | Chicken-tea, 2 oz. |
| 7.30 P.M. | Medicine. |
| 8 P.M. | T. 100° |
| 9.15 P.M. | Beef-tea and Murdock, 2 oz. |
| 11.10 P.M. | Medicine. |
| | Slight action of bowels, full of bile. |
| | Passed water. |

| | |
|---|---|
| | Medicine to be taken every 4 hours instead of every 2 hours. Says she has no headache now. |

*Wednesday, 25th.*

| | |
|---|---|
| 1 A.M. | Chicken-tea, 2 oz; slept 1 hour. |
| 3.25 A.M. | Medicine; slept 2 hours. |
| 4 A.M. | Chicken-tea, 2 oz. |
| | Slept an hour and a half. |
| 7.20 A.M. | Medicine. |
| 7.45 A.M. | Beef-tea and Murdock, 2 oz. |
| 8 A.M. | T. 99.8°. |
| 10.45 A.M. | Chicken-tea, 2 oz. |
| 11.15 A.M. | Medicine. |
| 12 A.M. | T. 99.6°. |
| 1 P.M. | Beef-tea and Murdock, 3 oz. |
| 1.15 P.M. | T. 98.6°; passed water. |
| 3.15 P.M. | Medicine. |
| 3.45 P.M. | Chicken-tea, 2 oz. Very thirsty. |
| 4 P.M. | T. 100.8°. |
| 5 P.M. | T. 101°. |
| 1.15 P.M. | Beef-tea, Murdock, 3 oz; passed water. |
| 7 P.M. | Medicine (New Pyrogenium, No. 12). |
| 8 P.M. | T. 100.8°. |
| | Slept off and on. |
| 10.55 P.M. | Medicine. |
| 11.30 P.M. | Chicken-tea, 2 oz. |
| 12 P.M. | T. 99.4°. |
| | *Pyrogenium*, No. 12, to be given every three hours in five-drop doses. Asks constantly for claret cup. A juicy plum. Drank a great deal of water, lemon water, and apple water. |

*Thursday, 26th.*

| | |
|---|---|
| 2 A.M. | Medicine. Slept. |
| 4 A.M. | Chicken-tea, 2 oz; passed water. |
| 5 A.M. | Medicine. |
| 6 A.M. | Chicken-tea, 2 oz. |
| 6.50 A.M. | T. 99.4°. |
| 8.20 A.M. | Medicine. |
| 8.20 A.M. | T. 97.2°. |
| 8.50 A.M. | Beef-tea and Murdock, 3 oz. |
| 9 A.M. | T. 98.2°. |

| | |
|---|---|
| 10.50 A.M. | Chicken-tea, 2 oz. |
| 11.20 A.M. | Medicine. |
| | Asleep 1 hour. |
| 12.30 P.M. | T. 99.4°. |
| 12.50 P.M. | Beef-tea and Murdock, 3 oz. |
| 2.25 P.M. | Medicine; passed water. |
| 2.50 P.M. | Chicken-tea, 2 oz. |
| 4 P.M. | T. 101°; little chicken and rice. |
| 5.25 P.M. | Medicine. |
| 6 P.M. | Beef-tea and Murdock, 2 oz.; bread and butter. |
| 8 P.M. | T. 100°; chicken-tea, 2 oz. |
| 8.50 P.M. | Medicine. |
| | Slept 2• hours. |
| 12 P.M. | Medicine. |
| | Craving for bread and butter. Has ceased to use the Eau-de-Cologne and rags to her forehead, and sponging face and hands — hitherto she used them constantly. A smaller quantity of water passed. |

***Friday, 27th.***

| | |
|---|---|
| 12.30 A.M. | Chicken-tea, 2 oz. |
| | Slept 2 hours and 1 hour. |
| 5 A.M. | Medicine. |
| 5.30 A.M. | Chicken-tea, 2 oz. |
| 7.15 A.M. | T. 98°. |
| 8.10 A.M. | Medicine; passed water. |
| 8.30 A.M. | T. 97.4°. |
| 8.45 A.M. | Beef-tea and Murdock; bread and butter. |
| 10.15 A.M. | T. 97.4°. |
| 11 A.M. | Brandy, raw egg, and milk in all, 2 oz. |
| 11.30 A.M. | Medicine. |
| 12 A.M. | T.99.8°. |
| 1 P.M. | T.99.4; chicken-tea, 2 oz.; bread and butter. Slept. |
| 3.15 P.M. | Beef-tea and Murdock. |
| 4 P.M. | T.100.4°; passed water. |
| 5 P.M. | T. 100.4°. |
| 6 P.M. | Chicken-tea, 2 oz. |
| 7 P.M. | Medicine and compress. |
| 7.40 P.M. | Beef-tea and Murdock. |
| 8 P.M. | T.99.8. |
| 11.15 P.M. | Medicine. |

| | |
|---|---|
| | Telegram from Dr Burnett to take off compress and discontinue medicine till he arrives at 6.15 P.M. No thirst to-day, has not once asked for a drink. |

*Saturday, 28th.*

| | |
|---|---|
| 12.5 A.M. | Chicken-tea, 2 oz. |
| | Slept 4 hours. |
| 4.35 A.M. | Medicine. |
| 5.5 A.M. | Chicken-tea, 2 oz. |
| 7.30 A.M. | Medicine. |
| 7.50 A.M. | T. 98.4°; compress. |
| 8 A.M. | Beef-tea and murdock; bread and butter. |
| 8.15 A.M. | T. 97.4°. |
| 10.30 A.M. | T. 97.4°; Medicine; passed water. |
| 11.30 A.M. | Beef-tea and Murdock; bread and butter, 3 oz. |
| 12 A.M. | T.97.2°. |
| 1.30 P.M. | Medicine. |
| 1.45 P.M. | T.97.8°. |
| 2 P.M. | Brandy, raw egg, and milk, 1 1/2 oz. |
| 3.30 P.M. | Chicken-tea, 2 oz. |
| 4 P.M. | T. 98.4°. |
| 5 P.M. | T. 98.6°; grapes; bread and butter. |
| 5.30 P.M. | Passed water. |
| 5.40 P.M. | Beef-tea, Murdock, bread and butter, 3 oz. |
| 6.30 P.M. | T. 99°; medicine; compress. |
| 8.30 P.M. | T. 98.4°; chicken-tea, 2 oz. |

***Sunday, March 1st.***

| | |
|---|---|
| 12.30 A.M. | Chicken-tea, 2 oz. |
| 3.10 A.M. | Chicken-tea, 2 oz. |
| 6.45 A.M. | Chicken-tea, 2 oz. |
| 8 A.M. | T. 97.2°. |
| 8.15 A.M. | Egg., brandy, and bread and butter, 1-1/2 oz. |
| 9.30 A.M. | T. 96.6°. |
| 10.10 A.M. | Beef-tea, Murdock 4 oz; bread and water; passed water. |
| 11 A.M. | T. 96.8°. |
| 12 A.M. | T. 96.8°; chicken-tea, 2 oz.; chicken sandwich; water, 2 oz. |
| 1.30 P.M. | T. 97°; came out in a rash on the left arm from the shoulder to the wrist. |
| 2 P.M. | Beef-tea and Murdock, 4 oz.; bread and butter; water, 2 oz. |

| | |
|---|---|
| 4 P.M. | T. 97.6°; chicken-tea, 2 oz; chicken sandwich; water, 2 oz. |
| 5 P.M. | T. 98°. |
| 6 P.M. | An apple. |
| 6.45 P.M. | T. 97.8°; beef-tea and Murdock, 4 oz.; bread and butter; water, 2 oz. |
| 7 P.M. | Passed water, natural in colour. |
| 7.30 P.M. | T. 97.6°; egg, brandy, and milk, 2 oz. |
| | Sunday — Slept all last night; gave chicken-tea twice without rousing her. Urine high coloured and quantity much less. Urine passed at 7 o'clock, a pale natural colour. Asked if she might get up tomorrow as she feels quite well. Passed 20 oz. urine. |

***Monday, March 2nd.***

| | |
|---|---|
| 12.15 A.M. | Has slept since 8 o'clock. |
| 1 A.M. | Beef-tea, 2 oz. |
| 6 A.M. | Beef-tea, 2 oz. |
| 7 A.M. | T. 96.4°. |
| 7.10 A.M. | Egg, brandy, and milk, 2 oz. |
| 8 A.M. | T. 97.2°. |
| 9.10 A.M. | Beef-tea and Murdock, 4 oz.; bread and butter. |
| 10 A.M. | T. 96.6°; passed water. |
| 11.30 A.M. | Chicken-tea, 4 oz.; bread and butter. |
| 12 A.M. | T. 97°. |
| | Slept 2-1/2 hours. |
| 3 P.M. | T. 97.4°; beef-tea and Murdock, 4 oz.; bread and butter. |
| 3.30 P.M. | Medicine, *Hydrastis* Q 2 drops. |
| 4 P.M. | T. 97.2°. |
| 5.30 P.M. | Chicken-tea, 4 oz.; chicken sandwiches. |
| 6 P.M. | T. 97°; medicine. |
| 7 P.M. | T. 97.4°. |
| 7.30 P.M. | Egg, brandy, and milk, 2 oz. |
| 8 P.M. | T. 96.2°; medicine passed water. |
| | Began *Hydrastis* Q 2 drops doses. Urine clear. At 8 o'clock complained of being very tired, and asked to go back to her bed. |

Tuesday, 3rd.

| | |
|---|---|
| 1 A.M. | Chicken-tea, 2 oz. |
| 5 A.M. | Chicken-tea, 2 oz. |
| 7 A.M. | Medicine. |

| | |
|---|---|
| 8 A.M. | Beef-tea and Murdock, 4 oz.; bread and butter and apple. |
| 8 A.M. | T. 97.4°. |
| 9.30 A.M. | Medicine. |
| 10 A.M. | Egg, brandy, and milk, 2 oz; bread and butter. |
| 11.30 | A.M. Medicine. |
| 12 A.M. | T.98.2°. |
| 12.15 P.M. | Chicken-tea, 4 oz., and sandwish. |
| 1.30 P.M. | Medicine. |
| 2 P.M. | T.98.2°. |
| | Asleep for 1/2 hour. |
| 3.15 P.M. | Beef-tea and Murdock, 4 oz. |
| 3.45 P.M. | Medicine. |

I will now tabulate the temperature markings, not in the form of a curve, but in figures according to days :-

| A.M. | Fri. | Sat. | Sun. | Mon. | Tues. | Wed. |
|---|---|---|---|---|---|---|
| 8 | 104° | 103.6 | 101° | 98.2° | 99.8° | |
| 12 | 103.2° | 104.4° | 102.4° | 100° | 99.6° | |
| P.M. | | | | | | |
| 4 | 103.6° | 104.4° | 103° | 102.4° | 100.8° | |
| 8 | 104° | 104.4° | 104° | 101.6° | 100° | 100.8° |

| A.M. | Thurs. | Fri. | Sat. | Sun. | Mon. |
|---|---|---|---|---|---|
| 8 | 98.2° | 97.4° | 97.4° | 97.2° | 97.2° |
| 12 | 99.4° | 99.8° | 97.2° | 96.8° | 97° |
| P.M. | | | | | |
| 4 | 101° | 100.4° | 98.4° | 97.6° | 97.2° |
| 8 | 100° | 99.8° | 98.4° | 97.6° | 96.2° |

*REMARKS* — The febrifuge and otherwise the curative action of the *Pyrogen* was soon manifest, and the normal temperature was reached within a week, and then came the subnormal reaction. Whether others will believe that *Pyrogen* here acted curatively I do not know. I personally am satisfied that the remedy broke up the fever, and humanly speaking, saved the young lady's life. That is also the opinion of the mother, who has large experience.

Case II. — Subsequently a middle-aged gentleman had an attack of fever, but it was complicated with, or arising from an enlarged liver with old peritonitic adhesions and adhesions of Glisson's capsules. In this case the hepatic and other remedies of a more constitutional action did not seem to act, and so I fell back upon *Pyrogen*, with the result that the other remedies then acted well, and patient made a quick recovery. Looking now back on this case, I am disposed to think that it was a mild septic fever supervening upon chronic hypertrophy of the liver, and the liver was not able to right itself till the continued fever had been quelled by the *Pyrogen*. This case I will not dwell upon, as the evidence it affords does not count for much. (XII 44)

**CASE III.** — This case, K. W. A., occurred subsequently in the same house as Case I., and the patient was at the time about 13 years of age, and he is brother of the subject mentioned in Case I.

I will also not dwell long on K. W. A.'s case, or give any particulars further than to say, that the giving of *Pyrogen* was followed at once by a distinct drop in the temperature of nearly three degrees, and it did not again go up, but remained at about 99° for many weeks, when the patient got well, and is now a strong fellow.

For the sake of making the case comprehensible, I will just add that from the course of the case, from the remedies that helped, and from those that did not, I am of opinion that patient had continued fever which started mesenteric mischief, and that the pyrexia 102.6° was cured by *Pyrogen;* whereas the slight febrile movement that went on for so many weeks — nearly nine — was consequent upon chronic inflammation in the mesenteric glands. There was much obstinate diarrhoea. However, whatever the nature of the case was, the exhibition of *Pyrogen* was followed by a drop of three degrees in the temperature.

Still I would not attach much importance to this case either. (XII 44)

**Case IV.** — William R.A., aet. 19, oddly enough also of the same family as the foregoing, but residing at Kensington. He came home (to Kensington) early from office, complaining of neuralgia, on the afternoon of Wednesday, and 17th of February 1886. Did not sleep that night, and so did not get up to breakfast next morning, when his temperature was found to be 100.6°.

As he seemed to have a feverish cold, complained of pains in his bones, he was ordered *Aconite* and *Bryonia*. Temperature at 5 p.m. 101 degree, when Dr. ____ was sent for, and patient was got upstairs : he had been sleeping in the smoking room adjoining the W.C. since February 2nd. The doctor ordered *Aconite* and *Bryonia*. Did not sleep much on Thursday night.

*Friday* — The doctor saw him in the morning, and changed the medicines to *Merc. viv.* 3x. trit., as much as would lie on a six-pence, every four hours. On Saturday, *Aconite* was alternated with it every hour.

Slept indifferently.

On *Sunday*, patient was removed to higher ground, viz., close to Cavendish Square. Patient bore the removal well, but profuse perspirations broke out from time to time, great aching in his limbs, headache from time to time all over forehead, great thirst, breath foul, tongue not much coated but brownish, gets depressed if left alone, and breaks out in perspiration; pain in the stomach at times, bowels rumble a great deal, nose bleeds readily, throat sore and congested, gum ragged where wisdom tooth has lately come through, gets a pain if he drinks cold milk, jaws very stiff, so much so that he cannot separate his teeth but a very little.

The physician in charge was very positive that it was a case of true typhoid, and I may say that the gentleman in question has had special experience of typhoid, and knows it better than many physicians. There was a regular staff of hospital nurses in attendance experienced in fevers, and they were quite sure it was real typhoid.

The young man's mother having seen the effects of *Pyrogen* in continued fevers — the cases I have already related — told the physician in charge about it, and wanted him to give *Pyrogen*, but he refused, saying that it was quite impossible to stop typhoid fever, and that, therefore, this case would have to run its course. But the lady was so sure that she had seen *Pyrogen* break up fever, that she did not feel it would be right to go on without at least trying it, and the doctor thereupon withdrew from the case. And as I had long been the ordinary medical adviser of the family, and being, moreover, the foster parent of *Pyrogen*, I was asked to take up the case, which I was sorry to do on the one hand, but rather keen to try my friend *Pyrogen* again all the same. This was Monday morning, February 22. 1886. Up to this date the temperature-markings were : —

| A.M. | 18th. | 19th. | 20th. | 21st. | 22nd. |
|---|---|---|---|---|---|
| 8 | 100.6° | 100.2° | 100.8° | 100.1° | 100.4° |
| 12 | 100.8° | 100.6° | 100.1° | 100.1° | 100° |
| P.M. | | | | | |
| 4 | 101° | 100.4° | 101° | 100.6° | |
| 8 | 100.8° | 100.2° | 101° | 100.6° | |

At two o'clock on the afternoon of 22nd *Pyrogen* was begun, five drops of No. 6 in water every two hours, and I saw the patient in the afternoon for the first time. The very pose of the patient, his mode of lying in bed, spoke clearly in favour of wanted food; kidneys and bowels and skin all told that the fever was not being treated merely by it, but jugulated, snuffed out, if I may so say.

No doubt I may be inclined to think too much of it, but my duty is done when I give my evidence and my opinion.

I had to wait some time after this before suitable cases of fever presented themselves for a further and more extended trial of *Pyrogen*, and I felt somewhat disappointed at not seeing any clinical results obtained by it brought to the notice of the profession either by Dr. Drysdale himself or by other colleagues. So I determined to wait till such were forthcoming, but I waited in vain, nothing came. However, *tout vient a celui qui sait attendre*, and in December 1887 I had the good fortune to be called in to treat two young ladies in London both with continued fever, the temperature in one case being 104° to 105°, and in the other ranging from 99° to 101°. (XII 46)

**Cases V and VI.** — The young ladies had been under allopathic treatment, and the fever would not lessen. Having them both in adjoining rooms, and both cases being clearly of common origin, whatever that may have been, I gave the worse patient *Pyrogen* as in the last case, and *Baptisia* to the less bad one. In three days the patient taking *Pyrogen* was feverless; and the one on *Baptisia*? Her temperature had gone on steadily rising, and was 104° or thereabouts. Why did you not give them both *Pyrogen* said the mother ?

I did not enter into the question, but ordered *Pyrogenium* then for the other, and down went the temperature as in the previous cases.

This is my experience of *Pyrogenium*, not, indeed, all of it, but the bulk of it.

Now, let those who have more fevers to treat than I have put it to the test, but not in low dilutions, or hypodermically, but in the 6th centesimal by the mouth, as I have done.

But the *Pyrogenium* should not be diluted or preserved with glycerine, but the matrix fluid should be forthwith run up to the 6th centesimal dilution, as is customary in homoeopathic pharmaceutics. In other respects it must be prepared as directed by Dr. Drysdale in his paper already referred to. (XII 50)

## 219. DIPHTHERITIC SORE THROAT

"In August 1887 I was attending a little boy for a diphtheritic sore throat, and the boy was not racing his way to recovery. Indeed, matters were at a standstill, when I thought of *Pyrogenium*, and gave it in the sixth dilution — centesimal. But let me first say, by way of parenthesis, that the boy's temperature was 102•° F. There were patches on both tonsils, the breath was offensive, the tongue thickly furred, and the complexion was muddy. The *Pyrogenium* was given on Tuesday, and by Wednesday morning there was a marvellous change for the better.

"The temperature had fallen to 99° F., the throat was less inflamed and less covered with membrane. The tongue was cleaner, and the complexion was less muddy.

"The next day matters improved still more, and by Friday I had taken leave of the patient.

"This was not all. (XII 53)

## 220. BLOOD POISONING

"The little boy's sister was seized with chills, headache, aching in the limbs, and soreness of the throat. The clinical thermometer marked 102•° F. in her case. Suspecting that I had another case of blood-poisoning to deal with, I gave *Pyro.* 6, and by next day all these uncanny symptoms had vanished like a dream. (XII 54)

## 221. SORE THROAT

"I fear, my dear Burnett, I weary you, but at the risk of being thought a dreadful bore, I will add one more experience.

"The mother of my little boy patient nursed her son, and was infected by the same blood poison. False membrane was deposited on both tonsils, the patient had a foul breath, a furred tongue, and a look of weariness and illness that betokened serious trouble. But she only remained in bed two days after having taken the first dose of *Pyro.*, and made a good recovery.

"My first patient, the little boy, was taking the traditional *Belladonna* and *Merc. biniod.* in low dilutions, and was not making progress till *Pyrogenium* came to the rescue.

"I had treated the little patient for a similar attack of sore throat in June, and *Belladonna* and *Merc. iod.* had acted well, so that this masterly inactivity on the part of these medicines made me look for fresh help, which I found, thanks to your previous suggestions, in *Pyro.* 6.

"I gave this medicine in a scarlet fever case just before Christmas on the second day of my attendance, and certainly I had a fall of temperature and a case free from complication, but the results were not so striking as in the diphtheritic cases.

"I shall look forward with great interest to your own experience of this strong power for good.

With friendly greetings, believe me to be —

"My Dear Burnett,

"Yours very truly,
"E. B. Shuldham" (XII 54)

## TUMOURS OF THE BREAST

### 222. TUMOUR OF EYELID

The very first tumour I had to treat was a small hard one of the eyelid of some years' standing. The patient was a young lady from Canada. She had consulted an eminent physician of the homoeopathic school, and he had advised *an operation*. "Have it cut out," said he, "medicines cannot cure it." She was sent to me by a mutual friend to see if I could cure it with medicines, and so avoid the dreaded operation. The tumour was but a small affair, about as big as a very small marble, but on a girl's lower eyelid that is a good deal. I used a number of remedies, but the two that seemed to be really curative were *Argentum-nitricum* 1, in one or two drop doses three times a day, and *Hydrastis-canadensis* applied freely to the tumour with a camel's hair brush.

The little tumour completry disappeared, the patient and her people were enthusiastically grateful. (XIII 3)

Some of the little tumours of the eyelids that one commonly meets with are from a wrong condition of the stomach, the state of the pancreas seems distinctly answerable for a certain number of them, some are apparently a sequel of vaccinia, and odd articles of food are known to cause them in certain people, *e.g.*, roast pork. Often such swellings will rapidly disappear, but not infrequently they become hard, insensitive, and chronic. A few months of proper constitutional treatment will cure them. The remedies most commonly indicated are *Thuja-occid., Argentum-nitricum, Natrum-sulphuricum, Pulsatilla-nig., Hepar-sul., Calc., Hydrastis-canadensis.* In very obstinate cases one has at times to call in the aid of certain nosodes. One of the last cases of *tumours of the eyelids* I have had to treat, has only just got well after many months of persistent treatment with medicines, the patient being a young married lady whose husband's friends were very anxious for her to have them excised, but the lady would not listen to their entreaties, having been told by me that such tumours are of a constitutional nature, and must be treated constitutionally by internal medication. She was jeered at and ridiculed by the wiseacres of her husband's family for "being so silly." said they (*they* knew!) "Of course, you *must* undergo an operation, no medicines can touch *that*."

For some months they seemed to be right, for my remedies did but very little good, and my poor patient had to bear a good deal of banter and "did not I tell you medicines were no use?"
However, after a month of *Chionanthus-virginica* in small material doses, the tumours waned and went.
Said I, "What do your husband's friends say now ?"
"Nothing !"
"Do they believe now that tumours of the eyelids can be cured by medicines ?"
The lady passed out of my consulting room laughing. (XIII 4)

## 223. PARALYSIS AND ATROPHY — RIGHT LOWER LIMB

Less than two years ago, a child was brought to me suffering from paralysis and atrophy of portion of the right lower extremity, that the local doctor said would end with the child's death in about a year or less. The most eminent London opinions, both special and general, confirmed this view. When the parents informed the local doctor that the child was to come under my care, he piously expressed the hope that it might avail, adding the rider : "If that homoeopath cures him, I will believe in homoeopathy."
When, however, the child was well and was running about on two straight, equal limbs, the said doctor looked very wise (what an easy task!) and stern, but would on no account have any conversation on the subject. (XIII 5)

## 224. CRACK — ANGLE OF MOUTH AND TUMOUR BREAST

In the spring of the year 1875 I was treating the children of a family of my *clientele*. While chatting with the children I noticed that their nurse, a woman of about forty, had an ugly unsightly *crack in the left angle of her mouth*, about the fourth of an inch deep, and surrounded with warty exerescences, the whole covered with a nasty secretion I considered it commencing epithelioma. I offered to treat the woman for it, but she did not believe in homoeopathy, and she was using a salve to it prescribed by her own doctor. At this period I was myself still suffering from my proving of *Cundurango* (see *British Journal of Homoeopathy*, July 1875), and I had repeatedly proved that the crack in the angles of the mouth was a very characteristic symptom of the drug. Altogether I have seen it produced pathogenetically four times, and I have cured along many times. It apparently finds no favour with the profession, but its importance will be recognised.

Some little time elapsed, and the before mentioned nurse was confronted with the chance of losing her situation, as her mistress was getting afraid lest the disease might be communicated to the children. The nurse was now willing to be treated homoeopathically, and her mistress accordingly sent for me. On inquiring I found the warty ulcer in the angle of the mouth was only a little worse; it was very *torpid,* had remained for many months, pretty much the same. This is also characteristic of *Cundurango.* The pustules and other cutaneous manifestations of this drug are *torpid* (see the proving in the *British Journal of Homoeopathy* and the Symptomatology" in *Allen's Encyclopaedia of Pure Materia Medica,* vol, iv., p. 1 *et seq.*) Once while using an ointment this ulcer had almost disappeared, but it soon returned to the condition I have described.

But what alarmed both mistress and maid (the former on account of the children, no doubt) was a *tumour in the patient's left breast i.e.,* on the same side as the epithelionatous ulcer of the angle of the mouth. On examination it was found to be about the *size of a small hen's egg, and very hard* and very painful at times; at other times painless. It had been there for several years, and was on the increase, but only very slowly. The odour from the axillae was very offensive indeed, but not from lack of cleanliness. Speaking generally, patient did not look ill-nourished or cachectic, though her teeth were very badly decayed, which gave an old appearance to the face from the falling in of the cheeks, and the dilated small cutaneous blood-vessels showed that she had probably been a florid subject.

The *history of the tumour* was this. She had four years been in the habit of sleeping with the youngest child, a bonnie boy, with a very large, heavy head, and he lay with his head against this breast. To that she attributed the lump. And she was probably right, for the boy would at times restless at night, and hit about with his head a good deal, hence we may fairly conclude that the breast had been mechanically injured very many times. Patient complained that he very often hurt her thus.

There was nothing to account for the ulcer of the angle of the mouth; it was idiopathic, as the phrase goes. There could be no reasonable doubt of the connexion existing between the tumour and ulcer. Was it cancer? I think so now, and I thought so then. I do not *call* it a case of cancer, but simply a tumour of the breast, hence my diagnosis cannot be called in question, whereas if I were to *call* it cancer it might be objected to. Still I will say I think it was cancer, — 1st, From the appearance of the floor and edges of the ulcer; 2nd, From the concidence of the ulcer and of the tumour; 3rd, From the hardness of the tumour; 4th, From its origin.

It is needful to state this view of its pathological nature, as it influenced the treatment.

The medicine I decided on was *Cundurango,* and for these reasons :

1. *Cundurango,* produces cracks in the angles of the mouth, and also cures such.
2. *Cundurango* is in my opinion, an antipsoric, and case appeared to be a psoric manifestation from injury.
3. *Cundurango* has beyond any doubt cured cases of cancer, and this seemed such a case.
4. It seemed to me that the ulcer in the angle of the mouth that started more crack-just supplied the phothogenetic differentia requisite for knowing whether to give *Hydrastis, Conium,* or what not.

The first prescription is dated July 16, 1875, and is

R$_x$ Pil. *Cundurango* 1, zij.

One four times a day.

This was taken until December 4, 1875, when I could perceive only slight amelioration of the ulcer and none of the tumour. I then remembered that the cures reported had been with material doses, and that Goullon, jun., and another writer on the subject on the continent, whose name has escaped me seemed to incline to that view. Now, I would rather cure a patient with a big dose than leave him or her *uncured* with a small one. And, of course, conversely.

Moreover, my patient rather objected to pilules; the *size* of the *means* seemed so *inadequate* to the *end*. Therefore I gave the following prescription, in December 1875 :

R$_x$ Tc *Cundurango* Q zij.

Aq. ad. zvj.

C. C. med. ter in die.

This was taken till September 1, 1876 with slight interruptions. At this date I certainly noticed much improvement in the ulcer, and the tumour seemed a little smaller, but still I felt very much disappointed. Then *Bryonia-alba* 1, two drops in water four times a day, was given till November 10, 1876 when, no further progress being apparent, I gave a short course of *Sulph.* 30 one pilule at bedtime. This is very old practice, and has been verified a great many times. In all about one drachm of the pilules was taken. Then at the end of 1876 I again went over the case and felt justified in reverting to the old prescription of *Cundurango* but I gave the tincture of the first centesimal dilution three times a day with occasional omissions, that the organism might not get insusceptible of the action of so small a dose. This was continued during the whole of the year 1877 during the first five months of the year 1878, and during the first five months of the year 1879 that is just about two years and a half.

I saw the patient at, intervals during this period, and was able to observe the course of the cure. In a few words it was this. At first the ulcer of the angle of the mouth became dryer, cleaned and less rugged, while the tumour went smaller and a little. About a year and a half the ulcer had entirely cleaned and remains so; nothing happened but a very slight puckering, of that angle of the mouth and faint streaks of scar-tissue. But to a casual observer these objective symptoms have no existance, it is only when examining it critically in the light of its past history that one can detect even these trifling rests.

Already towards the end of the year 1878 the tumour had nearly disappeared, and in the spring of 1879 it was gone. In sending a Report from Princes Park, Liverpool on September 2, 1879 the patient says : — "The lump has completely gone out of my breast," Further she goes on to state that she gave up taking the medicine. This case is very important from various standpoints; it shows the utility of proving a remedy that has an empirical reputation in order to find out the variety of a disease that it will cure. Thus *Cundurango* has undoubtedly cured a number of cases of cancer; but we may say the same of *Sulphur, Thuja, Arsenicum, Conium, Hydrastis, Carbo-animalis, Bryonia, Bufo,* of *Galium Aparine,* and hence the point to find out is ***what characterize*** or species. The greatest characteristic yet observed of our *Cundurango* is the crack in the angle of the mouth, and hence on theoretical grounds we may say that a case of cancer with a manifestation in the angles of the mouth calls for *Cundurango.* NINE YEARS LATER. I published the foregoing case in the *Homoeopathic World,* November 1, 1879, and I have just made inquiries regarding this woman, who was thus cured of her tumour, notwithstanding it declared impossibility, and find that she still continues in perfect health and free of tumour. (XIII 27)

## 225. TUMOUR : UPPER JAW

A gentleman at the prime of the life, or a little beyond, some might think, came to me at the end of 1887 with a hard tumour in the right upper jaw of about two years' standing. It had come on slowly. His dentist thought it was due to a set-up tooth in the wall of the jaw. An eminent surgeon had seen patient with the dentist, and was not of the dentist's opinion, believing it to be a new formation, for which he prescribed an ointment containing *Iodie* (*la vieille histoire* !) The ointment dutifully applied, and did no good.

The right half of face between eye, mouth and beard was notable swelled hard, and with glistening, shiny skin over it. Regarded front within the cavity of the mouth, it appeared as if the outer

wall of the antrum Highmore were pushed out, constituting a tumid mass.
All things considered, I thought the dentist right and the surgeon wrong, and on the mechanico-traumatic hypothesis, gave *Bellis per.* Q, five drops in water night and morning, and two months of this brought the jaw back pretty well to the normal, and patient did not think it needed any further special treatment. (XIII 18)

## 226. TUMOUR OF RIGHT BREAST ; TUMOUR OF RIGHT ARM ; ARM-PIT; SEVERE CUTANEOUS AFFECTION.

The case I propose now to narrate has taught me much in respect of the amenability of mammary tumours to drug treatment, indeed more than any other one case in my whole experience, and I may, perhaps, be therefore permitted to dwell upon it a little fully, more particularly in regard to its causation. The subject of it came under my medical observation in the year 1878, and she was then verging on 40 years of age. An examination disclosed several lumps in the right axilla about the size of a goose's egg, and all hard.
It appeared that the tumours in the arm-pit had been there for two years, and came after a successful vaccination; and simultaneously therewith, the face had broken out all over with an eruption of ruberous inflammatory elevations, with pustular stop technically termed acne variolae formis, and this eruption has also presisted for two years in this very aggravated form, like chronic small-pox. In the year 1877 there was an epidemic of variola in the neighbourhood, and patient was again vaccinated, so her vocation brought her into contact with it, and this time it was followed by the lump in the right breast. I did not then regard vaccination as a causal factor in the genesis of chronic disease, but I see now clearly enough that it was a case of chronic vaccinosis, axillary and mammary swelling and the facial eruptions being clearly of common nature and origin. And operation was not thought useful by her rather open minded friends, and hence my help was sought. I treated the case for a long time with such remedies as *Silicea, Psorinum, Sulphur, Heclae-lava, Grauvogl's Lapis alb., Conium, Iodium, Phytolacca dec.*, but made no great headway. The lady was, however, very patient, and went on with my treatment, feeding principally on hope; but hope, though not a bad auxillary, is no remedy for tumours or skin diseases. I then used various so-called nosodes, sometimes utilized by homoeopathic practitioners with isopathic procivities, and we made a little progress, but not much. When however, I had obtained more correct views

of the long-lasting effects of the vaccinial poisoning, I prescribed *Thuja-occid, Sabina, Vaccininum* and *Variolinum* in varying dilutions (mostly medium and high), and patient slowly got quite well, not only of the adenomata in the axilla, but also of the tumour of the breast and of the skin affection.

When she was up in London for the May meetings in 1888, the lady called upon me, and thus I am able to say that she remains perfectly cured.

Never have I seen a case that so well exemplifies and justifies my principle in regard to the treatment of tumours — keep on passing away !

That this lady would have died long since had she been operated on for the tumours I have no doubt at all. Others may doubt this, but that she was cured of her tumours by medicines is open to no doubt whatever. Amongst the frequent causes of tumours I must, therefore, reckon vaccinosis, and on this subject I would refer the reader to my little treatise entitled *Vaccinosis and its Cure by Thuja* etc, in which this thesis is to some extent elaborated. Sometimes we have to do *with* trauma upon vaccinosic tissue, and then the just appreciation of the two genetic factors leads to a cure. (XIII 19)

## 227. TUMOURS OF LEFT BREAST AND OF RIGHT OVARY

On February 5, a married lady, 40 years of age, came to me borne down by the weight of her physical miseries. Her father had lupus of the nose, and her mother had died of cancer. Eight years previously a very small tumour had been excised from patient's left breast and now there is another in the same breast. In addition to their tender swelling. The right ovary and the left breast are, curiously alternate in painfulness, tenderness and several trouble sameness. Patient's first baby was born dead, after very protracted labour. She had also suffered from sore throat, leucorrhoea, piles, thick scanty urine, and then profuse and limpid; stricture of the sigmoid of the flexure at its lower end, much pain in the breast and side,rectum packed full of piles, sore throat, worse in the night, and by far the most distressing symptom of all, constipation of the most severe and obstinate kind.

Patient made two conditions to my being her physician — the first was that I should allow aperients; "Life is unbearable without them," said she and the second was that I should tell her what each given remedy was, "because I take so much interest in these things." I absolutely declined both conditions, and the patient yielded, but under a desperate running fire of sarcastic obstructiveness, consisting in diffusive and

effusive epistles, such as your clever lay *guerisseues homoeopathiques* so well know how to keep against a stiff-necked medical autocrat, little weening that mental obedience is an essential part of the cure of some cases. However, she did give way slowly, and was eventually rewarded by being completely cured. At her visit to me on October 20, 1886, she *well* of tumour, of stricture, of piles, of constipation, of all pains (and of all the other physical miseries formerly complained of. The treatment lasted over three years, and the remedies used were in the order named) :
*Aesculus hippocastanumt* 3* trit.
*Sulphur* 30.
*Nux-vomica* 30.
*Graphites* 4 trituration.
*Psorinum* 30.
*Thuja-occidentalis* 30.
*Lapis-alba* (Grauvogl's) 4 trit.
*Mercurius* (strength not noted).
*Silicea* 6.
*Graphites* 5.
*Silicea* 6.
Besides various well-known and less well-known nosodes, the cure was aided a good deal by diet.
And in regard to diet, I think I could hardly do better than quote a very apposite paper by a very gifted lady, the late Mrs. Nichols; it will be found further on. I will produce it, as it is almost unique in its scientific purity, and in dietetics the scientific spirit is almost entirely absent; most doctors, I notice, go by their own stomach or old wives tales, as witness the rubbish one hears and reads about vegetable diet. (XIII 21)

## 228. CANCER OF BREAST

In the year 1883, a London professional man was under my care, and in odd conversations he told me about his mother who had cancer of the stomach. Could I do her any good ? I did not know, probably not.
I saw him pretty frequently. and almost every time after I had prescibed for himself, he recurred to the said state of his mother and her terrible sufferings, dreadful pains in the chest and stomach, keeping her awake at night for many hours together."She had her left breast removed some time ago for cancer, and now it had come in the right breast and in the stomach.
Could nothing be done ?

I told him that I often succeeded in curing simple tumours with medicines, and also cancerous tumours of small size if taken early, but that when they had once been operated on I mostly failed, the operation apparently generalized the disease and intensified it, so I could not give him much hope. Had she come before any operation had been performed, it would have been very hopeful.

So time went on, and still my patient insisted on conversation with me about his mother, of whom he is very fond. He even stopped me at railway stations to tell me of the poor lady's sufferings. Finally, *en desespoir de cause*, he brought her to me for my opinion. I am now particularly pleased that he did so, as the course of the case taught me for the first time the vastly important lesson, that even after an operation we need not give up hope, — nay, more, that where an operation has been performed, constitutional treatment should be begun *at once*, to get at the root of the matter and prevent any further local expression of the disease, by attacking its cause or causes. I say *or causes*, for cancer is not a disease that can produce its like after the manner of, say syphilis of scarlatina, but is essentially a hyperlasia of a degraded type at the end of a chain that has many (causal) links. But to my case :

October 23, 1883. Mrs. ____, 47 years of age, had her left breast removed for cancer two years ago last. May by an eminent surgeon. In February 1883 she had had erysipelas of the face, and as she lay in bed therewith paresis of right foot, which passed off. She had variola at the age of three; is subject to winter bronchitis with much despnoea. On examining the chest, one sees a long but every neat scar where the left breast used to be. The other and inner ends of scar are a little tender, and the tissue at the other end is rather swollen of late. The patient cannot bear the part to be touched. The right breast is the seat of a hard painful tumour of the size of hen's egg. The pain, however, is worst in the stomach (the ventriculus), which pain is "cruel," like cramps, and worse at night.

$R_x$ Tc. *Cundurango* 1x,, four drams. Five drops in water three times a day.

November 16. Only had two attacks of stomach pain since she was here. Anorexia no better; much flatulence; "flying spasms."

$R_x$ Repeat.

December 12. Much better in herself; stomach pain gone; had it a year; pain in the toe no better; the mammary tumour is less hard.

$R_x$ Repeat.

February 6, 1884. Menses at first stopped, and patient gave up the medicine, as she attributed their cessation to the medicine; after leaving it off for a fortnight she got menorrhagia gets nocturnal dyspnoea;

wakes up with a coughj; stomach continues better; feet are sore; the appetite is now good.

March 28. Has been laid up with a cold and bronchitis, but the nocturnal dyspnoea is much better; digestion fair; feet less sore; the pain in the stomach has not returned; the tumour is very much softer.

$R_x$ Tc. *Silicea* 30, four drams. Five drops in water night and morning.

April 28. The tumour of right breast is decidedly less painful; there is now a hard painful portion of tissue over the site of the left breast, which pains most at midnight; patient feels ill.

$R_x$ *Psorinum* 30

May 5. Feet very tender; both breast and the painful tissue very much better.

$R_x$ Tc. *Hydrastis-canadensis* 1, four drams. Five drops in water three times a day.

June 11. Menorrhagia every fourteen days; feet very tender; *tumour softer*.

June 26. Has prolapsus recti, with constipation; dirty brown leucorrhoea; breast is painless; tumour smaller, no pain in the stomach; feet better, less painful.

$R_x$ Tc. *Thuja* 30.

July 23. Worse; very much pain in the stomach; last night it was most severe; tumour hard and painful.

$R_x$ Tc. *Cundurango* 1x, four drams. Ten drops in water twice a day.

August 20. The tumour is rather smaller, but more painful; severe pain in the stomach. Patient has gone back to the lemons which I formerly recommended, and which seemed to suit. There are now two painful nodes on the edges of the scar of left breast. Has had menorrhagia twice.

$R_x$ *Psor*. 30. and *Cundurango* Q.

September 5. About the same; feet very tender.

$R_x$ Tc. *Cundurango* Q and *Silicea* 6 trit.

October 15. Feet no better; stomach well; no pain in the scar; tumour in the breast is smaller and softer.

November 10. Tumour of the breast much softer; the vaginal discharge has now ceased. Pains are always at night.

December 26. Much better altogether.

$R_x$ *Repeat*.

January 7, 1885. Gone back very much; breast very painful; the submaxillary glands are swollen and painful; the pain is "cruel," and causes "vomiting by the hour;" vomits blood; pain keeps her awake at night; she has a taste of phosphorus in the mouth. She tells me now, for the first time, that she is an enormous pepper eater, which I forbid.

℞ *Repeat.*
February 21, 1885. Been to the seaside to pull up; the nocturnal pain is much better; the feet are tender and swell.
℞ *Repeat* et *Cund.* Q.
March 4. March better; right breast much more elastic; the nipple is still very much retracted.
℞ *Psor. c.* et *Cund.*
April 30. The pains wake her up; she shrinks from pressure on the chest.
℞ *Ranunculus sceleratus* 3x. Four drops in water night and morning.
May 14. Has now much pain under left arm, where there is some swelling and redness.
℞ *Bellis p.* 1.
℞ *Lapis alb.* 5 trit.
June 17. Tumour decidedly smaller and better both sides.
July 22. Parts very tender, and there is much acidity.
℞ *Acid hippuric* 6, four drams. Five drops in water night and morning.
August 28. Did her seemingly much good for three weeks, when she had a dreadful attack of a pain.
℞ *Repeat* (12).
October 21. Did her much good.
℞ Tc. Q *Kreatin* 12, three drams. Three drops in water night and morning.
November 20. Much better; in fact, nearly well, but has, whites now badly.
February 5, 1886. Has not been since November 20, 1885. She says the powders then given gave her cramp in the stomach, waking her up between 12 and 2 A. M., and causing nauseous risings, pains in the feet, which are sore and tender. Left them off, and the same phenomena recurred on resuming them. Has had no medicine for a month, and these symptoms persist. When she has a stool, the faecal mass slips backwards in the rectum.
℞ Trit. 6, *Silicea'* gr. vj., ter die.
March 17. The breast is nearly normal, but the womb and feet are painful.
℞ *Repeat.*
May 5. Womb and feet better; gums very spongy, much water-brash and vomiting of water.
℞ Tc. *Natrum muriaticum* 12, four drams. Five drops in water three times a day.
June 28. Says the drops have very much upset her; gums are very blue.
℞ *Aconite* and *Silicea.*

November 2. Breast well, gums still red and swelled and sore. Much abdominal pain from 2 — 4 A.M.

$R_x$ Trit. 4, *Urea* gr. vj., ter die.

Patient has paid me irregular visits off and not since, for gouty pains in various parts, but there is no return of the cancer.

I have given so many tedious details of this obstinate and difficult case to illustrate several points as clearly as I am able. In the first place, this case caused me to modify my previously oft-expressed opinion, that when once an operation had taken place, treatment by medicine is useless. I now know that this is not necessarily the case, but that a *cure may be obtained even after an operation, and after a recurrence has begun*. In the next place I again learn, and continue to insist upon, the importance of dogged perseverance in the medicinal treatment. And finally, it confirms my genarel practice of striking out new therapeutic lines when the old ones do not suffice. The influence of the late Dr. Ameke's, teachings will be readily recognised by the learned in pharmacologic and therapeutic offshoots.

Looking now back on the whole of this case, considering all its points, the remedies those helped and those that did not, I get a comparatively clear view of its nature, which helps me in other case. Were I asked to name its biopathology, I should say it was a hybrid union of psora, vaccinosis, chronic poisoning by pepper and tissue-gout, to which complexity there came the element of trauma. (XIII 22)

## 229. MAMMARY TUMOUR

On July 5, 1883, a lady of 73 years came under my observation for small hard tumour in her left breast. This breast had been injured thirty years ago, and gave her much trouble for long time. For some months she has noticed its swelling and hardening. It pains a good deal; worse at night, and on moving the arm. In the preceding November there had been an eruption on the patient's left leg, "large inflamed patches showed themselves." The principal remedies used were *Bellis-perennis* 1, *Psor.* 30, *Var.* 30, *Hydrastis* 1, and then finally *Bellis* 1 again; and on January 29, 1885, patient was discharged cured; and she remained well, and is, I believe, alive and well at the time of going to press.

I do not give the details of this case as it is badly kept in my diary, but the foregoing contains most of the essential points, and the fine pharmacologist will readily see that the prescriptions were all more or less *ex hypothesi*. I might add that patient is deeply pitted with small-pox marks. (XIII 28)

## 230. HARD PAINFUL TUMOUR OF BREAST

On August 13, 1878, Mrs —, a country clergyman's wife, about 40 years of age, came under my care for a tumour of the left breast in its outer and upper aspect. It is about the size of a very small hen's egg, hard and very painful. It had existed for some time, and she and her husband had become very anxious about it, the more so as her mother had died of vulvar cancer (an enormous epithelioma). Perhaps I ought to say that the mother died *with* the cancer, as she was 82 years of age at her death. The mother had been my patient, but she was, she averted, unable to persevere with my medicines (*Thuja* 2, 3 and 30) as they caused her so much pain.

Patient is married, has several fine children, and has been long subject to a very severe form of leucorrhoea.

It would occupy too much space were I to give all my notes of this interesting case in detail, for she was under my treatment for this tumour about three years.

My notes begin with August 13, 1878, and prognosis was a serious one unless medicines could be made to prevent the disease advancing.

I began with *Urkalkgneiss* 4th trituration, ten grains at bed-time, and soon got into trouble on its account, for my patient showed the prescription to the learned lay lady, who is the recognised stock-taker general of all the unfortunate leeches of the neighbourhood in which they dwell, and she said, "Oh, Mrs — know what the doctor thinks you have the matter with you. It is cancer!"

"How do you know?"

"Oh, the chemist told me it was the new German *cancer* medicine."

Naturally this caused my patient much and needless anxiety, but then the chemist and the learned lady must have their confidential little wise acreings about the doctor's doings — it is no inconsiderable part of their rather monotonous lives. But this and many other similar experiences have compelled me often to whithhold the name of the remedies.

Well, Mrs ____ took Grauvogl's *Lapis alb.* (4, 5 and 6 trit.) for a number of months without any noticeable effect; the lump went on growing, and the pain getting worse.

July 26, 1879. *Acid. acet.* 1.

August 28. No better; very weak. *Conium-maculatum* 3x.

This remedy was continued for about two months, and it took away the pain, but it did not lessen the size of the tumour. Then followed *Carbo. an.* 30, which was suggested by the profound adynamia.

November 28. No pain; and she is no stronger, but the tumour is no smaller.

$R_x$ *Sulphur* 30.

On January 6, 1880, I received a letter telling me that the powders were finished, and that in addition to some pain in the tumour, patient had a good deal of pain in the stomach. I sent *Cundurango* 1, and ordered her to take six drops in water three times a day.

February 24. "A good deal of pain and uneasiness in the whole breast and shoulder and down the arm."

$R_x$ *Repeat*.

April 10. No change in the tumour; for two or three weeks I did not feel it at all, and now I have a good deal of uneasiness, though no acute pain." *Hydrastis* 1. Five drops in water night and morning.

May 19, 1880. On this day the lady was brought by her husband to London, and they called to inform me that having continued my treatment ever since August 1878 their friends wished for another opinion. The lady herself did not wish for any further opinion, but the husband was rather needlessly loud in demanding the opinion of at least one other, and that of Sir James Paget.

To this I declined to assent, because, said I, "What is use of an *opinion*, or for the matter of that, what is the use of a barrowful of opinions? The tumour is there; you can feel it and see it; that it is *hard* you can also *feel*; that it pains your wife knows but too well, and what possible prognosis can the men of the knife give but the everlasting old story, "Oh, you must be operated upon as soon as possible." Truth to tell, I am sick and weary of the lying statements that the knife is even any, and least of all the only cure for tumours. Not only does the knife not *cure*, but *anyone having a tumour or lump cannot, as a rule, take a shorter road to the grave than via the knife* — that, is unless it be very large, and *unless the tendency to its recurrence be outrooted simultaneously with the operation, or soon thereafter*.

Oftener than not, cutting out a small tumour is like pruning a vine.

But to return to my patient and her choleric husband, I absolutely declined my second opinion.

Why?

Simply because a very considerable number of people with tumours literally die of the doctors' opinions, and then what is the use or value of the opinion of a never so eminent a pathologist on a therapeutic point? Just none.

Of course, I know it is said to be very unprofessional to decline an eminent colleague's co-operation in a given case. But I did it for my patient's good, *not* for my own; and moreover, they do the same to me when people want my opinion.

Under date of May 19, 1880. I find in my Case-book, "She has suffered for many years from white sticky leucorrhoea, very much like the white of an egg; the tumour is softer, and about one-half its original size; the whites are considerably better since the last medicine (*Hydrastis* 1x, gtt. v., night and morning). The tumour is more painful eight days before menstrual period.

July 20. Whites worse; more pain in the tumour; pain in the epigastrium, making her feel quite sick, especially when standing.

℞ *Thuja* 3, four drams., gtt. v., bis die.

*Thuja* 6.

November 16, 1880. Have been almost entirely free from pain until last week, when the breast pained me; I am much better in regard to the white. So far as I can judge, the last medicine has been the right one."

*Thuja* 12, four drams., gtt. v., bis die.

January 28, 1881. "I have taken the last medicine for two months. When I first began to take it, I had more pain in the effected part than I had had for a long time previously, but latterly I have been quite well, except a spell of toothache, which yielded to *Belladonna* and *Gelsmeium*. *The tumour is very much smaller.*"

℞ *Hydrastis can.* 1, four drams., gtt. v., night and morning.

March 25. "I am going on improving, indeed I am very seldom reminded of my ailment; the tumour is now so small that my husband cannot find it."

℞ *Hydrastis can.* 6, gtt. v., four drams. night and morning.

May 27. "After I began to take the last medicine I felt a good deal more uneasiness in the affected part that I had done for some time before, now I am much as I was while taking the previous medicine. I think my husband told you of the decrease in size."

℞ *Psor.* 30, four in twenty-four hours.

July 29. "My husband thinks the lump nearly gone I think it *is* gone. While I was taking the last medicine, and for a week after, I had a good deal of pain in the region of the womb, and at the time I had this pain I was also a good deal annoyed with the whites; now I am quite free."

July 29, 1881, is the last note of the case in my book, but I saw the patient on another matter on November 3, 1886 — more than five years thereafter — and learned that there had been no return of the tumour or of other ill-health, and she had enjoyed very good general health. (XIII 28)

## 231. TUMOUR OF LEFT BREAST

Mrs — 26 years of age, came under my care in February 19, 1883, complaining of the swelling in her left breast about the size of a small orange. It was hard, and had been first noticed in August 1882. Last spring she had squeezed out some fluid from the left breast. Slight leucorrhoea. She was the mother of one child which was then three years old. Patient had been twice vaccinated, and was subject to labial herpes.

I informed the lady that the tumour was, in my opinion, due to her use of modern preventive measures, that it was, in fact, due to reflex irritations from the hypogastric region. My wide experience teaches me that a large number of mammary tumours in comparatively young married ladies are due to hanky panky manoeuvers of various kinds, the organism being, additionally, dyscratic. Without any dyscrasia, the hypogastric irritation would in all probability not so easily suffice, unless indeed, it were very great and applied over a long period. I explained that Nature in the long run is very rarely insulted with impunity. Nemesis may tarry, but she inevitably follows the trail of wrong doing. Oh, how true it is that the way of the transgressor is hard.

$R_x$ *Psor.* 30.

March 3. The tumour is rather smaller. She says, "I find it decreased by about one-half."

$R_x$ *Repeat.*

March 19. The tumour is a trifle larger than it was last time. The old itching has entirely disappeared.

$R_x$ *Kali chlor.* 6 trituration, in six grain doses night and morning.

April 2. *Emansio mensium* : she is probably *enceinte*. Herself she feels rather weak, but the tumour has much diminished.

$R_x$ Tc. *Thuja occidentalis* 30.

Patient needed no further treatment, the tumour quite disappeared, and in due time a baby came. (XIII 33)

## 232. UTERINE FIBROID ; SMALL TUMOUR ON LEFT BREAST — DISEASE OF LEFT NIPPLE

An unmarried lady, 43 years of age, came under my observation on September 24, 1881, for a severe sprain of the left ankle. It was several months before she got well, it being complicated by gout, dyspepsia, and dysmenorrhoea. The accident was a severe fall down stairs, and, in falling, she struck with great violence against the low part of the body, causing for many months much vesical trouble with metritis. The case was further complicated with attacks of breastpang, and with fainting fits. Evidently the fall had given her a rude shaking, and disturbed many important organs, the liver and spleen giving at times much trouble. This lady remained under my care, and very slowly got the better of most of the just described ailments, when, on March 14, 1882, she took me so far into her confidence as to tell me she had, for the past four years a little red lump on her left breast that discharged something, It was about the size of a hazel-nut, and situated at the lowest outermost part of the left breast. With it there was much pain all down the left side. At her next visit on April 19, 1882, patient took me further into her confidence, and stated that she had been for some time getting very large in the uterine region, — in fact, the size had been noticed by strange ladies, who thought she was married, and was expectant. On this account alone the position was most painful. The case went on, the abdomen continued to increase in size, when, on November 23, 1882, I came to the conclusion, from an examination obtained with much difficulty, that it was a uterine fibroid. The mammae became greatly hypertrophied. I could never quite make up my mind whereat fibroid really sat, and sometimes, from the hard nodes of the cervix uteri, I opined it might be a kind of fibrous hypertrophy of the whole organ. Very many remedies were used — *Lappa major* Q, *Thuja* 30, *Merc. met.* 30, *Lapis alb.* 3, *Aurum met.* 100, *Helonin*, *Kali chlor.* 6, *Aur. mur.* 3x, *Silicea* 4, *Bovista* 3x, *Psor.* 30, but all with but little apparent effect. Moreover, the left nipple became the seat or most distressingly painful moist cracks, and which are particularly significant.

This brings the case down to August 1883, when patient appeared like a lady about seven or eight months gone in the family way. To make matters worse, a child ran against her (impinging on the protuberant abdomen), and hurt her a good deal, when I gave *Platin mur.* 3x, but also to no good purpose. Any wonder that patient was getting down-hearted? Two years medication and bigger than ever! And the doctor — Are a few guineas any adequate reward for such responsibility? Then came *Bovista* 3x, *Mer. cor.* 5, *Aur. mur.* 3, *Helonin* 3x trit., when the breast was a good deal better, the cracks of the nipples better, and the little tumour drying up. The excoriation between the legs was described by the patient as dreadful; pain in the back every bad; disagreeable taste.

$R_x$ *Lapis alb.*, 6 trituration.

January 10, 1884. About the same in a general way; complains dreadfully of her *back*. This dreadful back distress finds grand remedy in the virus of variola, which I have in the 30th dilution, and in very infrequent doses, and any one objecting thereto is answered thus : *Aux grands maux leg grands remedes.*

February 14. Seems to have done her back real good; left breast is much better; was so well that she absented herself for a few days. The same remedy was continued.

March 6. Maintains that this last prescription did her harm, while the privous one did her much good, which I can well understand, viz., *de*

*trop* of the right remedy. Back exceedingly bad; much frontal headache.
$R_x$ Trit. 6 *Calc. fluoris.*
April 5. Head better; back very painful when she walks. anorexia; bad nights.
April 26. Has had a good deal of pain at the menses and in the left side, nights much better.
$R_x$ *Var. C.*
May 29. The nights continue good; much easier in general; is getting thin; was very stout, notably mammary hypertrophy; is very *debile*, but the tumour is decidedly smaller.
$R_x$ Tc. *Aur. mur. nat.* 3x. Two drops in water night and morning.
July 10. "Dreadfull sicky," i.e., intense nausea; she feels very weak, tumour is much smaller.
$R_x$ *Psorinum* 30.
August 21. Frequently faints away, at times falling down; less nausea; vision is failing.
$R_x$ *Thuja occidentalis* 30.
September 6. Is still giddy, but does not actually faint away; has menstruated three times in eight weeks' sick feeling gone; dreadful pain in the left side; toothache.
$R_x$ *Argent. nitric.* 5, four drams. Five drops in water night and morning.
October 16. Much enlargement of the spleen, which pains a good deal.
$R_x$ Tc. *Ceanothus Americanus* 1x.
November 5. No better.
*Berberis vulgaris* Q.
January 9, 1885. Breast well; the tumour of womb still very large; and patient has every appearance of being *enceinte;* wakes very early, and cannot get off again. (This is a capital indication for *Bellis.*)
$R_x$ Tc. *Bellis perennis* 1.
January 29. She now sleeps well, and feels much easier in the abdomen.
I would here interpolate a rather important clinical tip in regard to *Bellis.* viz., it is often curative of the symptom, "Wakes early in the morning and cannot get off again;" and in cases of pregnancy and of uterine tumours (also enlarged heart), *Bellis* given great ease in many case, i.e., takes away the effects of mechanical pressure.
February 26.
$R_x$ *Variol* 30.
March 26. Back is on the whole better; tumour rather smaller; giddiness.
*Ib.* (C.C.)
May 9. Pain in left side.
$R_x$ *Ceanothus Americanus* 1.
June 8. Toothache and pains in the back.

July 23. Much pain in the left side, which is tender. Tumour is smaller, which is evident from general appearance.
$R_x$ Tc. *Chionanthus virginica* Q.
September 3. Side better; the left nipple is very sore.
October 2. The nipple is better, more comfortable; the tumour of womb about the same.
$R_x$ Trit. 4, *Hecla lava.*
December 5. Feels much free from pain, and more easy and comfortable in herself than for long. This remedy has cured her constipation.
$R_x$ *Repeat.*
January 26, 1886. Is very giddy; fairly comfortable in uterine sphere; left nipple has been gathering. She is so cold in her stomach.
$R_x$ Tc. *Kedron* 1.
March 9. Feels dreadfully sick.
$R_x$ Trit. 3x, *Hecla lav.*
May 29. Patient is so much better that she is getting very irregular in attendance. The diminution in the size of the tumour is considerable.
$R_x$ *Repeat.*
August 6. Continued marked improvement in the size of tumour, but there is a good deal of pain in her legs, worse on getting up out of bed in the morning.
$R_x$ Tc. *Bellidis per.* 1, four drams, five drops in water night and morning.
October 6. This is the date of my last note when patient presented herself normally menstruating, in blooming health, plump and ruddy, though still complaining of some tenderness of the left ovary and left nipple. One can see where the little tumour formerly was on the left breast by the deeper colour of the skin. I prescribed *Kali chlor.* 6, which, no doubt, has taken away the tenderness complained of.
This is the long weary course of my treatment of this terribly complicated case, lasting, as the notes show, just five years. During this long period my patient was very often importuned by her well-meaning friends and relations to undergo an operation but she steadfastly refused, wavering only once or twice when her homoeopathic friends also urged surgical interference. If patient should call again before this goes to press, I shall add a few words more. Patient subsequently came to know if she might accept an offer of marriage, which I answered in the affirmative. (XIII 34)

## 233. ON THE CURE OF A SMALL ADENOID TUMOUR OF THE BREAST BY SUCKLING

A lady of 32 had a little adenoid tumour in her left breast of the size of a marble. As she was *enceinte*, I recommended her to do but little for so small a thing, but to be sure to well suckle her child when it came. This she did with very praiseworthy preserverance, although she had but very little milk, and the process had to be materially supplemented by the bottle, and at the end of the 4th month of suckling the tumour had entirely disappeared. It is true I gave her few medicines also with reference to the tumour and for her ailings, still I conclude that the baby helped to draw off the tumour, casually of it waning; the mammilla of that side had always been retracted, which a small circumstance, deserves attention.

Personally, were I a woman with baby, I would suckle it from purely selfish motives, merely to departure my own blood and organism, for woman who had a family and does not suckle her offspring, is drawing a bill on the future of her organism which she is likely to be either unable to meet at all or to do so with great difficulty. Mother Nature suffers no tempering with her provisions; with her if simply and emphatically, Obey; or suffer disease or extinction. (XIII 43)

## 234. TUMOUR OF BREAST

The case I am about to tell is psychologically and sociologically interesting, as my readers will see.

On December 15, 1884, a married lady, 44 years of age, mother of one child, then 16 years old, came to place herself under my care.

She had noticed a swelling in her right breast, was naturally much frightened. An intimate friend of hers (in fact, her former governess) had been cured of a mammary tumour by me with medicines, and so Mrs. — came off to London to place herself under my care, but when arrived, her metropolitan friends quite laughed her out of it, telling her it was all nonsense to trust heself to my tender mercies, — first, because of my homoeopathic proclivities, which they adequately despise and actively hate; and then "it was well known that no medicines (and least of all, homoeopathic ones) were any good at all in tumours." The poor frightened thing of course yielded, was hurried off to what I suppose I must call eminent men, who declared it to be cancer, and urged immediate operation in order to save her life. The operation was duly performed in April, the whole right breast being compeletely ablated by Sir — . The wound healed up quickly and well, the lady was sent home to her husband's country seat CURED (!!) and the case, no doubt, continues to stand as one of the CURED (!) of the eminent operator. The social value of these quasicures by the knife is — baronetcy. The social value of medicinal cures of tumours is — slander and contempt.

However, the cutting-off process was worse than useless, as in a few months another tumour appeared in the remaining breast, which confirmed the opinion of the operator that it was a case of cancer.

Was it cancer? No, I think not, but an irritable tumour of uterovarian origin. Indeed, I am quite sure this is the correct diagnosis. Our operating surgeons are mad : the biggest and best are clean mad. No sooner does a poor woman get a lump in her breast than she is frightened out of her wits by consultations between these eminent and eminently ignorant of knife-people, whose diagnostics are confined to feeling, seeing, and the microscope.

My treatment of this recurrent tumour lasted three years, and the following remedies were used — *Psor.* 30, *Hydrastis canadensis* Q, *Bellis per.* 1, *Ranunculus sceleratus* 3x, *Psor.* C., *Thuja occidentalis* 30, *Bellis perennis* Q, *Solanum tub.* 6 and 12, *Aurum muriaticum nat.* 3, *Cundurango* 1; and on February 7, 1888, the breast was normal, and the remarkable thoracic hyperaesthesia had at last disappeared, and this had for years been so bad, that the gentlest touch of one's finger on patient's chest caused her to wince and shrink from contact.

To all the notes of these three years of treatment would fill a little volume, and so I am compelled to narrate in the few words. But I again state that it was not a case of cancer, but the lumps came in the breasts — first in the one that was cut off, and then in the remaining one — from a wrong state of the uterus and ovaries, and in precisely the same physiological way as the milk comes into the breasts after childbirth.

The origin of the first tumour was curious; the lady was getting out of their carriage when she fell against one of the buttons of her husband's coat. When I first saw the left breast it was red, hard and very painful. the lady had been vaccinated four or five times, the last twice unsuccessfully. She was very fond of salt. She had had much grief and worry. Her confinement was very severe, owing to size of foetus. She subsequently had a good deal of congestion of the womb and leucorrhoea, for which her surgeon and physician gave her local treatment. This is the usual thing : at first a poor lady's constitution is wrong; Nature, kind clever Nature, sets about righting it with leucorrhoea, ulcers at the os uteri, and uterine congestion; the doctor (poor brainless creature), cauterizes, gives injection, and cures (drives back); then it concretes in the breast as a tumour, which is cut off, and — *apres ca le deluge* !

I told the lady straight away that hers was not a case of cancer at all, but as she had the opinions of the greatest living authorities on tumours and cancers she did not believe me. (XIII 43)

## 235. MULTIPLE TUMOURS OF BREAST

An unmarried lady of 32 came under my observation on the February 24, 1885 for a number of hard tumours in both her breasts, which were otherwise of enormous size, yet shapely. She had also prolapsus uteri, leucorrhoea, an enormous liver, the left lobe of which reached down almost to the navel.

*Carduus Marianus* Q restored the liver to the normal, and so made more room for the dislocated womb, which soon took advantage of the altered topography of the abdominal contents; in fact, the prolapsus was gone. Quite a number of nosodes followed in high dilutions, and then *Cundurango* 1, *Chionanthus virgin* Q. *Helonias dioca* Q, *Hydrastis canadensis* Q, *Bellis perennis, Acidum fluoris* 6, *Fluoride of ammonium* 5, *Secale cornutum* 6, *Sarza* Q, *Solanum tub.* 6, *Scrofularia nodosa* 6; and, under date January 17, 1888, I find noted in my Case-book — The breasts are quite normal, with the peculiar resilient elastic feel of that organ when healthy.

I attribute the original cause (or at least one of the causes) to numerous cauterizations of the *os uteri* to which the unfortunate lady had been subjected by a fashionable lady's doctor of repute. I do not mean that the cauterizations of the womb alone produced the tumours of the breast, but rather that what was the cause of the ulcers, being denied an outlet at the *os uteri*, became vitally concreted in tumid masses in the breast, aided by the reflected mammary irritation from the *os uteri*.

I feel it is not fair to my subject to give a string of remedies that were used to cure this case, without the same time giving their diagnoses and indications, but space fails me. I might just add that the most striking, prompt and permanent amelioration wrought in this case was by the *Solanum tuberosum* and by the *Scrofularia nodasa*, both in daily doses of five drops of the tincture of the sixth centesimal dilution, though the last prescription was the former remedy in the tweflth centesimal. (XIII 47)

## 236. CANCER OF RIGHT BREAST

At the beginning of the year 1887, a lady friend and patient was consulting me on account of her health, and she was very depressed and frequently burst into tears, I pressed her to tell me the cause of her grief. "Oh," said she, "I have a sister who is coming home from Germany to be operated on for cancer of the right breast. We are very fond of dogs, and one of my sister's dogs jumped upto her and hurt her right breast very much, and now it has turned to cancer. She has been using ice compresses for over a year, and been under the Crown Prince's physician, and under Dr. ____, who is sending her home for the opinion of Dr. ____."

"Is there *nothing* in the world that can cure cancer?" said she.

My reply was — what I here solemnly restate — that most cases of cancer are quite curable by the remedies IF TAKEN EARLY, AND TREATED LONG AND CONTINUOUSLY BY INTERNAL REMEDIES, and that in this way I had myself cured many cases of cancer.

"Then," said she, "I suppose it is too late for my sister, for she has had it for more than a year and a half, and the doctors, say that the operation is her only chance."

April 2. I went to see the lady at her sister's house soon after her arrival from the continent, and found them all very naturally, in a sad state of mind. The patient had received a letter from Dr. ____ urging an *immediate* operation, as otherwise the cancer-juice in the milk ducts would infallibly poison her blood. Subsequently the other gentleman, Dr. ____, saw the lady and concurred, and went so far as to say that delay, even till the next day was most dangerous for fear of constitutional infection. My kind professional brethren impatiently scouted my views as mere senseless, not to say wicked, talk.

On examining the right breast and comparing it with the left, one was struck with the diminution in the size of right one. The nipple was deeply retracted, and from the little funnel-shaped opening in the nipple-region there oozed an ill-smelling fluid. The breast itself was puckered, and one raised ridge on its outer aspect was inflamed, swelled, and bluish at one part, — an unmistakable picture of cancer. I therefore agreed as to the diagnosis.

We had a very long conversation about it, and it was a terrible position for me to take up in face of almost all the experience of the world in face of the eminent authorities arrayed against me in the teeth of the sneering, jeering opposition of connexions, belongings; and their medical and surgical friends.

Nor was it easy for the responsible friends or the patient herself to decide finally either for my treatment by the medicines or for the operation.

To see the unfortunate lady looking at her sister, then at me, then at her poor breast, and then reading her doctor's letters urging the imperativeness of immediate operative interference, and then bursting into a flood of tears, and saying she did not know what to do, is a scene similar to others I have often seen; but it remains ever with me all the same. I concluded the deliberations by saying "Mrs —, the breast is *yours*; mark that; not your sisters', not your doctors', not mine, but *yours*; and if I were you I would *keep it*. I promise you nothing, but I tell you that in my experience, and speaking humanly, medicines can cure you, though the course of the cure will be *slow*; for that I find is almost invariably the case in treatment of tumours, whether malignant or benign, the mending by the help of medicines is *slow*."

"Well," said she, "I refuse the operation, and will do as you tell me." The breast being painful (the weight of a heavy dog by its paws), I ordered *Bellis per*. 1. ten drops in water every four hours. This was April 2, 1887. Nothing locally at all, now, or hereafter.

April 14. Vast improvement.

$R_x$ *Arnica montana* 1x. Five drops three times a day.

April 21. Better on the whole.

$R_x$ *Repeat the Arnica.*

April 28. Wakes with a nasty taste in the mouth.

$R_x$ *Repeat* and also give *Chelidonium majus* 1x.

May 5. Not quite so well, and the skin of diseased breast is red; more painful; has just menstruated.

$R_x$ *Bellis per* Q. Five drops in water three times a day.

May 12. Better a good deal; the covering skin is less red, and the nipple is not quite so much retracted.

May 18. Mending beautifully; breast is softer; nipple less drawn in; a portion of the cutaneous covering is still red.

$R_x$ Repeat.

May 26. Mending.

$R_x$ Repeat.

June 2. The mammilla is less retracted, and the breast begins to be slightly movable. Heretofore it was so retracted and held down by bridles of tissue behind it that it could not be moved as a whole at all. Is menstruating.

$R_x$ *Repeat* four times a day.

June 9. Still improving; nipple less retracted.

$R_x$ *Repeat*.

June 16. The breast is getting bigger (*i.e.* returning towards its previous natural size) and less immovable.

$R_x$ *Repeat* five times a day.

June 23. The breast is much less drawn in; the top of the nipple is now sunk only about half an inch from the level; all the discolouration has gone from the mammary surface; and patient is getting stouter.

$R_x$ *Repeat*.

July 2. Much running from the nose; runs like water ever since she took the *Bellis* (pathogenetic?). There is a little more tenderness of the breast; to-day the last day of the menses.

$R_x$ *Repeat.*
July 9. Some redness around the *Areola mammillac.*
$R_x$ *Repeat.*
July 14. The coryza is very bad, for which patient comes; bad cough; much green expectoration tinged with blood. The cold is like others she has had.
$R_x$ *Repeat.*
July 28. The breast not quite so well (Is menstruating).
$R_x$ *Repeat gtt.* x.
August 6. I learn to-day from the patient, for the first time that this right nipple has peeled at times for years with offensive discharge. In this state it is now.
$R_x$ *Repeat.*
August 16. No change in the nipple, which is still peeling.
$R_x$ *Repeat.*
August 25. The breast is slowly returning to the normal as to appearance, but there is still much discharge from the nipple.
$R_x$ *Repeat.*
September 8. There is a little redness of the areola.
$R_x$ *Repeat Sul 30.,* three drams gtt. v. ter die.
September 27. Much improved, but the redness is there still.
To take *Belladonna* 30 with the *Sul.* and thereafter return to the *Bellis* as before.
October 11. Mending; the breast is slowly resuming its former proportion, though it is still hard.
$R_x$ *Repeat Bellis* Q.
November 12. Not so well.
$R_x$ *Hydrastic can.* Q.
November 19. Slight improvement, there being less redness in the areola.
$R_x$ Repeat.
November 29. The *Hydrastis* seems to be causing diarrhoea.
$R_x$ *Arnica montana* 3x.
December 8. Has a cold.
To alternate *Aconite* 3x with the *Arnica.*
December 29. Brest continues hard, but there is less areolar redness.
$R_x$ *Chelidonium* Q and *Aconite* 3x.
But I need not go on with these wearisome details; some more remedies were needed, patient got better and better, and returned early in 1888 to Germany, and I have not since seen her; but in a letter to me, under date of May 8, 1888, patient says, "The hard lump is slowly decreasing." Perhaps before this goes to press I may be able to give the end of

treatment, but this will not much matter, as patient was practically well before she left for the continent. (XIII 28)

## 237. TUMOUR OF BREAST

At the end of the month of November of the year 1886, a married lady of 40 odd years of age came to consult me in respect of a hard tumour of the size of hen's egg in the lower third of her left breast, painful at times, and due originally, it was stated, to a hurt. I find no note to the date of the hurt. Patient was the mother of large family, and she had also flooded and married, and her menses had always been very profuse and long lasting, so that for years she had been barely ever able to completely recover from one period before she was overtaken by another, and hence she had acquired a weak heart from the chronic anaemia. She had suffered also for many years badly from leucorrhoea, and letterly her feet swelled. She was stated to have had scarlatina, measles, and mumps, each twice, and besides having had smallpox, she had been four times vaccinated, the last three times unsuccessfully. There were many little wartinesses here and there on the cutaneous surface, such as I have become accustomed to regard as pointing to cancer.

$R_x$ *Thuja occidentalis* 30.

December 18. Very great improvement was reported, and patient was well of the tumour and of herself by the spring of 1887.

Besides the *Thuja occid.* given repeatedly and over a number of weeks, *Magnesia sul* 3x was given for some little time. Over a year later the patient was reported to me as being well.

Here the medicinal and curative action was not only very remarkable, but also very remarkably prompt, which attribute to the fact that the swelling was merely a dyscratic organismic reaction to the trauma of such recent date that the swelling was not yet neoplastic. When the casual dyscrasia was extinguished predisposing cause of the swelling was gone too, and hence the swelled tissue constituting the tumour had shrunk shrivelled. I thought it would have taken much longer to cure the tumour than it actually did, because it seemed to me probable that neoplasia had set in to a greater extent than was evidently the case. (XIII 54)

## 238. TUMOUR OF LEFT BREAST

At the beginning of 1888 I was consulted in regard to a tumour of the left breast of a healthy young lady of about 20 years of age, and which had not been noticed very long. It was in its upper and outer aspect, but deep in the body of the breast. Of course, the young lady's mother and friends were greatly alarmed, and an operation was thought to be the only thing to do. It stands described in my account of case of the size of large orange, but I do not think it was quite so large. In four months the tumour had quite disappeared, the remedies having been, *Thuja occidentalis* 30, *Bellis perennis* Q, *Ceanothus Americanus* 1, and *Cundurango* 1x, and the last named being apparently *the* remedial force, and which was given because of the browny look of patient's skin.

The rapid cure of this tumour was evidently due to the fact that it was from reflected ovarian irritation, and not a neoplasm. Nevertheless it was only "an operation" that the faculty and family discussed together indeed, the ready way in which the operating representative carpenters, commonly called surgeons, recommend the removal of ladies' breasts in whole or in part is truly staggering. (XIII 55)

## 239. TUMOUR OF RIGHT BREAST IN A MAN

Although tumours of the breast are much more common in women than in men still they do also occur in the breasts of males, more particularly in later life. Such a one is the following :

On April 23, 1881, there came to me a rather tall, spare, hectic-looking gentleman, a London professional man, of about 70 years of age telling me that ever since the previous February he had been greatly worried, and this was followed by a sensitiveness in his left nipple, which soon passed off and went to right nipple, wherein it still was. On examining the part I found it the seat of a hard tumid mass of the size of pigeon's egg. Patient first noticed it was swelled a month previously. It is not actually painful, but there is a sensation of fulness and uneasiness, and he cannot lie on it, hence it arrests his attention.

℞ *Psor.* 30. mvj.; s.l.*q.s.*, ft. pulv., tales xij., j. nocte.

May 7. There is still a sensation of fulness in it; patient thinks it is softer, in which opinion I share. It is a little smaller. Since taking the powders he had had some bilious attacks.

℞ *Repeat.*

May 21. It is much smaller; there is much less sensitiveness, and patient can now sleep lying on his right side, which was previously not possible.

℞ *Repeat.*

May 28. The sensitiveness is now confined to the nipple alone, still he can sleep lying on it. He is constipated, and his tongue thickly furred.

℞ *Hydrastis canadensis* 3x, four drams.

S. gtt. v., nocte maneque.

June 14. The sensitiveness; tumour still continues, but it has very much distressed.

R$_x$ *Repeat*.

July 2. Less sensitiveness; tumour still decreasing in size; on the sternum, on a level with the nipple, there is a scaly eruption of the size of a three-penny piece, having a red ground, the rest being yellowish. He is still constipated.

R$_x$ Tc. *Hydrastis canad.* 3x four drams., s. gtt. v., n. m.

July 23. He has scabs on the scalp; a yellow scab at the middle of the sternum; also on his hands. The nipple is no longer sensitive at all.

R$_x$ Tc. *Thuja occid.* 30, in infrequent doses.

August 13. The tumour has disappeared, with the exception of one of the size of a hazel-nut. There is still some scaly eruption on the sternum.

R$_x$ *Psor.* 30 (two to a month).

Sep. 16. No trace of the tumour to be found. There is still a patch of reddish scaly eruption on the skin of the chest.

R$_x$ Tc. *Chelidon maj.* 3x. gtt. iij., nocte.

Oct. 13. No trace of tumour; still a circular patch at mid-sternum. Bowels a little relaxed.

R$_x$ Trit. 6, *Nat. sul.*

Oct. 27. Well; and has a healthy complexion, whereas it was at the beginning of treatment, quite earthy.

Six yars have elapsed since then, during all which time the patient has remained well of the tumour, *i.e.*, it has never returned. Two or three times or more in every year the gentleman is in the habit of coming to see me, "To be kept in repair." Before I began treatment I was importuned by his friends as to whether I was *quite* sure it was safe to forego an operation, "which, you know, Sir J — says is the only *chance*!"

What did the friend say *after* the tumour was cured by remedies? Were they grateful? Perhaps'they have so scrupulously avoided the subject ever since that I have no means of knowing.

Nevertheless the tumour remains cured, and that is the main point. (XIII 55)

## ON NEURALGIA

### 240. NEURALGIA OF THE HEART

In connection herewith one may remember the known neurotic *origin* of certain cutaneous affection.

One Sunday morning, some ten or twelve years ago, a gentleman ushered his wife into my consulting room because she had been taken with an attack of *angina pectoris* in the street, on her way to church. Though only a little over thirty years of age, if so much, she had been subject to these attacks of breast-pang for several years : they would take her suddenly in the street, nailing her, as it were, to the spot, and hence she no longer went out of doors alone, lest she should faint away or fall down dead, as was apprehended.

An examination of the heart revealed no organic lesion, or even functional derangement, and I could not quite see why a comparatively young lady should get such anginal attacks. She had been under able men for her *angina*, but it got no better, and no one could apparently undrstand it. I prescribed for her, and saw her subsequently at her home, to try and elucidate the matter. I let her tell me her whole health-history from her earliest childhood. She said she was getting to the end of her teens, and was preparing to come out, but she had some cracks in the bends of her arms that were very unsightly; these cracks had troubled her from her earliest childhood. Erasmus Wilson was consulted; he gave her an ointment which very soon cured her skin, and the patient came out socially, made a hit right off, and got married in due course. She had always been very grateful to Erasmus Wilson for curing her arms, for otherwise, "How could I have appeared in short sleeves?"

But there soon followed dyspepsia, flatulence, dyspnoea, and palpitation, and finally the before-described attacks of *angina pectoris* threatened to wreck her life. Moreover, she had borne one dead child. As I have already said, there was no discoverable cardiac lesion, and from the lady's health-history I gathered that this cure of her skin (though to me the one important point) was of no causal importance.

I gave my opinion that her skin disease had never been *really* cured, only *driven* in by Wilson's ointment, and that her angina was in reality its internal expression or metastasis. No on believed it, however. I began to treat her antipsorically, and very soon — I think it was less than a month from the Sunday morning visit — the old cracks reappeared in the bends of the elbows, *and from that time on she had no problem.* (XIV 6)

## 241. FACIAL NEURALGIA

Mrs ____, aet. 24, came under treatment in 1876, in the early months of pregnancy, with very severe neuralgia of the face. The case proved itself very obstinate, and many drugs were fruitlessly tried, but eventually it yielded to *China* given in the form of pilules saturated with the matrix tincture, which drug was chosen because of *perspiration breaking out* when the pain became very bad. The neuralgia costantly re-appeared, and finally *China* ceased to have any effect. Then *Populus tremuloides* was given simply because of its being a congener of *China*, and did good — in fact, quite cured for the time.

This pregnancy passed, and my patient consulted me again, being again *enceinte* early in 1877, for the same kind of neuralgia, and this time its obstinacy nearly reduced her and her physician to despair.

The case was treated in the old Hahnemannian fashion according to the totality of the symptoms, which were very few and apathognomonic, the neuralgia being always bad and always worse, and apparently not ameliorated by anything.

After many weeks of fruitless endeavours to cure this neuralgia with medicines chosen from the repertory, I turned to *Guernsey's Obstetrics* (2nd edition), and found I had already tried all those given in his list at pp. 372, 373, 374, except two; these two I then fairly tried, and again failed. So my patient had received *Aconite, Belladonna, Bryonia, Calc-c., Cocculus, Cimicifuga, Coffea, Gels., Glon., Ignat. mag. c., Nux-v., Puls., Sepia, Spig., Sulph., Verat-a., China, Populus,* and some others. Besides which she had applied, often in almost frantic despair, nearly every known anodyne, so that the soft parts of the face seemed almost macerated.

Here I suggested change of air (what should we poor practical physicians do without this *ultimum refugium*), but circumstances prevented her from leaving the place for more than a day or two; so she took little outings to sea-side places and inland, when it was observed that the *neuralgia was worse at the sea-side* and better inland.

A happy thought struck me, that this might be due to the *salt* in the air at the sea-side, and being, moreover, absolutely at the end of my tether, I acted on it, and gave *Nat. mur.* 30, one pilule very frequently.

The neuralgia at once began to get better, and in a day or two was quite well. It subsequently returned at intervals much less severely, but promptly yielded to the same remedy in the same dose. The 30th dilution was chosen simply because some pilules of this strength were in patient's chest.

The patient was quite satisfied that the *Nat. mur.* 30 effected the cure, and so was I, and so will many others be; but, in a general way, the case will not carry conviction to unprepared minds, and still less so to prejudiced ones. (XIV 21)

## 242. FACIAL NEURALGIA

Not many years ago, the daughter of a London alderman was suffering from fearful neuralgia of the face; at intervals she had had it for years, and no trouble or expense had been spared in endeavouring to cure it. Their ordinary family adviser was a homoeopath, but he had not managed to cure this neuralgia, not-withstanding several consultations with colleagues, and other men of eminence had been consulted, but to no avail.

I found that the pain was worse in cold weather; worse at the sea-side; better away from the sea — inland, i.e., not so frequent or severe; and when the pain came on the eyes watered. A pinch of the sixth trituration of *Natrum muriaticum*, in water three times a day, cured my young patient in about three weeks. This anti-neuralgic action of *Nat. mur.* had the great advantage of being permanent curative, as the pain did not return, and patient herself continued otherwise well. (XIV 28)

## 243. NEURALGIA

A patient of mine once went to the sea-side, where then practised Dr. Harmar Smith, now of Guildford. I had in vain treated the lady's fearful ovarian neuralgia, but Dr. Smith cured it very quickly with *Arsenicum*. This very day I saw in the *Homoeopathic World* that the same gentleman still cures neuralgia with this faithful antiperiodic. I will not quote the whole case, although it tallies with my own views, that neuralgias yield best to higher dilutions, but will just say that Dr. Harmar Smith was treating a case of *acute gastrodynia* that yielded to *Ars.* 12x trit. after the *Liquor arsenicalis* (F.), the 3rd trituration of *Arsenicum, Trisnitrate of Bismuth* 1x, and *Apomorphia* 3x, had all more or less failed. The one weak point in this case is that the after-history of the case is only of a few days' duration. But neuralgia of all parts with arsenical symptoms has been so often cured dynamically by *Arsenicum*, that its anit-neuralgic reputation is firm, and needs no prop. (XIV 33)

## 244. ANGINA PECTORIS

A short time since, it was my duty to see a lady in Belgravia with *angina pectoris* : unwonted domestic drudgery, loss of loved ones, fright, loss of fortune, had led up to it.

Apart from the anginal attacks, there was a chronic constant pain across the praecordia, running away under the left breast. For years blisters had been applied at intervals with temporary relief, till they could no longer be borne. Patient was very depressed, sulky, and morose. The menses suppressed. *Aurum metallicum*, 3 trituration, six grains every four hours, cured the constant pain in a week, and the anginal attacks have thus far not recurred, and patient smiles now, and is bright. The menses have, however, not appeared, and for this she remains under treatment.

Since this was written a year has elapsed, and the lady is quite well of her angina.

What led me to use *Aurum* was its known affinity for the heart, and the profound melancholy of the patient.

As I said, the cure has been maintained, but the lady keeps some of the *Aurum* powders in the house *for fear*, and thus unconsciously testified to its therapeutic efficacy. The lady had for years used the *nitrite of amyl* with temporary and prompt easement, but the attacks returned just the same, though rather less violently she thought. Although the *nitrite of amyl* will not often cure genuine angina, it does temporarily stop the agony, and may therefore not be despised. Unfortunately, it is too superficial in its action.

I will now pass on to and draw somewhat from my little book entitled *Vacinosis and its Cure by Thuja, with Remarks on Homoeo-prophylaxis*. (XIV 35)

## 245. POST-ORBITAL NEURALGIA OF TWENTY YEARS' STANDING.

This case (which came under observation on January 9, 1882) is one of considerable interest on various accounts. Its subject, a lady of very high rank, over fifty years of age, had been, in turns and for many years, under almost all the leading oculists of London for this neuralgia of the eyes, *i.e.*, terrible pain at the back of the eyes, coming on in paroxysms and confining her to her room for many days together; some attacks would last for six weeks. Some of the neuralgic pain, however, remained at all times. Her eyes had been examined by almost every notable oculist in London, and no one could find anything wrong with them structurally, so it was unanimously agreed and declared to be *neuralgia of the fifth nerve*. Of course, no end of tonics, anodynes, and alteratives had been used. The oculists sent her to the physicians, and these back again to the oculists. The late Dr. Quin and other leading homoeopaths had been tried, but "no one had ever touched it."

Latterly, and for years, she had tried nothing; whenever an attack came on, she would remain in her darkened bedroom, with her head tied up, bewailing her fate. To me she exclaimed, "My existence is one life-long crucifixion!"

I should have stated that the neuralgia was preceded and accompanied by influenza. In the aggregate, these attacks of influenza and post-orbital neuralgia confined her to her room nearly half the year. In appearance she was healthy, well nourished, rather too much *embonpoint*, and fairly vigorous. A friend of hers had been benefited by homoeopathy in my hands, and she therefore came to me "in utter despair."

These are the simple facts of the case, though they look very like piling up the agony! Now for the remedy. The resources of allopathy had been exhausted, and, moreover, I have no confidence in them anyway; homoeopathy — and good homoeopathy too, for the men tried knew their work — had also failed. Do nothing, now much in vogue, had fared no better. I reasoned thus : This lady tells me she has been vaccinated five or six times, and being thus very much vaccinated, she may be just suffering from chronic vaccinosis, one chief symptom of which is a cephalalgia like hers, so I forthwith prescribed *Thuja* 30. It cured, and the cure has lasted till now. The neuralgia disappeared slowly; in about six weeks (February 14, 1882) I wrote in my case-book, "The eyes are well !"

As I have not heard from the patient for some time, I am just writing a note to here to know where the neuralgia has thus far (December 30, 1882) returned. The reply I will add.

Of course, it does *not* follow that because *Thuja* cured this case of neuralgia of some twenty years' standing that *therefore* the lady was suffering from *vaccinosis*; that *Thuja* DID cure it is incontrovertible, and my vaccinosis hypothesis led me to prescribe it. More cannot be maintained. At least, the case must stand as a clinical triumph for *Thuja* 30 — this much is absolute.

In reply to my inquiry, I received the following :

"Jan. 1, 1883.

. . . "I have been in very much stronger health ever since I crossed your threshold, and excepting one or two *attempts* at a return from the enemy, I have been quite free from suffering." . . .

This lady continues well of her post-orbital neuralgia at the time of going to press. After the disappearance of the neuralgia she had several other remedies from me for dyspeptia symptoms.

I shall probably never have a more severe case of what I conceive to be vaccinosis than the one just narrated, or one that had lasted longer. Twenty years may be considered enough to declare it *en permanence*, and its gradual cessation within six weeks from the time of commencing with the *Thuja* stamps it as an undoubted drug-cure.

## 246. NEURALGIC HEADACHE OF NINE YEARS' DURATION.

Miss G ____, aet. 19, came under my care on March 12, 1881, complaining of bad attacks of headache for the past nine years. She said it was as if the back of her head were in a vice, and then it would be frontal, and throbbing as if her head would burst. She was very pale, and her forehead looked shiny and in places brown.

These "head attacks" occurred once or twice a week.

Tendency to constipation; menses regular; and old sty visible on left eyelid; poor appetite; dislikes flesh-meat; liver enlarged a little; had a series of boils in the fall of 1880.

Feet cold; used to have chilblains. For years cannot ride in an omnibus, or in a cab, because of getting pale and sick; skin becomes rough in the wind; lips crack' gets fainty at times.

To have *Graphites* 30.

April 13 — Appetite and spirits better, but otherwise no change; questioned as to the duration of the head attacks, she tells me the last but one continued for three weeks — the last, three days. Over the right eye there is a red, tender patch; *has two or three white-headed pustules* on her face.

Was vaccinated at three months, re-vaccinated at seven years, and again at fourteen. Had *small-pox about ten years ago.*

Thus here was a case that had had small-pox ten years ago, or thereabouts, for she could not quite fix the date, and had been vaccinated three times besides, once subsequent to the small-pox.

$R_x$ Tc. *Thuja occidentalis*, ziv. 3x.

To take five drops in water twice a day.

May 13 — Much better; has only had one very slight headache lasting an hour or two; the frontal tender patch is no longer tender; no further faintness at all. Lips crack. The pustules in the face gone and skin quite clear.

To have *Thuja* 12, one drop at bedtime.

June 17 — Was taken ill yesterday fortnight with soreness of stomach; fever; nausea and perspiration. Subsequently spots broke out like pimples, — eight on the face, one each on the thumb and wrist, one on the foot, and two on the back, — they filled with matter, were out five days, became yellow, and then died away. Her mother says the symptoms were just the same as when patient had the small-pox. Her headaches were well just before this bout came on.

July 1 — Continues well.

July 27 — The headaches have not returned.

February 24, 1882 — The cure holds good, for she has had no headache and is otherwise well. She had subsequently some other remedies for the little tumour on her eyelid and for a small exostosis on lower jaw, but she had received nothing but *Thuja* when the cephalalgia disappeared, and it was two or three weeks before the next medicine followed.

Some months after this date this young lady was brought by her mother merely to show me how well she was, and to take final leave of me. Two years later I learned from her mother that she continued well; so the cure is permanent.

An interesting feature in this case is the curious attack which came on at the beginning of June. My reading of it is that it was really a proving of *Thuja*, or a general organismic reaction called forth by it; and this sent me often up to the thirtieth dilution in my subsequent use of *Thuja*, though I have occasionally found the third decimal dilution answer better than the thirtieth.

But this is not the point of my thesis, for this case was evidently cured by the low dilution, and when the low dilutions cure, and cure promptly, even though not very agreeably, but well, it cannot be necessary to go up any higher, especially as one's faith is sufficiently on the stretch without it. (XIV 44)

## 247. NEURALGIA OF RIGHT EYE

Mr. — , a gentleman of position and means, about fifty years of age, came to consult me on June 28, 1882 for a neuralgia of the right eye. He had come in consequence of the cure of an already recorded case of neuralgia.

He complained of almost constant pain in right eye ever since Christmas 1881, *i.e.*, just about six months. Had had neuralgia in head and shoulders in 1866, and so much morphia had been injected in his shoulders by a doctor in Scotland that it almost killed him : for seven or eight hours it was doubtful if he would recover.

Has a brown, eczematous, itchy (at night) eruption on both shins and between the toes. The neuralgia of right eye, and for which he comes to me is bad both by day and night, but rather worse at night. Mr. (now Sir William) Bowman had examined the eye, and declared it to be neuralgia, the eye being normal. Mr. White Cooper had done the same.

On my inquiring when he was last vaccinated, he seemed completely frightened, and stammered out rapidly, "I should not like to be vaccinated again."

"Why?"
"I was very seedy the last time I was vaccinated; in fact, I felt awfully ill for about a month," and he again hurriedly protested that he would not like to be vaccinted again. The vaccination that had made him so ill was either in 1852 or 1853.
This seemed to me to be a case of vaecinal neuralgia, and therefore I ordered *Thuja* 30 in infrequent dose. This was on the 28th of June 1882.
July 8th — But very little pain after the first powder. To have the same medicine again.
The cure proved permanent, and is interesting as proof of the rapidity with which the *most like* remedy can cure a neuralgia. And, considering how "awfully ill" he had been after his last vaccination, I think it rather probable that this case is an example of vaccinosis. (XIV 49)

## 247. NEURALGIA OF EYES OF NINE YEARS' STANDING

Miss. — , aet. 20, came to me on January 18th, 1883, with various ills. The constipation for which I had treated her had been cured by *Nux* 30 and *Sulphur* 30, but the *Fluor albus* was no better. "But then," said she, "there is the neuralgia in my eyes, which I have had for nine years; nothing has ever touched that." The neuralgia complained of was worse in the morning and at the menstrual period.
*Thuja* 30 (4 in 24). One at night.
I saw her no more till the 8th of December 1883, when she called, complaining of too frequent and too profuse menstruation.
"What about the neuralgia?"
"Oh ! that is cured; I have not had it since those powders."
Was this a case of vaccinosis?
Patient had been twice vaccinated, and the second time was when she was 15 years old, when it did *not take*. I do not feel so sure that this was a case of vaccinosis, because patient was re-vaccinated unsuccessfully *after* this neuralgia began, and, besides, her mother died of epithelioma, so it may have been merely a case of *sycosis Hahnemanni*. The only certain thing about it is that the neuralgia had lasted nine years, and disappeared after the giving of the *Thuja*.
This strikingly curative action of the *arbor vitoe* in vaccinosic neuralgia is sometimes prevented from being effective by being masked with another taint, as the following will exemplify, and this will also show us why a series of remedies may often be needed before the neuralgia will depart. (XIV 53)

### 249. NEURALGIA OF EYES OF TWENTY-FIVE YEARS' STANDING, CHRONIC HEADACHE, CONSTIPATION, AND DYSPEPSIA

On July 16, 1882, a lady, 68 years of age, wife of an eminent allopathic physician came (importuned by some of her lady friends, I believe) to see if homoeopathy could cure her neuralgia and dyspepsia. The headaches were life-long; she could not remember ever being without them on and off. But she did not come on their account, regarding them as absolutely beyond medical art. She, however, hoped the dyspepsia, the constipation, and, maybe, the neuralgia might be helped in some measure. The neuralgia was violent, was very violent in the eyes, wave-like in intensity, rarely entirely absent, so that her life was a torture. This ocular neuralgia had sent her to Liebreich, Bader, and Bowman, who all agreed that it was "from her general state." This eye neuralgia began twenty-five years ago after worry and trouble; is worse at night, reading for two minutes bringing it on, and hence she has not read for seventeen years. She had been vaccinated as a child successfully, but her mother, not trusting it, had her subsequently inoculated for small-pox, but it did not take, and neither of the three subsequent vaccinations took, the last one being twenty-five years since. The neuralgia is deep in and screwing, the pain going back seemingly into the brain. Her headache is right across the forehead from temple to temple.
*Thuja occidentalis* 30, infrequently.
July 29 — No change.
*Cyclamen Europ.* 3x. Five drops in water three times a day.
August 19 — Has now a rash on her skin, and there is much acidity.
*Nux. vom.* 30 and *Sul.* 30.
September 21 — Rash very bad and severely itching. Constipation and dyspepsia a good deal better. *Thuja* C.
October 12 — Neuralgia *much* better; constipation well; is tormented and irritated most unbearably with the skin eruption; "the itching is intolerable, it is a torment !" exclaimed the lady. So bad was it that patient did not wish to go on with the treatment.
Omit all medicine.
October 24 — Bowels normal; skin better. The eruption had been deep-seated, in clusters of raised lumps, some the size of half a pea. The skin remains discoloured.
No medicine.
November 21 — Headaches are better; the neuralgia vastly improved; more appetite, but still a good deal of dyspepsia. *Thuja* C. And thus the treatment went on intermittently till September 1, 1884, when patient

was practically well. I say practically, and by that I mean that patient did not consider herself in any real need of further treatment for her now relatively trifling suffering. (XIV 56)

## 250. THE NEURALGIA OF THUJA OCCIDENTALIS

*By Robert T. Cooper, M.D., Phys. Dis. of Ear, London Homoeopathic Hospital.*

On mentioning to Dr. Burnett that I was at one time in the habit of prescribing *Thuja* for neuralgia, he asked me to report any cases by me. This I am extremely delighted to do, if for no other reason than that it will be a testimony to the accuracy of Dr. Burnett's observations, so admirably and scientifically laid before us in his little work on *Vaccinosis*.

**Case I** — Elizabeth Thomas, a woman of 72, came to me, September 22, 1868, in Southampton, with *face-ache,* attended with much soreness of the face after the pain had gone away. Pains have continued night and day for the last two months : come in paroxysms at never more than an hour's interval. Unable to masticate food from the pain occasioned; gums are very sore, and side of the face is very sore when she attempts to lie on it; feels then a throbbing in it. Pains are aggravated by lying on the other side as well; the slightest pressure causes a feeling of soreness. The pain extends all over the *right* side of the face and head; when very violent, it shoots to the opposite side. Is worse in a very cold or very warm room; does not dare to venture into a draught. Her teeth are decayed, and the pains shoot up from these; are equally violent when sitting or standing; they come "all of a sudden," and leave her equally suddenly; sometimes they shoot into the ear; attempting to read or think brings them on. Had much fatigue while nursing her sick husband last year; has taken calomel, ginger brandy, and various kinds of herbs.

*Thuja Occ.*, 12th dec., a pilule three times a day.

Sept. 29 — Has been much better; can now rest all night; occasionally a few twitches, but nothing like it was, although the weather has been unusually cold.

The above we may fairly name *neuralgic alveolar periostitis*. As the teeth were in no way interfered with, nor any change prescribed in her mode of living, we may fairly ascribe the assuagement of the pain to *Thuja*. (XIV 61)

**Case 2** — On the same day (September 22, 1868), Harriett Sheppard, a woman of 54, came to me with violent pains under her right shoulder, going through to the breast and down to the elbow; worse in the

morning, getting out of bed, and when walking. *Soreness in the hepatic region; urine very fetid*. Has had these symptoms a week.
*Thuja Occ*. 3, seven drops to go over a week.
September 29 — Has had diarrhoea the last few days. Pains in the shoulders and soreness of liver gone, Continue.
October 7 — Still relaxed; urine not so fetid; much pain in stomach after meals, with passage by bowel of undigested food. This last symptoms yielded at once to *China* Q. In this case, it is possible the diarrhoea may have been spontaneous, and, alone, may have relieved the congested liver; at any rate, the pains ceased upon her taking *Thuja*.
As to whether these, or the next case, had anything to do with vaccination, I am not in a position to determine. (XIV 64)
**Case 3** — Anne C., aged 21, neuralgia for three weeks, came to me Sept. 17, 1869. Complexion florid and clear; hair dark; sclerotics yellowish. Complains of great weakness, with pains in the right side of the face and head — begin in decayed teeth, and extend up the side of the head and down the neck. She feels feverish when the pain is severe, and the parts throb; is worse on meditation. Relieved by application of hot things — mustard, for example.
Much tenderness in different parts of the face and behind the ear; aggravation from drinking anything cold; is worse at night, but keeps on in the day as well.
Four weeks ago, weaned her baby, and menorrhagia set in, which ceased just before these pains set in.
In this case, *Nux vomica* 30x, *China* 12x, *Merc sol*. 3x, *Sulph*. Q, *Silicea* 30, and *Staphisagria* were given at different times, but without any positive relief.
It is unnecessary to reproduce each report, but that of 1st Dec. had better (taking *Silicea* 30); last monthly natural. Facial pain very bad, in fact worse — worse now in day-time; teeth very painful; gums pale, with inflamed dental margins; pains come from the teeth.
*Staphisag*. 3x.
Dec. 17 — Was better for a time, but last two days and nights pains very severe and continuous; same side, gums painful.
*Thuja Occ*. 12x.
Jan. 5, 1869 — Has not been so well as at present the pains in face have left her; has some pains in chest when inspiring, and legs ache towards evening.
Appetite wonderfully improved, and can drink anything without inconvenience. This last case we may term *Rheumatic Alveolar Periostitis*.
It is true that Dr. Cooper does not vouch for the vaccinosic origin of his cases, but his cures corroborate my statement that the working out of

the homoeopathic equation and my theory of vaccinosis alike lead to *Thuja*. (XIV 65)

## 251. NEURALGIA OF LEFT BROW OF OVER THIRTY YEARS' STANDING CURED BY CUPRUM ACETICUM

I have lately cured a lady of fifty years of age of a very severe neuralgia of the left brow, which had plagued her for thirty-four years. For years I had seen this lady for metrorrhagia and other ailings, and with much acknowledged benefit. *Juglans regia* and *Juglans cinerea, Sanguinaria canadensis, Heloninum, China, Arnica, Thuja, Psorinum,* and *Nat. mur.*, I find noted as those remedies which had confessedly been of more or less benefit. But it was Rademacher's tincture of copper that *cured* the old neuralgic enemy that at times was described as boring, screwing, but more generally the lady spoke of the pain as *awful*. Whether the *Cuprum* here acted on the basis of the Paracelsic Universalia, of which it is one, or by reason of its homoeopathicity, I am unable to say. (XIV 69)
The first, Mrs. E., a woman over 40, whose mother was gout crippled, and died of gouty peritonitis. She has had many attacks; now they are few, slight, and medicine has remarkably controlled them. I have seen her in some; the face is pale, head thrown back, pulse feeble, surface cold, neck stiff and painful. Her state is nearly one of insensibility. On one of these occasions she was nauseated, and phlegm threatened to choke her. *Ant. tart.* 2x, trit., second dose, at a few minutes interval, relieved her, and allowed her to resume the recumbent position. Her younger sister has gout in the hands. Her mother was drugged to death years before I attended her, and after electric baths ptyalism set in. For a time Mrs. E. was relieved by *Amyl nit.* 1x and olfaction of the crude; but her marked distress was precordial coldness, frightful pain, stiffness of the neck. She had *Juglans cinerea* 1x; the 2x did not do the same, and twice she proved it; two-drop doses at short intervals; and when relief came, which was speedy, a dose night and morning for a few days. Her restoration to health, vigour, and good action of the heart from a weak, miserable one, is a great change to her, and astonishment to friends. Her life is now enjoyable; she takes her medicine with her, and goes to Devonshire without fear." (XIV 71)

## 252. NEURALGIA AFTER SHINGLES

This is often extremely tedious, wearing, and difficult of cure indeed, outside of homoeopathy it can hardly be said to be curable at all. Some years since, I was hurriedly summoned to the country house of a middle-aged lady, who had finally decided to "give homoeopathy a chance!" This was done not for the sake of homoeopathy all the same, but because said lady had had *herpes zoster*, and the sequential neuralgia was atrocious, and unyielding to all her various physicians' more or less violent means. *Phosphorus* made very short work of the neuralgia, and thus brought about a violent conversion of the patient to homoeopathy. She became a homoeopath because the pathy of the homoeopaths was the means of curing her neuralgia. And in my judgement a very sound reason too. That is just my reason for being a homoeopath. I like homoeopathy because it affords a splendid *means to an end*, and that end a ____ cure. (XIV 73)

## 253. CASE OF ANGINA PECTORIS.

A good while since, an old patient of the late Dr. Hilbers, 62 years of age, came under my care for painful spasms of the heart (*neuralgia cordis*), running principally down or up the left arm, often after walking quickly. He was wont to pass a great quantity of water, having to rise many times in the night for that purpose. His tongue was cracked, which is a capital clinical indication for the horsetail, and positive indications from the heart itself being absent, I gave *Equisetum hyemale* 1, ten drops in water three times a day. This seemingly rather unlikely remedy did him so much good that he continued to take it on his own account for three months, and then I put him under *Bellis perennis*. So pleased was my patient with the result of his treatment that he sent me a well-known book, for which he is responsible, as a token of gratitude, though himself I have not since seen. This gentleman had long been taking antispasmodics to no avail. (XIV 85)

## 254. SICK HEADACHE

Mrs. H., a very fleshy lady, aet. 50 nearly passed the climacteric, complained of a distressing "sick headache" hanging about her for years. In some degree the symptoms were almost always present. A typical headache would commence in the forenoon, gathering violence with the hours until sunset, when it would quiety subside, or else would confine her to her bed for a day or two. The pains, which originated low in the occiput, drawing upwards in rays, located over the right, sometimes the left eye, attended with vomiting, often of bilious matter. She was subject to sudden flushes of heat, burning of the soles of the feet, and that singular symptom noted in Hale's third edition, "a quickly diffused transient thrill," felt at the remotest extremity. At times she had sensible throbbing of every pulse in the body. The urine was generally scanty before and during the severe headache, but quantities of clear urine would pass away when getting better. Prescribed *Sanguinaria* 200, six pellets night and morning, for a week. Eight months afterwards patient reported relief from the first dose, during the week complete relief, and from that time until now not a vestige of the old complaint has shown itself. — *Dr. J. P. Mills.* (XIV 107)

## 255. SUN HEADACHES

Dr. Mills regards what he calls "sun headahces" that is, those increasing in violence with the sun's ascent, decreasing as it declines, when preceded by *scanty urine* and pass off attended by *profuse flow of clear urine*, as indicating *Sanguinaria*, and the *urine symptoms* as its *keynote*, giving the following case as an additional illustration : Mr. W., railroad engineer, was taken early in the morning with headache and nausea, the symptoms increasing hour by hour. At 4 P.M. the pain and distress had reached such a height that, fearing "brain fever," I was summoned. I found the patient on the bed groaning and writhing in agony, face very red, head hot, injected eyes, sensitive to light. The arteries about the head and in the scalp were distended like whip-cords, the blood coursing through them at a furious rate, giving a sensation to the head as if the scalp and temples were alive with irrepressible pulsations. The pain was over the whole head; paroxysms of retching occurred every few minutes, with such violence that I feared rupture of blood vessels. I prescribed *Bell.*, *Glon.*, and *Bry.* in succession, but without benefit, not thinking at first of *Sanguinaria*, though I was aware that the headaches passed off with free flow of clear urine, and that he, being an engineer, would be subject to kidney trouble. At midnight a messenger came, saying that Mr. W. was wildly delirious, with no abatement of symptoms. I sent *Sanguinaria* 200, to be given in water every half hour. Fifteen minutes after the first dose, symptoms began to abate; in an hour and a half, he fell into a quiet slumber for a little time, awaking quite relieved from the acute pain, but an intense soreness continued for two or three days, which compelled him to keep quiet or to walk with great circumspection. — *Idem.* (XIV 109)

## 256. NEURALGIA

Miss. T., aet. 36, had suffered from periodical attacks of left-sided hemicrania for upwards of nine years. The attacks set in early every summer, and continued to recur regularly about every two weeks, lasting each time about three days, and compelling her during that time to exclude herself from society. The paroxysms, which set in just after sunrise in the morning, were of the most violent character, causing severe pulsating pains in the left temple and eye, and reaching their greatest intensity about noon, when they were attended, with vomiting and retching, after which they gradually declined, and at sunset gave place to anxious and disturbed sleep. The slightest motion or noise greatly aggravated the headache; even the movement of the eyes would increase it. After the paroxysms subsided the scalp felt sore to the touch, and the brain confused. After trying two or three other remedies without any marked benefit, I placed her upon *Spigelia* 30, five pellets every night and morning for one week. No more paroxysms occurred until July of the following year, when the remedy was repeated : four years later she remained quite well. This is a brilliant cure. (XIV 112)

## 257. TRIFACIAL NEURALGIA

Some years ago, a patient who had long been the victim of obstinate trifacial neuralgia had all the affected nerves excised by Nelaton. The operation only gave temporary relief, and the patient declared she would commit suicide. By the advice of Debout *Aconitia* was tried, and after five milligrammes had been taken, she was permanently relieved. In another patient, who had suffered agonies night and day, six milligrammes completely dissipated the disease. (XIV 121)

## 258. POST HERPETIC NEURALGIA

"Mrs. S. ____, an old lady of 70, suffered from herpes zoster a year ago. She avers that she is still never free night or day from a distressing aching pain in the parts which were affected (ear, neck, and shoulder). The pain does not now shoot and sting as it used to at first, but is rather an unbearable ache. Her nerve pains did not begin with any severity till the herpes spots were healing. This statement applies only to her skin, for the first symptom which drew her attention to the eruption was a severe pain in the ear. She asserts that she has had earache ever since. I saw her in the first instance on June 16, 1889, at her own house, when she was just recovering from influenza. She was then in bed, and suffering so much from the herpes after pain, that she could not bear to be examined, and could scarcely speak to me. Since that she has visited me several times. She is a cheerful person, inclined to make the best of things, and she has now regained very fair health, but her complaints about the pain are incessant, and she will sit and weep during her visit to me. She says that it entirely prevents sleep at nights, and compares it to a gimlet boring into the ear. From the ear it passes down to the clavicle and tip of shoulder.

"This is perhaps the most severe case that I have seen, but I have observed not a few which closely approach it. I have known several in which herpetic after-pains made the remainder of the patient's life a state of misery. They were all in old persons. *Qunine* and *Aconite* are the most useful remedies, but I have had no triumphs. (XIV 134)

## 259. LIGHTNING PAINS

On the June 28, 1892, a London clergyman, fifty-five years of age, of rufous constitution, came to consult me in regard to certain pains in the left foot and left thigh. These pains were irrespective of period, had existed for "a long time," *i.e.*, months, and were getting worse. While sitting before me in my consulting room he repeatedly twitched with his leg, and writhed with the pain, his face at the same time becoming contorted. These pains he described as "awful agony" and "like lightning." Otherwise patient was fairly well; a patch of erythrasma on left thigh.

*Bacill*. 30.

July 15 — There was at first furious exacerbations of the pains, and now they have gone altogether.

August 9 — No return of the lightning pains.

January 5, 1893 — Coming on this date in regard to his son . . . "Oh, no ! thank God, these pains have never returned."

What led me to such a prescription as *Bacill*. for foudroyant pains? Well, not tradition at any rate. My reasons were these : 1*st*, Total absence of any venereal historic datum. 2*nd*, Patient is of rufous constitution. 3*rd*, Collaterals of patient have died of phthisis. 4*th*, His descendants have been treated by me for phthisis. 5*th*, Patient had already had the advantage of our usual remedies from his own homoeopathic physician, and hence it was desirable to go out of thc beaten track. (XIV 140)

## 260. SEVERE INTER-COSTAL NEURALGIA OF SEVEN YEARS' DURATION

A lady, sixty-two years of age, came under my observation on November 26, 1890, for a terrible neuralgia of the left side of the trunk, just behind the spleen and the base of the left lung. The pain was most severe, and described as of a screwing character. During the past seven years patient has been going from one doctor to another, and finally on this day came to me most unwillingly and in sheer despair, driven hither by a severe attack then on. These attacks were not well defined as to time, but they were distinctly intermittent, and started as a small pain, going on *crescendo*, and eventually passing off *decrescendo*. Patient had been three times vaccinated; and, moreover, she tells me she once had true cow-pox, caught from a cow. Patient has been about a great deal in the world, and though very strong she has had a great many diseases, she enumerating to me measles, whooping-cough, chicken-pox, scarlet fever, South American fever (ague cured by *Quinine*), yellow fever, jaundice, and rheumatic fever. All things considered, I was of opinion that it was a malarial splenalgia, and so prescribed *Urtica urens* Q, 10 drops in water three times a day. This was November 26.

December 16 — Only one attack of pain; appetite much better. "The medicine roused me and made me tremble." The patient looks quite a different woman.

January 16, 1891 — No attack; considers herself quite cured. "I am also not so cold, and do not feel the cold so much as I did."

There was no further attack of neuralgia till the month of November 1891, which was, however, not very severe, and the same remedy in half the dose was quickly efficacious, Then in July 1892 there was a threatening again but it came to nothing, and there has been no further return of the neuralgia whatever.

I name this in the headline Intercostal Neuralgia, because that was what her numerous other physicians had treated her for. My own conception of the nature of the case is expressed in the name *Malarial Splenalgia*. (XIV 142)

## 261. SPLENALGIA OF TEN YEARS' DURATION

An army man, retired, fifty-three years of age, came to consult me in August 1891 for a pain at the same place as in the last-named case. The spleen was very slightly enlarged. There was a very slight endocardial bruit, best heard at apex — best during the diastole; sensation of pins and needles down the left arm. Cold water drunk caused fearful pains across the chest (angina pectoris — neuralgia cordis), Patient suffered from ague for years. The same remedy as in the previous case quite cured him, and he was discharged cured on October 21, 1891. There were two small relapses several months apart, but the *Urtica* promptly cured them, and patient continues well. The endocardial murmur, however, remains. (XIV 145)

## 262. ANGINA PECTORIS WITH CARDIAC INADEQUACY CURED BY STARVATION-DIET

A London merchant of forty odd years of age, came under my care some three years ago for angina pectoris and blood-spitting, starting a few weeks previously from violent exertion when he was romping with his children. Patient was plethoric. Blood oozed up constantly into his mouth from his bronchial tubes. Lungs quite sound. Heart floundering rapidly and without rhythm. My remedies did no good; allopathic remedies did not better, and all hope was abandoned. At this stage his business partner came to me to know if I could think of anything further that might yet offer a chance of saving the patient's most valuable life, I having formerly told him of a heart case I once cured by semi-starvation. I gave as my opinion, based on some experience, that a starvation-diet offered the only remaining chance of saving the patient's life. His heart had become absolutely inadequate, only just keeping up life by fearful overwork, and as there was no means of making it adequate to the bulk and blood-mass, the only conceivable outway was to starve down the bulk and blood quantity till the heart had a chance of recovering itself and doing less work adequately. He clearly saw the point, and hastened to convince patient and his surroundings. My starvation plan was carried out, and by the time the patient had become much reduced in bulk, and had much less blood, the angina and haemorrhage quite disappeared, and the heart completely recovered itself, though very slowly, and patient returned to business, and there continues, "as well as he ever was." (XIV 154)

## 263. ANGINA PECTORIS CURED BY PHYTOLACCA DECANDRA Q, ETC. - 1

A gentleman from the north, aged about sixty years, consulted me for angina pectoris on June 28, 1891. The left lobe of his liver being enlarged, I gave him a month of *Carduus marianus* Q.

August 11 — Pain not so acute : the pain runs across the chest into the right shoulder; he is puffy, and walking and talking bring on the pain.

$R_x$ *Bellis perennis* Q, ten drops in water at bedtime.

September 7 — So much better; all pain gone. His wife wrote : "I believe it (the *Bellis*) has done my husband a great deal of good, as he has not complained of pain for some time now."

October 13 — There is again some pain.

Repeat the *Bellis*.

October 27 — No angina, though he has been walking a good deal, even uphill.

November 17 — No angina; but there is a constant pain near the right clavicle, and some under the left ribs, and the spleen is somewhat swelled.
*Urtica urens* Q, eight drops in water night and morning.
December 22 — The angina has returned badly.
Repeat the *Bellis*.
January 28, 1892 — Much better all along the line, but he still gets a good deal of pain behind the breast-bone.
*Arnica* 1.
March 2 — Gone back, and has the angina now every day, and at times badly at night right behind the sternum.
$R_x$ *Bacill.* CC.
April 1 — Certainly feels better, but complains of getting so fat.
*Phytolacca decandra* Q (from the berries.).
May 13, 1893. — Almost well of his angina.
*Rep.*
August 18 — Been quite well.
May 19, 1893 — Continues well.
May 1894 — His son tells me his father continues quite well, and is abroad on business. (XIV 158)

## 264. ANGINA PECTORIS - 2

The wife of the foregoing patient went last year to a certain wellknown hydropathic establishment and had Turkish baths, and finding that the attendant or masseuse was a sufferer from angina pectoris, and was thus very painfully incommoded in her daily work, told her of her husband's cure of the same affection by the writer. Said masseuse very shortly afterwards came to consult me on her own account; her sufferings were considerable, and all the more serious considering the nature of her occupation. Patient had no discoverable lesion, but she was fleshy, somewhat stout, and of laxfibre. I ordered her the *Phytolacca*, and two months' use of it has seemingly cured her. The case is recent, so I cannot tell whether it is only relieved or lastingly cured. In any case she has now no pain, and her health and spirits have very notably improved. (XIV 161)

## 265. ANGINA PECTORIS OF LONG STANDING

Years ago — eight or nine — a staff-officer brought his wife to me for angina pectoris that had embittered her life for years. None of the means tried had done any good, and a cure was not asked for or expected. I found both spleen and liver swelled; patient had lived long in India, and had had fever and liver trouble there off and on. At first I made no headway with the case, as I used *Aurum* and other cardiacs and our usual myotics. I then used splenics on account of the malarial history, and because of a pain under the left ribs. The angina was notably relieved.

Noticing one day that her soft palate was very icteric, I gave hepatics,— the one that acted promptly and brilliantly being *Hydrastis canadensis* in small material doses. After its use the angina receded into the background, being complained of only occasionally, and now for sometime not at all. In this case the angina seemed a synalgia starting at one time from the spleen, at another from the liver and spleen, at another from the liver, and once in a way from the pit of the stomach, and in the last case *Prunus virginiana* Q promptly cleared the matter up. I saw the case many times and prescribed various remedies, and thus satisfied myself of the synalgic nature of the angina, and that its point of origin was always below the diaphragm, sometimes in the right hypochondrium and sometimes in the left, and occasionally from the pit of the stomach. *Viscum album* is a notable remedy, and has its place in the treatment of angina pectoris. There are certain cases of angina that are synalgiae, starting from given points in the abdomen, sometimes from one ovary, at times from both ovaries, and at others from *beneath* the spleen, rather than from the organ itself. In several of such cases *Viscum album* 1x has helped me. (XIV 162)

# ON FISTULA

## 266. RECURRENT CIRCUMANAL ABSCESS

On May 22, 1882, a married London merchant, thirty seven years of age, called to consult me in regard to recurrent fistula and circumanal abscess. He related to me that eighteen months previously he got an abscess at the seat, which his surgeon lanced and treated, and in the end pronounced as cured. Cured it was, in the surgeon's opinion; he was quite honest in this expressed opinion, but you might as well say that when you have plucked the apples from your apple-trees in the autumn, you have cured the said apple-trees of apple-bearing, for, although the surgeon had "cured" the abscess he had not cured the patient of his power to produce more fistula-leading absceses, inasmuch as the disease had returned each subsequent spring and fall. And this is really the point I am contending for, viz : The abscess at the seat with its sequential fistula is not disease in its real essence, but only its local expression in the anal region. Not being satisfied with his "cure", patient had consulted other surgeons, in all three, for his anal trouble, and all three alike lanced and poulticed, and still it came afresh. On examination I found he was suffering from an incomplete external fistula that had also just been diagnosed by a noted specialist for diseases of the rectum who had lately seen it, and urged the imperative necessity of cutting it at once.

Patient had a good deal of acne on his shoulders and neck, the eruption often showing white, mattery heads. He had only been vaccinated once, and that as a baby. Has had often and many little indolent boils in the nape.

$R_x$ *Kali carbonicum* 30.

June 12 — He is much better; the opening of the fistula is now about the size of a split pea.

$R_x$ *Psorinum* 30 in very infrequent doses.

July 16 — He is not so comfortable at the anus, and the fistula seems more active.

To have *Thuja occidentalis* 30 in very infrequent doses.

September 19 — There is great improvement in the anal trouble and the skin of his neck and shoulders and nape is much healthier and clearer.

To have *Mercurius corrosivus* in the same strength as the Kali, Psorinum and Thuja.

Jan. 15, 1883 — Fistula well, but there are still blind boils in his skin.

To have *Aqua silicata,* which finished the cure.

But in the autumn of 1883 another abscess formed, when the same kind of treatment, together with *Arctium lappa., Calcarea carbonica,* etc., was helpful. And finally, in the spring of 1884, patient paid me three visits with what might be called the last faint flickerings of his fistula disease. Since then ten years have elapsed, and there has been no return, and no attempt at a return, and patient continues otherwise in excellent health. This I know, because he lately brought his wife to me for another matter relating to her health, when I gathered the fact just narrated. (XVI 8)

## 267. SIMPLE FISTULA

The most simple form, however, in which fistula comes before one is where the subjects are seemingly in good health, and in whom the whole thing can be cured by medicines in two or three months. Thus a gentlemen of some forty-six years of age, hale and hearty to all appearance, consulted me for fistula-in-ano that had plagued him for a number of months. An operation had been decided upon, and assented to by the gentleman, but as he was not exactly ill, and was, moreover, over head and ears in big affairs, he constantly put it off.

It never occurred to him even that medicines were any good in such cases; his own surgeon said they were not, and that was enough. The fouling discharge was the only thing that really inconvenienced him, with a certain amount of local irritation, and a little blood once in a way. But it did not heal, and one day he met with a gentleman, an old friend of his own, and whom I had cured of severe fistula several years previously; the result was that he came to me. Under *Hydrastis canadensis* Q he got quite well in a little less than two months. No local application of any kind was used. He was the more pleased at his rapid cure as he was about to marry at the time, and a fistula is not desirable under such circumstances. (XVI 12)

## 269. PERENNIAL ABSCESS

I shall not easily forget a gentleman I once attended for perennial abscess, in which the pains were extremely severe. Troubles about the anus are, in my experience, for the most part distressing ones, even if only slight. Well, this gentleman, in my judgment, was ridding his organism of a tuberculous tendency by means of this perennial abscess, i.e., the organism was brimming over at the part to save the lungs, so I was particularly anxious not to have the abscess interfered with, for I have noticed that cutting open immature abscesses is no gain; they simply go on "sweating", for double the time it would have taken to heal had the abscesses been allowed to mature in their own way. But he really could not bear the pain; when I applied limewater rags, with the result that the pain became a mere nothing, and patient forthwith had a beautiful sleep. He made a capital recovery, and fistula was prevented. The principal remedies used were *Aconite, Silicea, Hepar, Calc. sulphurica,* and *China;* with one or two subsequently given constitutional remedies, foremost being *Kali carb.* 30 and *Lappa major* Q. (XVI 15)

## 270. GASTRITIS

For the relief of the pain of acute gatherings I have very great confidence in limewater rags. I have often felt very thankful to this excellent practical tip that I first learned of Dr. George Wyld, of London, and if my reading memory does not deceive me, it was a favourite little clinical knack of no less a man than Theophrastus Von Hohenheim, commonly called Paracelsus, and splendid friend in need it is. I once had a case of gastritis near Hyde Park that resisted all my remedies, and began to look very ugly

indeed, when I applied abdominal compresses, saturated with *Liquor calcis*. P. B. and frequently changed.
Patient had a good sleep within two hours, and returned home to her friends in the country within a week. (XVI 16)

## 271. FISTULA IN ANO

Dr. Kidd ("Laws of Therapeutics", p. 174) shows that whether we profess homoeopathy or not, we require its teachings to cure our patients. He says : Fistula-in-ano cured by dilute *Nitric acid*. Mr. B., of a dark sallow complexion (note the unhealthy skin), aged 42, applied to me for a fistula-in-ano, which had existed for nearly a year, and which two of the best London surgeons agreed must be operated upon, saying it could not be cured without operation. He complained of soreness and burning pain in the lower bowel; a thin greenish discharge flowed freely from the fistula. I (Dr. Kidd) prescribed eight drops of dilute *Nitric acid* in a wine-glass of water three times a day, without any local treatment. This perfectly and permanently cured the fistula in two months. (XVI 17)
Then Dr. Kidd gives (p. 175) the following : Fistula-in-ano cured by *Hydrastis canadensis*. — Mr. L., aged 46, a Greek merchant came to me suffering from fistula-in-ano, which had existed for three months. A well-known specialist and the family medical attendant assured him that he could not be cured without operation. Unwilling to submit to this he came to me. I prescribed ten drops of the tincture of *Hydrastis canadensis* in water, night and morning, also a compress over the fistula of four drachms of tincture of *Hydrastis* to four ounces of water, applied on cotton wool, night and day. To his great delight this perfectly cured him in a month." As our author gives no data or dates we cannot judge of the cases for ourselves, but they serve my purposes for quoting them, viz. to show that homoeopathy enables her followers to cure fistula medicinally. And *Hydrastis* (as well as Hydrastin) is well known in the United States as possessing power over fistula-in-ano, and it is thence that we have both the remedy and our knowledge of it. (XVI 18)

## 272. FISTULA

A stout, middle-aged merchant came to me on April 20, 1887, for fistula-in-ano. His local medical man had got the fistula to heal by local and topic measures, but the uneasiness of the anal region was even greater than before. Patient had for long been subject to boils, but had had no complaints, except measles and scarlatina in his childhood. From the fact that he had a good deal of pustula acne on certain parts of the body and also taking into account the fact that he had been twice vaccinated, I thought it likely that vaccinosis lay at the root of the disease expressed at the anus.

The first remedy given was *Thuja occidentalis* 30, which was followed by a small lump at the part where the fistula had healed up : really it evidently was not. And there was another abscess just beginning. I then gave him *Bellis perennis* 1, five drops in water night and morning, and he thereafter had *Hepar sulphur* 3x, *Silicea* 6th trituration, and *Kali carbonica* 30, was then discharged perfectly cured. All the sclerosed circumanal tissue had become quite healthy, and his old eczema had also disappeared.

And I would remark that the consentaneous disappearance of the eczema stamps the cure as like the disease, i.e., general and constitutional. (XVI 20)

## 273. FISTULA

In Ruckert's "Klinische Erfahrungen" I find *Silicea** takes a very high rank.

1. A boy, two years and half old, was to have been operated on for fistula, but two doses of *Silicea* cured it within three weeks — Altmuller.
2. A tender-skinned, fair-haired young man, in whom scabies had been twice got rid of with ointments, and who had been twice rid of gonorrhoea by injections, got an abscess in the perinaeum, near the anus that had been opened surgically, but this would not heal up. The consequence was a fistula of the anus, accompanied with debility, emaciation, cough, and fever. Large doses of *China* were given him in vain. His general condition was much ameliorated by *Sulphur*, and in about a week there was a tickling sensation at the aperture of the fistula, with an increased discharge of pure pus. *Sulphur* was repeated every sixth day. Afterwards three doses of *Silicea*, whereupon the fistula was completely cured within three weeks from the time of its being first administered.

Here again we have the causal treatment in the first place — the prime antipsoric for psora. (XVI 30)

* Silicea was a favourite remedy with Hahnemann himself for fistula.

## 274. CASE OF FISTULA-IN-ANO

On May 17, 1889, an unmarried city gentleman, thrity years of age, came under my observation for fistula-in-ano. Four or five years previously he had an abscess on the edge of the anus. It burst and healed. Fourteen months ago another one in the same spot. It burst with the aid of poulticings, and healed up (?), some moisture and blood ooze thereforom ever since. Patient is dusky and delicate looking. On examination, I found a small opening

to an incomplete fistula. He also complained of "feverishness" and indigestion.
$R_x$ Tc. *Pyrogenium* 5, five drops in water night and morning.
May 31 — "I am much better." How do you know?
"Because the sweating at my seat that I had had so many years has gone."
Complains that in warm weather he is apt to get dry eczema of the hands.
Since taking the *Pyrogenium* his skin has assumed a cleaner aspect.
*Thuja* 30 in infrequent dose.
June 29 — Discharged thick matter and blood soon after beginning with the powders. The fistula still discharges, and there is a good deal of sclerosed tissue at its bottom and around it. Patient is dusky and drowsy.
$R_x$ *Nux vomica* 1, five drops in water night and morning.
August 7 — Perfectly well of ihe fistula, and of the circumjacent telar sclerosis. Just before the fistula began to heal up definitely, a small calculus — hard and sharp size of a pea — was passed from it with much pain, or rather it pained very much, and on feeling the part he discovered the calculus formation and removed it, and brought it to me. (XVI 38)

## 275. FISTULA IN ANO AND CHEST

A city gentleman, single, thrityfive years of age, came to me on March 4, 1889, for fistula-in-ano and chest. He informed me that he had had much expectoration of phlegm all his life, but for the past two years the same had become bloody. For a number of years, under homoeopathic treatment with benefit, he had maintained his ground, and even gained a little in strength and bulk. Present weight ten stone. I found his throat studded with tubercles, his lungs very flat, vocal resonance much increased at both apices, and all down the left side of the throat; he is very short-winded, coughs and expectorates almost incessantly; his skin is dingy, dusky and greasy; the glands of his neck hard, though small; the phlegm is thick, yellow-green. For the past two years has been suffering from fistula. Under my treatment the old fistula dried up, but then (Ap. 9) a new one formed on the other side. Previously he had been twice cut for fistula. This needless torture I was able to spare him.
April 29 — "Perineal abscess reopened, burst, discharged very freely, and has now all healed."
May 13 — Fistula quite well.
August 9 — Fistula continues well. Patient himself much better and stronger, and remains under tretment for his throat and chest. Patient received some nosodes — *Thuja* 30, *Hydrastis can*. O, *Nux vomica* 1x, and *Dulcamara* Q. (XVI 40)

## 276. FISTULA IN AN INFANT

On June 23, 1879, a country gentleman brought his little six-year old son to me for fistula-in-ano. At its birth the nurse discovered a lump at the seat. A little time afterwards this gathered and burst like a boil, and had continued ever since to gather and burst at intervals, The right eye had no lashes; he had severe ophthalmia tarsi of the same eye — also ever since he was born.

An examination of the anal region showed a fistula external and incomplete, and numerous scars where others had healed.

The right nostril was also chronically inflamed. If he gets a thorn or splinter in his flesh, it festers as does equally the tiniest scratch or prick. A connexion between eye and fistula is noticed, for when the eye is very bad the anus gets better, and conversely.

$R_x$ Tc. *Phos* 30, three drops in water night and morning.

July 24 — The eye-lashes are beginning to grow.

$R_x$ Tc. *Kali carb.* 30

October 20 — Fistula cured. His nose bothers him a good deal, becoming very much inflamed. There is considerable mattery discharge from the eye.

$R_x$ *Aurum foliatum,* 3 trituration, four grains dry on the tongue twice a day.

January 15, 1880 — Fistula continues well; nose well; eye better; lashes perceptibly growing.

Repeat the *Aurum foliatum,* but in the fourth centesimal trituration, four grains at bed-time only.

July 25, 1881 — Fistula and nose continue well; there is now quite a show of eye-lashes; still some ophthalmia tarsi, however. Around the meatus of the left eye there is some eczema.

$R_x$ *Psorin.* 30 in frequent dose, and there after *Thuja occidentalis* 30 in like manner.

Discharged quite cured.

Four years later he was again brought but this time for enlarged tonsils, which our ordinary remedies slowly (not rapidly) cured, and then he was reported well, and I again ascertained that he was well in all respects in February 1894. (XVI 41)

## 277. PILES, PERINEAL ABSCESSES, AND FISTULA

One certainly meets with a goodly number of cases of fistula in portly men about forty years of age. Such a one, a dark gentlman, forty-one years of age, came under my observation on November 26, 1887, complaining of his liver and perineal abscess, and also haemorrhoids. Patient suffered

also from pains in the stomach, coming on in the early morning about six or seven o'clock. Both liver and spleen were swelled; tongue and fingers gouty; slight eczema of anal region; and there was much depression of spirits, attributed to business worries.
$R_x$ *Nux vomica* 1x, five drops in water night and morning.
February 4, 1888 — Much better in almost all respects; only had the stomachic pains once lately. Complains of anal irritation on getting warm in bed at night. Sleeps badly; has much business worry, and is in consequence depressed; weight on the top of the head.
$R_x$ *Sulphur* 30.
May 5. — Not very materially improved; has indigestion, anal irritation, insomnia, depression of spirits, some uncomfortable feelings about the heart, and he has grown very stout of late.
$R_x$ Tc. *Vanad ammon*. 12.
Feb. 16, 1889 — Has had another perineal abscess and there is now an incomplete external fistula with much mattery discharge.
Two months of *Phytolaccin* 3x, six grains at bed-time, cured him of the fistula, and he was otherwise so far well that he did not want my further treatment. (XVI 45)

## 278. SYMPATHETIC RELATIONS BETWEEN THE ANUS AND THE HEAD

One very frequently observes an intimate sympathy between the anal region and the head. Let me relate a case in point. A gentleman of sixty was under my care for haemorrhoids and nocturnal pruritus ani that at times was maddening, and which had worried him for many years, and for the cure of which an almost endless array of local applications had been used in vain. He used to have attacks of giddiness and faintings, and he also had a small lipoma in the poll. What distressed him most was the pruritus ani, due, he thought, to threadworms. My treatment cured his giddiness, but the anal itchings grew rather worse than better. I will here interpolate the remark that whisky often causes itchings at the seat at night, and then the cure consists in leaving off the whisky. But this gentleman did not take whisky, being a teetotaller for many years.
The only time in his life he had ever obtained a respite from his pruritus was from the cure at Kissingen, so to Kissingen he would go, though I tried to dissuade him from it.
The Kissengen cure was effectual, for he returned without the pruritus ani. However, not very long after his return from Kissingen, cured of the pruritus, he had a "fit", consisting in a long fainting attack, evidently cephalic, and he became very giddy and habitually unsteady in his gait,

so that he was afraid to go about. Moreover he then got partial ptosis, notably of the left side. In this state he returned under my care. *Zincum aceticum* put his head quite right, and he feels now perfectly well and sure of gait, and free from faintings, and the ptosis is better, but the nightly itchings at the anus have returned. For these and for the lump in the neck (which, however, is decreased) he remains under my treatement, I should say that patient carries on an enormous business, and often sits up half the night intensely occupied with intricate calculations, while on Sunday he takes a complete rest in the form of preaching and Sunday-school teaching. He is a grand man, but whether the Master's work, at this time of day, needs such a sacrifice may be questioned. My own opinion is that a labourer is worthy of his — rest.

But my point here is the sympathy between the anal region and the head. By the way, for a fagged brain *Zincum aceticum* 1x, five drops in water night and morning, is indeed mighty for good (see Rademacher's experiment in "Erfahrungsheillehre") (XVI 47)

## 279. PROLAPSUS AND THREATENED FISTULA

A gentleman consulted me last summer in a very agitated frame of mind for fistula. An examination of the parts disclosed slight rectal prolapse, and a certain amount of inflammation of the projecting folds of the mucous membrane lining the rectum, in which the haemorrhoidal vessels were very prominent. He had been operated on for fistula, and also for piles and prolapse; but notwithstanding all this beautiful rectal surgery, the unfortunate patientt is never comfortable at the seat, nor do I think he ever will be, as the anal region is puckered with the crookedly healed tissue, and a blind funnel has been produced more than half an inch deep; this funnel is lined with common integument, and would otherwise be an incomplete fistula. There was blood at the anus almost every day. His nerves had received a grave shock from the operations, for notwithstanding the ten years that had elapsed since they were performed he still suffers from the effects. I have often been struck with the grave head symptoms that occur at the same time as rectal troubles, and these former are made much worse by all surgical interference. Thus this gentleman lives in a constant state of daze and fright lest a further operation should be needful for piles, prolapse, or fistula; his so-called nervous headaches are at times so bad that he thinks he will go out of his mind. The very mention of the words "fistula" or prolapse quite horrifies him.

A close examination showed so little to account for his state, that I was led to conclude that his very numerous vaccinations might have caused his trouble : he had been vaccinated five times.

Remedies greatly improved his condition, and so far that there was no further fear of fistula : *Thuja* was the principal remedy; infrequent doses of the thirtieth dilution administered during two months. He is not comfortable at the seat, nor do I think he ever will be, — a fact due, I think, to the bungling way in which he had been operated on. I see evidences of bungling after operations in this region so very seldom that I am constrained to admit this much in common fairness to the surgeons, that they believe in the operations I do not doubt; that they do their work well I can testify; but that their views are erroneous and their practice bad I am certain. (XVI 49)

## 280. URINARY FISTULA - A REMARKABLE CASE

Some seven years since, a London professional man came under my observation for an ordinary gonorrhoea. He is otherwise a good, conscientious fellow, but harvested the wages of sin at the very start, and was in a great state of mental perturbation. I was, after careful examination, enabled to assure him that he had a gonorrhoeal urethritis, and nothing else; there was absolutely no sign or suspicion of anything beyond that. *Aconite, Hepar, Hydrastis* and *Cynosbati* were administered, and in some six or seven weeks I thought were out of the wood there only a little urethral suintement left. But one day, without any concern whatever, he told me he thought he had caught a cold, and was getting a boil in the fork, that he also had some lumps in the groin, and nettle rash on the body. The experienced may judge of my utter amazement when I discovered a typical roseola syphilitica all over his body, notably on the chest and abdomen, and all the superficial glands of the body enlarged and indurated ! Moreover, on the undersurface of the member, some two inches or more from its extremity, and just in front of the prostate, there was in the very deed a "boil" of the size of a gooseberry, and very hard. I set to work vigorously with antisyphilitic treatment, and in a few weeks the roseola and other prominent symptoms had much abated, but his hair came out, and the nuchal glands were very prominently enlarged. During all this time the urethral discharge, which had returned, persisted. Just as I thought I was mastering both the gonorrhoea and the syphilis, he called one day and informed me that he had a "leak" in the region of the "boil", as said boil had burst. *Horrible dictu*, I found a fully established urethral fistula, with a thick hard wall surrounding and lining it. Several further months of persistent treatment finally resulted in a cure of the gonorrhoea, and of most of the manifestations of syphilis, but the terrible fistula persisted, notwithstanding *Merc., Aurum, Acid. nit., Stillingia, Iodatum,* and *Silicea* and some other seemingly likely remedies. I do not easily despair of a case, but when distinct consumptive symptoms began to show themselves, I certainly felt very anxious indeed, and I deemed it my duty to tell my poor patient that I feared he would have to undergo an operation for the urinary fistula, as it seemed to be wearing him out. However, I thought the matter over a few days, and finally came to the conclusion that the fistula was not only syphilitic, but also tuberculous, though how the infection could have been communicated within the urethra some three inches from the orifice I cannot even now understand. I then alternated *Mercurius solubilis Hahnemanni* 3x with very infrequent doses of *Bacillinum* c. (six grains of the former, and as many globules of the latter to the dose). At the same time I put him on very full diet with a generous wine.

Result — In a few months the patient was quite well in every respect; the indurated glands all returned to the normal, the hair grew again, the night-sweats ceased, the fistula completely healed up, the sclerosis around it disappeared, and patient put on flesh and reassumed his old healthy appearance.

I will finish this long story by remarking that the amelioration, that set in as soon he was put on the last-mentioned double prescription, was truly remarkable, and for weeks and weeks whenever it was discontinued for other remedies, the amelioration at once ceased, so that I had to recur to it over and over again. The *Bacillinum* was, however, never given more than one dose in four days. The *Merc. sol.* three times a day. To look at this gentleman now no one would suspect what he has gone through. *Aux grands mau les grands remedes*, they say over in France. This case forcibly reminds one of Hunter's famous experiment on himself. We have here a case of urinary fistula, a very bad one too and its having been perfectly and permanently cured with medicines, should encourage us all to treat urinary fistulas also with medicines only — a thing I believe never even attempted. Perhaps I had better add, to prevent mistakes or misapprehension, that absolutely no local applications were used, not even a bit of lint or charpie. (XVI 53)

## 281. HEREDITARY FISTULA

The gentleman whose case is first narrated in this book sent me a friend of his suffering from fistula, as does also this latter's father. This friend came to me on November 2, 1891, telling me that he had a perineal abscess, which broke six weeks ago, and left a fistula which at date is again gathering. He early seeks advice because of his father's chronic condition. Patient has, besides, a chronic winter cough, very hard; otherwise he is in excellent condition, — a trifle stout, perhaps. There are no indurated glands anywhere to be found, but he gets a little acne here and there. He suffers a good deal of pain during defecation.

In December 1892 the fistula had quite disappeared and had not since returned, though I think it very probable that he may have a few more flickerings here and there yet, though of course he may not.

The chief remedies were *Bacill, Thuja, Sabina, Levico, Hydrastis, Hepar, Acidum nitricum*. There were numerous gatherings of pus before the cure was accomplished. (XVI 81)

## 282. FISTULA

An unmarried gentleman came to consult me for fistula just before Christmas 1890. Originally there appears to have been a fall, and then an abscess. Patient was operated upon for his fistula in 1886, and again in 1887 but without avail. He was in fairly good health all the time, and though he still had his fistula when he came to me, notwithstanding the two operations, he did not come because he was ill, but because he was desirous of getting married. He complained only of one thing, viz., he was always very chilly.

I examined him with very great care, and apart from the fistula itself I could find nothing wrong with him except that he had a very greatly hypertrophied spleen.

About two ounces of *Urtica ur.* Q, spread over a number of weeks, seemingly cured him, for he reported himself as cured in the early summer of 1891. In July of that year he went up the river, and reported some swelling of the old fistular region. The *Urtica* was repeated, and I believe cured him : I am not quite sure but he had previously reported himself cured, then he reported the swelling, and a few weeks later he got married. I think he must be cured, because he passes my door about twice a month to see a mutual friend of us both, and this mutual friend is in the habit of referring to this cure of fistula by medicines. Still I have not examined him, and thus do not vouch for its being a complete cure. I regard it as a fistula of splenic origin, and hence the fistula would heal as soon as the spleen was cured. (XVI 82)

## 283. POST MALARIAL FISTULA IN THE BACK

The following case of fistula is unique in my experience, and not far from being absolutely unique in the annals of fistulae.

In the fall of the year 1890 a gentleman brought his wife to me; they were just returned from India. In June 1890 the lady had a fall in Bombay, whereupon she miscarried and before she could recover she developed malarial fever. Then abscess formed in the womb and also in the back, about the region corresponding to the part lying between the left-hand end of the pancreas and the lower part of the spleen. On inspection I found a freely discharging fistula, with much inflammation around it, occupying the first described region of the back. The spleen was very much enlarged. Patient is a large woman, 30 odd years of age, very bloodless and washed-out looking, and very ill in herself. As I find that *Urtica ur.* has a strong affinity for the spleen, I thought I would just bring that organ back to the normal therewith (which I have very often done before), I gave her twenty drops of the *Urtica* tincture daily. This was on September 12, 1890.

October 20 — Patient continues to improve. The fistula has closed; a little throat cough, seemingly from a cold.

$R_x$ *Phosphorus* 3 and *Chelidonium* Q.

November 19 — The fistula has healed up, patient has had her second period since the miscarriage, and there was very much uterine pain at the time. There has been a slight attack of malarial fever with night sweats. *Helianthus annuus* Q, six drops in water night and morning.

December 10 — Menses normal; a lump — flat — of the size of a baby's open hand, has come in the left breast. Regarding this as from the uterus, I gave *Bursa pastoris* 1x, six drops night and morning.

January 7, 1891 — Breast normal, some pain in the liver, much less pain at the last period; a bit of a cough.

$R_x$ *Carduus Marianus* Q, five drops night and morning.

February 6. One bad bout of fever, and since then very well. The fistula remains perfectly healed. I heard from the husband a good while subsequently, telling me there had been no relapse. (XVI 84)

## 284. FISTULA PROCTALGIA — GRAVE DEPRESSION OF SPIRITS

A city merchant, about 50 years of age, came to me in the month of March 1890, in very great distress of mind on account of his fistula, or rather, on account of the fact that three different surgeons — one an eminent specialist for diseases of the rectum — had declared an operation imperative. The idea of being operated upon had almost unhinged his mind, and he was seemingly neglecting an important business; he could talk of nothing but his fistula and the impending operation. The fistula was very small, very painful, and had made his life miserable for about three months. During the past six weeks he has lost 16 pounds in weight. The proctalgia he described as "terrible, day and night". At first *Hydrastis can.* took the pain away, and it returned; *Var.* C. I thought indicated, but it did no good. *Hydrastis* was again resorted to, but it did not help, and patient literally ran about wildly from the pain, often standing with legs apart with much bearing down.

On April 23, my note runs thus — "No amelioration. The tongue is gouty; he compares the pain to that caused by nettles. His sufferings are awful."

$R_x$ Tc *Urtica ur.* 1x, ten drops in water every four hours.

May 9 — These drops cured the burning pain in three days.

$R_x$ *Phytolaccinum* 3x,.

June 4 — No return of the pain at all. Patient has regained much of his lost weight, and is now as hilarious as he was previously depressed. At the seat there is nothing observable save a flap of flesh at the side of the anal mouth.

$R_x$ *Sodium silicate* Q.

July 2 — Not happy at the seat; mentally apprehensive; a close inspection shows, hidden behind the before-named flap of flesh, a small wart with a bleeding fissure athwart it.

$R_x$ *Sambucus* Q.

Patient was discharged quite cured and in fine physical and mental condition just fourteen months from the beginning of his treatment. During the remaining part of his treatment he received from me *Chelidonium majus* Q, *Urtica ur.* in several differing strengths. *Hecla* 30, *Kali iod.* 30, *Calc. carb.* C, C., and finally *Silicea* C.

In this case I did use one local application, viz., powdered *Thuja* applied direct to the bleeding comb-like processes behind the fleshy flap, and of this flap its shrivelled remains are still in situ. (XVI 86)

## 285. FISTULA — VERRUCOUS GROWTH AND HAEMORRHOIDS

Early in the year 1890 a gentleman verging on 70 years of age came from the country to consult me for anal trouble characterized by a sticky, gummy discharge. An examination of the part disclosed a wart-like growth of te size of a walnut, and also a pile. I could not find any fistula. A month later I found the mouth of the fistula leading into a funnel-shaped discharging cavity.

He remained under treatment the best part of a year, during which time the fistula healed and patient greatly improved in health. *Bacillinum* C. *Hydrastis can.* Q, *Phytolaccin* 3x, *Sodium silicatum* Q, *Sambucus* Q, were the chief remedies. The growth was much smaller when patient discharged himself, and was wishful to continue the treatment longer, but he was comfortable in himself, the anal region being dry since the fistula healed up. His digestion so very much improved that he "would not be bothered with any more physicking." (XVI 88)

## 286. FISTULA IN A LADY

A married lady, 33 years of age, was brought to me by her husband in the spring of 1891 to be treated for fistula-in-ano, that had been a source of annoyance and trouble for a little over two years, seemingly starting from the retention of a dead foetus at that period, which was then thought to have been three weeks dead. At a previous confinement there had been considerable laceration of the perineum, the sequel of which had had to be remedied by the electro-cautery, and thus a somewhat imperfect closing of the sphincter ani has come about, and loose stools being the rule, the poor lady had a sad time of it. A fistula alone is a humiliating possession, but when faecal incoontinence is added, the condition becomes fearful. The fistula was situated at the back, and was in the habit of closing for a few days, and then it would burst and discharge. Besides the fistula and an inadequate sphincter muscle, there were piles; that, however, did not cause very much inconvenience.
Patient was put upon *Thuja occidentalis* 30 in infrequent doses for one month. The case was seen from month to month, and required some pretty careful differential drug diagnosis before it was permanently cured, patient being discharged quite well in the month of July 1892. The chief remedies used were *Bacill.* M. and CC. given altogether during four separate months, *Helianthus annuus* Q, *Bursa pastoris* Q, *Kali iodicum*. 3 trit. and 30, and *Bovista* 3 trit, have come into play in between as indicated. In this case I was guided to the use of the remedies from the state of the cervical glands and the circumscribed flush of the cheeks, and by the patient's various symptoms. (XVI 89)

## 287. PRE-FISTULAR CELLULITIS DISPERSED

Sometimes one is fortunate enough to get cases of pre-fistular gathering soon enough to prevent both abscess and fistula. Thus a middle-aged merchant from the Midlands came under my care in the fall of 1891, with a "lump at the seat" that was giving rise to inconvenience and anxiety to the patient, partly because he was quite familiar with fistula in his own family. He was well in three months; during the first half of the time he was taking *Arnica montana* 1, twenty drops a day in water. This took away much of the swelling and nearly all the hardening, and then I gave *Chelidonium majus* Q on organopathic lines.

That we here prevented both abscess and fistula hardly admits of any doubt. (XVI 91)

## 288. RECTAL ABSCESSES AND FISTULA

In the month of January 1892 a London professional man came under my care. Two months previously he had had a very large abscess of the rectum which had been freely incised but would not heal, and a fistula state remained, with much discharge; or, rather, I should say that there remained a hole in the flesh fully two inches long, discharging matter profusely. And notwithstanding the profuse discharge from this gash, there was another large gathering on the other side of the anus, which the surgeon was on the point of operating on.

Patient's father and one of his sisters had died of phthisis. I began the treatment with *Ignatia amara* 1, alternated with *Hydrastis candensis* Q, because of patient's low nervous anorexial condition. This was continued for a fortnight, much to his comfort and feeling of well-being, when early in February gout broke out in his right foot. This was met with *Aconite* 6 and *Bryonia* Q. With the outbreak of the gout the activity at the seat lessened, and the gash in the flesh began to heal from the bottom. I had applied nothing to the wound, but rather encouraged its activity.

The treatment was continued — patient all the while attending to his professional duties — with some ups and downs, till May 25, 1893, when the patient was discharged cured, and in capital health and spirits. Many remedies were needed and used, and of these the chief were : *Bacill.* CC. and C.; *Bryonia alb.* Q; *Chionanthus virginicus* Q; *Nat. mur.* 6 trit.; *Levico* (strong); *Thuja* 30, and *Lycopodium* 6. To give the reasons for giving the various medicines would occupy more space than I can here afford, but there were three leading ideas underlying them viz. :

1. The hereditary phthisic taint.
2. The enlarged unhealthy liver.
3. The gout; and then we had to meet —

a. The debility
b. The anaemia.
c. The anorexia.
d. The neurasthenia, the last-named being a potent factor in the sum; at any rate, neurasthenia cannot be operated away. (XVI 91)

## 289. GRAVE CASE OF RECTO-VAGINAL FISTULA

A childless lady, many years married, 42 years of age, came to consult me for recto-vaginal fistula early in the year 1890. Both of her parents died about 80 years of age, — in fact her mother lived to be 82; and all her brothers and sisters being still alive and well, and patient herself being of very fine build, I was quite astonished to hear the following narration of her health-history and present state : formerly had a fearful cough, remaining as a sequel of a pneumonia, the cough, being so bad that some thought it from a form of asthma. Formerly very thin then stout (large, not obese), i.e., polysarcous, and now losing flesh. It is noteworthy that when she began to get perineal abscesses her cough entirely disappeared.

In childhood she had had measles, whooping-cough, and sclarlatina in the proper way, — since then a carbuncle on her right arm. Menses copious; she is weary and tired; tongue gouty, with no "strawberry" pips ( a very important point); considerable leucorrhoea; she is very chilly. Notwithstanding the history of pneumonia, and notwithstanding the very bad cough that disappeared as soon as the pre-fistular abscesses began to appear, I still could not regard the fistula as in any sense indicative of a phthisic taint, but I came to the conclusion that it was a case of genuine vaccinosic manifestations; the chilliness, the leucorrhoea, the polysarcia, the pithy tongue, the sterility all, in my judgment, pointing at any rate to the hydrogenoid constitution of Grauvogl.

The fistula was sequential to abscesses at the spot, and patient stated that it had gathered twelve times.

Patient had been operated on by a distinguished surgeon three months previously but without success, and a further and very much more serious operation was in prospect, and hence the lady's visit to me. Now it happened that this lady's house was, and is, the rendezvous of quite a number of medical men all sincerely attached to this lady's husband. "Nearly all our friends happen to be medical men," said she, and my husband has discussed the question of the possibility of my fistula being cured with medicines, and they all declare it to be absolutely impossible, and my husband is so sure that it is impossible that he has refused to come with me."

Still, in an aside, she gave me to understand that he privately hoped she would come, on the off-chance of a cure, and so avoid the alarmingly radical operation in contemplation.

It is to be remembered that an operation for fistula depends a good deal on the kind of person to be operated upon as well as its position. In this case the position was most awkward, and the quantity of tissue through which the incisions would have to be made very considerable.

In the left groin glands are indurated and enlarged; moreover, they become tender just before each gathering, and remain so till it has burst and discharged.

Inasmuch as many medical men had declared this case absolutely unamenable to medicinal treatment, and two of them watched the progress of the case, inasmuch as one operation had already failed (it was performed in a well-known hospital, it being considered too considerable to be conveniently done at home), and inasmuch as my diagnosis will be unacceptable to almost all medical men, even to many of my best friends and colleagues, I am going to enter into very full details of the case, to motive my diagnosis and the line of treatment such diagnosis compelled. If any one of my readers takes an interest in the question of the constitutional effects of the poison of vaccination, I refer such a one to my little treatise on the subject, entitled "Vaccinosis and its Cure by Thuja".

In this case patient had been vaccinated four times. From this fact, and for the reasons already given (symptoms negative and positive), I considered I had to do with a genuine and severe case of vaccinosis.

I began the treatment on January 10, 1890, with the matrix tincture of *Hydrastis Canadensis*, giving eight drops in water three times a day.

February 3 — The leucorrhoea is not so bad; the place is angry, but the swelling is less. Patient feels better. "I am picking up." Feels very cold always, and she is also cold to the touch. Sleeps lightly, and gets the fidgets in her legs.

$R_x$ *Thuja occidentalis* 30, infrequently.

February 17 — Markedly better; no trouble with the gathering whatever; no discharge from the fistula worth while; no menses for six weeks. still feels very chilly; parts no longer swelling! no tenderness of inguinal glands; much better of the tiredness and weariness.

No medicine, to allow the remedy already set up to continue undisturbedly.

March 7 — No pain, and no gathering; one scanty menstruation; she is always cold. the enlargement of the inguinal glands has disappeared; not so tired or weary.

$R_x$ *Vaccininum* C., very infrequently.

March 26 — No gathering; not so cold; leucorrhoea better; has a cold, with a little cough; is gaining flesh.

$R_x$ *Ceanothus Americanus*, ten drops in water night and morning.

April 12 — No gathering; feels less cold; and the left hypochondrium is less uneasy.

$R_x$ *Hydrastis Canadensis* as before, but in a smaller dose.

May 22 — Menses set in three weeks ago, and still continue; left ovary is tender.

$R_x$ *Juniperus Sabina* 30, very infrequently.

June 30 — Fistula quite gone, and almost well in herself.

$R_x$ *Cupressus Lawsoniana* 30, very infrequently.

I heard no more of the patient till the followig November, when she came, telling me she had continued quite well, but the last week or so she had felt slight tenderness where the fistula used to be, and it seemed as if it might gather.

$R_x$ *Thuja* 30, as before.

February 9, 1891 — Has been quite well, but the old fistula is again active and gathering.

$R_x$ *Silicea* 30, ten drops every three hours.

This was followed by complete cure and capital health till.

July 13 — When patient again called, telling me she felt as if it were going to gather again, but objectively there was absolutely nothing abnormal.

$R_x$ *Thuja* 30, as before.

At this point I ceased keeping notes of the case, although patient called to see me on two or three occasions for little threatenings and flickerings, but these have now long ceased.

On May 19, 1893, patient told me that she had been quite well in all respects for nine months, and she was in blooming health.

In this case I made the diagnosis of vaccinosis, and base the treatment thereon. As soon as the blood disease was much lessened the fistula healed up, and as soon as the blood disease was quite cured the flickerings in the old fistula ceased entirely. The healing process shows itself also in this case, as in so many others, as gentle, gradual, and with candle-like flickerings until the disease becomes quite extinguished.

Could any more conlusive proof be given of the constitutional nature of fistula?

I used no local measure whatever. (XVI 93)

## CURE OF CONSUMPTION

### 290. HYDROCEPHALUS, ECZEMA, LATENT VACCINOSIS

**Case I.** In the early part of the year 1885, I was requested to see the only surviving child of a country clergyman, who had been given up by three medical men, as it had water on the brain. The child's head was of the usual hydrocephalic type; he was alternately wakeful and delirious at night, and he talked nonsense by day at intervals. Their local doctors had taken a consultant's opinion, and they agreed that the boy was suffering from tuberculosis of the meninges with effusion, of which a little brother had previously died. The child's life-history was told to me, and I underlined the facts that he had had eczema, and had been twice unsuccessfully vaccinated. After the unsuccessful vaccinations (want of organismic reactionary power) the eczema almost disappeared, and very soon the present disease began. I treated the case thus causally *ex-hypothesi*; a severe pustula eruption, and then patches of lepra and eczema appeared, and at the end of about six months' treatment I was able to dischrge the little patient, cured of his water on the brain and of his skin diseases. I saw him the other day, and learned that he continues well and has grown a good deal.

When said essay was sent to the proper quarters for the opinions of medical experts, one of the reviewers called attention to the fact that I had not named the remedies which cured the boy, and called upon me to make them known. Well, *the* remedy of the case was the poison of consumption; after taking this in a high potency and infrequently, the head went smaller; the delirium ceased, as did also the nocturnal hallucinations and fright, and the pyrexia entirely disappeared. I happen to know that the cure holds good to date, now nearly six years, though a certain amount of irritability of temper remains.

I did not mention the remedy then, thinking the world not ripe for it; but now that Professor Koch's large dose injections of the same substance are the order of the day, my harmless infinitesimals will hardly meet with any objectors, rather shall I expect to incur ridicule. Anyway, it was the virus of consumption that cured the case, and nearly six years testify to its genuineness and lastingness. (XVIA 21)

## 291. INCIPIENT TUBERCULOSIS

**Case II.** About two years ago I was called to a boy of 3 years of age in the night, with diarrhoea, furious fever, burning hot skin, great heat in the head, red flushed face, and eyes turned upwards, quivering and rolling. Patient had been ailing a little, and ordinary homoeopathic remedies had been given in vain. Considering the case to be one of incipient tuberculosis, I gave one dose of a high potency of its virus; within an hour patient quited down, went to sleep, burst into a free perspiration and awoke in the morning greatly improved, and very soon completely recovered, and is now a very fine boy. (XVIA 25)

## 292. FEVER WITH TUBERCULAR FAMILY HISTORY

**Case III.** I was called last year, also in the night, to a bairnie of some 20 months of age, who had been ill for days with "something in the head," high fever, restlessness, and constant screaming. I had seen him from his first ailing, and prescribed our usual remedies, but they took practically no lasting effect. I had seen the child in the evening and prescribed for it, and did not apprehend any mischief, although there had been no sleep for some forty hours, but when called in the night I was greatly alarmed at the child's fallen-in and collapsing state, and I feared the worst. There was the peculiarly fetid smell of the child's body, such as I had noticed in the previous case. Moreover, he was the brother of Case II., and of both very numerous near relations had died of consumption at different periods, and one young cousin had died of tuberculosis of the brain coverings. I gave an infinitesimally minute quantity of the phthisic virus on sugar of milk dry on the tongue .... and the result?

I hardly like to pen so remarkable a result, as it looks so strangely improbable ........ Patient fell asleep within ten minutes, and uttered thereafter no further screams. He made a rapid and complete recovery, though his forehead still gives him a rather old-mannie look. (XVIA 26)

**Case IV**. In the early fall of this year, 1890, I was called upon to prescribe for a tall girl of 12 years of age, of a distinctly phthisic habit. She had a tedious little hack of a cough that had lasted for months, and refused to yield to the common homoeopathic remedies. As before stated, she was tall for her age; she had long fingers, almond-shaped nails, a long neck, indurated glands in the neck. Infrequent doses of the phthisic virus in high potency rapidly altered the entire face of the case, the cough went in ten days, and in a few weeks she was reported "perfectly well and getting quite fat". Many of this young lady's relatives have died of tuberculosis. It is in just this early stage of consumption that the virus acts with such promptitude and brilliancy. And I will add that the action of *Psorinum* is often very nearly equal to it in old cases, whereof I could cite some very notable examples, but here they would not be apposite. (XVIA 28)

**Case V**. In the early spring of 1887 a young lady of 15 years of age was brought to me from the North, for her age she was very big. She had very large tonsils, chronic running from the nose, worse in the early morning on rising; her speech was thick; her thorax, the so-called *pigeon-breast*; she menstruated freely; she has moist palms, and she perspires across the nose a good deal; she gets chilblains. She feels very chilly and I find her spleen a good deal swelled. Distinct dullness on percussion at the apex of the right lung.

As patient had suffered badly from vaccination, I ordered my favourite **arbor** vitae. This brought no change for the better; her perspiration of chest, armpits, palms, nose and feet became very bad.

The virus of consumption was here administered; the thirtieth at twelve days interval, and after one month of this the perspirations had greatly diminished; after two months the dulness on percussion at the right apex had gone, the chest took on a much better shape (the depressed right side stood out much better). In another two months of the same medication she was in capital health, and her mother wrote me at te end of October, 1887, "She is so well."

And now, two years later, I am able to say that she has never looked back, and is a bonnie person — just a wee bit stout, perhaps. Patient had altogether forty-eight globules of the virus, of the thritieth potency, spread over four months. (XVIA 29)

**Case VI — Recurrent Cough.** It is nearly four years since, the exact date being February 25, 1887, that a married lady, then 38 years of age, mother of seven children, came to me for a bad cough, that troubled her all the more as she was then enciente. This cough was worse on going to bed and on getting up. She had been four times vaccinated, and three out of the four were unsuccessful. She had suffered from leucorrhoea a good deal, and from coughs. As she had had three sisters die successively of consumption (at 28, 32, and 40 years of age, respctively), her husband was much concerned about her future. Considering her family history, and the fact that the apex of the right lung was consolidated, though I did my best to cheer him up, I had sad misgivings myself. She had from me in succession, and with very striking benefit, the following remedies in the order named, *Thuja* 30, *Pulsatilla* 3x, *Bellis perennis* 3x, *Sepia* 12, *Hepar sul.* 6, *Thuja* 30 (a second time), and *Nux vomica* 3x. We found patient after these remedies, at the end of the month of October 1888, in a pretty bad way; there was the same dulness on percussion at the apex of the right lung, the same little hacking cough continuing all day, and exacerbating at bedtime and on rising, and patient was very thin. I then determined to try the phthisic virus. After being under it for a month she did not trouble to report herself till March 15, 1889, and then she only came because she had a cold, and therewith some cough again. She had been so well all the winter that she considered herself quite cured. Here I repeated the October prescription of the virus, and I discharged the patient cured in one month and two days therefrom, viz., on April 17, 1889. She has never looked back, and is now a stout woman. (XVIA 32)

**Case VII — Consumption.** At the beginning of July, 1887, a young woman of about 30 was brought to me, far gone in consumption. She was very, very emaciated, the menses had ceased. Her two sisters had died in the same way, and all hope for her recovery had long since been abandoned; but hearing, or rather having observed, a youg lady in the same neighbourhood get well of consumption under my care, her mother accompanied her to me. Having used *Thuja* (the poor thing had been vaccinated four times, the last three unsuccessfully), *Calc., hypo-phos.*, and *Cardius*

*Marianus*, with decidedly good results, I felt encouraged, and thought it almost possible yet to save her if we could only get rid of the fever. With the virus I succeeded in doing this after a few months; patient lost her cough to a very large extent, the expectoration came down to a mere nothing, and she put on a few pounds in flesh, and lived for nearly two years free from consumption, or rather, free from the ordinary symptoms of that disease, such as fever and cough. Her mother said to me one day, "You seem to have cured the consumption, and yet my daughter gets weaker and weaker every day, and the dropsy goes on getting worse and worse." And so it was; and of the dropsy she died, nearly two years after the consumptive process seemed cured. This case is unique in my experience. The phthisic virus cured the phthisis so far as I could tell. I used a good many remedies then to meet the varying symptoms with, at times, very good effects, but the effects did not last. To give some idea how persistently I treated her, I will name the remedies she had from me — *Fragaria vesca* Q, *Chelidonium majus* Q, *Ceanothus Americanus* 1, *Scilla maritima* Q, *Iodium* 3x, *Aconite, Baptisia* 3x, *Pyrogenium* 5, *Calc. Phos., Rubia tinctoria, Fer. acet., Cholestearin, Arsenicum, Phos., Iodoform* 3x, *Pancreatin*, and *Spirit. glandium quercus*. Still in the end I failed, and she died of hepatic dropsy, due to hopelessly far advanced granular atrophy. When I say the phthisis was cured, I, of course, do not mean that to be taken literally; on the contrary, I mean that though the fever, etc., were quite extinguished, and patient's condition was for some months relatively comfortable, still, the frequently recurring haemorrhages showed that occult processes were still going on within the closed circle of the economy. (XVIA 34)

**Case VIII — Case of Profound Debility and Dyspnoea and Evening Fever.** I will now briefly narrate the successful case through which Case VII came under my observation :

The patient was 17 years of age, and her sister had just died of consumption of the lungs.

Patient was very anaemic, sickish, pale almost to whiteness, profound debility, dyspnoea, cannot mount or hurry, menses very irregular.

"She is going just like her poor dear sister, she has the same fever every evening."

Of the diagnosis there could be no doubt, and the sister's fate determined me to use the virus 30. This was on the 4th of October; on the 1st of November then next following, I find in the case a record : "Certainly better, the evening feverishness has gone."

I then used the virus in higher potency (and at all times and in all cases at certain intervals). She got quite well of all the consumptiive symptoms, but remained neuralgic and anaemic; but these ailings having been righted by *Mangan. acet.* 1, *Zincum acet.* 1, *Fer. acet.* 1, I discharged her cured. She is a fine, bonnie woman now, and anything but consumptive looking.

Here I conclude that the phthisic virus acted, and acted adequately, curatively — its stop-spot being on the offside of the disease as expressed in this damsel.

As to the use of the other remedies, I would specially insist upon the fact that the phthisic virus only acts within its own sphere, and that this sphere is very sharply defined as to time, and what it does not do soon and promptly it does not do at all. Its action is, if I may so express myself, acute : its chronic equivalent is *Psorinum.* (XVIA 38)

**Case IX — Bronchitis.** "I have come to town again for the purpose of preparing to go abroad. You will remember that you advised me to go south last year, and that I spent the winter and spring at Cannes. You sent the powders to me there. Those white powders did me a great deal of good — almost set me free from bronchitis. Since I last saw you I have had but very little bronchitis. I look well, and people tell me I was looking very much better than I did last year."

The complaint was dependent upon a phthisical taint in the constitution, and it was the phthisic virus that cured the case. At first it was given over two months, and later on for six weeks. The one-hundredth potency in very infrequent dose. Patient's brother had died of consumption. (XVIA 41)

**Case X — Fistular Anaemia & Consumptiveness.** A city merchant, married and father of a family, came under my observation in the spring of 1888 for phthisis and fistula, or, I would rather say, for fistular anaemia and "consumptiveness", for the consumption was not declared, though the experienced eye was not to be misled. The whole circumanal surface was red; glands of the left side of the neck very much indurated. The gentleman's poitrinary constitution may be accounted for, seeing that his father was dying of consumption when patient was born.

I treated him with much success with *Kali carb.* 30, *Nux vomica* 1, *Hepar sul.* 3, *Silicea* 6, and *Hydrastis canadensis* Q, with two intercurrent courses of, each one month of the phthisic virus, and in seven months — end of 1888 — discharged him quite cured, and, so far as I could tell, sound, in all respects. I have never seen him since, and I believe he has never looked back. (XVIA 42)

**Case XI — Tuberculosis of Brain.** The following case is striking. On April 23, 1888, a lady and gentleman brought their only boy, 2 years and 8 months of age; he was their only child, because their other two had died of tuberculosis of the brain, and this one was going the same way, and with the same symptoms, and at about the same age. The parents told me nought of all this till I had given my diagnosis. these were the symptoms. He is fretty and ailing, whines and complains, feelably indurated glands everywhere, hottish, drowsy, urine red and sandy, much given to be frightened, particularly by dogs. Has been vaccinated, and had thereafter a dreadful arm for four months. He would not smile for or at anyone or anything, and when spoken to forthwith began to whimper. His skin was dingy, his skull hydrocephalic.

*Diagnosis* : Tuberculosis.

When I had fenced awhile with the anxious mother's questions, she broke down and begged me to be candid, and then told me of their sad troubles and loss of their two previous children. I then stated the diagnosis, but stated that I hoped I should cure it. Of course the parents tried to believe the welcome prognosis, but could not, and went home in terrible distress of mind.

I began with *Aconite* and *Chamomilla* 30.

April 30th — Better a good deal; sleeps very well; less drowsy, urine better. *Pulsatilla* 1 was then given.

May 14th — Urine normal; no longer drowsy; but the glands and anatomical condition no better. I had often treated such like cases with steady, general, and particular amelioration of symptoms, but I had by this time grown wiser, and fully recognized that the stop-spot of such remedies as *Aconite, Chamomilla* and *Pulsatilla* was a long way on the hither side of a cure. Said I to myself, .... this sort of remedy only goes up to the tubercle, and the tubercle sphere is their stop-points ..... But it is the tubercles that kill! I therefore began with phthisic virus.

June 11th — Not sleepy; sleeps quietly at night; he is wasting; frets and whines; urine normal.

Mindful of the vaccinosis, I thought it probable that as that was the more recent, and planted upon the tuberculosis, the vaccinosis would have first to be cured.

*Thuja* 30

July 11th — Was better, but yesterday was at a flower show, and he now screams a good deal.

$R_x$ *Glonoin* 2 and *Aconite* 2.

18th — He has got over this attack, and the glands are a trifle less. He now sleeps badly again. The previously administered one-hundredth (centesimal) of the phthisic virus not having acted as well as I anticipated, I came down to very infrequent doses of the thirtieth.

August 22nd — Appetite better; nights good; not drowsy by day; urine red and brick-dusty a week ago; is still mum and fretty; he is stronger; can walk further; glands of the neck much worse, notably those on the left side.

*Pulsatilla* 3x and *Calc*. C. 12.

October 17th — He is worse, and screams dreadfully in his sleep. I then put patient again steadily upon the virus alone as our only chance, and the patient was discharged cured on January 7, 1889. At the end of the year I received this letter :

"4th December 1889.

"Dear Sir, — I feel I must thank you for your kind advice and trouble you have taken in curing my litte son ..... I am happy to say he has taken a change for the better for some time past; he has made flesh, and has so altered that you would scarcely know him. Hoping he will keep so; and should anything happen that he is not so well .... I shall fly off to you," etc.

Since then I have heard nothing, and so conclude that the cure is permanent.

The striking amelioration in the boy which filled the mother with gratitude, and impelled her to write the above, I take to be the natural healthy growth of the boy, which set in after he was cured of the tubercles.

This case greatly impressed me, and, moreover, much encouraged me. Evidently it has only been taken just in time; a little later and the phthisic virus (at any rate in my homoeopathically prepared infinitesimal quantities) would have been unavailing. (XVIA 45)

**Case XII — Case of Fever, Wasting, Abdominal Pain with Enlarged Glands.** A little girl of 6 years of age, daughter of a country squire, being under almost ideally perfect hygienic surroundings, her father, however, suffering from chronic pulmonary consumption, fell ill in the spring of 1888. There was fever, wasting, abdominal pains and discomfort, and restless nights. the glands of both groins and on both sides of the neck enlarged and indurated, some were visible on simple adspection. Except that she had been vaccinated in the usual way, she had had no illness. The local family doctor considered her case a very anxious one, and had small hope of her ultimate recovery.

I gave the virus in the thirtieth potency, and at intervals of nine days. This was on July 27th.

On August 27th I find noted in my record of her case : "Was nearly well, but is now feverish again; cries out in her sleepl strawberry tongue; very feverish." I then repeated the virus, but in the one-hundredth potency, and at the same intervals (to allow of undisturbed action, see Hahnemann).

November 2d — is better decidedly; has quite ceased crying out in her sleep all the glands are nearly well.

*Thuja occidentalis* 30 also at like intervals.

She remained well for some months (from September, 1888, till May 1890), when, on

May 28th, 1890, I thought it was wise to repeat the virus, as on August 27th, 1888, and this set her right; and after three months she continued well, except for a slight stomach derangement; which *Pulsatilla* 1 and *Arsenicum* 5 put right. She is now well.

Her younger sister I treated for a much minor degree of the same constitutional state with *Iodium* 3x and *Glonoin* 3x, with seemingly complete success, and therefore I did not need to have recourse to the bacillic virus. (XVIA 50)

**Case XIII — Consumptiveness.** There are certain cases of what may, perhaps, be termed CONSUMPTIVENESS, but where the patients, through being fed largely and richly, manage to get stout, even very fat, and who yet are distincly afflicted with the tuberculous taint, and who in the end get diabetes, or go into common consumption. Such a one was a very big, stout, provincial gentleman, of bright, florid complexion, who came under my professional care in the spring of this year. His mother died young, of phthisis, and his only sister is stated to be going the same way. He gets pneumonia very often in the cold weather, and hence he now goes from place to place to avoid cold. He coughs much, and brings up much phlegm. As his father died of pnuemonia, and, as I have just observed, his mother of consumption, he regarded his own outlook with reasonable apprehensiveness. He perspired very profusely, drank huge quantities of fluids, some of them alcoholic, and had wretched, sleepless nights, with almost constant fever. The glands of his neck were very much enlarged. He was three months under the bacillic virus, and was then a very different man; he now sleeps well; the glands are well (i.e., cannot be felt); the temperature is now normal; no cough; no phlegm; and his tissues are much less watery. He is, therefore, not so huge, and much more active. (XVIA 53)

**Case XIV.** I have had another case so much like the one just narrated that I will merely note it shortly. There was a similar unhealthy parentage, the same liability to pneumonia, the same watery hugeness of body, the same sort of cough and wet phlegminess, the same excessive perspirations and thirst, and restless nights. But no fever as a rule.

The treatment was mixed; the bacillic virus had not the same decided effect, but under it he went smaller in bulk, but did not lose weight, from which I conclude that he really gained in proper flesh, but lost in water from his tissues. In this case *Pulsatilla, Spiritus glandium quercus*, and the *Acetum lobeliae* greatly aided in his cure. When I lately saw him, and passed the time of day, he cried after me, "Oh! I am splendid." (XVIA 55)

**Case XV — Pulmonary Tuberculosis.** A young lady, unmarried, aged 19, was brought to me by her father at the beginning of the month of July, 1889. The hectic flush of the cheeks announced the dreadful diagnosis; shortness of breath for long, much worse the past three years; little hacking cough; a number of strumous scars of various dates in the neck; dusky skin; there are large moist rales in both lungs; amphoric sounds in the right lung; increased vocal resonance of right lung; there is a large soft-feeling gland in the left side of the neck; a very pronounced endocardial bruit, best heard at the apex beat; and the before-mentioned hectic flush.

July 12th — Trit. 3x *Iodoformum* in four-grain doses.

Two months of this treatment effected very pronounced improvement, and patient had gained in flesh, but the hectic was not touched.

October 9th — At this date I began with the bacillic virus (C.) Always in very infrequent dose, and, in future, this is always to be understood, so I need not again state this all-important fact. Thereafter the same remedy (C.C.)

Recovery complete, and she remains plump and well. As patient lives 150 miles away from London, I have never been able to see her to percuss and auscultate with the view of ascertaining the physical state of her thoracic organs. They were under a promise to come, but as she is so evidently well they do not see the need of incurring the expense and taking the trouble of a journey to town merely for my satisfaction. (XVIA 57)

**Case XVI — Incipient Phthisis.** A little boy of 7 years of age was brought to me at the end of the spring of 1890 for symptoms of incipient phthisis; he had had an ill-defined sort of fever, and then the Russian infleunza. Consumption being in the family, his parents had become anxious about him principally because of his loss of flesh and great prostration, together with a morbid timidity. The glands of his groins and both sides of his neck were very much enlarged and indurated, particularly the glands over the apex of the right lung. As he had suffered much from vaccination, I first gave *Thuja* 30, and *Sabina* 30,and then the *bacillic virus* (C.) "He has gained in flesh, weight, and spirits; his nerve is also better, as he has taken to riding, a thing he was afraid of before."

He got quite well, and remains so to date. (XVIA 59)

**Case XVII — Tubercular Synovitis — Left Knee.** A lady of 56 years of age came to me, with what I considered tubecular synovitis of her left knee, in the fall of 1889. She walked in with difficulty with the aid of a stick. The thing was evidently *de souche tuberculeuse*; she was florid; her mother died young of conumption, and six of her brothers and sisters had succumbed to the same malady in different forms. After two months of the bacillic virus (C.), she reported herself as quite well, and free from pain and inconvenience, and "able to walk slowly without stick for an hour and a half at a time."
She is quite well now. (XVIA 60)

**Case XVIII — Nocturnal Perspiration, Indurated Glands and Recurrent Cold.** A boy of 8 years of age, whose mother is in consumption, and of whose ancestors quite a number have died of consumption, was brought to me on Septmber 6, 1889, for these symptoms : nocturnal perspirations; (notched incisors); indurated glands everywhere very large and very numerous; drum-bellied; grinds his teeth in the night; great susceptibility to taking cold; perspirations worse at the back of the lungs and of the head; big head with bulging forehead; subject to attacks of fever and diarrhoea.
Two months of the virus (C.) cured all these, and he is now well and thriving. (XVIA 61)

**Case XIX — Consumptiveness.** On September 9, 1889, a young merchant, 26 years of age, of pronouncedly phthisical habit, both of whose parents had died young of lung disease, came to me telling me he had been under nine physicians, and also in a well-known hospital for what may be collectively termed consumptiveness : severe piles; constipation, and a brown cutaneous affection on the abdomen, that, I think, has been termed erythrasma. He is tall, thin, long thin neck, and bends forward. He was three months under the bacillic virus, got quite well, and has since married. He is altogether a different man. He had subsequently *Thuja* for his vaccinosis, and then *Hydrastis canadensis* Q five drops in a tablespoonful of water twice a day for some time. And here I wil allow myself to interpose the remark, that *Hydrastis* given as just named fattens up patients after the cure with the bacillic virus in an often truly wonderful manner. The bacillic virus has a well-defined and limited sphere of action, and very frequently needs to be followed by other remedies, as so few cases are quite simple. (XVIA 63)

**Case XX — Menorrhagia and Emaciation.** A married lady, 35 years of age, mother of three consumptive children; her only brother died of rapid consumption. She had miscarried three times, and was dying piecemeal of excessive menstruation, and had become alarmingly emaciated.

She had the virus (C.) and this was followed by *Chelidonium majus* Q and *Thuja* 30, and she was discharged cured at Christmas, 1889.

She is now well and in good condition. (XVIA 64)

**Case XXI — Thin Legs and Indurated Glands.** Daughter of the foregoing, 7 years of age, with limbs like sticks; right lung very flat; ribs of the right side fallen in; indurated cervical glands; stawberry tongue; spleen swelled; irritable and restless.

She had the virus for two months followed by *Calc. phos.* 3x, and was discharged cured on May 14, 1890. (XVIA 65)

**Case XXII — Chronic Diarrhoea.** The baby brother of the foregoing was brought on September 11, 1889, in an emaciated state suffering from chronic diarrhoea, and evidently without the intervention of medical art not long for this world. In my case-notes he is described as "all glands," i.e., the cervical and inguinal glands feelably indurated and visible. Without doubt his mesenteric glands were the seat of the same consumptive process and the real cause of the diarrhoea. He had *Elaterium* 3 (the motions went off "pop"). *Iodium* 2 and *Thuja* 30, when he was considerably better, but still had the diarrhoea and excessive perspirations. After a month of the bacillic virus, however, his mother reported "Very much better; no diarrhoea; no perspiration; we consider him quite well."

I gave him, however, two months of *Calc. phos.* 3x. (XVIA 66)

**Case XXIII — Headache.** An author of eminence, well known in theological circles, a little over 50 years of age, came to me in the fall of 1889, complaining of terrible pain in his head, almost absolute sleeplessness, and profound adynamia. Most of his brothers and sisters had died of water on the brain; his own right lung is solid, probably from healed-up cavities, as he used to have blood-spitting for years, and after much good treatment and foreign travel he "grew out" of his pulmonary consumption. His own friends, on advice, were having him "shadowed," as he was thought to be on the verge of insanity. The pain in his head he described as if he had a tight hoop of iron around it; his hands tremble; but what distresses him almost more than anything is a sensation of damp clothes on his spine.

It sounds hardly credible, but in less than a month after beginning with the virus the pain in the head had gone, the sensation of damp clothes had gone, and his sleep was very fairly good.

As a matter of prudence, I gave it him at long itervals for another month, and then he needed no further treatment. He continues, I believe, in good health, and is hard at work finishing a forthcoming publication. (XVIA 67)

**Case XXIV — Black-eyed, Fattish, Restless Boy.** An anxious young mother brought her fifteen months' old baby boy to me at the beginning of October, 1889. He was dark, sullen, taciturn, black-eyed and fattish (the kind of fat that I regard as hide-bound). He is irritable, costive, screams in his sleep, and he is very restless at night.

"His little sister died at 2+, of consumption of the brain, and she was just like he is."

He had at first some *Thuja*, with benefit, but we had not cured him by any means, then I gave the *bacillic virus* (C.), which his mother said made him at first "terribly ill," and thereupon amelioration set in. Here I gave *Calc. phos.* 3x, and he was thought well. But in May, 1890, he had a slight, relapse when I again gave the virus but this time in the two-hundredth potency. He got quite well and is now thriving. (XVIA 69)

**Case XXV — Consumption.** A young married lady, 28 years of age, one child, was recommended to me by her clergyman, and I first saw her on October 21, 1889. She had been under their very able and careful family physician for consumption, and then, said she, "I have been to all the physicians." She had formerly been very plump, but is now very thin, and has lost ten pounds in weight during the last two months. "No one can do me any good, and I want you to tell me if I am to die, or whether there is any chance for me, all my mother's people died of consumption."

As she had had typhoid very badly, so badly that she never quite throve since, although that was eleven years ago, I began with *Pyrogenium* 5, five drops in water, three times a day. the same principle that guides me in the exhibition of the bacillic virus guided me in my choice of the *Pyrogenium*.

Under the *Pyrogenium* she gained 3+ lbs. in weight.

I should have mentioned that she had no cough, though the apex of the right lung is solid, and the part pains very much, as does also the region of the base of the left lung. The vocal resonance was unequal. Besides gaining thus in weight, the top of the right lung is not so dull, and the vocal resonance seems pretty equal.

She then had *Nux vomica* 1 for her indigestion. She is what the homoeopaths call a nux subject.

On Nov. 18th she had gained another 2 lbs. in weight, and scaled 8 st. 11+ lbs. (She is a tall woman). She begs for the *Pyrogenium* again, but instead,

seeing the very pronounced hectic flush, I put her upon the bacillic virus (C).
December 4th — She weighs 8 st. 13 lbs. or 1+ lbs. more than last time. the hectic flush is gone. I continued with the virus.
January 1st, 1890 — She weighs 9 st. 2 lbs. Is weak, much indigestion, worse at 6 p.m.
*Thuja occid*. 30, as I considered the virus had done its work, and her two vaccinations had to be reckoned with.
January 29th — Weight 9 st. 7 lbs., and her indigestion is much better. But there is a little hectic flush again, and hence I hark back to the virus (C).
Feb 12th — She weighs 9 st. 9+ lbs., and is vastly improved. "That medicine tried me a good deal, but I am quite another woman." *Hydrastis* Q.
March 14th — She weighs 10 st. but still has dyspepsia, which I think may be from the old typhoid, and hence ordered *Pyrogenium* 5 as before.
April 8th — She weighs 10 st. 2 lbs. and is doing well. (XVIA 71)

**Case XXVI — Dyspnoea and Loss of Weight.** A single lady of 26 came to me in November 1889, in the first stage of consumption; both her sisters and her mother are said to be in consumption, and both parents of her mother died of consumption.
Beyond dyspnoea and rapid breathing the physical signs were but few : just loss of flesh and a greasy, dingy skin. She had two months of the virus followed by *Hydrastis canadensis* Q, etc., and was discharged cured in the following May. She is now plump, well, and thriving, so her brother tells me. (XVIA 75)

**Case XXVII — Incipient Consumption.** A city merchant, single, 28 years of age, came to consult me early last summer for incipient consumption. His mother had died of consumption; his brother is far gone of the same malady. He had an eruption in the skin over the larynx, and his general state was so distressed that I began the treatment with *Zincum aceticum* 3x, five drops in a tablespoonful of water every three hours. this cured the eruption, and I then noted that his skin was very dusky; he had long had chronic diarrhoea. Moist rales all over the chest, with pretty free expectoration. For the state of the bowels I gave *Iris versicolor* 30, and that cured the chronic diarrhoea, but the expectoration was very profuse. He had been formerly operated on for fistula. The bacillic virus continued for two months quite cured him, and he put on some 8 or 10 lbs. in weight. He continues well, and with my approbation has now married.
*Second Edition* : He continues well, and his wife has presented him with a fine healthy boy. (XVIA 75)

**Case XXVIII — Incipient Consumption.** A country gentleman brought or rather sent, his little 7 year old daughter to me on October 4, 1889, for treatment for incipient consumption; the cough was at its worst at 6 a.m. Notched incisors; very thin and puny; her cervical and inguinal glands very much enlarged and indurated; strawberry tongue. She was three months under the bacillic virus, the doses at 8 days' intervals, and got quite well. She continues thriving. She also had *Thuja* afterwards. (XVIA 77)

**Case XXIX — Consumption.** A young clerk, 34 years of age, was sent by his employer to me in the early spring of 1890 to be treated for consumption. He was dusky, pigeon-breasted, and ill-conditioned, but had only been acutely ill for three weeks. The haemoptysis was very bad; repiration rapid. His father had died of lung disease. He was put on *Acetum lobelia*, which did good palliatively, and then on the bacillic virus (C.), which did no good whatever, and he died in a very few weeks. This is quite in accordance with my other experience, *when the consumptive process is in full blaze the virus is unavailing*. (XVIA 78)

**Case XXX — Attacks of Feverishness, with Slight Cough.** An Oxford student of 22 years of age was sent by his widowed mother to me two years ago, for a little insignificant cough, rapid respiration, and attacks of feverishness. He was not emaciated, but listless, apathetic, and always tired; withal of a very sweet disposition, and had all his life been timid and retiring. I treated him to the very best of my ability, and with great care, with our usual remedies, and with the bacillic virus, and sent him to places which are supposed to be good for this malady. He did not suffer, but slowly died; his life went out, as it were, from utter weariness. I have his photograph before me, taken just before he died, and he, in it, does not even look ill. Perhaps it was thus to be. (XVIA 79)

**Case XXXI** — A gentleman, well over fifty years of age, whose only brother had died of phthisis pulmonalis, and whose father's three sisters had also succumbed to the same malady came to me early in the year for severe haemorrhage from the bowels, cough and emaciation. It was the great loss of flesh that alarmed him. Under the virus he put on flesh, the cough and haemorrhage ceased; he looks years younger, and is now well up to work and actively engaged in his profession. He ceased to lose flesh after the second dose of the virus. He continues under my care for a skin affection, and for prolapsus recti. (XVIA 80)

**Case XXXII — Tuberculosis Swelling — Right Knee.** A city gentleman, married, 30 years of age, came to me at the beginning of April, 1890, for an affection of his right knee. In 1877, he was kicked on the knee by a horse, which knocked him over. The knee remained swelled, and ever since he has had intermittent attacks of pain in it. He had been to a London hospital, and preparations were being made for an operation. A friend persuaded him to come to me as one known to be averse to operations. The operation was considered to be imperative, because of the supposed tuberculous nature of the knee swelling. This was pretty certain as most of his brothers and sisters had died of tuberculosis — in fact, of fifteen, ten had thus died; and he himself has expectorated clots of blood, and suffered from exhausting sweats.

Two months of the bacillic virus cured him completely, the last vestige of tenderness and swelling, however, disappearing under *Bellis perennis* Q, six drops in a tablespoonful of water continued for a month. (XVI A 81)

**Case XXXIII — Consumption.** A married lady, about 30 years of age, came under my care some six years ago, sent to me by a colleague in the north. She had long been in consumption, and her husband had taken her to almost all the renowned health resorts in Europe, but the disease progressed. Finally a warm house was built for her on the Surrey Hills, and I paid visits to her at short intervals for some four years, With the aid of the bacillic virus, and *Phosphorus, Bryonia, Scilla, Ceanothus, Iodium, Calc. Phos., Calc. Sul.*, the *Hypophosphites, Ant. tart.*, and some others, including Churchill's inhalations, *Terebinth*, etc., I several times thought to win. I got two successive cavities to heal up, but the third, deep in the base of the left lung, refused to heal, and the poor lady, weary and worn, died of exhaustion. (XVI A 83)

**Case XXXIV — Consumption.** An unmarried lady, 29 years of age, whose sister had just died at the age of 30 of consumption, and whose mother had also died of the same malady at the age of 39, was brought to me by her father early in April, 1889. She was considered a hopeless case, and my hopeful prognosis was not credited. The disease was principally confined to the right lung, and the cervical glands on this side could be felt like marbles. She is thin, skin dingy and dirty looking, ill smelling and greasy, and there was a good deal of acne of the chest. The bacillic virus, with *Thuja* and *Hydrastis*, enabled me to discharge her cured in four months. (XVI A 84)

**Case XXXV — Tuberculosis.** The little son of a distinguished clergyman, 2 years old, was brought to me on May 9th, 1889, for feverish attacks that were clearly pointing to tuberculosis, evidenced by the strawberry tongue, the indurated glands, and pining state generally. The bacillic virus, followed by *Thuja* and *Baptisia*, was followed by perfect recovery and in three months he was discharged in rude health. (XVI A 85)

**Case XXXVI — Nocturnal Restlessness with Pallor.** A babe of 18 months, whose sister I had formerly cured with the bacillc virus of a tuberculous affection of the eye, was, in consequence thereof, brought to me in May, 1889, for soft bones and nocturnal restlessness, with pallor and thinness. I knew the family well for years, and thus was quite sure that the child was necessarily born with a tuberculous tendency. And the virus cured her right off in six weeks, and her poor digestion was then righted by *Pulsatilla*, and she continues ever since to thrive, and her bent bones have hardened and become straight.

A first cousin was formerly under me with tuberculosis of the meninges, but as I then knew nothing of the virtues of the bacillic virus, she was cured by me of her symptoms, and then died of the disease, viz., tuberculosis. (XVI A 86)

**Case XXXVII — Scabs Scalp, with Bulged Forehead.** A lady brought her baby boy to me at the beginning of May, 1885, She had had four children. One died at birth, and the other two died of tubercles of the brain. Patient's scalp was the seat of a good many scabs; his forehead bulged; very bad nights all his life, and he is peculiarly fond of salt. I had him rubbed with oil, after the manner of the old practitioners of renown; *Psor.* 30 did him much good, and rather ameliorated the nocturnal diarrhoea, and his head seemed to bulge rather less. And after he had also been under *Calc. Carb.* 30 a very severe pustular eruption came out on his scalp, with much relief to his general condition. But very suspicious pyrexia occurred at frequent intervals. Here followed *Thuja* 30, but nothing was really adequate till I gave the virus 30 in infrequent doses, by which he was metamorphosed into a healthy boy; fever, feverishness, calling out in his sleep, and grinding his teeth, all disappeared. He pined a little in 1888 in the spring; a fortnight of the virus quickly righted that, and beyond *Calc. Phos.* he has needed nothing else.

Thus we have in this case five years of good health to prove the genuineness of the cure. (XVI A 87)

**Case XXXVIII — Consumption.** In the year 1885 a young lady of 20 was brought to me to be treated for the form of consumption commonly known as decline. She had a strumous scar in the neck, and her sister had just died of decline.

Patient's weight was, in June, 1885, 7 st. 8 lbs. Had had diarrhoea for nearly three years, and her tongue was raw-red. The full record of the case would occupy more space than I can here afford; suffice it to say that I gave her many remedies with very slow and varying success, but she took a distinct turn after a course of the virus, and I finally got her up to 8 st. 9 1/2 lbs. in weight.

She continues well now, but her digestion is easily upset. It will be noted that the aggregate increase in weight was 15 1/2 lbs. (XVI 89)

**Case XXXIX — Consumption — Of Left Lung.** A married lady, 29 years of age came to me just four years ago for consumption of the left lung, She was very pale and neuralgic, and was greatly distressed by her cough. All her friends knew her to be in consumption and she had of late years spent the winters abroad and by preference in Malta. I treated her with slow, bit-by-bit ameliorations with the remedies symptomatically homoeopathic, and thus passed just two years, when it was very clear that we had not got to the root of the matter. After a couple of months of the virus she got rapidly quite well, and, so far as I can tell, entirely free from any sign of consumption.(XVI A 90)

**Case XL — Consumption.** An overgrown girl of 13, of phthisical habit and parentage, and then lately under Sir — for her lungs, was brought to me for treatment in the month of August, 1886.

The top of the right lung gave no respiratory sounds at all, and the vocal resonance was slightly increased. Her constitution was said to have been broken by one of the infectious diseases of childhood. Pain in the left side and profuse perspirations. After a month of the virus 30 : "Has done her a great deal of good, the perspirations were chiefly on the hands, feet and armpits, but these have nearly ceased." After a pause of a month or two it was again given, and patient was discharged cured nearly three years ago. She continues well. (XVI A 91)

**Case XLI — Emaciation.** A girl of 10, daughter of a country squire, was brought to me in March, 1887, to be treated for *decline*. There was great emaciation, but not of the feverish consumptive kind. She had a number of remedies from me. *Thuja*, *Ceanothus*, *Quercus*, *Chelidonium*, *Ferrum*, and *Carduus*, and on, the whole, every one was more than satisfied with the general progress and increase in weight and *intelligence*. But not one of the remedies had influenced the indurated glands in the slightest degree, and hence I put her on the virus 30. This was in February, 1888, and the same remedy had to be repeated once subsequently.

She is now a thriving person. (XVI A 92)

**Case XLII — Emaciation, Hepatomegaly & Dyspepsia.** An unmarried lady, about 30 years of age, was accompanied to me by her mother, in the month of August, 1887, so that I might treat her for decline. Her father had died of consumption at about the same age, and her steady and ever-increasing emaciation had resulted in a fixed belief that she was just doomed to follow her father. She had a huge liver, and severe and long-continuning dyspepsia. Her father's was also the wasting form of consumption. She had some fever at times, with a hard, dry, deep cough. On account of the liver I began the treatment with *Chelidonium* Q following it up with *Carduus Marianus* Q and this again with *Argentum nit.* 1. These remedies did decided good, and were followed by *Cimicifuga, Coccus cacti, Thuja,* and *Iodine,* but notwithstanding bit-by-bit ameliorations, relief of the symptoms, and all that, the "consumption" was not gripped, as the evening fever clearly proved. Three months of the virus wiped out the whole thing, if I may be allowed to use such an expression.

A year has elapsed, and the cure holds good, notwithstanding the wearing, burdensome life she is obliged to lead, and still, this notwithstanding, she has gained a good deal in flesh and healthful appearance. (XVI A 94)

**Case XLIII — Consumption.** A young lady of 14, daughter of a staff officer, was brought to me at the end of the year 1887, in the month of November, She was distinctly in consumption, and very tall for her age, and very thin. Twice, lately, there had been a good deal of bleeding from the lungs. The outer portion of the apex of the right lung was dull on percussion, indeed, it had barely any respiratory sound of any kind; scaly eyelids; very large tonsils; emansion of the menses. I at first treated her with *Phos.* and other pulmonary remedies, but I needed the virus to extinguish the fever. She had inter-current pleurisy once, and a good deal of bleeding, but has made a complete recovery, and is now thriving. I quite lately very carefully examined her chest, both the old seat of the mischief at the apex of the right lung, and also the seat of the inter-current pleurisy at the left side, near the top, but failed to find any evidence of disease what-ever. (XVI A 96)

**Case XLIV — Consumption of Bowels.** A lad of 10 was brought to me by his monther in the early summer of 1888, with mesenteric disease, commonly called consumption of the bowels. "My little boy has a swelling on his left side, I think there was a swelling also of his right side, and he complains of a stitch in his side after running, but he seldom runs much. He is often languid and indisposed to talk; sometimes he is very nervous and irritable; he talks in his sleep and grinds his teeth; his appetite is small; his hands blue."

I found indurated palpable glands everywhere; a drum belly, the spleen region bulging out.

What rendered the case of importance, was the fact that a sister of his a year or two older had just died of tuberculosis of the brain, and many of the family had died of consumption. I treated him for a year, three separate months of which he was under the virus, and in June, 1889, or just a year from the beginning of the treatment, the note in my record is ..... "Well and fat," and that he is now, I believe. (XVI A 97)

**Case XLV — Incipient Tuberculosis.** A little girl of 6 was brought by her mother, Lady X., in the month of August, 1888, for evident symptoms of incipient tubercular disease : restless nights; sleeplessness : grinds her teeth; tendency to diarrhoea; want of appetite; foul breath; notched teeth; pain after food; vomiting of food; indurated glands; strawberry tongue; naughty; very irritable temper; puny growth; very thin.

After being four months under the virus, and having one or two tissue remedies, she was discharged in nine months in capital health, and without any morbid symptoms of any sort or kind. And the cure holds good to date. (XVI A 99)

**Case XLVI — Case of Evening Fever, Cough, with Hepatosplenomegaly.** A young unmarried lady, 22 years of age, of delicate habit of body, was brought by her mother to me in October 2, 1888, for the following symptoms : — A nasty little cough these seven weeks; a good deal of expectoration; pains in the right lung; evening fever; liver and spleen both enlarged; cough worse in the morning after breakfast; her neck is slightly goitrous. Her brother has consumption of the bowels. She had first *Chelidonium majus* Q, and *Scilla maritima* Q, as spleen and liver remedies respectively, but there was but very slight amelioration, the cough being very bad after her breakfast, or, perhaps, I should say breakfast *time*, as she eats hardly any breakfast. So I went to the root of the matter, gave the virus (C.) for six weeks, and then discharged her cured, now ten months since, and I learn from her mother that she continues quite well. (XVI A 100)

**Case XLVII — Consumptiveness.** A married lady of 40 came to me in November, 1888, for grave consumptiveness, not to say actual consumption; almost all her people have died of consumption, indeed, I believe she is the only survivor of her own generation, and now she is clearly going the way of the rest. She has a good deal of fever, worse in the evenings;

she is restless and terribly irritable; she is much depressed, and in almost constant agitation; her tongue is very red; she has chronic diarrhoea. She has lost 14 lbs. during the past six weeks, and she has no appetite. Six weeks of the virus 30 quite cured her, the fever went after the second dose, the diarrhoea quickly followed, and she soon became quite plump. The mode of exit of the motion from the bowels in this case was, "pop," as it were out of a popgun; this I have several times noticed. It has often been noted that the phthisical are wonderfully hopeful, but this does not hold good when there is tuberculosis of the brain, but, on the contrary, they are mum, taciturn, sulky, snappish, fretty, irritable, morose, depressed and men-lancholic, even to insanity. When, however, they are cured, they become sweet and charming. So it was in this case, and still more so in the one I am about to narrate. (XVI A 101)

**Case XLVIII — Old Pleural Effusion After Pleuro-Pneumonia.** A young lady, 18 years of age, was brought by her mother to me in the fall of 1888 for an old effusion into the left pleura remaining after severe pleuro-pneumonia; the ribs of that side bulged a good deal; respiration acceler-ated, and also the pulse; her teeth are very foul and discoloured (not from want of the most scrupulous care); the heart is a good deal disturbed, probably mechanically; patient sleeps but very little, and that little is very distressful; she is painfully conscientious, depressed, and suffers greatly from spiritual melancholy. Her period comes very seldom. She is sub-ject to lichen ruber, and gets feverish. She was two months under the virus C., and this effected an essential cure, but other remedies were needed for the non-consumptive part of the case, for, as I have before stated, and here again expressly point out, the tubercular virus acts *within its own sphere only*. Thus, in this case patient had been twice vaccinated, she had *Thuja occidentalis* 30 for a month; *Bryonia* 1x was used for getting the pleura better; *Pulsatilla* 1x brought a good deal of comfort to the ovarian region, as did also *Cimicifuga* 1, *Bellis perennis* Q, *Rubia tinct*. Q, and *Ceanothus* 1, did much to restore the sympathy of the left costal region, and *Ignatia amara* 1 was of real service in the emotional sphere — and yet, for all that, the actual consumptiveness was wiped out pleasantly and promptly by the virus. She is now quite well these seventeen months. (XVI A 103)

**Case XLIX — Tuberculosis Left Knee.** A little girl of 7 was brought to me in the month of December, 1888, with tuberculosis disease of the left knee. For eleven months she had been limping; the knee is much enlarged and very tender; her teeth are tuberculous; there are numerous cases of consumption in the family, and her father had spine disease. After one month of the virus 30 the swelling of the knee had gone down one-third, the joint had become more movable; the strawberry condition of her tongue had gone, and her teeth had cleaned. She had thereafter two months more of the virus C., and got quite well; the remaining enlargement of the knee yielding to a course of the third decimal trituration of the *Perlarum mater*. (XVI A 106)

**Case L — Hip Joint Disease.** This is one of severe hip-joint disease of a severe type and of long-standing, who was long under Dr. Drysdale, and who handed the case on to me when the family removed to London. The child eventually quite recovered, and is now a fine girl of 16, but of course the leg of the diseased side is shortened. Dr. Drysdale, and the orthopaedic surgeon who kept patient in his very excellent apparatus for several years, will be both interested in hearing that the *essential* remedy in the case was the virus of which we are here treating. (XVI A 107)

**Case LI — Consumption.** A young gentleman of 20 was accompanied to me in February 1889 in fully developed consumption. There were all the usual symptoms, and haemorrhage from the lungs for many months. He was tall, good-looking, and weighed 9 st. I lb. I treated him with the virus, and in a few months got his weight up to 10 st. 5 lb., when he, in August 1889, went to the seaside as I thought safe and nearly well. He returned, however, in October voiceless, phthisis of the larynx set in, and he eventually died. Over the acute laryngeal process the virus had no power whatever. (XVI A 108)

**Case LII — Consumption.** A lady of 40, unmarried, came under my care on October 26, 1885. "I am almost in a consumption, and have been so for many years." She was very thin and "consumed with fever." All that one could say of the lungs was that they were very flat, and the respiration almost imperceptible. It is not easy to understand such cases, they are evidently in a chronic state of feverishness, they cough, they are thin, they eat very little, they suffer much, and vegetate forth and on languidly. The virus cured this lady; all the fever left her — she had had it "very constantly for years." She no longer takes cold as formerly, and has become plump and thriving. Now amongst her friends and relatives she is generally supposed to have at last "grown out" of her constitutional delicacy. (XVI A 109)

**Case LIII — Ringworm, Cough, Enlarged Lymphatic Glands & Rudimentary Teeth.** The influence of the virus upon the teeth and their growth and appearance is very striking. What I regard as tubercular teeth are those — often more or less rudimentary — with holes in their external surface

. Whether this is a recognised pathological fact I do not happen to know, perhaps it is not. But it is an important clinical observation. I recognised it clinically some three years since, while treating a highly strumous lady with many scars and glands in her neck. While under the virus I noticed an extraordinary improvement in her teeth, they became a nice colour, and the numerous superficial holes cleaned and partially disappeared. It was even more apparent and striking in the following case : A girl of 11, with ringworm on the scalp; the lymphatic glands everywhere palpable, and her ribs very flat; strawberry tongue; a bad cough, worse at night; although 11 years old she had practically no teeth, that is to say, they were rudimentary and not above the level of her gums. *All* her mother's brothers and sisters had died of consumption ; after three months' treatment with our ordinary remedies we had made but small progress, and then I kept the patient altogether five months under the bacillic virus, with the result that her palpable glands ceased to be palpable; her ringworm disappeared; her ribs took on a better form; her breathing was notably better; and, *mirabile dictu, her teeth had grown*. She is now well, and has a mouthful of teeth which are quite passable. It may be noted that the ringworm has disappeared, and in respect to this nasty thing I find it generally disappears under the influence of the virus. I learned this very important fact also purely clinically in the following manner :- A whole family of children of different ages had had ringworm for a full year, and the mother told me on bringing them that she had already spent over £60 on medical fees for its cure, but in vain. All known remedies had been applied by the local doctors in two neighbourhoods, and several skin specialists had worked hard at their poor heads, but to no avail. Their heads were shaved and their scalps were well scoured night and morning, but *still* the ringworm persisted. Finally, a distant cottage had been hired, and the afflicted ones were there isolated, and the services of a noted ringworm curer of the non-qualified variety had been secured; but these also failing, they were put under my care. I have had no great cause to complain of the homoeopathic treatment of ringworm with our antipsorics — indeed, quite the contrary -- but it is apt to be a bit tedious at times. Now their mother had been cured by me of incipient tuberculosis with the virus, and it occurred to me that ringworm might be a manifestation of the tubercular kind, and so I forthwith put the whole lot under the virus, administered in the usual way, internally in dynamic dose; this I did all the more readily, as they all had numerous superficial palpable glands. And the result? In a very few weeks they were all well of ringworm and of the glands, and have thriven splendidly ever since. Something like a dozen bad ringworm cases have come to me since then, and they were *all* quickly cured by the virus, and in each case the general state has been greatly improved. No doubt some bacteriologist will cultivate, some fine day, the germs of the ringworm, and astound the world with his subcutaneous injections. *It is well that medical men should approach each subject from a different standpoint as they serve to correct one another.* (XVI A 110)

**Case LIV — Consumption.** This shall be my last case in illustration of my "Five Years" Experience in the New Cure of Consumption by its Own Virus." A young lad of 14 was brought to me in July, 1884, for treatment for consumption. For about a twelve-month he had had a bad cough, with spitting of blood, and one of the apices was audibly diseased. He had previously had pneumonia. His chest was flat, and respiration accelerated. After the use of the virus he got quite well, and nearly four years of subsequent good health, free from any consumptive symptom, testify to the genuineness of the cure.* There was one feature in his case to which I desire to call attention, viz., he tanned unduly in the sun before the cure, but not since. For many years I have regarded the *rapid* darkening of the skin in the sun's rays as indicative of a consumptive tendency; and as I have verified it many times, I have no doubt about it. I know a little boy who was brought to me for a *bad temper* : he is the scion of a consumptive family. I noticed that he was very much pigmented where the sun's rays impinged upon him, but not on the covered parts of his body, and his teeth were dirty-greeny. After he had been two months under the virus, his teeth went clean, and he no longer tanned in the sun, and finally he had become amiable and good tempered. (XVI A 115)

*He has just successfully passed the medical examination for service in the British army. — Second Edition.

## 293. CONSUMPTIVENESS

A young man of about twenty years of age was tall, big-made and from his bulk ought to have been very strong, but this he was not but on the contrary very weak indeed, and he had a number of indurated glands in the neck.

Three months of the *Bacillinum* has seemingly quite cured him and his cervical glands can no longer be felt and patient feels quite well and is now employed as an electrical engineer here in London. (XVI A 147)

A younger brother of the foregoing, about 12 years of age, was in a similar state and in addition to indurated glands his skin had a very dusky brown aspect, he tanned unduly in the sun.

He also has quite recovered under the *Bacillinum* and his father not long since reported of him from the country as quite well and hearty. (XVI A 148)

Young Lord X. just verging on his teens came under my professional care in the winter of the year 1890 for a group of symptoms that I have already ventured to lump together under the designation of *consumptiveness;* he was pale, spare, neck long and thin, and in the neck his glands visible from their very considerable enlargement and induration, and his temper most miserable. He had *Thuja occid.* 30, *Phytolacca dec.* 3 and *Psorinum* 30 all with some benefit, but the really radical improvement set in after the use of *Bacillinum* C., under which I kept him for about three months. Lord X. was discharged cured in nine months in quite a different physical state. No glands in his body can be either seen or felt and his neck must be fully half an inch thicker. The experienced know well what I mean when I speak of the long thin neck of the consumptive and consumptively-disposed, and if they will treat these thinnecked ones as I here relate they will slowly get a very weighty change. (XVI A 153)

## 294. INCIPIENT PHTHISIS

On the 29th October, 1890, a country gentleman brought his twenty-four year old daughter to me. Himself one of those experienced semi-professional lay homoeopaths, he had treated his daughter with almost all our usual remedies but their effects did not last. Said he : "The worst feature is that she gets fits of rapid respiration, 45 to the minute, and she lost flesh so." Objectively the cicumscribed redness of her cheeks at once struck me, and the breasts were very soft and flabby, in fact shrivelled and this is a weighty symptom in an English girl of twenty-four years of age. Patient complained of feeling very tired in the evenings; pains through the right half side of the neck feeble and even visible; the right mamma stringy and tender.

The bacillic virus in the one hundredth potency produced some improvement, but not very striking. The rush of blood during an attack of hurried breathing reminded me of the action of *Urtica* and hence the prescription of *Urtica urens* Q five drops in a tablespoonful of water night and morning. This seemingly cured the patient and she was verbally reported well on January 5, 1891. But the symptoms soon returned; the pains through the right lung became severe and the respiration very rapid. This acceleration of the respiration being pronouncedly worse in the evening I ordered *Psorinum* 30. March 6, 1891, — The breathing was normal after the *Psorinum*, but it has again returned seemingly from a slight cold. She is less tired in the evening, very depressed, lachrymose; the glands in the neck only very slightly improved. *Bacillinum* C.C.

April 29 — The remedy has acted promptly and decisively; the swelling of the glands has gone; the respiration is normal as is also the appearance of patient's cheeks. To continue with the *Bacillinum* C.C. in the same manner, viz., six globules dry on the tongue at bed-time every eighth day, Placeboes being administered on the intervening days.

June 19 — Discharged quite well.

November, 1891 — Patient continues well.

Patient's father is being successfully treated by me for an osteoma; her mother is asthmatic and was formerly under my care. And what I would specially refer to is the fact that patient's environment is and always has been specially favorable to health and in no way conducive to consumptiveness.

In the first edition I stated how I came to discover that our *Bacillinum* cures ringworm; this discovery I regard as of very great importance; the cure is sometimes rapid, at other times it takes some months, but amelioration soon set in all the cases that I have treated. I may add that I used in all my cases of ringworm no external applications whatever, merely directing the head to be washed with soap and water two or three times a week. I will add just one more case of ringworm. (XVI A 157)

### 295. RINGWORM

In the first edition, as just stated, I communicated the important fact — many smaller things are called great discoveries — that ringworm yields readily to *Bacillinum,* and that I therefore regard this cutaneous eruption as a tubercular manifestation.

A little girl, five and a half years of age, was brought to me at the end of January, 1891, to be treated for ringworm. There was only one ring on the back of the neck — but this was well defined. *Bacillinum* C. was ordered and the whole thing disappeared within the month, and the little lady has been very thriving ever since.

So far as I am concerned in this work the curability of ringworm by *Bacillinum* is an established fact, and I therefore take leave of the subject so far as this work is concerned, but in view of its doctrinal and practical importance, I am contemplating a separate essay on "Ringworm." (XVI A 161)

### 296. LICHEN RUB. DISCOLORATION OF TEETH, NOCTURNAL RESTLESSNESS

A young lady of fifteen summers and winters came under my observation this summer to be treated for frequent eruptions of red lumps on her skin, much rolling and tossing about in her sleep and a greeny-yellow discoloration of her irregular but otherwise sound teeth. Her younger brother was formerly cured by me of a chronic hydrocephalic condition and blackish teeth. Her mother was strumous and many members of her family have succumbed to phthisis. I ascertained that the nasty colour of her teeth was in no way due to lack of cleanising care. Two months of *Bacillinum* brought me a written report of her good health, winding up thus : "Her teeth are now a very good colour." Patient is of that fat strumous habit which some mistake for health. (XVI A 163)

## 297. ARRESTED DEVELOPMENT

Dr. John Young formerly of Brooklyn and now residing in Switzerland came over from the Continent to see me in regard to a very peculiar case of arrested development in a lad. He had no teeth, he was stunted in growth and his skin was very dirty dingy-looking — having read the first edition of this work Dr. Young remembered what I say in regard to the influence of *Bacillinum* on the teeth and the tawniness of skin as an important indication for its use. Acting upon these indications Dr. Young gave *Bacillinum* in high potency for some time with the result that the patient took to growing and his teeth sprouted, and altogether he was very remarkably changed under the bacillinic influence. (XVI A 165)

## 298. CHRONIC PILES

In the month of June, 1891, a married man of about thirty years of age, known to me from his boy-hood almost, came to me for chronic piles of a most distressing nature that were making him almost an invalid. He had attacks of pain *about an hour after stool*; he was also a chronic sufferer from hay fever, and his teeth were tubercular (indented in dots) and the pains were greatly aggravated by coughing and sneezing, both of which he indulged in very freely.

*Bacillinum* 1000 cured him right off in a fortnight both of the piles and of the just - described pains after stool, and today, December 7, 1891, he continues quite well and has had no relapse. His hay fever was also seemingly cured in the same rapid way, but hay fever has an ugly knack of returning again and again after you have cured it ! Two or three successive summers must pass before we can rely upon a cured case of hay fever being really cured to return no more. From the remedies I have found useful, and also useless, in the therapeutics of hay fever I have come to the conclusion clinically that what nosologists and clinicians call hay fever includes several aetiologically and pathologically totally different ailments or diseases. In some, I think hay fever very distinctly a manifestation of a phthisical taint, — about the others I have not yet made up my mind. The pollen of grasses has the same relationship to hay fever as the north wind has to a phthisical cough — the cough is hardly a north - wind cough in a pathological sense. (XVI A 167)

## 299. PRE-PHTHISICAL DYSPEPSIA

A married gentleman twenty-four years of age came under my care on the 2nd of March, 1891, to be treated for most distressing and inveterate dyspepsia of three years standing. He had the characteristic symptom "as if a tight rope were bound round his stomach." Debility, paleness, acidity; nervous, a kind of dead-all-over feeling. He had from me at first *Argentum nitricum* 3 x with a certain amount of benefit, but he was not cured by any means, and complained very bitterly. The dyspeptic generally know well how to grumble and their descriptive talents are by no means inconsiderable. But after I had had him a few weeks under *Bacillinum* CC. he turned all his talents at graphic grumbling into persuasive recommendations to his sick friends to journey forthwith to see the writer.
One of his friends came a long distance — some 200 miles — to see me and burst forth : "You have made a great cure of Mr. — -, etc." I was ultimately led to give *Bacillinum* CC. in this case because of th numerous peripheral glands that were visibly and feelably enlarged and indurated; by the fact that he had had blood-spitting and because his mother had died of phthisis at 49 and one of his sisters had also died of phthisis.
He considers himself quite well these three months; I put it in this way as I have not *seen* him, he living so far away. (XVI A 169)

## 300. COUGH WITH CHRONIC PULMONARY CATARRH

A London gentleman just turned fifty years of age came under my professional care in the first days of January, 1891. He was subject to a chronic cough with much catarrh of both the lungs; his cough was very distressing indeed, and no wonder considering the awful fog then on. But, though the cough was much aggravated by the fog, it was by no means due to it. There was some wheezing all over the chest, much worse of the left side, and patient gets feverish atacks which he terms his "heats and sweats." Cough worse at night, wakened by it. Said he : "I was always a 'coughing' man, my father died at my present age of consumption, and I have lost a brother and also a sister from consumption."
Two months of the *Bacillinum* C. quite cured him and he was really a different man, and his friends hardly knew him without his cough so frequently had it been to the fore. (XVI A 172)

## 301. INCIPIENT GENERAL ATROPHY

A boy of ten years of age was brought to me by his mother at the beginning of the year 1891 for wasting weakness. Rather tall for his age, he presented the following symptoms a glum, ancient face, thin, almost cheekless, hollow eyes, neck long, thin, studded with "waxen kernels," i.e., peripheral hypertrophic glands, thorax almost like a skeleton, and its cutaneous covering very full of wee veins ; abdomen thin and yet pot-like, the so-called drum-belly ; extremities long and thin ; groins full of feelably indurated very small glands. He is mum always, gives no replies to my enquiries and his mother tells me he will hardly ever talk ; he takes no interest in strangers or in general surroundings, and seemingly has no very special desire for anything or anybody, and hardly ever wants either to eat or drink, "And yet, : exclaimed his mother, "he is not ill !"

Five months under our *Bacillinum* C. and C C. (in infrequent dose I will here again reiterate) with an intercurrent month under *Thuja* 30 and followed by another month under *Calc. Phos.* 3x and now he is bright, chatty, nearly a stone heavier, enjoys his food and is full of interest for his surroundings ; the old shrivelled-up joylessness has gone and given place to cheerful thrivingness. I ordered no alteration either in diet or place of abode ; the boy lived before the treatment, and during the treatment and now after the cure, in the same house in a London suburb. (XVI A 173)

## 302. HYDROCHEPHALISM OF TWENTY YEARS' STANDING

A gentleman forty-six years of age came to see me in the month of November, 1890, for pains at the back of the left side of his head that had worried him for over twenty years. He complained also of a pain in his right foot. His tongue coated, frothy and quivery. Deep-brown eyes. Although married he gets at times nocturnal emissions. His pains are worse in the evening, no pains on awaking. He tells me he has been subject to pains in his head (*Bacillinum* produced severe long-lasting headaches in the writer) all his life and that he had water on the brain as a child. His mother died at 73 of carcinoma ventriculi. He is depressed.

He had the *Bacillinum* C., altogether thirty globules spread over a month and twice repeated, and then reported his pains as cured, and his spirits much brighter. I saw him six months later, and thus know he continues well. "I have been in splendid health and well up to my work all summer," said he the other day. (XVI A 176)

## 303. CEPHALIC SUFFERING IN LATER LIFE PRIMARILY DUE TO OUT-GROWN HYDROCHEPHALUS

This part of my subject may be regarded as new, and deserves more than a passing consideration. In the first edition of this work I narrated a case in point (Case XXIII, Pp 470). Let us enter upon the subject somewhat.

We have all met with cases of oddly-shaped more or less piled-up or bulging-out heads, and these people really bear about with them a cephalic misshapenness (perhaps very trifling, but still peculiar) as the permanent expression of the hydrocephalic states of their early lives. Such people are frequently gifted, their children are very delicate and apt to die of consumption ; and although they have grown out of their hydrocephalus and may be gifted and distinguished members of society, they generally suffer more or less in various ways ; they are apt to be a bit peculiar in their sexual spheres and their ways — glum sort of folks, by no means excelling in amiability. I know one gentleman whose skull is drawn up somewhat sugar-loaf fashion or rather as if the skull had developed while it was hung up by its top ; his periodical haemorrhoidal bleedings indicate, I think, a tubercular taint.

I will further explain what I am trying to express by narrating a case in point which has been all the more instructive to me because he was a faithful patient before I knew anything about the virtues of *Bacillinum*. He first came under my observation in the year 1880 in some distress of mind because he was childless ; I found the urethra gleety and this I thought was the anatomical cause of his wife's barrenness. He had a course of treatment from me to cure this sticky urethritis, and got in succession *Thuja occidentalis* 3x, *Hepar sul.* 3x, *Natrum sul.* 4, and *Cynosbati* Q. These therapeutic measures were followed by his wife getting in the family way, and patient there upon ceased attendance. There were three or four points in the case at the time that struck me, viz., the peculiar bulging state of his skull, certain brown patches on the skin and head suffering, and finally his frequent nocturnal emissions notwithstanding the fact that he was happily married. I did not see him again for nearly ten years, when on Janurary 30, 1890, he again put in an appearance and complained of insomnia, headaches, and the fact that he still suffered pretty severely from nocturnal emissions, *worse* after the exercise of the marital function. The peculiarity of his insomnia was that he awoke in the very early morning and could not get off again. I have before explained that this symptom is characteristic of *Bellis perennis*, and as this drug is an excellent restorative from sexual fag I ordered it him, five drops of the matrix tincture night and morning.

His own estimate of the prescription was : "I have never had such a good tonic in my life."
By this time I had read this gentleman's constituion in the light of his head and other symptoms as what I for convenience sake will call "hydrocephalism." His hearing troubled him a good deal ; the aurists called it "internal congestion," but his hearing did not improve under their treatment ; he suffered from great depression and life-long constipation and his nocturnal emissions added very much to his irritable melancholy. Here I gave him *Bacillinum* C. and thereafter C.C.altogether during about two months.
And the result? For the first time in his life his bowels acted normally, his hearing greatly improved, and, unless both he and I were and are mistaken, his head altered in shape quite perceptibly. So it seemed to us, but his seeming change in shape may have been due to his changed expression from a kind of sour glumness to one of smiling brightness. I may add that the patient knows nothing of my theories or of what remedies he had.
A year has since passed and the great change wrought in him still holds good — this I know because he has had his daughter under my care. (XVI A 177)

## 304. PELVIC CONSUMPTIVENESS

Consumptiveness may show itself not merely in the lungs, in the glands, but also in the brain ; we have cited enough examples of all these manifestations of the tubercular diathesis. But it shows itself, perhaps almost as frequently, in the pelvic region ; as disturbances of the menstrual or sexual functions : in the young men as more or less furious incoercible nocturnal emissions, masturbations, or excesses in venery, that if not cured run the sufferer to ground. The excessive fecundity of the tuberculously disposed needs no dwelling upon. The girls develop very quickly and ripen perhaps unduly in the bust. Such a case came under my care very early in the year 1889. She had had profuse and too frequent periods for long though she was then but twenty years of age. In bust, large ; in colour, white, waxen almost amyloid. Her breathing very distressing and debility profound. Her father has spinal curvature, and a little brother has died of tubercular meningitis.
I regarded the dyspnoea as from the anaemia ; the anaemia as from the excessive monthly losses and want of appetite, and the menorrhagia as from a consumptive state of the pelvic organs. Two months of *Bacillinum* C. cured the pelvic consumptiveness, the period becoming naturnal, whereupon the anaemia and dyspnoea began to mend in equal pace; the

remaining painfulness of the menstruation disappeared under *Thuja* 30, and patient was well. With some difficulty I got her to take *Hydrastis Canadensis* Q, five drops in water night and morning, for a month, and the subsequent two years of capital health testify to the soundness of the curative work then done. I have before pointed out my fondness for *Hydrastis* in small material doses as an aftercure to the bacillinic treatment. Here I gave it for a month, but at times I give it for two, and I sometimes use it intercurrently between two courses of *Bacillinum* with much advantage, not that it has any relationship to tuberculosis as such, but it increases the appetite, and patients under its influence put on flesh of good quality. (XVI A 184)

## 305. HEPATIZATION OF LEFT LUNG

A gentleman of sixty years of age consulted me on October 13, 1888, for a cough, consolidation of left lung and albuminuria; the vocal resonance of the left lung is very pronounced; pains in the back, dreadful perspirations. There was a curious point as to the colour of the hair on his hirsute body : that on the chest exactly down to the diaphragm is white; below the diaphragm his body-hair is black.

*Bacillinum* 30 soon cleared up his lung, but patient refused to go on under my care; said he : "The medicine is awful, I was seized in the stomach with pain accompanied by diarrhoea and perspirations; it loosened all my teeth, made my gums sore, set up dreadful vomiting, : but the left lung seems well.

But I am not sure he rightly ascribed all this to the remedy, and the less so as he had been salivated with mercury long before. I only cite this case to show the violent action of the remedy even in the thirtieth dilution, and because it rapidly cleared up the left lung, the cough becoming much more active. One of his daughters died of consumption of the bowels, so he informed me. (XVI A 187)

## 306. TABES MESENTERICA. CONSUMPTION OF THE BOWELS

In the early summer of this year, 1891, a lady and her asthmatic husband brought their eight year-old boy to me to be treated for chronic diarrhoea of four months' standing, pretty extreme emaciation, a dark mahogany-like discoloration of the skin (all over, not in patches), feelable induration of glands in both sides of the neck and even more so in the groins. "He is nothing but skin and bones, and won't eat anything, and the doctor has been treating him for worms but he gets no better." Hereupon the mother burst into tears and was not to be pacified for several days, she

seemed to feel he would die. "His grandparents are sure he will die." Indeed I at first gave a bad prognosis and was only inducted to modify it by the mother's distress.
Three months of *Bacillinum* slowly and completely cured the boy, and a letter reached me this day to say, "R. is so well and bonny," and a fortnight ago the governess wrote me, "R. is as well as ever, and needs no more medicine." The boy himself I have not seen since his treatment, but it is pretty evident that he is now quite well. He had no other remedy at all to account for the cure. (XVI A 189)

## 307. OFFENSIVE OTORRHOEA & SWOLLEN GLAND

April 5, 1889, — Leonard
X., aet. 4 ; has a strawberry tongue and a very offensive chronic discharge from the left ear; behind the left ear there is an indurated swelled gland, and there are some hard feelable glands in the neck." And what was the remedy in the powders the mother wanted again for her little Leonard? *Bacillinum* 30; one dose of six globules on sugar of milk every 12 days.
In my judgment there is not any higher testimony to the eficacy of a remedy than that of a mother when she remembers and picks out a given prescription of two years and a half ago. The little man's sister had pyothorax after pleurisy last winter, but she is quite well now. (XVI A 192)

## 308. CONSUMPTION

One, a young woman, aged 28, came here last March in the second stage of consumption; had spent one winter in the home at Ventnor. The doctors said no more could be done for her, and I did not think she would ever be any better, but had just come here to die. The kind friend who lent me your book administered the virus, and the patient so far recovered as to be able to take a situation near Liverpool, and by a letter received a day or two since is evidently fairly well. The sister, who has resided with me many years, aged 26, was looking very pale and feeling languid, no energy ; suffered, too, at monthly period. These young women are orphans - both parents died of consumption. She, too, began taking the virus once a week for eleven weeks, and the change was wonderful; does not suffer monthly now. All who knew her said 'how well she looked'. She discontinued it the middle of July, and one reason I write you is to ask if you think she had better resume it?
"The second case was a young person far advanced in consumption; left lung affected; could not lie on the left side. After taking the virus was certainly better, and could sleep on the left side.

"Third case, a child, wasting away, and poor appetite. She is now looking bonny and gaining flesh.

"I ought to say the first-named patient had the right lung affected ; cavities in it, and the left very weak. Her sister had lost flesh, but has gained nearly six pounds since taking the virus. (XVI A 193)

## 309. ACUTE PHTHISIS

I have rarely been impressed with any case more than with the following one of acute phthisis, and I think it would be very difficult to find a more direct proof of the simple art-cure of a very dangerous malady.

A single gentleman, from a very healthy part of Kent, aged 24, had been ordered abroad in the month of October, 1891, for acute phthisis, and so severe were his symptoms that he came straight away up to London in that month to arrange for some one to take over his business previous to starting. The merchant to whom he went in the city urged him to come and get my opinion before disposing of his business and going abroad. He came, and I found his condition indeed one of intense anxiety, and had he come to me before I knew of the virtues of *Bacillinum* I should have advised hasty departure from our fogs and damp. But I thought we might possibly cure him with the said remedy, though I did not feel very sure that he was at all curable on any means whatsoever, so very ill was he. His throat was studded with tubercles, and for two months he had been consuming with fever. He had expectorated masses of matter and blood for weeks past, in bouts, but not continuously. Sleep very bad; says he has had none for a week. Much phlegm in the morning, but not always with blood; spleen and liver much swelled; respiration accelerated; morning and evening exacerbations, and very tired out of a morning, so that he is unfit to rise. His parents and brother alive; one of his sisters died of hip-joint disease, and one of pulmonary phthisis. The case being so severe and acute, I used the one-thousandth of dilution of the remedy every fifth day.

Towards the middle of November his sleep had greatly improved; nearly all the tubercles had disappeared from the throat; no further blood spitting; much mattery expectoration; still had fever, but only in the evening; all cough gone, and his appetite had begun to improve.

By Christmas he was practically cured, and business being brisk, he ceased attending.

Four months later, May 2, 1892, he called to say that he had been quite well, but had had a little expectoration streaked with blood the past few days. I did not readily recognize him, so greatly had he improved. "I have gained quite a stone in weight, and everybody wants to know what sort of treatment I have been having."

He had another month of the remedy, and only a few days ago I inquired of the before-mentioned merchant who sent him to me how his friend was. "Ah," said he, "I never thought he would get well; he looks first rate now; I have told ever so many people about it, but they won't believe it, because they don't believe in Homoeopathy; I don't understand them."

If this patient had gone away as he was ordered, I am of opinion that he would have succumbed to his malady. "Going away" is by no means synonymous with"being cured." Not a few go away dutifully enough, but the return? Ah! they commonly enter upon a long journey whence no man returneth.

October 16, 1893 — I heard today from the said merchant that this gentleman continues quite well. (XVI A 203)

## 310. ANOTHER WITNESS FOR THE CLINICAL VALUE OF TUBERCULINUM (BACILLINUM)

"On April the 17th I (Dr Chas W. Roberts, M.D.) was called to see Adele L., aged about two years; found her in a convulsive condition with twitching and spasmodic contraction of the muscles, great hyperaesthesia of the skin, photophobia, nausea and vomiting; temperature 103° F; great cerebral excitation; nervous temperament; prominent roundish forehead, small face and slightly downward look of the eyes. Bowels constipated, attacks of colic, grinding of teeth, terrible thirst for water; very slightly open fontanelles and sutures. With these symptoms and many others less prominent my prognosis was, of course, very guarded, the chance of recovery being extermely slight; but with the powerful guns that homeopathic remedies furnish, I was not willing to announce to her loving parents that their only little one could not live, and I therefore mustered all the courage I possessed, and said that, while I considered their little one very dangerously ill, still I had hopes that she might pull through, and went into the fight with a determination to win if possible. To make a long story short, my first prescription, on account of the intense thirst and small,rapid, tremulous and intermittent pulse, sensitiveness to touch about the head, was *Helleborus nig*. 30; this remedy seemed to control the eagerness for water, and the pulse, but stopped there.

"My next prescription was *Apis mel*. 30, dil. Continued this remedy forty-eight hours with improvement. I was then taken sick myself, and did not see the patient for four days, but recommended a physician who carried out my line of treatment, and when I again saw my little patient she had lost flesh so rapidly that it sent a shudder over me as I viewed her tiny limbs and body. I prescribed at once *Calc. carb.* 30, dil., and asked for a sample of urine, which I received in twenty-four hours, and to my horror it seemed to me almost solid albumen. I thought then my little patient was doomed. After thinking over the history of the case, and from what I knew of the family history, and the prodromal symptoms, the irritableness, swollen abdomen and constipation, great and rapid loss of flesh, etc., I concluded to prescribe Boericke & Tafel's 200 dilution of *Tuberculinum*, one dose every three days, with placebo every hour.

"From this day began rapid and permanent improvement. Oh, what a relief to mother, father, friends, my little patient, and myself! I know that under any other treatment, and I might say remedy, this interesting little child could not have survived. Great credit is due to her mother, whose good judgment never forsook her for a moment. (XVI A 211)

## Dr. John Young's Cases
## (Cases 311 - 324)

### 311. SYPHILITIC ERUPTION

"A mother brought a child of 12 months, covered from head to foot by a syphilitic eruption, the eyes like raw flesh. I gave the child on her tongue 15 small pellets of *Bacillinum* 200. A week after, the change was more than could be expected. Again the same dose; eight days later the child could see well, and the eruption more than half gone. Two weeks longer treatment in the same manner, the child was perfectly healed — a proof that *Bacillinum* has curative effect on syphilis. (XVI A 231)

### 312. CONSUMPTION

'2. A Miss E.,of 27 years, having spent the winter of 1890-91 in the hospital at Basel, being sent home in April,'91, pronounced incurable, suffering with consumption, sent for me, May 15, 1891, Examination pronounced both lungs in an advanced state of phthisis. She began with 20 pellets of *Bacillinum*; every eighth day the same dose. In July after, she called at my house in Herisau, and in truth I was astonished to see her so well. Kept on taking *Bacillinum*, when in September, visiting Basel, I found her very well. (XVI A 231)

## 313. DYSPEPSIA

"3. A Miss S., teacher, of 38 years, in Basel, suffering for years with bad stomach, not able to keep food in her stomach, had the symptoms of a beginning cancer of the pylorus.This lady received *Bacillinum*, one dose every eight day, and after six months was totally cured. (XVI A 232)

## 314. CONSUMPTIVENESS

"4. A merchant in Basel, 32 years old, consumptive for several years, received from his doctors, as the last resort, *Kreosotum* in capsules. Getting worse from month to month, the family desired he should consult a homoeopathic physician. Was consulted, and examination showed the upper parts of the lungs badly affected, covered by tubercles; also had chronic bronchitis. Received *Bacillinum* 200, 20 pellets every eighth day, keeping on for three months the medicine, and to the astonishment of his friends he became a healthy man. (XVI A 233)

## 315. CONSTANT COUGH

"5. A *dessinateur* here in Herisau, suffering from weak lungs, constant cough day and night, under-went a so-called 'Knipps' treatment at a place in Germany. Six weeks after he came back a skeleton, emaciated, miserable. Examination proved the whole upper part of the lungs covered by tubercles. *Bacillinum* cured him perfectly in two months. (XVI A 234)

## 316. CONSUMPTION

"6. A young girl of 16 years, of Lofingen. Over two years ago she had scarlet fever, was neglected, and lost appetite and sleep; her menses ceased more than eighteen months. All appearance was that she was in the decline (consumption). I gave her of the *Bacillinum*, every week 20 pellets. The result was indeed beyond my expectation. The menses returned and the other complaints disappeared, sleep came back, and after three months she became a blooming girl. (XVI A 234)

## 317. SPINAL IRRITATION

"7. This is a very remarkable case. A maiden lady of 37 years, residing at Lichtensteig, being more or less sick for sixteen or seventeen years. The first cause was hysterical spinal irritation; grew worse from year to year; her spine curved over 1 inche; her left hand inflamed, which led to amputation of her index (fore-finger). Over two years ago she became helpless in both legs.

The doctor at Wattwyl (city hospital) thought (it was then just the fury of Dr Koch's lymph system) to inject in her the lymph. This he did eighteen times. After this had been done her legs, from hip to foot, became as dead, without any feeling. It was on December 2, 1891, I found her in that condition I left her *Bacillinum* 20 pellets, every week one dose. After four weeks some feelings returned; also became able to move her toes, keeping on for some time more in the same manner. In May last she was able to sit up. In June she was strong enough to get up and walk alone in her room. Now it is August 9th. Her legs are perfectly normal, and with the exception of the curve on her back and the sore hand she is as well as she had been in her younger days.

"This lady had been pronounced incurable, and the people of Lichtensteig, with their doctors, are enchanted over such a cure. Bacillinum has done its work perfectly, and many such so-called incurable cases would yield under the blessed influence of this wonderful medicine. (XVI A 235)

### 318. RHEUMATISM

"8. Another case where old and new school doctors have more or less failed. A butcher's wife, about 58 years old, residing in Lichtensteig, has been for years complaining of rheumatism, but more especially a stiffness and redness in her arms, hands, legs, and feet, which resulted slowly into arthritical, gouty contractions of the joints of fingers, toes, even on the knees, so as to become unable to shut the hands, and walking only with great difficulty. She received *Bacillinum* in the above-named order, and in less than three months all her stiffness was removed, and she is now very well. Here it was evident that *Bacillinum* absorbed the chalky substance in the joints. (XVI A 237)

### 319. IDIOTISM & CRETINISM

"9. A case of *idiotism* and *cretinism* which made a great stir. In August, 1891, I was called by telephone to go to a place near Neuchatel, about 150 miles from Herisau, and found there a 10 year old girl, a perfect idiot and cretin. The history of the child was about this : Until after vaccination (she was 1 year old), was very well; from that time she began to act as having no sense, growing worse from months to years Her parents consulted in different cities, as London, Paris and Vienna, with out the slightest amelioration. They heard of me from a doctor of Basel, that I had attended there a 16 year old idiot, whose reason returned partially. I found the girl in the following condition : height two feet and five inches; age, 10 years; the teeth hidden in the gums : could hardly stand on her feet, unable to walk and talk; head, front narrow and large on the back; several smaller and larger elevations on the skull, some soft, others hard; nose, eyelids and lips extremely large; type of an idiot and cretin.

"A careful examination, especially of the deformed head, with its elevations, disclosed nests of tubercles. Her eyes without life, no desire for anything; in fact, the most ungrateful expression! Now what to do? My thoughts settled soon on one point - to give an antidote to these colonies of tubercles, and decided on *Bacillinum* as the only means to being on a change. She received on the 10th of August, 1891, 20 pellets, to continue every week the same dose. Visited her in October said year; great change; she began to talk and walk, the teeth sprouting out of the gum, the head a better form, and the general condition of the whole body was changed. Kept on by the same medicines. In November it was decided that I should go to London to a conference, to confer with Dr. Burnett. (Dr. Burnett mentioned my visit to him in his second edition of 'Cure of Consumption,' pages 151 and 152.) After this, every month brought some new change. It is just a year since the child came under my attendance, and what a change has *Bacillinum* 200 operated! The child talks, walks (even runs), has grown 3 inches, intelligence restored, enjoys her life extremely, being so cheerful and bright. (XVI A 238)

## 320. BACILLINUM : ITS CURATIVE POWER IN DIFFERENT DISEASES.

"**Case 1.** — Another case of lameness, in which *Bacillinum* has shown its decided power to subdue and destroy the hindrance of growth and harmony in the whole body : "Was called to examine a youth of about 18 years, in a city 20 miles distant from my residence. It was on July 9th this year . Found him sitting in an arm-chair. His upper limbs, lame, especially the left arm, his legs crossed under the chair; positively impossible to move, either forward or backward; very little feeling in his legs; had to be carried from his bed in the morning to his chair in the sitting-room, and again, at night, to his bed. This had been his condition for about 18 months. His sleep was very heavy and profound; appetite was rather ravenous, especially for pickled things. His mental faculties very unsteady and heavy; unable to think much. On examining his leg, I found some hard knots around both knees and ankles, and also on the wrists, of the size of small nuts, tender to the touch. Studying the case very carefully, I came to the conclusion that those knots were colonies of tubercles, hindering the activity of the joints and deadening the feeling.

"The history runs as follows : He was working for several years in a factory, exposed to water and dampness, as his shop was underneath the factory. The constant dampness brought on in a slow way some stiffness in the limbs, especially the joints of the knees. At last, be was obliged to stay at home, was attended by several physicians, until he became perfectly helpless and lame. It was in this state I found on the 9th of July, 1892. Prescribed *Bacillinum* 200, 25 small pellets every eight days. End of July, received news of some amelioration of the whole condition. Contiuned *Bacillinum*. Saw him on August 27th. He was able to use his arms a little, and move his legs. Again *Bacillinum* 30. On September 30th, received word of very great improvement. October 22nd, saw him again; his arms were all right, could move his legs forward and backward, and even stand on them; and no doubt in two or three months he will be as well as before his lameness. He was also troubled with enlargement of the glands of the neck and under the ears. Under the effects of *Bacillinum* this condition was alleviated, some of the enlargements opening and discharging a thick matter and afterwards healing. (XVI A 243)

## 321. CONSUMPTIVE CASE

"**Case 2.** — A consumptive case. On June 20, 1891, a gentleman brought his 13 year old daughter for treatment. Examination revealed : Very weak lungs; isolated tubercles on both upper lobes of the lungs; pulse variable, from 95 to 100; strawberry tongue; brownish spots or blotches on the face; short breath; all appearance of quick decline, running into galloping consumption. Her patents were both of a scrofulous diathesis; I had attended her father for ophthalmia scrofulosa, and her mother for general weakness. Prescribed *Bacillinum* 200, one dose every eight days; also gave orders to feed the girl well, and for her to exercise in the open air; especially to be much in the sun, keeping her head well covered. From week to week the change became visible; her thin limbs rounded out, her face became fuller, and had a healthy color. In six months all the alarming symptoms had disappeared, and the child was healed. (XVI A 247)

## 322. CONSUMPTION

"**Case 3.** — Another case of consumption. Was called on June 9th, 1892, to a village four miles from here, to see a girl of 20, low for several months with consumption. Found her very feeble; pulse hardly perceptible; visible vibration on both lungs; constant short, dry cough; face bloated; as also the rest of the body. The skin resembled parchment, but was moist and deadly-smelling; eyes haggard. The whole expression as one doomed to die! — indeed, a hopeless case! Left *Bacillinum*, one dose of 25 pellets every eighth day. Three weeks later her mother called at my house, telling me of a change for the better; the patient's appetite had improved, and she rested better at night; was able to sit up and had become more cheerful. Contined *Bacillinum*. End of July, she was so much better, able to walk a little in the sun, to get warmed by its heat. The improvement would have gone on more rapidly, but her parents were very poor, and were unable to feed her properly. This case speaks loud enough of what *Bacillinum* is able to do, even in advanced cases of consumption. (XVI A 248)

## 323. CONSUMPTION

"**Case 4.** — Another case of consumption from the same village. On July 1, 1892, a mother brought her 16 year old daughter to my office. The girl was a true type of the consumptive. Pulse 105; face brownish; strawberry tongue; eyes without any expression; cough more or less constant; very tall for her age, but very slim, weak, unable to walk, even to stand on her feet. Prescribed *Bacillinum* 200, 20 pellets every eithth day. September 8th, she came alone a long way on foot. What a change after eight weeks of taking *Bacillinum*! My astonishment was great. Fleshy and stouter; rosy cheeks; cough completely gone. In this case the conditions were different from the case last related. Her parents fed her with nutritious food, so that in weight she gained several pounds; this wonderful and quick cure of that girl made quite a stir up in her village. (XVI A 250)

## 324. CONSUMPTIVE CASE

"**Case 5.** — Again another consumptive case. On July 30th, 1892, a farmer's wife of the same village, aet. 42, made her appearance at my office, wishing to be cured of what she complained, having consumption, or what people and her husband called decline. Her skin was of a grayish-brown color; thin, emaciated, and very weak; completely exhausted by constant dry, hacking cough, often with purulent expectoration. She attributed her ill feelings to over-work in the fields and not sufficient suitable nourishment. Prescribed *Bacillinum* 200, every eighth day 25 pellets. On September 10th she came again and asked for more, as she said, 'of the same little pellets. Indeed, there was a great change. Her whole countenance had changed. She had gained flesh, looked better, and a real brightness shone in her face. Towards the end of October her husband came for medicine for himself, telling me of his wife's perfect cure, and by her cure he had become converted to Homoeopathy. (XVI A 251)

### 325. RACHITIS

**Case 6.** — *Bacillinum* triumphant in rachitis. Early in June, 1892, a lady brought her little five year old girl to be examined and attended, as the girl was very sick. Questioning the lady concerning how long the disease had troubled the child, she answered, "Since childhood!" Examination revealed a quite advanced state of rachitis; spine curved inwards (lordosis); the belly and stomach pressed out, very large and hard, especially the lower part; skin of the face deep yellowish, and of the body brownish color; the front part of the head narrow, pointed out, while the back part was very large and rather square. No appetite; no sleep; and more or less diarrhoea of putrid, strong-smelling excrement. As several quite eminent physicians (Allopaths) from different places had attended her, but without avail, the child getting from time to time weaker, unable to stand on her thin legs, I hesitated at undertaking the treatment of such a forlorn and apparently hopeless case. But the clamor of the distressed mother decided me to try *Bacillinum* 200, 20 pellets every eight days. End of July the mother wrote me of the effect of the pellets in the following terms : 'My child begins to walk, belly and stomach smaller and less hard; diarrhoea subsiding; appetite and sleep good. Send more medicine!' Continue in the same manner. September 25, child improving, runs and jumps around the rooms. Keep on the same dose of 25 pellets of *Bacillinum* 200. October 29, child all right; she has grown taller, gained flesh on chest, arms and legs; and to the astonishment of all, her head has become its natural shape, as also the stomach and belly. This peculiar case greatly occupies my mind concerning the possibility of the curative power of *Bacillinum* on rachitis, and strengthens my assertion that in many so-called incurable diseases the main causes are parasites of a peculiar nature. (XVI A 253)

## Dr. Robert Boocock's Cases
## (Cases 326 - 329)

### 326. CONSUMPTION

"**Case 1.** — I had at this time coming to my dispensary Mrs. O., aged about 40, slowly recovering from confinement; has a very severe and racking cough; no appetite; copious night sweats; very acrid and copious leucorrhoea; not able to nurse her baby, no milk. She presented the picture of a woman in the last stages of consumption. A careful examination revealed a great dulness in two or three parts of the right lung, with some rales in other parts, and much pain. I was not able to make a complete examination, and the bulk of this was what she told me. However, it was a nice case on which to try the new remedy, so I gave her one powder of *Bacillinum* 30th, ten globules, and a bottle of *Aqua d. and Glycerine* as a placebo, one teaspoonful three or four times daily or when her cough troubled her; and seeing her every three or four days, so that I might watch her carefully (for we have to give something in order to win their confidence). To my joy, she at once began to improve; appetite returned, night sweats ceased, cough was relieved, and so cure was completed in less than two months. She received sixty globules of 30th. (XVI A 258)

## 327. TUBERCULOSIS

**Case 2.** A car driver's wife. Tall, thin, fair skin, high cheek bones, hectic flush, 34 years old, mother of several children; has a hard life to live — a drunken husband and insufficient food, and the care and worry of a large family. When she bared the upper part of her body she was a perfect skeletion. Every bone could be counted, and the interostal muscles were very severely shrunk. Tubercles in all parts of lung. Cough; sputa raised in great quantities, yellow and like oysters as if floated in water, or partly so much sinking, heavy with gray particles. She looked like a physical wreck. What could *Bacillinum* do for her? Well, it was given in 30th, ten globules and placebo. In four weeks a steady gain. She then stopped coming, and after four weeks' waiting I went to find her, but could scarce believe it was she. I asked her for Mrs. B., and when she said, 'Why, doctor, did you not know me?' you may judge of my surprise. She was fair and good-looking; her cheeks had filled out, and she was well; I could see she was. What a rapid change? Thank God! A woman saved to her family. (XVI A 259)

## 328. COUGH, WEIGHT LOSS & NIGHT SWEAT

'**Case 3.** — Mrs. T. A., about 37 years, was given up, or she had given up doctoring, as she believed it was no good. History : had two attacks of what her doctors had called *la grippe*, and had not been well since. Lost her voice; continuous severe, racking cough, which all the medicine she took did not relieve. Losing flesh constantly; night sweats; no appetite; cold feet; sweat, clammy hands and feet, burning at times. Bluish purple face; aphonia. She had been under the care of two specialists for her throat, but they told her that her vocal cords were paralyzed, and she would never speak a loud word again. With the cough and this form of aphonia there is always a gushing from the bladder. For this I began treatment from her husband's description. Gave *Caust.* in 3d. At the end of a week report very much better; cough, voice, and urine. So continued giving the same medicine, but in 30th diluton; still improvement. At the end of the week she was able to come and see me, and was very much encouraged. Gave *Bacillinum* 30th, ten globules and placebo powders nightly. To report in a week. Very much better; said, 'I have been able to do my household work, which I thought I should never do again.' She came weekly during July; still gaining. In August she went to the mountains; the running down had been stopped, for she had lost twenty-nine pounds in three months previous to my taking her in hand. Now she said, 'I believe I am gaining;' which was true, and in her month in the mountains she gained two pounds weekly, and has kept up gaining in weight and strength. She is now happy, and preparing for her confinement in February next. She coughs some in the morning yet, and there is some huskiness of the voice, but she eats well sleeps well, and is able to work well, and come to see me every two weeks. To gain strength and healing and support an unborn baby must be considered a grand triumph for any remedy. (XVI A 261)

## 329. CONSUMPTION

**Case 4.** — Mrs. M., aet. 41. Knowing that she is of a consumptive family, having attended her sister when in the last stage of consumption, while she was visiting at this lady's house, I was anxious about her, and upon inquiry, found that she was weakly; cold legs, a feeling as if she had on wet stockings; hands and feet hot at times, with clammy sweat; some night sweat, but no cough, only when she took a cold, and then it hung on in spite of anything she took. I gave her two powders of *Bacillinum* 30th ten days apart, but she got rid of all her bad feelings, so that both she and her husband thought there was no need of going through the three months' course I had asked for. (XVI A 264)

## 330. TUBERCULOUS PHTHISIS

"James K., a carman, age 40, was admitted into the hospital October 17, 1892, The following notes are taken from the case-book of Dr. Vincent Green, junior resident medical officer. The family history is excellent, there being no history of phthisis. The patient's present illness dates from an attack of influenza three years ago, the attack being followed by cough, expectoration, night sweats and emaciation. These symptoms continued for a year until the patient could hardly get out of bed on account of weakness. He was in the North London Hospital six weeks, where he improved, but during the next six weeks he bacame rapidly worse, having two sharp attacks of haemoptysis. When admitted to the Homoeopathic Hospital he was emaciated, suffered much from dyspepsia, and had a poor appetite. He had an irritative hacking cough, but not much expectoration, but the sputum contained tubercle bacilli. At the apex of the right lung there was a crack-pot note, tubular breathing and abundant coarse crepitations. In the infraclavicular region there was some dulness, with prolonged expiration and fine crepitations; posteriorily, there was audible prolonged expiration and fine crepitations; posteriorily, there was audible prolonged expiration with crepitations all over the lung. At the apex of the left lung expiration was prolonged, but there were no accompaniments. The heart sounds were clear; pulse 110. The patient complained of a feeling of weight in the right chest, sleeplessness, and cough for several days, and then he began to improve; constipation was one of his chief troubles.

"On November 9th, as he still complained of the weight in the chest, he was given *Tuberculinum* (Heath) 100, gt. iii., on the tongue, and this was repeated the following week.

"By November 20th he had gained one and a quarter pounds in weight; the sensation of weight in the chest was better; there was very little cough, no expectoration, no night sweats, but he was troubled a good deal with flatulence. *Tuberculinum* was repeated on the 30th, and again on December 10th; by this time he had gained another pound and a half in weight.

"December 19th. — He complains of pains in the joints without swelling; there is a return of the sweats and cough, with frothy white sputum. Under *Merc. vivus* 12 the rheumatic symptoms perfectly subsided.

"*Tuberculinum* was repeated on January 4th and 25th.

"On February 2nd it was noted that he had gained four and a half pounds since January 18th,; he had no cough, and felt quite well. There was a prolonged expiratory murmur and increase of vocal fremitus, and resonance at the right apex, but no abnormal physical signs at the left apex. — *The Journal of the British Homoeopathic Society.* (XVI A 267)

## Dr William Lamb's Cases (Cases 331 - 333)

### 331. LUPUS EXEDENS

"**Case 1.** — I had prescribed for some time for an elderly lady suffering from Lupus exedens over the left superior maxilla, with very unsatisfactory progress. I then advised *Bacillinum*, which she had in the two hundred and first potency. One drop of this caused such medicinal aggravation, that she first thought of taking no more; but after a few days (I think five) she ventured upon half a drop, which agreed and two more doses healed the part up completely. Her general health has improved wonderfully. (XVI A 273)

### 332. TUBERCULAR ULCERATION OF INTESTINE

**Case 2.** — Another instance is that of a boy about 11 years old, who was reduced to the last extremity by tubercular ulceration of intestines. His disease had resisted three allopathic doctors before I saw him, and he was so very far through that the parents asked for a consultation with another doctor (allopathic), which I assented to. His verdict was to give the boy all the nourishment he could get, but that there was no hope for him. Just then Dr. Young's article (see cases 311 to 319) came before me, and I decided to give *Bacillinum* 200 mj. every eighth day. His recovery took place steadily, and from being skin and bone, with constant abdominal pain and vexatious alvine discharges of blood, faeces and pus, he has become well-nourished, and has lost his pains, etc., entirely. (XVI A 274)

### 333. CONSUMPTION OF BOWELS

A third case was that of a baby 14 months old, who had been unsucccessfully treated at the Dunedin Hospital. It was emaciated to a degree, and was evidently not long for this world, and was another example of consumption of the bowels. I gave *Bacillinum* 200 mj. every eighth day, with such perfect success that the father told me afterwards that the child had never been so well since its birth. (XVI A 275)

## Dr. John H. Clarke's Cases (Cases 334-345)

### 334. CONSUMPTION

"**Case 1.** — One of the first cases in which I proved its (Bacillinum's) curative power was that of a little girl, R. W., whom I had practically 'cured' of consumption with ordinary homoeopathic remedies nearly three years before. At the first time I saw her she was 7 years old, and was reduced almost to a skeleton. Right lung dull all over. Rattling sounds over both lungs. Breath short and noisy — audible almost all over the house. Cough distressing and breath most fetid.

"After a severe attack of scarlatina six months before, these symptoms developed, and the progress of the case had been so rapid that two allopathic medical men had pronounced her case hopeless. She had had her farewell photograph taken; everybody (including the small patient herself) was waiting the end with sufficient resignation, when I happened to be consulted somewhat incidentally. Under *Iodide of arsenic*, to the astonishment of all, there was decided improvement. The fetor of the breath 'with every cough' disappeared under *Capsicum;* but much more markedly when I gave it high. (I m.) than when given low.

"I saw her first in May, 1888. She gained steadily, put on flesh, grew strong and ruddy, and in few months was able to go to school.

"But though the lung dulness cleared up (leaving, however, evidence of a cavity at the right apex), and the cough left her, the breathing remained short and noisy. Creaking sounds were heard all over on auscultating, and she required treatment from time to time.

"On January 8, 1891, there was wheezing respiration; rattling on chest; cough in morning. Otherwise she was well.

"Bacil. 100, two globules.

"January 12. — Wheezing much less.

"January 20. — Very much less wheezing.

"For the next week she had much heat, with perspiration at night. The wheezing still continued less marked; but the chest was a little tight, and she got up a little phlegm in the morning.

"January 27. — *Bacil* 100, glb.ii.

"February 5. — Keeping very well.

"February 19. — No wheezing since.

"Since this date, at long intervals, she has required treatment, and *Bacillin* has never failed to relieve her. I have not seen her now for about a year, but I often see her father. The last time I prescribed was in August last, when she was reported to have more rattling on the chest and a little cough.

"*Bacil.* 30, four globules in a powder; four powders, one to be taken each week.

"September 5. — Report, very much better. Chest very different soon after the powders.

"October 19. — Keeping much better.

"She is now, I understand growing into a strong, hearty girl. (XVI A 280)

## 335. RHEUMATISM & COUGH

**Case 2.** — Mrs. W., aged 38, first seen in November, 1888. She was fair, extremely thin, had suffered from rheumatism all her life, and had had a cough as long as she could remember. Eighteen months before she had had a severe illness (pleurisy, I gathered) after exposure, and was at one time given up for dead. Still had pain in left side of chest low down in front on taking a deep breath or coughing. There was prolonged expiration in both sides of chest, and a systolic bruit heard all over the cardiac areas. She was exceedingly sensitive to cold air.

"I attended this patient through many an illness, including several attacks of influenza, the last of which, in the summer of 1892, gave such an impetus to the tubercular process that she eventually succumbed to it. The only reason for my mentioning her case now is that in January, 1861, I gave her two doses of *Bacillinum* 100, at an interval of a week. After the first dose there was very little change, though the appetite was not so good. After the second she was seized with a 'a spasmodic pain in the chest, going up to the throat.' This lasted, though diminishing till the next morning. She got up much worse. This attack (which I attributed to the *Bacillin*) was of such an alarming character that I did not venture to repeat the medicine, especially as it was not followed by any evident amelioration. (XVI A 285)

## 336. BRONCHITIS, POTT'S DISEASE & SCROFULOUS CONDITION OF EYE

"**Case 3.** — Sydney W., the youngest child of Mrs. W., seen first on July 2, 1888, aged then 12 weeks. He was suffering from bronchitis, from which he recovered. Afterwards he had commencing Pott's disease of the spine, which was checked by ordinary homoeopathic remedies — *Silica* and *Sulphur* chiefly.

"On February 22, 1891, he had a scrofulous condition of the eyelids, the margins inflamed and somewhat eczematous. *Bacillinum* quickly made a change for the better in these. Whenever this condition has since threatened to recur, *Bacillinum* has at once put him right and improved him in general health. He is now a strong, sturdy child. (XVI A 287)

## 337. ECZEMA CAPITIS

"**Case 4.** — This eczematous condition of eyelids calls to mind another case in a boy of 12, who had had eczema capitis severely as an infant, healed up by local applications, but not perfectly, the right eyelid being left eczematous; the eczema spreading to the face when specially active. One direct consequence of the local method of treatment was facial paralysis, which came on when the eruption disappeared under the ointments, and has left the boy disfigured for life. The condition of eye had been ameliorated by several remedies, but nothing acted so promptly or so satisfactorily as *Bacillin*, given at rare intervals. (XVI A 288)

## 338. REDNESS OF EYELID MARGIN

"**Case 5.** — My coachman, a young man of about 30, also suffered from redness of the eyelid margins, and he asked me to give him something for it. This condition was also eczematous. A few doses of *Bacillinum* permanently removed it. (XVI A 289)

## 339. LUPUS

"**Case 6.** — This was a case of lupus. Miss., W. 26, consulted me July 17, 1891. She was a member of a very consumptive family, and one sister was insane a long time, and eventually committed suicide. The patient lived in Scotland, and consulted me whilst on a visit to London.

"She had been affected with lupus for ten years, the affection having begun in the eye, the right being the worst. It then invaded the right cheek, and finally nose. The right wing of the nose was ulcerated and scabbed. The face is much disfigured.

"*Bacil.* 200 every ten days.

"July 24 . — Marked improvement in nose.

"On examining the throat I found a small clean-punctured perforation in the soft palate near the uvula. No appearance of inflammation round it. Has left the throat a little sore the last few days. Never had a sore throat before. (I conclude there must have been a tuberculous nodule in the palate which the *Bacillin* caused to ulcerate out.) Can breathe much more freely through nose.

"On September I, she reported (having left England) that there was much improvement.

"*Bacillin*. 1 m. (F. C.).

"October 9. — Face keeps on improving, but is at times very red. I now gave her Koch's preparation — *Tuberc. Koch.* 200 (F. C)

"March 4. — Face very much better. She has had an attack of influenza since last report, which left her with her legs and feet swollen and pitting. The doctor (allopathic) who attended her said she had Bright's disease; and further added that the medicine she had taken 'had cured the face, and driven it to the kidneys.' As the same authority had pronounced her face incurable before, I did not accept the latter part of this statement as final. I got her to send me specimens of her urine from time to time. The first I examined was pale, alkaline, contained some mucus, slight cloud of phosphates, but no albumen. Subsequently I found a slight deposit of albumen, but no tube-casts. Under indicated remedies she soon recovered, and sent her last report on April 30, 1892. I have heard of her since as having kept well. (XVI A 290)

## 340. PAIN RIGHT KNEE JOINT

"**Case 7.** — A young lady of very good physique, but coming of a scrofulous family (her mother's sister suffering from tuberculous ulceration of the nose, and her own elder sister having died after amputation of the thigh for scrofulous disease of the right knee), was taken last spring with pain in her right knee-joint. Being subject to rheumatic pains, she at first thought little of it; but as it persisted, I was asked to see her. Several remedies were given with but little success, and considering that her sister's illness had begun in a similar insidious way, her friends became somewhat anxious, and, to some extent, so did I.

"I gave her one dose of *Bacillinum* 100, four globules on the tongue.

"Seeing her the next day, she asked me if I intended to make her knee very much worse? She said the dose 'went' straight to the knee' — at least, within half an hour after taking it. she had violent pain in the joint, as after overwalking. This lasted for over four hours; then it went to the ankle on the same side, and then got better. From this time the knee began to mend, and in a few weeks was perfectly well. I gave other medicines afterwards, and did not repeat the *Bacillinum* till a month after the first dose. This time it produced no aggravation, and was again followed by general improvement. (XVI A 294)

## 341. DEAFNESS

"**Case 8.** — The mother of the last patient, who was in good health, had for some time consulted me about deafness of her right ear. I had removed an accumulation of wax wihtout giving relief to the deafness, and remedies had had little effect. She could only hear my watch on contact.

"In view of her family history, I gave on June 27, 1893, *Bacillinum* 100, four globules on the tongue.

"July 4. — Hearing 3 inches off contact.

"July 13. — 3 inches. Repeat dose.

"July 20. — Hears 5 inches.

"July 31. — Hears 18 inches.

"At this date she told me of a symptom which may have been due to the last dose. On the 28th, suddenly, had pain in right upper teeth. This lasted all evening. She wrapped a stocking round her face, and the pain was gone in the morning.

"August 4. — Hears only 5 inches. Repeat.
"This was the last dose I gave her.
"On August 9, she heard 19 inches.
"On October 24, the hearing was practically normal; she heard 25 inches away. (XVI A 296)

## 342. PNEUMMONIA

"**Case 9.** — A well made young man came into the Homoeopathic Hospital suffering from right-sided pneumonia, which rapidly cleared up under *Bryonia*, which was well indicated in the case. But long before he got the pneumonia he had suffered from loss of voice and pain in the throat, due to the presence of tubercles in the larynx, as was demonstrated by the laryngoscope.
"Shortly before he left, I put on his tongue a few globules of Koch"s *Tuberculin* 200 (F.C.).
"He experienced the greatest relief from this dose, and in a few days returned to his work, exceedingly pleased with himself. I begged him to come again as out-patient, and he promised to do so, but failed to keep his promise. No doubt he was unable to get away from his work, and too well to risk losing it. (XVI A 298)

## 343. BRONCHITIS

"**Case 10.** — A well-known *prima donna* had a severe attack of influenza last spring, the form taken being that of bronchitis. Two winters before she had had peritonitis from the same cause, and before that, right-sided pneumonia, following immediately upon an 'orificial' operation in the United States. When I first saw her there was incessant cough; rales all over the chest; pains in the chest, right side chiefly; and dulness in right apex. Under *Sanguinaria* the chest cleared and the violence of the symptoms subsided; but induration signs of a cavity at the right apex remained. *Bacillinum* in occasional doses materially aided her recovery, and she has since passed through a very arduous season with great success.
Many cases of indurated glands have been cured by *Bacillinum* in my hands; also cases of ringworm. One of the latter cases I will now mention. (XVI A 299)

## 344. RINGWORM FACE

"**Case 11.** — Master C ____, aged 8, returned from school in December, 1891, with ringworm pretty well covering face, scalp and neck. There is a strong scrofulous taint in the family. Under *Tellurium*, and then *Sulphur*, he did well for a time, but on February 5th the eruption had spread all over his back, and was very irritable. *Calcarea* did much good, and afterwards *Psorinum*; but he was not quite clear by July 23, 1892.

"$R_x$ *Bacillinum* 30, four powders — one a week. *Calc. Phos.* 3, one tablet three times a day.

"August 10. — Head a good deal better. After this I did not see him for many months, his mother believing him to be quite well.

"On April 3rd he was brought to me again that I might sign a certificate of health, as he had a nomination for a new school. On examining him closely I found still a scurvy spot of undoubted ringworm. It was now a case of curing to time, for the certificate had to be given in a fortnight, or he would have lost his chance.

"I again put him on *Bacillinum* 30.

"On the 18th the dose was repeated, as the spot was still visible.

"On the 27th the head was perfectly clear, and I was able to give him a clean bill of health. (XVI A 300)

## 345. TUBERCULOSIS

"**Case 12.** James K., aged 40, a carman rather dark, shortish, but of fairly strong build, was admitted to Hahnemann Ward of the London Homoeopathic Hospital on the 17th of October last, giving the following history. There was no consumption in his family. Three years before admission he had an attack of influenza, which left him with a slight cough. His occupation entailed much exposure, and after Christmas, 1891, he gradually became weaker and weaker, until at last he was hardly able to rise in the morning, and he had not strength enough to lift anything at all heavy. He went to Hastings, but returned worse; he felt the air too bleak. After this he attended the North London Hospital as out-patient for a fortnight; then he was taken in, and discharged at the end of six weeks (in accordance with a rule of that hospital) improved. Whilst he was in the hospital he had two attacks of hemoptysis, spitting almost half a pint of blood on one occasion and a few spoonfuls on the other.

"About the end of August he again began to get worse, and steadily lost ground until the time of his admission. For over a year he had suffered from indigestion, a catching or shooting pain from the right mamma to the left shoulder, with a feeling of a lump at the root of the neck.

"Physical examination showed that there was consolidation of upper part of right lung with formation of a cavity, with slight indication of the left apex also being affected. The heart and other organs were normal.

"The cough was worse on rising in the morning, and in the evening.

Expectoration scanty, hanging about throat and difficult to get away. An examination showed it to contain tubercle bacilli. The cough caused pain in the right side. The irritation which caused the cough seemed to be in the chest. Movement or any exertion aggravated it. He could not lie on his right side. At times he felt as if he could hardly breathe. Was very weak. Had night perspirations. Appetite fair; bowels regular.

"Under *Bry.* 1 the pain in the side improved; under *Nit. ac.* 12, and afterwards *Ars. iod.* 3x, there was some improvement. Later he became troubled with constipation, feeling of nausea and mental depression. Nux 3 and *Sulph.* 30 did good in these respects. *Phos.* 6 had no particular effect.

"On November 9, as he was still complaining of the weight on the right side of the chest, the cough symptoms continuing, I gave him on his tongue three globules of *Tuberculin* H. 100. Improvement was noted on the 14th. On the 16th the dose was repeated. He then reported himself as feeling better. He had gained 1 lb. in weight since October 27th. He now complained of a lump at the chest coming on when he had eaten a little; much flatulence passing downwards, so he was put on *Lyc.* 6, and continued on this for a week, during which time the flatulence and other symptoms of disordered digestion improved much. At the end of the week a sharp attack of diarrhoea supervened, stools sudden, watery, light brown, with much wind. *Colocynth* 3 soon put this right.

"On the 30th of November another dose of *Tuberc.* was given, and again on the 10th and 17th of December.

"Up to the 17th of December there had been steady improvement. On that day the patient was feeling less well. More cough, tickling and wheezing on chest, tongue rather dirty, no appetite. On the 19th a rheumatic attack began to develop, with pains in ankles and wrist. There was fever and heavy night sweats, with night aggravation of the cough. The pain was chiefly in left ankle and across instep, and under left knee. There was also pain in right great toe (which he had had before). Under *Merc. sol.* 12 these symptoms passed away by December 30th; but the cough continued to be troublesome, occurring between 12 midnight and 3 A.M., first thing on waking. Sinking sensation on getting up. *Kali carb.* 12, *Arsen.* 30, and *Bry.* 30 were given in succession without producing any observable effect, and on January 4th *Tuberc.* was repeated. After this he made rapid progress, but the cough still troubled him a good deal. There was a tickling behind the middle of the sternum. The cough came on in the afternoon. He was put on *Lachesis* 12, one drop every two hours, on the 12th of January, and by the 23rd the cough had left him completely, and did not return. He regained the flesh he had lost, and was quite free from all symptoms referable to the chest.

"The condition of the right lung on February 2nd was as follows : Tympanitic note on percussion above and below right clavicle; tubular breathing. Expiration prolonged and harsh over the upper lobe anteriorly, and as far down as the sixth rib at the back. No moist sounds.

"The patient left the hospital, looking and feeling quite well , on February 3d. The consumptive process was completely arrested and the patient practically cured. Of course the lung tissue that had already been destroyed could not be restored, hence the physical signs of a cavity remained But the cavity was a healed cavity, and not an ulcerating one. (XVI A 303)

## DISEASES OF THE LIVER

### 346. CATARRHAL JAUNDICE

A good many years since I was summoned to see a country gentleman for sudden indisposition. It was a rather tedious railway journey, and a humble friend of the family, anxious to enlighten me, told me that the squire had the "Yeller Janders." Yellow the patient was, indeed, and the colour was from janundice! There were the usual symptoms — constipation, scanty urine of a dark yellow browny colour, and debility with depression of spirits. *Chelidonium majus* in small material doses, put matters right in a few days, leaving the patient, however, weak.

"What medicine have you been giving my husband?"

"A new remedy."

"What's it's name."

"*Chelidonium majus*."

"What's the English of that?"

"The greater Celandine."

"Then it is not by any means a new remedy, for it is in my old Herbal, in which it is recommended for jaundice."

And so it was : the use of the greater Celandine in jaundice has trickled down to us through the ages from the primary source of the doctrine of signatures.

Of *Chelidonium majus*, I would say that it is in this country the greatest liver medicine we have and there is, in all conscience, no lack of hepatics. Some of my early success in practice was due to my use of *Chelidonium*. (XVII , 29)

## 347. HEPATALGIA

It came about thus : I went to see an important lady for a well known physician in the north, he being too busy to attend, but said lady strongly objected to new doctors. She took a look at me — as I subsequently learned — from a position where she herself was invisible to me, and did not like the look of me. So I was sent away with many apologies from the daughter. Her hepatalgia was easier just at that moment : she would wait till her own physician would come.

A few days later the pain in her right side became unbearable, and the said physician again sent me. This time I was admitted and found her in very great pain in the hepatic region : she had had it at intervals for very many years — about thirty years, if I remember rightly. The liver was very much enlarged and the pains very acute; there was no jaundice, the tongue mapped.

I mixed some *Chelidonium majus* and had it given pretty frequently : it eased the pain more promptly than ever the pain had been relieved before, and finally cured it altogether. Her whole life was changed. To make amends for having refused to see me on my first calling upon her she presented me with a peice of plate, and sent me subsequently very many of her suffering friends.

So *einflusserich* was this venerable dame that I feel her practical influence to this very day.

This cure, and its gratifying results to a struggling young doctor, fixed my attention a good deal upon *Chelidonium*, and upon liver affections, which are everywhere so common; and it has been my lot to relieve or cure a very large number of liver diseases — and from this wide experience I now write. My first real acquaintance with *Chelidonium* was from Dr. Richard Hughes' "Pharmacodynamics," a work which I owe so much, and which I sincerely commend to all who wish to understand the actions of drugs.

I would not be too sure of my botanic knowledge, but I have an idea that *Chelidonium* is the only plant, indigenous to this country, which possesses a yellow juice, That the colour of this juice led to its use in liver diseases on the lines of the doctrine of Signatures the historically competent will hardly deny. That it has a specific affinity for the grat gall-organ anyone may verify for himself if he will take a few drachms of the mother tincture in divided doses. It is kindly and gentle in its actiòn which action is fully set up with only a very minute dose, but in as much as my more intimate knowledge of it comes to me from the Rademacherians, I have generally used it in small material doses.

It will be interesting to give Rademacher experience with *Chelidonium*. He used it as an organ remedy, or in other words on the homoeopathic principle in its elementary form of specificity of seat. (XVII 31)

## 348. ENLARGEMENT OF THE LIVER WITH JAUNDICE

A lady of seventy, stout, and given to very little exercise, came under my observation, and on examination I found her severe and frequent right-sided pains were due to a swelled liver, which was tender in pressure. Skin and conjunctivae subicteric, motions containing but very little bile; urine on the contrary loaded with it. She was at the seaside and this it was, she said, that had upset her liver. Tongue coated, giddy, lowspirited, pulse intermittent, insomnia, lethargic, loss of appetite, fear of death.

*Chelidonium majus* in smal material doses resulted in complete recovery in ten days, when she returned home with a regular pulse, clear eyes and skin, and all the functions normal, and very decidedly of opinion that life, even at seventy years of age, is not at all a bad thing.(XVII 44)

## 349. ENLARGED LIVER AND CONGESTION OF THE RIGHT LUNG

A young officer in the Army was invalided home from India for liver and lung disease and came to me. I found his liver large and tender, the right lung engorged, his skin very muddy, bowels costive, and he was dreadfully depressed and weak. He was quite sure he was in consumption. The lung affection I regarded as consecutive to the engorgement of liver. there being, in the words of Rademacher, a primary affection of the "inner" liver. *Chelidonium* in small material doses quite restored him to health in three weeks. In due course he returned to his regiment. (XVII 45)

## 350. PRONOUNCED JAUNDICE

A middle-aged gentleman, a merchant, returned from the East Indies with very severe jaundice, which had resulted in considerable emaciation. The voyage home and a stay of some duration in the north had not mended matters. He was very depressed in spirits, almost the colour of mahogany, and the urine was very scant and brown-yellow. His bowels very constipated.

How quickly and pleasantly he was cured, he even now never tires of telling his Manchester friends.

I might tell of a lady who had severe and long lasting jaundice and who was speedily cured by *Chelidonium*, and of a notable number of other cases of liver affections cured by it, but it is needless. What I have already narrated will suffice.

I would, however, just dwell upon the fact that *Chelidonium* will very frequently cure engorgements of the right lung even when it is a concomitant of true phthisis, but it has no influence over the general phthisical state, other than what pertains to, and results from, the lower half, of the right lung and liver. As an intercurrent remedy in the hepatic complications of phthisis it is capable of rendering important service.

Likewise as an intercurrent remedy in gall-stones it is useful, as is also *Myrica cerifera*, but both stand far behind *Hydrastis* in this affection.

My own conception of its true seat of action is that it affects the liver cells : Rademacher's "inner" liver.

There are numerous affections of the liver that *Chelidonium* will not touch curatively at all, and therefore it must not be regarded as a liver cure all, which it is not.

For instance, it affects the left lobe of the liver much less than does *Carduus Marianus*, to a consideration of which we will proceed after having first given a short account of Rademacher's use of a combination of *Chelidonium* and *Calcarea muriatica*.

**Rademacher's Use of Chelidonium and Liq. Calcarie muriat.** Our author tells us he is convinced that there exists in nature a liver disease that can only be cured by a mixture of *Chelidonium* and *Liq. Calcarie muriat.*

This is his formula :

R. Liq. *Calcariae muriat.* 3ii.

Tinct. *Chelidonii*, 3i.

M.

He administered fifteen drops in half-a-cupful of water five times a day. With this he cured many cases of grave fevers and hepatic affections that did not mend with either remedy by itself, but he tells us he knows of no reliable or characteristic indications for its choice.

I might add that muriatic acid once had a seemingly well-founded reputation as a liver remedy; and some still esteem it highly. (XVII 47)

## 351. ENLARGEMENT OF LIVER AND SPLEEN

A young lady, of sixten summers, was brought to me by her mother on the seventh of September, 1887, for servere attacks of vomiting that had lasted for three months. She was often roused rudely from her sleep in the morning with an attack of vomiting. Her constitution had been damaged by diphtheria, and eighteen months previously she had had varicella. I treated the case symptomatically with great relief to the vomiting, but the pains in the abdomen became rather worse than better.

After I had given her my old favorite *Nat. Mur.* 6 she was still further improved, but there the thing still was : I had relieved the symptoms but I had not cured the real primary seat of the same. I then did what might with advantage have been done before the treatment was begun, viz : I made a careful physical examination of the bare epigastrium and of the two hypochondria. With what result? The note in my case book taken at the time will enlighten us .... "Liver and spleen both very much enlarged so that they seem almost to fill the abdomen."

Here I had to do with the severe and long lasting vomiting which yielded partially to close symptomatic treatment but would not get quite well .... (Oh, how often are we in this unsatisfactory state); and a physical examination revealed the reason of my failure I had treated the case with remedies that were homoeopathic to the superficial symptoms, but NOT homoeopathic to the cause of those symptoms; the degree of homoeopathicity was not adequate though it went a long way towards it.

Here I fell back upon my Rademacherian experience with *Carduus* and gave five drops of the matrix tincture in a tablespoonful of water, night and morning, and this cured the enlargement both of Spleen and of Liver, and as this enlargement was the cause of the pains and vomiting, of course pains and vomiting likewise disappeared.

The only further abnormality which I could discover in the young lady after taking the *Carduus marianus* for about five weeks was an indurated condition of a few of the cervical glands of her left side : the side on which she had been vacinated : *Thuja occidentalis* 30, in infrequent doses, cured these and patient has had no vomiting or any of its concomitants since. She continues well to date. Although my own prescription of *Carduus* was from pure experience, there can be hardly any doubt that an adequate proving would shew its homoeopathicity to the case, inclusive of the enlargements of liver and spleen.

Riel's proving of *Carduus* shows it to produce pathogenetically : "nausea, uneasiness, pain vomiting, with inflation of the abdomen, etc."

The generally improved appearance of the young lady after she had been a month under the *Carduus* was very striking, and repeatedly remarked upon, by friends who were not acquainted with the circumstances of her ill-health and its treatment at all.

The kind of liver enlargements which *Carduus* cures is in the transverse measurement.

By way of comparison I will now quite shortly exemplify the kind of enlargement of the liver which is cured by *Chelidonium*; it will be seen that the comparison is crude and mechanical, yet withal, I submit, not wihout practical value. (XVII 53)

## 352. ENLARGEMENT OF THE LIVER IN THE PERPENDICULAR LINE

An independent gentleman of thirty, usually resident in Paris, came over to London to cosult me in the early part of the year 1886, and that for this liver and for dyspepsia. He had twice had jaundice in previous times. His symptoms were waterbrash, indigestion, constipation, attacks of intra-abdominal chilliness; he was very dusky, his urine had a strongly urinous smell. His liver reaches almost up to the right nipple.

An ounce of the tincture brought the liver back to the normal; the dose was five drops in water, two or three times a day, and sometimes once a day. But altogether he consumed nearly an ounce.

This is the kind of hepatic enlargement which *Chelidonium* rights in small material doses. But it did not restore the patient to complete health; why? For the simple reason that the increase in the perpendicular measurement of the liver was only a part of his complaint, the other bearings of the case being foreign to my present thesis. Suffice it to say that his liver was cured by the *Chelidonium*, and patient contiunes well in these (and now in the other) respects to the present time. (XVII 59)

## 353. USE OF ORGAN REMEDIES

I treated a young lady for a liver disease and gave her successively *Carduus*, *Chelidonium*, *Natrum sulphuricum*, *Taraxacum*.

She had a mapped tongue and vomiting, with headaches and squinting. The liver was reduced to its right dimensions and the vomiting was cured, but the mapppiness of the tongue remained, and patient did not feel well. But the tongue became normal after a month of *Thuja* 30. She had headaches which she herself termed bilious and the others neuralgic, and there was a third kind of headache called by another name and which seemed distinctly connected with the squinting. The bilious headaches ceased after the use of the before - mentioned hepatics; the neuralgic headaches continued till after the *Thuja*, and disappeared simulataneously with the mapped state of the tongue. The squint headaches she still gets, and remedies like *Glonoin* and *Gelsemium* do them good.

From these considerations it is manifest that *there are cases that cannot possibly be cured by one remedy* and inasmuch as the symptoms form part respectively of groups of different causations, covering the totality of all the symptoms present in the patient would be a useless and fruitless task. Hence it is that Rademacherian organ testing helps me so much in my every day practical clinical life; for, if I cure an organ with its *Appropriatum Paracelsi*, and certain symptoms go while others remain I am enabled slowly to unravel the most complex groups of symptoms and finally find a simile or even the simillimum of the ground-evil.

The adage *Naturam morborum ostendunt curationes* also comes in here as an auxiliary. With me it is an axiom to relieve uncomfortable or dangerous organ states with simple organ remedies as promptly as possible, leaving the more remote and deeper going to be afterwards considered, and treated, if possible, with its pathological simillimum, or else aetiologically, say according to Hahnemann in his Coethen phase. (XVII 61)

## 354. ENLARGED LIVER, CARDIAC AFFECTION WITH STERNAL ERUPTION

I will narrate is that of a mayor of a large town in the north : - He had a patch of brownish eruption on the sternal portion of thorax of the size of a woman's palm. with it were associated an enlarged liver and a cardiac affection evidenced by palpitation, systolic murmur, and general uneasiness. He came to town to see me at odd intervals for about two years, and was then discharged cured. He has passed under my observation since, but though his liver gives no trouble the same cannot be said of his skin, and he has moreover *pyorrhoea alveolaris*.

I treated him antipsorically and organopathically, the most notable benefit being derived from *Carduus marianus* in five drop doses of the strong tincture given three times a day. (XVII 67)

## 355. STERNAL PATCH, HEART AFFECTION WITH ARCUS SENILIS

The second I remember was a Manchester merchant, with the same kind of cutaneous patch on the sternum, and very notable heart trouble with arcus senilis as a concomitant. Here the case and comfort brought by the *Carduus marianus* were very striking. Under date of January 31, 1883, I find in my case book these words of the enthusiastic patient — "It had a most marvellous effect, soon made me right; the patch went away in a fortnight; had had it for years."

This gentleman has remained under my care, calling upon me at odd times when in town and during the past two years has had besides the strong tincture of *Carduus*, *Bellis perennis* 1, *Aurum Metallicum* 4, *Vanadium* 6, and *Acidum oxalicum* 3x, and some other remedies, and I consider him vastly improved, and his life — speaking commercially — worth 40 per cent. more than previously. (XVII 68)

## 356. ENLARGED LIVER & STERNAL PATCH

The third case was that of a New York merchant, who suffered from liver and had come over to Europe to consult a physician, as he seemed to get no better from the treatment of his New York advisers. I found his liver very much enlarged, and also the before mentioned sternal patch of skin disease. I gave him *Carduus* in like dose to the foregoing, and he came in a week declaring himself quite well. I advised him to remain awhile under observation, to see if the cure proved permanent, but he hurried out of my room in great glee, and I never saw him again. (XVII 69)

## 357. STERNAL PATCH : INDICATOR OF LIVER AND HEART TROUBLE

The fourth case in which I found the sternal patch and enlarged liver, giddiness and palpitations of the heart was that of London Lawyer. Here the liver was weak and heart too, together with the giddiness, but it needs a course of antipsoric treatment to finish the cure of the patch of diseased skin. I might say the same of a fifth case, an officer in the Royal Navy, where this patch co-exists with hypertrophied liver, and in which the affair has a specific air about it, probably inherited, and it may be that when Sarcognomy is better understood, and when the relations of the various cutanous regions will be recognized as constituting the very base of medical and medicinal diagnosis, this sternal patch will be understood to indicate "liver and heart."

But the following CASE CURED BY *Carduus* is also instructive in considering its relationship to skin and liver. (XVII 70)

## 358. DYSPEPSIA HEPATOSPLENOMEGALY WITH SEBACEOUS CYST

A city merchant, thirty years of age, unmarried, came to me in May, 1888, for windy dyspepsia, the probable ground-work of which proved to be an enlargement both of liver and spleen, and he had amongst other things very numerous sebaceous cysts strewn about his body, looking for all the world like the malva seeds (cases), children call cheeses.

At first, I gave *Ceanothus Amercicanus*, believing it to be primarily a spleen affection, and then *Pulsatilla*, but they did no great good; when *Carduus*, given for a little over a month, brought the liver back to the normal and all the wee wens were gone.

The enlargement of the liver and the wens disappeared simultaneously, but the genuinely causal nature of both was neither hepatic nor cutaneous : That was scrofula. But as scrofula can only be treated in its manifestations, he who treats such manifestations successfully cures it. The general improvement under *Carduus* was most striking and lasting : patient got quite well and has since happily married.

E. Stahl speaks in his Dissertations most highly of *Carduus* in those inflammations of the chest which are accompanied by gall fevers, and it was from him that Rademacher first learned its use and never ceased to prize it, notably in blood spitting from liver and spleen engorgement. No remedy, he declares, in our whole drug store can compare to *Carduus* when there are stitches in the side with bloody expectoration. He recommends his readers to note well where the last trace of pain is felt as it dies away, as that is likely to be the primary seat of the real disease. (XVII 72)

## 359. JAUNDICE IN A NEW BORN BABE

An able accoucheur attended a lady who bore a jaundiced babe; said he, "I cannot give that wee thing any medicine, so you had better send for your homoeopath (meaning me), as he can give some of his 'pips'!" This was done and pilules of *Myrica cerifera* 3x (crushed into a powder and rubbed on the baby's tongue) rapidly cured him, and he at once began to put on flesh, and has thriven ever since. Before taking the *Myrica* he was very weedy, thin, and leathery looking.

*Myrica cerifera* is one of the very valuable additions to our materia medica that have come to us from America. I have often used it in liver disease, notably in bad cases of jaundice, with striking success; it produces jaundice in the healthy pathogenetically, and is very searching in its action. It was the great American Samuel Thomson, the botanic practitioner, who brought it into notice. A pale green wax is obtained from its berries, and hence it is called *ceriferus*, or wax - bearing. Its powdered bark was Thomson's "canker powder," and he advised it in all discharges from the mucous surfaces, especially in leucorrhoa, dysentery, and nasal catarrh. Dr. Leland Walker's proving, as given in "Hale's New Remedies," shews an accurate picture of severe catarrhal jaundice; we are, therefore, on indisputably scientific ground when we prescribe *Myrica* for catarrhal jaundice. No wonder that the old American botanists practised with so much success. That Thomson was a close and accurate observer may be seen from the fact that he commends it to "disengage the thick viscid secretions of the mucous membrane," for we find Walker's pathogenetic *Myrica* catarrh was of the same viscid quality; he says : "throat and nasal organs filled with an offensive tenacious mucus." (XVII 75)

## 360. *PODOPHYLLUM* — LIVER REMEDY

*PODOPHYLLUM PELTATUM* is a great liver remedy, and has been greatly abused. Its use in "torpid liver" is not good practice, and has done much harm. Its true scientific homoeopathic use is in diarrhoea from overflowing bile, with much irritation, and even inflammation of the gut. It once stood me in good stead in a case of diarrhoea that threatened to end fatally — at any rate the allopathic family adviser had informed the lady's husband that he considered the patient would not recover, as nothing would check the diarrhoea, and the lady was seemingly sinking. I was telegraphed for and had to travel nearly 200 miles. On arriving, the family physician, although he had given the patient up as past recovery, declined to meet me because of my homoeopathic creed, and this although he professed to be a friend of the family, and only lived two doors off. The stools were foul smelling, hot, bilious, excoriating, and passed out of the anus in a constant dribble. The patient had become too weak to be raised or even adequately helped, and things had to be just left. I studied the case a short time, and finally decided upon *Podophyllum* 6. The next evening patient was convalescent, and I returned to town. The cure was complete and permanent. (XVII 79)

## 361. GALLSTONES AND ORGANIC DISEASE OF LIVER

A lady of fifty years of age came under my observation early in the year 1888 with a very muddy complexion, subicteric whites of the eyes. She suffered very much from acidity and also from vomiting.

She told me she had been a sufferer from her liver for many years; severe bilious headaches and dyspepsia. She had been merculized for her liver till all her teeth fell out. and now her digestion had given in almost completely, and she had become so thin that her appearance was quite cachectic. She had got so frightened of anything bringing on her attacks of gall colic that she avoided almost every article of food.

Owing to her emaciation and trim build I was able to make the diagnosis of gallstones from actually feeling them, a thing I am very rarely able to do myself. The region of the gall-bladder was, however, so tender that a very little feeling with my hands was as much as she could bear. I treated her for close upon two years, and then she was a plump, bonny woman, enjoying her life and dining out with her friends. Her skin had become comparatively healthy looking, though not as clear as a healthy English lady's generally is.

I chose the remedies on homoeopathic indications, and here and there as Rademacher would have done; and, when I the last few times examined the region of the gall-bladder, I entirely failed to find any stones.

She had the following remedies seriatim, *Ignatia amara* 1x, *Chelidonium* 1x and Q, *Nux vomica* 1x, *Cholesterine* 3x, *Hydrastis Can*. Q, *Thuja occ*. 30, *Sanguinaria Can*. Q, *Carduus mariae* Q, and *Bilirubin*. 5. All these remedies did their portion of the good, and were given as they were indicated. (XVII 87)

## 362. HYPERTROPHY OF LEFT LOBE OF THE LIVER ; SLIGHT HYPERTROPHY OF THE HEART; STERNAL PATCH

On January 27th, 1885, a young gentleman, twenty-one years of age, and who had long been ailing of no one seemed to know what, was sent by his father to me "to be thoroughly overhauled and put right." The overhauling disclosed slight enlargement of the heart, considerable enlargement of the left lobe of the liver, and a very prominent sternal patch. Patient complained of suffering a good deal from giddiness.

R. *Carduus mariaanus* Q, five drops in water night and morning.

He was discharged permanently cured in six months. During a considerable portion of the time he was taking the *Carduus*, which quite set heart and liver right, but the sternal patch I had to cure nosodically, of which . . . *une autre fois*. I often see members of this gentleman's family, including his parents, and know, as I said just now, that he has continued well ever since. (XVII 91)

## 363. GALLSTONES

An elderly lady came under my observation early in the summer of 1888, for gallstones, characterized by frequent recurrent attacks of jaundice, colic, and vomiting, with the usual agonizing pains. She was under me a good many month — about eighteen, if I remember rightly — and then discontinued her treatment, and has since continued well. I strongly urged her to go on longer, lest there should still be present the remains of the old colic-causing stones, but to no avail. Why should I continue taking medicines when I am well?

She had in succession (and several repeatedly), *Kali bichromicum*, *Carduus mariaanus*, *Hydrastis Canadensis*, *Prunus Virginiana*, *Cholesterine*, *iodofor-*

*mum*, and finaliy *Ferrum picricum* 3x. The last named medicine does capital service in bilious debility.(XVII 92)

## 364. COLIC FROM GALLSTONES

A middle-aged gentleman brought his wife to me three years since to be treated for gall - stones, and the usual attacks of colic with vomiting, that came on at odd intervals, from known and unknown causes. Patient had been long under their own doctor in the country, but to no good purpose; in fact, a chronic pain in the right side had been superadded to the before - mentioned colic attacks, and patient had lost flesh a good deal. She paid me visits once a month for many months, until she was quite well and in a thoroughly thriving condition.

However, I told the husband that I did not think the biliary calculi were really entirely gone, and that I thought it would be wise to continue with the use of gentle gall medicines till we had sounder ground for believing that there would be no further relapses.

But patient seemed and looked in such capital health that there really seemed, from their standpoint, no reason for continuing my treatment, so my warning was not regarded.

The remedies that helped so brilliantly in this case were *Hydrastis, Carduus, Chelidonium* and *Berberis*, and two or three other which I have not noted. It must be fully a year since I saw any of the family, but this morning I was prescribing for her brother-in-law, who told me that she is now lying in the country very ill with gallstones, and her attending physicians consider her case hopeless. So all experience goes to show that the after treatment of gallstones should be carried on for a very long time, so as to get rid of the disease altogether. Long delay at the printers' enables me to add that after having been thus given up, this lady again placed herself under my care, and has at last completely recovered her health, *Euonymin* and *Thlaspi bursa pastoris* Q having helped most.

*How* the biliary calculi are disolved I am unable to say; that they *are* eventually really and truly got rid of by dissolution I infer from the fact that the sufferers get well and remain so.

It might be asked : What is your indication for *Bursa pastoris* in Gallstones? Answer : When the original liver ailing started primarily from the womb. I will refer to this again. (XVII 94)

## 365. CHRONIC BILIOUSNESS AND EMACIATION CURED BY CHELIDONIUM

A strumous gentleman, about thirty years of age, came over from Ireland to consult me with regard to loss of flesh, dyspepsia, and biliousness. He was over six feet in height, and only weighed ten stone. Hair reddish; thorax flat; pronounced venous zig-zag; digestion very weak; poor appetite; a brownish rash across the epigastrium; cannot digest vegetables.

The state of the liver led me to prescribe *Chelidonium* 1; five drops in water night and morning.

Under this prescription (with the same diet, occupation, and place of abode as previously), he increased five pounds in weight in thirty two days. In six months he had reached 10 stone 12 lbs. in weight, and he long after reported to me that he had "remained in very good health, indeed."

Besides being for some months under the influence of *Chelidonium*, he had inter currently also *Badiaga* 3x and *Psorinum* 30, each during one month.

The state of the skin caused me to interpose *Psorinum*, and some symptoms of indigestion led me to give the *Badiaga*.

But the strikingly great amelioration set in first under the sole influence of the *Chelidonium*, but this remedy did not extend its influence far enough or wide enough, and hence it had to be supplemented by the other two, but with the spheres of action of them we are here not concerned. (XVII 98)

## 366. ENLARGEMENT OF LIVER, PRODUCING SHORTNESS OF BREATH AND PALPITATION

Some years since a retired merchant, sixty eight years of age, consulted me for a supposed affection of his heart. He complained of obestiy, fulness in the stomach, violent perspirations on moving about — so much so that he was in the habit of changing shirts during the forenoon already; feels puffy on going up a hill; loses his breath from the stomach on the least hurry. Has a fresh healthy look. No arcus senilis. Is very active, and takes a good deal of exercise.

After taking twenty drops of *Chelidonium maj.* 3x per diem for a few weeks I noted, at his dictation : "The puffiness is much better; I can walk with greater ease; I feel as if something were gone from me." That is to say, his swelled liver had gone down and there was more playroom for his lungs and heart.

He weighed 15 stone 9 lbs., and under the action of *Chelidonium* this came down to 15 stone 6 lbs.

Here afterwards had *Chelidonium* I, and also *Euonymin* 3x, and after 15 months' treatment he had gone down one stone in weight, and was able to go up hill and upstairs with comfort.

I saw him a year ago for neuralgia, when *Silicea* 200 was followed by the disappearence of the neuralgia. (XVII 100)

## 367. GALL COLIC

In the year 1889 a lady of some 30 odd years of age came to consult me for her liver. She seemed healthy and bright, but severe pains in her right side, pyrosis, and certain brown patches on her skin clearly implicated the liver. Patient took for a month *Chelidonium* Q with distinct benefit. She afterwards had *Ignatia amara* 1 and subsequently *Hydrastis Can.* Q, and both with some considerable benefit.

She came then to town to see me, when I again failed to find anything to account for her dyspepsia, though the pain I could trace clearly to the gall bladder.

After taking *Myrica cerif.* 3x, five drops in a table spoonful of water, for some weeks, I received a very grateful letter from her, in which she says : "That medicine has done me a great deal of good; I have lost all pain in my side, and have had only one headache, and no indigestion, and I walk six miles a day."

What the exact state of the gallducts was of course I could not tell; I could not feel any calculi; none had ever been passed, she thought.

Although *Chelidonium* and *Hydrastis* both did much good, it was the *Myrica* that really hit the mark curatively. (XVII 103)

## 368. TAWNINESS OF SKIN, BRONCHIAL CATARRH, AND COUGH.

The tawny skin is met with in greatest perfection in those who have lived in hot countries ; and where this dirty looking dinginess of the skin is not from constitutional disease, or inherited from phthisically disposed parents (see Cases 290-345) it is quite amenable to treatment. The tawny discoloration can be more or less removed. This tawniness I regard as chronic subicterism, and, indeed, the anti icteries cure such cases beautifully. They generally take a good deal of time to be really and permanently cured, and a whole series of such remedies have to be brought into play in succession, one after the other, together with here and there an inter current nosode; but at times they will mend quickly from one or two remedies only.

Thus at the beginning of the current year a city merchant, fifty five years of age, came to consult me for a cough, with a bronchial catarrh. The tawniness of his skin was very marked, and this he attributed to a twenty years' residence in Africa. The cough was habitual, and worse in the evening. There are a good many crescentic cutaneous efflorescences on his chest.

Two months of *Hydrastis Canadensis* Q.

He took altogether just an ounce, in small material doses. Cured the cough; reduced the catarrh of the bronchial lining to a minimum; and very materially lessened the tawniness of his skin; many of his friends remarking upon the very striking improvement in his seemingly dirty complexion. I should have followed up with some three or four other anti icterics, but the gentleman considered he was well enough, and would not come any more, even "to please his wife." (XVII 106)

## 369. VARICOSE VEINS - UPPER LIMB

At the beginning of 1889, a young lady was brought to me by her mother for a large varicose vein running from her right shoulder, over the right clavicle, and across the upper half of the right side of the chest. It varied in size somewhat, and at its largest was about the size of an ordinary quill. Being great society people this vein cast quite a shadow over their lives, it being "quite impossible, you know, to dress."

One sees the oddest things in the way of varicose veins in the lower half of the body, but not very often in the upper, as gravitation is enough to empty them when they are higher up.

All kinds of treatment had been applied, or applied to, and quite lately the vein had been treated by that wonderful cure-nothing — electricity.

I reasoned thus : Veins that dilate in that manner, steadily, slowly, increasingly, must do so from an obstruction in their progression heartwards, just as the little rivulets higher up the stream must fill up when the stream is dammed up lower down.

From a rather careful physical survey of the parts involved, I found the liver very large — indeed huge, which was probably accounted for by the fact that patient had thrice had ague. or else three attacks of the same. Her skin was dirty dingy looking, and the portion covering the lower end of the breast bone studded with wee flat warts, and the degree of anaemia was considerable. Moreover, she had a disagreeable cough, and her sleep was not good.

An ounce of *Chelidonium* Q, spread over eleven weeks, restored the liver to its normal size, and the varicosis had almost entirely disappeared, so that patient had again taken to evening dress — respectively, undress. Her skin at the same time became clearer and her blood of evidently better quality. (XVII 112)

## 370. DYSPEPSIA DUE TO GALL STONES

The wife of a well-known clergyman came under my observation on the 12th of June, 1889, for gall stones. Competent medical men had attended her in these attacks, and had diagnosed gallstones. Patient had turned fifty, and is the mother of many children. Her attacks began with sharp agonizing pains in the pit of the stomach, extending to the arms, and with them severe vomiting; her breath is very short; her bowels are costive, and she is a martyr to flatulent dyspepsia.

Being a rich woman, she had sought the best advice in London, but to no avail. Her physicians had stated that nothing more could be done. Her lower extremities had begun to swell, and this, coupled with a loss of flesh, dyspnoa, and a very darkly icteric coloration of the skin, seemed to corroborate the given prognosis, and the more so as patient's able physicians had long tried their best with such remedies as are current in the orthodox school of medicine.

But knowing well their poverty in remedies, and in knowledge of remedies, I set about treating this lady precisely as if she had never had any medical treatment at all.

Thirteen months later, while I am actually writing these notes, she is plump, healthy looking, and touring with her husband in Scotland and she has had no pains at all for just eleven months. Friends who have not seen her for some time barely able to recongnize her because of her changed appearance.

Her remedies were *Hydrastis Canadensis, Bryonia alba, Thuja occident., Helonium, Strophanthus,* and intercurrently, for far-reaching constitutional effects, two common nosodes in high dilutions.

The change in this lady's disposition is rather remarkable, as from being dull, taciturn, unengaging, and almost socially uncivil, she has become bright, affable and chatty. *The fact is, our brightness and chatty sunniness in our social life do verily depend much upon the liver.* (XVII 115)

## 371. MALIGNANT AFFECTION OF LEFT LOBE OF LIVER

Sometimes one meets with cases in which there appears to be a semi-malignant affection, involving the left lobe of the liver, and what lies between it and the pylorus and the pancreas, and here *Cholesterine* 3 and *Iodoformum* 3, in four-hourly alternation, have several times rendered me sound service.

I may relate one such. Summoned 60 miles into the country late one afternoon, to a supposedly dying lady of 60 odd years of age, I found her icteric, vomiting, bathed in cold perspiration, very thin, debile; the pulse small and weak, and patient seemingly almost moribund. Nothing would stay on the stomach. The seat of the affection was the left lobe of the liver, extending to the left and towards the navel. That there were gallstones is probable, but, quite outside of the acute attack, there was a chronic affection of some kind in the region just named, evidenced by swelling and tenderness.

*Kali bich.* 5 relieved; *Cholesterine* 3x and *Iodof.* 3x cured in a month, and, the case being of long standing, the cure converted several families to the contemned pathy of Samuel Hahnemann.

But, allowing for all doubfulness and vagueness in what I here relate, *Cholesterine* is my sheet-anchor in the organic liver disease in which the commoner hepatics — *Chelid., Carduus, Myrica, Kali bich., Merc.,* and *Diplotaxis tenuifolia* have failed.

I do not think that *Chlosterine* has any influence upon the "disposition" to cancer, but it acts by reason of its elective affinity for the seat of the disease; it effects therefore not a cure in the Hunterian sense, in as much as it only gets rid of the product of the disease, but that is something, as there is then a temporary cure, which under favourable circumstances may become permanent, proof of which permanence of curative results I will presently adduce. In this case the cure has proved to be permanent, as now (two years since the lady is in capital health, and on a visit to her daughter in the North of England. (XVII 120)

## 372. *CHOLESTRINE* FOR HEPATIC CARCINOSIS

On January 30th, 1889, an American gentleman, confessing to sixty-five years of age, and on a visit to his daughter, married to an English clergyman in the north, was accompanied to my rooms by the said daughter, so ill was he that had I thereafter heard of his immediate demise I should have been not in the very least astonished.

The note taken at the time stands thus in my case book under the above date . . . Thin, weak, debile; yellow conjuctivae, insomnia : very nervous and apprehensive. Been treated for enlarged liver and had lots of calomel and chloral. His skin is tawny, cachectic. There is a swelling of the liver or of the pancreas — probably malingnant disease of the left lobe of the liver. Always suffered from dyspepsia. Been a great ocean traveller. "I am very fond of salt, and eat a great deal." Is a practical teetotaler. Bones of the fingers very knobby. He is a spring-and-fall ailer. Has lost a stone weight since November. Never been ill but ailing, and has taken much medicine : bromides and chloral, urethran. Very chilly. He is very ill. Urine normal. Has had ague, and been twice vaccinated.

I ordered him six grains of the third decimal trituration of *Cholesternium* every four hours, and requested him to call in a few days. The married daughter demanded my candid opinion, and I said it was, in my judgement, cancer of the liver, when she informed me that that was the unamimous opinion of all their medical advisers the most trusted of whom were quite sure the lethal end was not far off.

That would also have been my opinion had I not seen *Cholesterine* bring back hope in several desperate cases of cancer of the liver. I therefore, felt warranted in stating that I thought our remedies carefully and persistently applied might yet cure him. In a few days patient returned to me in company with his daughter, and I hardly like to say that the change was, so great was the amelioration. he looked vastly improved and walked firmly, and indeed already considered himself on the high road to recovery, almost wondering what all the fuss had been about.

When Mr. D.R. had retired, his daughter very anxiously said, "What do you think, now?" I said I had not altered my opinion; and that the improvement was due to the remedy and not natural recovery, and that the said improvement would have to be followed up with close scientific treatment which might, and indeed most likely would, result in a positive and direct art-cure. I also tried to explain that we had begun successfully and rapidly to deal with the product of the disease, and that done we could proceed to deal with the disposition thereto. I ordered patient to go on another few days with the prescription which I had given to him at first (Cholest.,) and then to report himself to me.

In about half an hour thereafter the daughter returned with her husband, and the latter almost flew at me in very rage, "What," said he, "do you mean to tell me that my wife's father has cancer?" "Yes." "And that you are going to cure him?" "Yes. I think I shall, but I am not sure." Hereupon he raised his voice somewhat and repeated his questions so offensively that I turned away from him and he left. I have never seen or heard of any of them since; nor have I ever since seen the wife's sister, Lady __, whom I cured in 1886 of a thickening of the Cardia, but Lady __'s cure was a truly Hunterian one, and she has been quite well for long, I have been so often amazed at the insolence of ignorance that I not infrequently find it hard to bear with equanimity. Thus here I was postively insulted, essentially becuase I knew more on a given point than certain others, viz., that *Cholesterine* will at any rate curatively modify some cases that seem to be hepatic carcinosis. (XVII 125)

## 373. TUMOUR OF LIVER OF GREAT SIZE

A country squire nearing seventy years of age came under my observation in the early part of 1889 for a very large tumour clearly connected with the left lobe of the liver. Patient was so ill that he reached town with difficulty, and became so weak that it was impossible for him to return. Orthodoxy well represented had given him up; and his profound adynamia and cachectic look warranted me in stating that I had but small hope. But he was a plucky fellow — a type of the British aristocrat (born to govern and fit therefor : because living out of doors and not reading books — Becaonsfield) and he was willing to obey to the letter.

I advised him to go to the Grand Hotel and quarter himself in the sunny front high up out of the dirt and din, and there abide. He did so, and a very pleasant abode that is : the sun streaming in; the quiet; and yet the outlook upon the seething mass below, which keeps from stagnation.

A homoeopath for half a century he had boundless faith in *Nux vomica*, but I told him that I was sure *Nux* would not cure him, and as this visibly depressed him, I said I would give him my medicine, but in alternation with it he should have his *Nux*. Hence this was given in alternation with *Cholestrine.* The tumour slowly disappeared, the liver went down to the state it had been in for forty years i.e. the left lobe somewhat bulging, and patient returned to his country seat in about two months, and ever since he is not, as a rule, conscious of possessing a liver at all, though once in a way he feels a little uneasy in the hepatic region. This I know, as patient has long been worried with vesical catarrh, and for this I am now treating him, keeping all the time a certain amount of attention directed to the hepatic region in case of any further explosion; for I do not imagine that the cure thus far is a truly Hunterian one. (XVII 133)

## 374. AMEKEAN TREATMENT OF HEPATIC TUMOURS; HEPATIC CANCER

About five years ago, a gentleman of 67 or thereabouts came under my observation for a swelling under the right ribs that competent authorities had diagnosed as of a cancerous nature. It had come a good many months subsequently to an accident : a cab wheel having gone over the body at the part mentioned. He had been under a good West-end homoeopathic physician who had agreed, after a close examination to the diagnosis, and declared positively to the gentleman's wife that he had no hope whatever of curing the case, and he thought it his duty to say so.

The whole thing was quite cured with the remedies in about a year; the most striking, palpable result being observed after the use of *Cholesterine* in different dilutions, though numerous remedies were needed as well, notably *Carduus marianus* Q, *Chelidonium majus* Q, *Myrica cerifera* 3x, *Iodium* I, *Kali bich.* 5, and *Nat. mur.* 6 trit.

Five years have elapsed and there has been no recurrence of tumour, and during the whole of the five years the gentleman has only been away from his business for three weeks and that was to go to the seaside last August.

A few days since I saw his wife on her own account, when she reported him "quite well." (XVII 137)

This certainly looks like a Hunterian cure. I can now report on another and very similar case, as follows : —

## 375. ANOTHER *CHOLESTERINUM*

Nearly six years ago, indeed a little longer, as it was early in the year 1876, I was required to treat a liver case almost exactly like the foregoing one. But patient was not much over fifty years of age then, and it arose primarily, it was thought, from adhesive peritonitis of long before. For years this gentleman, a county man, had felt the jolting in a carriage at first uncomfortable, and latterly so painful that he had got into the habit of holding his hand against the swelled part to support it and prevent its feeling the effects of the shaking.

With the sole addition of *Medorrh*. C. the treatment was as in the last case, and of about the same duration, viz., about a year, and with an equally satisfactory result : he got well, and has remained well to date, working very hard almost all the time. This I know, as he has come about four times a year to be assured that his old enemy had been, not merely scotched, but killed.

In this case I myself originally gave a bad prognosis to the gentleman's wife, and it was the *Cholesterine* that brought life and hope into the matter. *It is very difficult to cure a tumid mass of any kind with one remedy : one needs Organopathy, Homoeopathy, Amekeanism, and empiricism, together with theories no end, if the full extent of the possible is to be attained.* (XVII 139)

## 376. GALLSTONES AND ASTHMA

It must be nearly ten years ago that a widow lady from abroad came to consult me for asthma and biliary calculi : and I will relate her case, not only becuase it is apposite as a cure of a liver affeciton, but because the lady has been more or less within my professional ken ever since, and at this present time she is in very good health, and for long has had neither Asthma nor Gallstone attacks.

Another point of interest for me lies in the fact that four well-known homoeopathic physicians had treated the case during over three years with only indifferent success. They treated the symptoms without any physical diagnosis, and after having prescribed for the symptoms and temporarily cured many of them, the patient remained pretty much where she was before. Had they gone into the case they would have found that the bronchial asthma, retching and vomiting had their *point de depart* in the gall bladder.

No doubt this had again its origin in the constitutional crasis of the individual, and hence I began the treatment with very infrequent doses of *Psorinum* 30. This much lessened the pain in the right side, and it greatly relieved the cough. Then during about five weeks patient was under the influence of *Chelidonium* 1, and pain and cough quite disappeared.

In a fortnight the pain starting from the gall bladder returned, and was accompanied with much retching. Patient was of opinion that the side pain had originally come from taking such quantities of *phosphorus* for her cough years ago. At any rate, she affirmed that she never felt pain in this region before.

There is no return of asthma since she let off the *Chelidonium*. I next prescribed *Terebinthina* 3x, four drops in water three times a day. The *Tereb.* rather upset her at first, and then she got better.

After this an attack of gall colic came on from exertion.

The duskiness of the skin, and the big brown patches on the forehead, led me to give *Nux*. It did much good, and under its influence patient's skin became lighter and cleaner. Then followed *Thuja* 30, and subsequently at odd intervals, according to the symptoms, *Mercurius vivus*, *Antimon. tart.* 3, *Pulsatilla* 3x, *Cholesterine* 2, *Ipec.*, *Alnus rub.*, *Nat. Sul.* 6, and *Calc. carb.* 30.

But these were mostly for the gallstones, as there had never been any return of the asthma after the *Psorinum* followed by the *Chelidonium*, and that is more than nine years ago.

This I consider the more remarkable, as both her own mother and her own son had asthma; and an asthmatic lady, daugher and mother of individuals similarly afflicted, would hardly have a transitory or spurious kind of asthma. (XVII 151)

## 377. CHRONIC ENLARGEMENT OF THE LIVER

In the month of June of the year 1883, a widow lady came under my observation for diarrhoea. It was clearly of hepatic nature, and patient felt as if she were sinking into the earth; icy cold feet; pains in the abdomen; has piles; last year nearly had jaundice. A physical examination revealed chronic enlargement of the liver; the patient looked ill, and in very ill-health. With an enlargement of the liver, tenderness of the hepatic region, pains in the abdomen, piles, diarrhoea, and evident *Angegriffensein* of the organism, I think the ordination of *Podophyllum pelt.* 6x may be fairly called

scientific; in fact, I maintain that the prescription was demonstrably and strictly scientific.
It cured the patient slowly — seven weeks — surely, and permanently and not only subjectively but objectively, for her improved appearance was very pronounced. (XVII 168)

## 378. JAUNDICE OF NINE YEARS' DURATION GALLSTONES OF LARGE SIZE

I will now go on to this case by narrating that patient, a married lady, mother of a family, was brought to me by her husband with some difficulty, owing to her great weakness and loss of flesh.
I noted as follows : — Mrs. X., 38 years of age, eleven years married, mother of seven children, came under my observation on September 29, 1890. During the past three months intensely jaundiced, and is given up as past all hope of recovery.
During the past nine years her doctor has been giving her morphia to ease the pain in the right side, left side, and in the stomach, abdomen, and hypogastrium respectively. At the present time she takes about a dozen quarter-grain pills of morphia a day; she is emaciated to a painful degree. The spleen is very much hypertrophied, and extends across to the mesial line and inferiorly down to the crest of the ilium; in fact, it practically fills the left half of the abdomen. It is very tender, and the contours of the big spleen can not only be felt but readily seen, as it rises above the surface. The liver is only very moderately enlarged, about an inch and a half beyond the ribs, towards the epigastrium.
While I am examining her, patient appears very weak and faint, and hardly able to bear the undressing. Her eyes are lustrous, her tongue raw red. Urine is scanty; loaded with bile; bowels costive. The region of the gall-bladder and ducts very tender, but the greatest pain is in the pit of the stomach. Catamenia always scanty, and at present stopped. The motions are without bile, and moved with the very greatest difficulty. No appetite. In almost constant distress from the agonising pains at the pit of the stomach.
Patient had been twice vaccinated, and years ago had severe ulceration of the womb, for which she lay in bed for three months, and during that period was six times cauterised. The cuaterizations, aided by many introvaginal injections and much lying-up, were followed by the disappearance of the said ulcerations.
I did not really know where to begin at in this formidable case, but in view of the severity of the epigastric pain, jaundice, constipation, etc., I ordered

*Hydrastis Can.* Q, four drops in a tablespoonful of tepid water every four hours. This was the last day of September, 1890.

October 6th — The urine has begun to improve; it is more watery, and not quite so full of bile; the motions more natural, but the liver is very distinctly bigger than it was six days ago. I therefore, feel justified in going on with the *Hydrastis*.

13th — Patient's jaundiced skin is not quite so intensely black yellow; the pain has altered. There is very distinct, though not great, improvement; for the first time for very very long her period is full and free, which has much relieved her. The spleen is a trifle smaller; the tongue dry and glazed.

I find on reference that a few doses of *Thuja* 30 were given inter-currently on the 6th instant. Continue with both *Hydrastis* Q and the *Thuja* 30.

20th — There is no longer any pain in the region of the gall-bladder; patient complains of cold shivers; liver has gone down in size while the spleen is more swelled and very painful, and patient complains very much of chilliness.

$R_x$ Tc. *Urtica urens* Q, seven drops in water three times a day.

27th — No "spasms"; pains in the spleen worse; the spleen is, however, softer to the feel; liver larger. To alternate *Carduus mar.* Q with the *Urtica*, every three hours.

November 3rd — Spleen and liver both bigger, which I take to mean that they are being acted upon by the remedies, particularly as patient is not so chilly and is in less pain. Patient has never ceased to take about a dozen morphia pills every day; some days many more.

To continue with the *Carduus* and *Urtica*.

12th. — The jaundice is much worse; the pains in the region of the gall-bladder are atrocious. I try to persuade the patient to leave off the morphia, so as to give the remedies a chance, but she appeals to me not leave her unhelped in her agony; I could not resist, and so consented to the morphia pills being continued.

We had made a little progress in the case, but not much, and so I made a further and very careful survey of the aetiological history of the case, and came to the conclusion that the whole thing was of *uterine* origin.

As I have had a good deal of clinical experience of *Bursa pastoris*, tending to shew that it is a remedy specifically affecting the womb in like manner as *Chelidonium* does the liver, I at once determined to test for the right *appropriatum uteri*, as I conceive Paracelsus or Rademacher might have done.

I reasoned from the clinical data taken in historic sequence that the primary affection years ago was uterine, and the hepatic affection consecutive thereto, and starting therefrom. I saw clearly that the old ulcerated condition was at the bottom of it, or rather that was as far back as I could get for the present. For although the cause of the ulcers was presumably the *fons et origo mali*, yet the real disease *at present* to be grappled with was the jaundice, the gallstones, and the colic.

In this case getting rid of the primary constitutional cause would not necessarily have mended matters, therefore I started with *Bursa pastoris* Q, five drops in warm water every five hours.

That was on the 12th, and by the 17th there was a very extraordinary change come over the face of the case; indeed it was at first blush almost incredible. There was much less jaundice, the liver had gone down in size almost to normality, and the spleen was fully an inch smaller. Moreover, there was no pain in the liver at all.

My inkling that the start of the disease of the biliary apparatus was in the womb being thus confirmed, indeed, rendered certain, I continued with the *Bursa* as before.

November 24th — Although there has been no further spasms, there has not been any further progress; patient does not sleep so well; the liver has again begun to enlarge, and there is no further diminution in the size of the spleen. Still, I did not feel justified in leaving off with *Bursa*, and hence I alternated it with *Chelidonium* Q.

December — Patient was very ill, and everybody gave her up, excepting myself. I did not see my way out of the wood, but still *I hold that the physician who gives up a case before the patient dies is on a par with the soldier who runs away from the enemy*. So here, though I was absolutely alone in my view, I refused to surrender.

The bowels had ceased to act; there was more jaundice again, and patient could no longer rise from her bed.

I then gave *Euonymin* 3x, six grains every two hours, just as a liver remedy. Under very great agony patient in the course of a week or two passed a handful of gallstones by the bowels, and her jaundice was gone!

A number of the largest were obtained from the stools, and on account of the great interest of the case I now present my readers with a photogravure of them, taken by Sprague, of London, and which gives them in their natural size.

I have shewn these biliary calculi to certain medical friends, and amongst them to Dr. Robert T. Cooper, of London, as a curiosity.

I should explain that these biliary calculi were very much larger than here represented they were first passed, but their outer layers were friable, and were washed, picked, and rubbed off before the calculi were brought to me; it is really only the hard kernels of the calculi which are given in this photogravure.

Notwithstanding the disappearance of the jaundice, and the passage of the gallstones as just described, patient had got very low, and the spleen did not seem to be any better subjectively, and not much smaller, and there was no period.

Here I gave *Ceonothus Am.* I, five drops in water four times a day.

15th — Patient has had severe rigors, seemingly caused by the *Ceanothus*, which is therefore discontinued. She has no appetite, and the menstruation has not appeared.

To have *Pulsatilla* 1, three drops in water every three hours.

20th — Liver nearly normal; has just mensturated; the spleen has gone down a little; the entire abdomen very tender all over; has again had an awful attack of gallstone colic, and passed a number of stones, one very large. There is still bile in the urine.

To have *Bursa pastoris* Q, and *Nux vom.* I.

29th — Another attack of colic; a further passage of biliary calculi — three large ones; patient is low and weak, and prefers death to so much pain. It is to be remembered that large numbers of morphia pills are being taken all this time. To relieve the effects of the passage of the calculi, and the almost general feeling of bruisedness and tenderness, I ordered *Bellis perennis* Q, eight drops in water every four hours.

1891, January 12th — Great general improvement from the use of the *Bellis perennis*, but her liver and spleen are more swelled and greatly distress her.

$R_x$ Trit 3x *Cholesterin*. Six grains dry on the tongue every four hours.

19th. — Spleen and liver seem larger than ever. No jaundice, however. No menses.

Five drops of *Pulsatilla* Q three times a day.

26th — Has normally menstruated; liver smaller; spleen very tender.

$R_x$ *Bursa pastoris* Q. Five drops in a tablespoonful of water three times a day.

February 3rd — Has passed some more calculi; region of gall duct very tender; no jaundice; urine normal; is gaining flesh; the spleen is very large.

$R_x$ Tr. *Ceanothus Americanus* 1. Five drops in water every four hours.

13th — There is further improvement; she feels better; is beginning to go about like other people, has passed one gallstone small size, and a number of lumps of "sooty stuff." Feels that this medicine has done her much good. Rep.

23rd — The spleen has gone down about one inch and three quarters; has menstruated again normally; is increasing in weight. Rep.

March 16th. — By letter I am informed that the spleen is not so well; and that there is a good deal of pain in the right side again.

$R_x$ Trit. 3x *Leptandrin*. Six grains dry on the tougue, three times a day.
31st — No improvement from the *Leptandrin*, and generally not so well, though the jaundice is entirely a thing of the past, and she is now of a very clear white complexion, and getting no longer to appear to be particularly thin.
$R_x$ *Bellis perennis* and *Bursa pastoris* in alternation.
April 15th — Liver, spleen, and womb are described as "all blown out;" much pain in the region of the gall bladder.
$R_x$ *Puls.* and *Byronia*.
May 4th — Patient is doing well; liver normal, or nearly so; spleen now only reaches half way down the crest of the ilium, and is well defined. Patient has now the old symptoms of ulceration of the OS UTERI — the forcible healing up of which started the whole thing years ago!
And here I think I may resume, and conclude this already too long narration.
We see in this case the importance in Paracelisic organ-testing to find out the *point de depart* of the series of morbid phenomena; hepatics and splenics had no adequately curative action till the uterine medicine (*Bursa pastoris*) had touched the place of origin of the liver affeciton, and as soon as this was done (see Notes under date November 17th, 1890) immediate improvement began!
We have now cured the jaundice; the gallstones have been got rid of through the natural ways; the liver is well, and patient is going about her business; and our interest in the case in this treatise on "The Diseases of the Liver" is at an end.
*THREE MONTHS LATER*
August 10th, 1891. — Having this day seen and carefully examined this patient I am enabled to say that she is in excellent health, plump and pleasing, and equal to and performing the usual duties of an English housewife with a large family. (XVII 180)

## 379. ENLARGEMENT OF LIVER REMAINING FROM HEPATITIS AND PERITONITIS

The wife of the Vicar of St. B. brought a young lady, about 24 years of age, to me on February 20th, 1893, for considerable swelling of the abdomen and such severe varicosis of lower extremities that the patient had been confined to her couch for nearly a year. Patient had had thrombosis of the veins of her lower extremeties repeatedly and the swelling in the right side of the abdomen dates from a severe attack of peritonitis and hepatitis. All idea of a cure had been abandoned. Percussion and palpation revealed an enlargement of the left lobe of the liver and a painful lump

lying between the liver and the navel about the size of a small fist. Glands in the groins feel like marbles, lower extremities lårge and unshapely, clearly the remains of the original thrombosis. In as much as the whole series of phenomena — thrombosis, peritonitis, hepatitis — began with getting a chill (cold, wet) six years ago, I ordered my old friend *Bellis perennis* ten drops in a tablespoonful of water night and morning.
March 20th — Very greatly improved, indeed, lump nearly gone and the lower extremeties are now shapely!!
The left lobe of the liver however remaining enlarged, I ordered *Carduus marioanus* seven drops in water night and morning.
Aril 28th — Patient at this date was walking about like other people, and the only thing that remained was a little transverse swelling of the liver and this was removed by a short course of *Chelone glabra*.
In the fall of the year 1893, a slight relapse occurred which was quickly righted by *Bellis perennis*.
The Vicar's wife was with me on October 15th, 1894, on another matter and mentioned incidentallly that Jessie's cure had proved complete and lasting. (XVII 208)

## 380. SWELLING OF EPIGASTRIC REGION

I have lately cured a stubborn case of a throbbing swelling in the pit of the stomach involving the left side of the liver and the spleen and the tissues lying between the two organs.
No defined epigastric tumours could be satisfactorily distinguised but the whole epigastric region was very tender on pressure and patient could not bend down without getting giddy and feeling much distress at the epigastrium. The particular interest in the case lay in the long duration of the ailment and the pulsating epigastric mass.
Patient took five drops of the matrix tincture of *Helianthus*, night and morning for some weeks when the only abnormal thing remaining was the very slight enlargement of the left lobe of the liver and for which he was put on *Chelone glabra*. The spleen was put right and also the epigastrium of which the pulsation ceased, together with the tenderness and distension and in view of the difficulties one encounters in dealing curatively with pulsating epigastric swellings I think this short narration worth penning and preserving. (XVII 212)

## 381. VARIX GROIN, WITH ENLARGED LEFT LOBE OF LIVER

A Commander in the Royal Navy, about two years ago, came under my observation for an enormous varix in the right groin, just on Poupart's ligament. The varix was about the size of a very small orange and the thing was certainly becoming alarming on account of the thinning of the wall of the dilated vein. And being in the bend of the groin it was almost impossible to apply mechanical support. The patient was a thoroughly healthy fellow and though I diagnosed him up and down and questioned him unto very weariness, still there was absolutely nothing findable beyond a slight enlargement of the left lobe of the liver. I first used *Chelidonium majus* with some advantage, and under *Carduus marianus* the varix certainly diminished somewhat, but under the remedy in question the varix disappeared and patient hastened off on active service. From this (and similar observations I have laid it down for my own future guidance that the *seat of action* of *Chelone glabra* is the left lobe of the liver and its line of action is in the direction of the navel, bladder and uterus. That this is really so the competent will have no difficulty in verifying whether *Chelone* acts upon the liver itself as a true hepatic I would not venture to affirm; perhaps it reduces the swellings of the left lobe of the liver by its action on the veins running up to the liver.

Many of the "New Remedies" have come and gone; *Chelone* has come to stay : its sphere of action is small, its action sharp and withal well defined. (XVII 214)

## 382. RIGHT-SIDED VARICOCELE FROM ENLARGED LIVER

A gentleman, who had long been under me, consulted me again in the spring of 1894 for varicocele of the right side. Casting about to find the primary dam I found the left lobe of the liver notably swelled, patient himself being however in capital health. There was besides the varicocele a moderate degree of varicosis of the large veins of the whole of the right leg. I prescribed *Chelone glabra,* five drops in a tablespoonful of water night and morning.

I did not hear from him for eleven months when he called to see me telling me had had gone on with the remedy steadily all the time as it seemed to be doing him good.

On examining him I found the varicocele had gone down about one-half and the varicosis of the leg had also notably diminished, so that he can now safely dispense with the elastic support. I was here led to prescribe *Chelone* because of its line of action from right to left and from above downwards.

The testimony afforded by this case is very high indeed because patient has been under me for years for his varicosis with but small benefit, and his being an officer in the Royal Navy rendered it very important that he should have his varicosis mended. He is not entirely cured now but the amelioration is such that in his own words "they (the authorities) will let me go now on any expedition." I had before made use of a number of vein medicines and constitutional remedies, but *Chelone* alone did ten times more than they all. (XVII 217)

### 383. LIVER DISEASE, STERNAL PATCH INSOMNIA & CHRONIC DIARRHOEA

A gentleman of thirty years of age came under my observation for liver disease, skin disease, insomnia, depression of spirits and chronic diarrhoea though, only thirty years of age, he has lost all his teeth from shrinking of the gums; they just fell out. His skin disease consisted in what I have elsewhere called the Sternal Patch, the liver affection in an enlargement of the left lobe and for this I ordered *Carduus marianus*, six drops in water, three times a day. In a short time he reported himself as sleeping well and his spirits notably improved. *Arsenicum* and *Thuja* followed but no further improvement worth while mentioning, when, on June 13th, I prescribed *Chelone glabra* in the same manner in which I had formerly ordered *Carduus*.

July 13th — "That medicine (*Chelone*) acted like a charm.

Patient remained well for a year or so and then returned with the old symptoms again — I have now come to the point of my case. *Carduus* was ordered as before. *Chelone* followed, but neither acted as formerly, that which a year before acted like a charm now acted not at all. The fact is in this case there exists a constitutional crisis quite away from the hepatic state, it is an organismic ailing and not merely one of the organ, and here I found it necessary to go in quest of the homoeopathic simillimum, the simple homoeopathic part-elective drug-effinity not sufficing. (XVII 221)

### 384. COLD HANDS — INDIGESTION DUE TO LIVER TROUBLE

Mr. X., a singer of world-wide fame, had been under me for some months with much advantage; under hepatics and renal remedies he greatly improved, but did not get rid of his "cold hands" and "I am so dreadfully nervous, I am frightened at everything, sometimes I dare not enter a cab or carriage, and feel it to be absolutely impossible to face the audience and my indigestion is pretty bad and I have a great deal of heartburn."

At the left side of the liver, deep in, seemed the faulty part.

$R_x$ *Calendula off.* Q, five drops in water, night and morning, was ordered and after a month of this I heard, "Oh, I am getting on splendidly; the heartburn is gone, my digestion is better, my hands have quite lost that nasty cold feeling and my nerve is so much better, I am quite a different man."

I had formerly won this gentlmen's confidence by materially improving his grand voice.

What with?

*Thuja occidentalis* 30.

Why given?

For Vaccinosis.

The number of people I have benefitted by *Thuja* 30 is really almost beyond belief; one dose of six globules every week is my rule. (XVII 227)

### 385. *CHELONE GLABRA* IN HEPATIC DROPSY

In a case of severe dyspnoea from hepatic dropsy *Chelone glabra* rendered me good service; the case was very complicated inasmuch as in addition to bradycardia, cirrhosis of the liver and Bright's disease of the kidneys there was seemingly a tumour lying between the liver and the navel : tense, tender and certainly of quite a different nature to the general ascitic swelling. By reason of its topographic position and in view of the line of action of *Chelone* as I have before pointed out, I gave five drops of *Chelone* Q in a tablespoonful of water every four hours and in less than a fortnight the lump between liver and navel had quite disappeared, and simultaneously therewith also the cardiac dyspnoea. I say cardiac dyspnoa as it lay in its origin between the liver and the heart, I could not trace any direct influence of *Chelone* on either the heart or kidneys though both were much influenced by the removal of the obstructive mass between liver and navel (XVII 230)

### 386. *QUASSIA* AS A LIVER MEDICINE

It is difficult to conceive of anything outside of one's own self and one's own experience and hence it comes to pass that I have never been quite able to realize that *Quassia* has any action on the liver worth while. *Und Doch.*

Very early in 1895 a gentleman sent me a young man from Hampstead who had been in vain operated on in University College Hospital and thence discharged as incurable. Incurable at twenty years of age !

This young man informed me that he left University College Hospital quite lately and showed me a long scar in the right axillary line where an incision would have enabled an exploration of the right kidney region, gall bladder and back of liver, which no doubt was the object of the operation. He himself stated that it was for stone in the right kidney but on reaching the kidney no stone could be found and so the wound was stitched up, and as soon as it had healed-up patient was discharged as incurable. Patient complained of attacks of severe pain at the back of the liver — just where the fresh scar is seen — coming on with vomiting at any time, any day and in any weather; these attacks average about one a week and the pain once on will last from one to three days. Has been subject to these attacks for five years and has had to give up all work for long and is now much reduced in health and strength. The vomiting comes on whenever he attempts to eat. As the attack comes on he swells and sems very tight in the girth. In the perpendicular the hepatic dullness goes right up to the nipple. I put patient at first on *Hydrastis Canadensis*, then on *Urtica urens*, then on *Chelidonium majus* with the sole difference that under the *Chelidonium* the dull percussion note of the liver in the mammary line was a trifle less.

On April 9th I ordered *Quassia* tincture Q, five drops in water every four hours.

23rd. There is very great improvement and the young man has quite a different look, his low whining complaining tone having given way to much greater mental and physical alertness, only one attack of pain. Rep.

May 7th. There have been two attacks of pain, but very much less severe and he feels much stronger.

To take the *Quassia* in five drop doses three times a day.

May 21st. Attacks are much less in severity and less frequent.

Patient has put on flesh, the previous dirty colour of the skin of his face has gone and given place to a clean, healthy looking face. Rep.

Remains under treatment so I am not able to say whether the *Quassia* is the real remedy in the case; but, assuming that it does no more than it has already accomplished, at any rate its record in the case is better than that of my allopathic friends at University College Hospital. So far as I see at present it is a case of neither liver nor kidney merely; but of the right supra-renal capsule, but into this dark continent we will now not penetrate. (XVII 232)

## RINGWORM

### 387. RINGWORM SCALP

A whole family of children of different ages had had ringworm for a full year, and the mother told me on bringing them that she had already spent over £ 60 on medical fees for its cure, but in vain. All known remedies had been applied by the local doctors in two neighbourhoods, and several skin specialists had worked hard at their poor heads, but to no avail. Their heads were shaved and their scalps were well scoured night and morning but *still* the ringworm persisted. Finally, a distant cottage had been hired, and the afflicted ones were there isolated, and the services of noted ringworm curer of the non-qualified variety had been secured; but these also failing, they were put under my care. I have had no great cause to complain of the homoeopathic treatment of ringworm with our antipsorics — indeed, quite the contrary — but it is apt to be a bit tedious at times. Now their mother had been cured by me of incipient tuberculosis with the virus, and it occurred to me that ringworm might be a manifestaiton of the tubercular kind*, and so I forthwith put the whole lot under the virus, administered in the usual way, internally in dynamic dose; this I had all the more readily, as they all had numerous superficial palpable glands. And the result? In a very few weeks they were all well of ringworm and of the glands, have thriven splendidly ever since. Something like a dozen bad ringworm cases have come to me since then, and they were all quickly cured by the virus, and in each case the general state has been greatly improved. (XVIII)

* *I find Tilbury Fox and Startin were of this opinion; so are, doubtless, many others.*

## 388. INVETERATE CASE OF HERPES TONSURANS OR RINGWORM

A lad of eight years of age was brought to me at the end of April 1891, to be treated for ringworm, under a very severe form of which he had been labouring for over a year. At the date in question it was nearly all over his body, scalp, neck, upper extremities, in large numbers of rings, varying in size from that of a six penny piece to that of a half penny. His scalp is one mass of scabs and scales extending all down the neck (said to have come from gunpowder). The scalp is at times moist. He has no feelable glands in his neck; but those of his groins are like so many very small marbles. Sparsely strawberry-like tongue, teeth yellow and decaying.

"What have you tried for your son?"

"Tried! everything, but he gets worse and worse, and since that gunpowder his head has gone like that."

I am sure that any experienced practitioner of medicine, who places his faith in the outside treatment of ringworm, recongnises the picture.

I am drawing as that of a type of ringworm cases that *will not* get well do what we will. I have had them myself in olden days, till I hated the very sight of them, with their closely shaven scalps that seemed to consist in a number of little exits of sticky, mattery ooze that then dried into scabs. Such was this boy's aspect, but some of its hideousness was covered by a natty, well-fitting skull-cap.

*Bacillinum* C. was given for two months, when on the 24th June, I find noted that the red pips of his tongue were nearly gone; the lower half of his scalp was clean and healthy; appetite better; teeth much cleaner and whiter. "He is much better in his health."

To continue with the same remedy.

July 29th, 1891 — He is quite well of his ringworm, though his scalp is slightly scurfy, and his teeth still rather dirty looking. He then had the same remedy (1000th), whereafter the only one thing wrong with him was the greeny state of his teeth, which presumably was from another aetiological source, and therefore not amenable to the bacillinic influence. A worse case of ringworm would, indeed, be hard to find — a prettier, cleaner, or more accurately scientific cure I do not ask for. When cured the boy was a picture, with his splendid crop of hair stubbles about an inch in length — and, moreover, in excellent general health.

I used *no* external remedies at all. (XVIII 22)

## 389. CONSUMPTION, AFTER RINGWORM

I remember years ago attending the family of a farmer, when several of the children were presented to me as having caught ringworm from the cows, and one of the boys afterwards became very distinctly consumptive, and was given up as past praying for, and then he was sent up to London to me. Four months of *Bacillinum*, high, quite cured him, and he is now thriving.

This all confirms me in my view, which is the underlying idea of this book, that there is some close relationship between tuberculosis and ringworm. (XVIII 36)

## 390. RINGWORM : BACK

A little girl, five and and a half years of age, was brought to me at the end of January 1891 to be treated for ringworm; there was only one ring on the back of the neck, but this was well defined. *Bacillinum* C. was ordered, and the whole thing disappeared within the month, and the little lady has been very thriving ever since. (XVIII 37)

## 391. FOUR CASES OF RINGWORM (SISTERS)

Miss Winnie X., aged ten, came under my care in the month of July 1891 to be treated for ringworm. There were several large patches on her scalp and numerous little ones; the largest was on the crown of the head, a trifle to the left, and nearly two inches in diameter. The child had a profuse mass of hair; is of fairly healthy parentage. I say fairly, because I formerly cured her mother of an abdominal tumour and her brother of very severe eczema. Winnie herself is small for her age, thin, and not robust looking, though she has been living in a fine healthy part of Yorkshire. Her neck was thin, and on both sides studded with feelable, large, hard glands. I put her on *Bacillinum* in my wonted way; in a month her glands were smaller and the herpes tonsurans was less active; and in three months the glands of her neck were well, she had grown, had taken on a healthy look — quite ruddy — and the ringworm was nearly gone, the hair all growing again. At the end of the fourth month she was in all respects normal, and a bright, bonny girl, and so she continues.

The three other sisters of Winnie had the same disease, and the same general conditions of non-thriving; numerous pretty large, hard glands on both sides of the neck, and patches of the ringworm on their scalps and necks, and, like Winnie, with the bald ringworm patches, great shocks of hair. They had the same treatment for the same length of time, and with the identical result; the ringworm quite disappeared, the indurated glands got well (*i.e.*, impalpable), the girls took to growing, and took on a ruddy, healthy appearance. The cure of the ringworm in these four cases — as also in my others — was effected solely by the internal treatment by high potencies of *Bacillinum*. The improvement was gradual, general, and all along the line, as one, indeed, should theoretically expect from any remedial agent that cures organismically and organically. (X 41)

## 392. CASE OF TINEA CIRCINNATA

A young lassie of eight years of age was brought by her mother to me on February 18, 1889, for a patch of ringworm on the left side of the nose and several others on the back of the neck, where the hairy scalp ends. She had from me *Morbillinum* 30.

March 20 — The old spots have gone, but she has quite a number of new ones on chest and arms; her tongue is pippy; she does not get off to sleep very readily. There is no ringworm on the body.

R Bacillinum C.
This quite cured the ringworm, and it never returned. I should have stated at the outset of this little narration, that patient had had ringworms for many months before she was brought to me at all.
Three years later — *i.e.*, April 11, 1892, — I again saw this girl with her mother, when I inquired whether there had been any return of the ringworm? Patient had almost forgotten all about the affair, but her mother exclaimed — "Oh ! Kathleen has never had any return of the ringworm, though fresh places had kept on coming for over a year when I first brought her to you." (XVIII 52)

## 393. RINGWORM

Towards the end of the year 1891, a lady was induced by relatives to bring her twelve-year-old son to me, because he had suddenly arrived home from school with a circular bald, scaly patch on the top of his head. The ring was about the size of a florin, and for the past three weeks had been treated most actively; one might say that said little ring-shaped patch had been attacked with venom, fury, and hatred by the surgeon, the mother, the governess, and by "uncle," the general impression conveyed by the onslaught was "we'll soon get rid of you!"
But in vain, though "uncle" is a general in the army. The indurated glands in the neck, the dusky colour of the skin of the neck, the dirt that would not wash off, showed quite clearly that the stroma was ill. Three months of the *Bacillinum* CC., and nothing else locally or internally, effected a very perceptible change in the boy : not only had the nasty horror-inspiring ring-shaped patch become covered with clean, healthy hairs, but the scurf had gone, and the boy had grown an inch; he looked fresher, brighter, and — "Doctor, his face and neck are *so much* cleaner."
The boy duly returned to school in capital health.
Said the boy's mother, "I am beginning to have faith in your treatment, but oh! what a life 'uncle' and the others have led me."
What does your uncle say, now that the nasty thing has gone.
"He says he always had his doubts as to whether it was a *true* case of ringworm." (XVIII 53)
The nephew of one of the best known dermatologists of this country was lately brought by his mother to me to be treated for an ill-defined pining condition and a trifling cough. "He has never been well since he had the ringworm," exclaimed his mother. An examination of the boy's scalp showed that we had to do with pretty severe scalp eczema, or Alder Smith's Diffuse Chronic Ringworm. There was anorexia, and restless nights had brought down patient's state of nutrition. His cervi-

cal glands were hard and visible : two months' *Bacill.* and the boy was discharged well, or rather the mother did not bring him again, as he was in her judgement "perfectly well." (XVIII 90)

### 394. RINGWORM SCALP

"But," said the mother, "I have come this time about myself; ever since my children had the ringworm last year my own head is covered with scurf, and my hair breaks off, and my hair has become quite thin and short, whereas I have always been so proud of my beautiful head of hair, especially as I have had so many children.

After being two months under the influence of *Bacillinum* in high potency and infrequently administered, the lady wrote to me saying, "My head is now quite free from scurf, and the hair is growing again beautifully." (XVIII 91)

## VACCINOSIS

### 395. A SEVERE CASE — A DYING BABY

Very early in the year 1881, I was called to see a baby in Harley Street, about ten weeks old; its mother thought it was dying. She had previously lost babies by death, and knew what a dying baby looked like. The wee patient had begun its life's journey on the bottle; but, being overtaken by the measles, it nearly died, when a wet nurse was obtained and the baby rallied and began to thrive. But a new wet nurse had to be obtained, as the first went dry from over-feeding. The new wet nurse was healthy and strong, but, having gone into the Marylebone workhouse with her own very fine boy, she was re-vaccinated the day before she was removed therefrom to take charge of the patient in question. The baby throve for two or three days, and the mother was just congratulating herselt on her success, when one afternoon it went very ill, and getting much worse towards the evening, the mother sent this message to me — "I think baby is dying." I visited the babe in the warm and airy nursery, and investigated everything. There was nothing to account for the sudden change. Baby was ghastly white, and in collapse. On questioning the wet nurse as to her own health and state, she remarked that she was quite well (and she looked it, and had a notably good appetite), but she said her re-vaccinated arm "was a little painful." The vesicular stage of the local vaccinial eruption was just at the point of turning to the pustular.

I thought the matter over a little, and came to the conclusion that the poor wee thing was, in point of fact, sucking the vaccinial poison from its nurse through the milk. There I gave *Thuja* 6, in pilules, both to babe and nurse, but whether every half-hour or every hour, I do not now remember. Calling later in the evening, I noticed baby was asleep and looking a little less ghastly. Next morning it was indeed still pale, but practically well; *and the vaccinial vesicles on the nurse's arm had withered*, and they forthwith dried up completely, in lieu of becoming pustular. That baby never looked back, and is now a bonny child.

It is not possible to prove, of course, that this apparently dying baby was suffering from vaccinosis. It lay apparently dying : I feared it would die. But *some* points in connection with this case are incontrovertible. For instance, it is a *fact* that the nurse had been re-vaccinated; it is equally a fact that she was suckling the baby; the baby was desperately ill of something; it got *Thuja* and began to mend forthwith. Moreover, and this point is significant, the vaccinial vesicles in the nurse's arm *withered* instead of going on to their usual development. Hence some disturbing influence must have intervened in her organism, and the only thing I know of was the *Thuja*. If the *Thuja* had no effect upon the suckling woman, what made the vaccinial vesicles wither?

Let us suppose that they withered because the milk drained off all the virus. But the baby sucked the milk, and very ill; and the withering of the vaccination vesicles was *synchronous* with the prompt and evident *amelioration* in the child. (XIX 14)

## 396. TRUE VACCINIA IN A CHILD FOLLOWING THE VACCINATION OF HER MOTHER

On the 13th of February, 1882, I called at the house of Mr. G.___, intending to vaccinate his two children, one about three years old, the other a seven months' babe at the breast, whose head, face, arms, and legs were covered with eczema, *Crusta lactea*, from which it was suffering severely. Fearing an aggravation of the humour from complication with the vaccination I declined to operate, giving as my reason that I thought the child was suffering already; that she would be more feverish, irritable, and would require greater care if vaccinated than at present. Although the three-years old child was troubled with the same form of humour, I vaccinated her, and also the mother. Both vaccinations took, and ran the usual course without much constitutional disturbance. The fifth day after the operation was Mrs. G ____'s sickest day. She then had headache, backache, fever, and chill. The vaccination developed normally, but more rapidly than usual.

On the first day of March the baby was more restless and feverish, requiring constant care. On the second day the mother noticed a number of little red pimples upon the child. These increased rapidly upon the face, arms, and legs. I was called to see the little patient on Saturday the 4th of March. The little pimples at this time were very numerous, had increased in size; the areola quite red; some swelling; baby feverish; temperature 102°. To the question, "What is it, doctor?" I frankly answered, "I do not know; it is not small-pox nor chicken-pox. I shall have to wait until it is more fully developed."

On Sunday morning, the fifth day of the fever, the vesicles were forming and more or less filled with lymph, and in the afternoon some were umbilicated. Fresh eruptions were also developing, and upon the face, arms, and legs — those portions of the surface most severely marked with the eczema — the new eruption had become confluent, the whole character of the eruption resembling that of small-pox. There were without doubt between four and five hundred well-defined circular vesicles upon the child during the course of the disease. I invited Dr. Miles to see the case on Sunday afternoon. After a careful examination we concluded that it was a case of vaccinia, communicated to the child through the mother's milk. That there should be no mistake, however, I called upon Dr. M. Cullom, the city physician, reported the case, and invited him to see the patient with me, which he did on Monday morning. Dr. Martin, of Roxbury, and Dr. Cutler, of Chelsea, also saw the case, and were much interested in it.

On Monday, Tuesday, and Wednesday, the sixth, seventh, and eighth days, there was much swelling of the face, arms, and legs, where it had taken on the confluent form. The little patient was quite feverish and restless. On the seventh, eighth, and ninth days was quite hoarse, and had some difficulty in swallowing. All the symptoms gradually diminished after the ninth day, and many of the scabs were rubbbed off. On the seventeenth day very few adherent scabs remained. *Acon.* and *Tart. emetic* were the remedies used.

At the present time May 14*th* the child shows pits, not deep, however. The parts where the eruption was confluent are still quite red. The eczema, however, seems to have left for good, and I am in hopes of seeing a good clear skin before many weeks. Although the diagnosis the first few days was obscure, all doubt was removed, and it was pronounced a case of vaccinia communicated from the mother. You will note that on the fifth day after the re-vaccination of the mother the paroxysm of fever occurred, and ten days after the baby was feverish and the eruptions made its appearance one day later. We can, therefore, call it fourteen days from the time the babe first took the milk impregnated with vaccinia from its mother. If the system can thus be so thoroughly impregnated with vaccinia, may we not also fear various and worse evils from the milk of unhealthy and unclean nurses?

My remark to this instructive experience of Dr. Harris is, that *Thuja occidentalis* was more homoeopathic to the case than *Acon.* and *Ant. tart.* It shews that vaccinia may most probably be sucked by the babe in the milk, though this is not conclusively shewn, inasmuch as it may have been a case of small-pox in the suckling.

The same transmissibility of disease through the milk has been observed more than once. (XIX 18)

## 397. ACUTE VACCINOSIS

Aug. 21st, 1881 — On the day there was brought to me a little boy, of five months of age, on the bottle, and I was informed that he had been ailing a week, beginning with violent vomiting, loss of appetite, and greenish slimy diarrhoea. The child looked very ill, pale; upper eye-lids drooping; tongue very thickly coated, moist; temperature high; throat severely ulcerated; deglutition painful; on the anterious aspect of uvula one saw an open ulcer of about the size of a large split pea. The greatest distress lay in the throat — the mother brought him on this account; it pained his throat, which was visibly and demonstrably severely ulcerated : so I gave him *Kali chloratum* 6, trituation, a dose every hour, and ordered him to be kept in a room with a good fire, and the windows open.

Aug. 22nd — I called and found him no worse; more could not be said. He had had a very restless night. He was profoundly weak, hence I gave *Kali phos.* 6 in alternation with the other medicine.

23rd — Not quite so weak, but the green, slimy diarrhoea continues. To have *Merc. iod.*

24th — The tongue had begun to clear a little on the left side, but otherwise there was no material change except that he could swallow a little better. Baby was very weak; his mother looked up at me, and the anxious father kept his eyes fixed on my visage, as I sat and studied the little mannikin : he looked very pale, very ill and weak; could not be got to notice anything, but perpetually whined in a piteous little way. I do not know when I ever felt the weight of responsibility greater. Previously I had carefully inquired about the drains, and had ordered the milkman to be changed, and was careful to seek for the real origin of the child's illness, but I could not trace it to anything. The dwelling was healthy, the bottle clean, and there seemed nothing to account for the illness. Suddenly it occurred to me to ask when the child had been vaccinated. The answer was, on the 12th July. I learned also that the child had a very bad arm, and that the present illness commenced on the day on which the last vaccinial scab fell off the arm. This shed a light upon the case, and allowed its true aetiopathology to be understood. The disease evidently was an en-exanthem, an eruption on the lining membrane of the throat and gut, due to the vaccination; and the vomiting, diarrhoea, and sore throat started just as these inside pustules broke and discharged their contents, and the feverishness was synchronous therewith. The child's organism had essayed to free itself from the vaccinial poison by an eruption on the internal mucous membrane. Had the child been stronger the eruption would probably have been on the skin in the form of an exanthem simply. I prescribed *Thuja occidentalis* 30, one drop powders, one every two hours, and no other medicine.

25th — Much better, began to mend (in the mother's opinion — and what more competent?) "very soon after the first powder." has slept better. To continue the *Thuja* powders.

28th — I called to say good-bye, and found the little one still rather weak, but well and cheerful and at play on his mother's lap.

Here, *Thuja* 30 brought health to the child and joy to the home.

## 398. PUSTULAR ERUPTION

I. Mr. J___, a hale-looking, middle-aged London merchant, came under my observation on November 3rd. 1881. Said he, "I am not a homoeopath, but twenty years ago I had eczema, and the allopaths could not touch it, so I went to a homoeopathic doctor, and he cured me." And he went on to say that he believed in homoeopathy for skin diseases. On the left leg he had a pustular eruption, due, he believed, to a bruise. He had also eczema of the ear, and he volunteered the information that ever since his second vaccination he had been subject to eczema. The eczema of twenty years ago was soon after the re-vaccination.

$R_x$ *Thuja occidentalis* 30. Four three-drop powders to the two dozen. To take one, dry on the tongue, three times a day.

He came in a week nearly well; the pustules had at once begun to wither. The *Thuja* was repeated, but in less frequent dose, and the patient subsequently sent word by his brother to say that his skin was well, and he himself too busy to shew himself as he had promised.

This case also proves nothing, because anyone might get a pustular eruption after a bruise, or without a bruise, and be quickly rid of it, without either suffering from vaccinosis, or getting *Thuja*, supposedly, to cure it. The fact is it is exceedingly difficult to absolutely prove anything clinically at all. The patient himself attributed his cure to the powders, knowing of old the very stubborn nature of all his cutaneous eruptions. (XIX 29)

II. Miss —, aet. 18, was re-vaccinated in July, 1881, at her parents' country residence, thirty miles from London, by the local surgeon, with "lymph" direct from the calf. The operation was very successful, and she had a very "fine" arm. But as the "arm" was just at its greatest perfection she got an eruption on her chin, covering its whole extent and involving the lower lip. The thing was very unsightly, and had a singularly ugly repulsive aspect. The gentleman who had done the re-vaccination was of opinion that Miss ____ had got some of the vaccine virus on to her finger-nails and inoculated herself by scratching. The sequel, however, shewed that the chin manifestation was from within. The surgeon had ordered applications, two of which were vaseline and zinc ointment, but the eruption on the chin was not to be got rid of. The young lady had to wear a dense veil to hide her face when driving out. She was brought to London for my advice, and I gave *Thuja* 30. In a fortnight she was out and about, and only some diffused redness of the skin remained, but no scar or thickened skin. Now, it might be objected to this case that the *Thuja* had nothing to do with the disappearance of the eruption, because it was just the history of the disease : it ran through its natural course and died. I thought that to myself at the time of prescribing it, but against this was the fact that the arm had healed already, and it had depassed the natural course of vaccinia by at least a fortnight when I first prescribed the *Thuja*. But to have a test I gave her brother, who also had a somewhat similar pustular eruption (and who had been re-vaccinated at the same time), but more spare, and instead of being on the chin, it was round the left nostril. I say, to have a test, I gave this brother of Miss — *Antimonium tart.*, which is also, as every one knows, apparently homoeopathic to such a pustular eruption. (XIX 31)

III. This is the brother of Miss ___. (*Observe. II.*)
The two eruptions were similar, though the boy's was comaparatively trivial, and of the same age, and from the same cause, *i.e.*, from the vaccine virus. The patients went into the country, and in two or three weeks' time the mother wrote that the young lady was quite well, "the medicine soon put her right" was her expression, but the boy had "a bad cold in his head; nose-bleed; left side of nose swelled and red; two little spots of matter, the size of a large pin's head, at the edge of the nostril, and below it, having something the look of —'s chin; his arm is also not well, and he has had four little pocks about the vaccination marks." I sent *Thuja* 30, and he was reported well in ten days.

If any one can account for the cure of these two cases independently of the *Thuja*, his ingenuity is greater than mine. That they were causally connected with re-vaccination admits of no doubt whatever. Nevertheless, it does not do to be quite sure of one's facts; sources of error are often occult. (XIX 34)

## 399. POST-ORBITAL NEURALGIA OF TWENTY YEARS' STANDING

This case (which came under observation on January 9*th*, 1882) is one of considerable interest on various accounts. Its subject, a lady of very high rank, over fifty years of age, had been in turns and for many years, under almost all the leading oculists of London for this neuralgia of the eyes, *i.e.*, terrible pain at the back of the eyes, coming on in paroxysms and confining her to her room for many days together; some attacks would last for six weeks. Some of the neuralgic pain, however, ramained at all times. Her eyes had been examined by almost every notable oculist in London, and no one could find anything wrong with them structurally, so it was unanimously agreed and declared to be *neuralgia of the fifth nerve*. Of course, no end of tonics, anodynes, and alternatives had been used. The oculists sent her to the physicians and these back again to the oculists. The late Dr. Quin and other leading homoeopaths had been tried, but "no one had ever touched it."

Latterly, and for years, she had tried nothing; whenever an attack came on, she would remain in her darkened bedroom, with her head tied up, bewailing her fate. To me she exclaimed, "My existence is one life-long crucifixion.!"

I should have stated that the neuralgia was preceded and accompanied by influenza. In the aggregate these attacks of influenza and post-orbital neuralgia confined her to her room nearly half the year. In appearance she was healthy, well-nourished, rather too much *embonpoint*, and fairly vigorous. A friend of her's had been benefited by homoeopathy in my hands, and she therefore came to me "in utter despair."

These are the simple facts of the case, though they look very like piling up the agony! Now for the remedy. The resources of allopathy had been exhausted, and, moreover, I have no confidence in them anyway; homoeopathy — and good homoeopathy too, for the men tried knew their work — had also failed. Do-nothing, now much in vogue, had fared no better. I reasoned thus : This lady tells me she has been vaccinated five or six times, and being thus very much vaccinated, she may be just suffering from chronic vaccinosis, one chief symptom of which is a cephalalgia like her's, so I forthwith prescribed *Thuja* 30. It cured, and the cure has lasted till now. The neuralgia disappeared slowly; in about six weeks (February 14, 1882) I wrote in my case book, "The eyes are well !"

As I have not heard from the patient for some time, I am just writing a note to her to know whether the neuralgia has thus far (December 30, 1882) returned. The reply I will add.

Of course, it does *not* follow that because *Thuja* cured this case of neuralgia of some twenty years' standing that *therefore* the lady was suffering from *vaccinosis*; that *Thuja* DID cure it is incontrovertible, and my vaccinosis hypothesis led me to prescribe it. More cannot be maintained. At least the case must stand as a clinical triumph for *Thuja* 30 — this much is absolute.

In reply to my inquiry, I received the following :

"Jan. 1, 1883.

. . . "I have been in very much stronger health ever since I crossed your threshold, and excepting one or two *attempts* at a return from the enemy, I have been quite free from suffering . . . "

The lady continues well of her post-orbital neuralgia at the time of going to press. After the disappearance of the neuralgia she had several other remedies from me for dyspeptic symptoms.

I shall probably never have a more severe case of what I conceive to be vaccinosis than the one just narrated, or one that had lasted longer. Twenty years may be considered enough to declare it *en permanence*, and its gradual cessation within six weeks from the time of commencing with the *Thuja*, stamps it as an undoubted drug-cure. (XIX 35)

## 400. CHRONIC HEADACHE OF NINE YEARS' DURATION

Miss G ___, aet. 19, came under my care on March 12, 1881, complaining of bad attacks of headache for the past nine years. She said it was as if the back of her head were in a vice, and then it would be frontal, and throbbing as if her head would burst. She was very pale, and her forehead looked shiny and in places brown.

These "head attacks" occurred once or twice a week.

Tendency to constipation; menses regular; and old sty visible on left eyelid; poor appetite; dislikes fleshmeat; liver enlarged a little; had a series of boils in the fall of 1880.

Feet cold; used to have chilblains. For years cannot ride in an omnibus, or in a cab, because of getting pale and sick; skin becomes rough in the wind; lips crack; gets fainty at times.

To have *Graphites* 30.
April 13th. — Appetite and spirits better, but otherwise no change; questioned as to the duration of the head attacks, she tells me the last but one continued for three weeks — the last, three days. Over the right eye there is a red, tender patch; *has two or three white-headed pustules* on her face.
Was vaccinated at three months, re-vaccinated at seven years, and again at fourteen. Had *small-pox about ten years ago.*
Thus here was a case that had had small-pox ten years ago, or thereabouts, for she could not quite fix the date, and had been vaccinated three times besides, once subsequent to the small-pox!
$R_x$ Tc. *Thuja occidentalis,* 3 iv. 3x.
To take five drops in water twice a day.
May 13th — Much better : has only had one very slight headache lasting an hour or two; the frontal tender patch is no longer tender; no further faintiness at all. Lips crack. The pustules in the face gone and skin quite clear.
To have *Thuja* 12, drop at bedtime.
June 17th — Was taken ill yesterday fortnight with soreness of stomach; fever; nausea and perspiration. Subsequently spots broke out like pimples — eight on the face, one each on the thumb and wrist, one on the foot, and two on the back, — they filled with matter, were out five days, became yellow, and then died away. Her mother says the symptoms were just the same as when patient had the small-pox. her headaches were well just before this bout came on.
July 1st — Continues well.
27th — The headahces have not returned.
Feb. 24th, 1882 — The cure holds good, for she has had no headache and is otherwise well. She had subsequently some other remedies for the little tumour on her eyelid and for a small exostosis on lower jaw, but she had received nothing but *Thuja* when the cephalagia disappeared, and it was two or three weeks before the next medicine followed.
Some months after this date this young lady was brought by her mother merely to shew me how well she was, and to take final leave of me; two years later I learned from her mother that she continued well, so the cure is permanent.
An interesting feature in this case is the curious attack which came on at the beginning of June. My reading of it is that it was really a proving of *Thuja,* or a general organismic reaction called forth by it; and this sent me often up to the thirtieth dilution in my subsequent use of *Thuja,* though I have occasionally found the third decimal dilution answer better than the thirtieth.

But this is not the point of my thesis, for this case was evidently cured by the low dilution, and when the low dilutions cure, and cure promptly, even though not very agreeably, but well, it cannot be necessary to go up any higher, especially as one's faith is suffciently on the stretch without it. (XIX 40)

## 401. ENLARGED GLANDS — APEX-CATARRH

Master C ___, aet. 11, came under my care on August 18th, 1881, complaining of a cough, worse at 7-30 P.M.; he also coughed by day and through the night, but it did not wake him. He perspired fearfully, worst on the head, and worse during the night. Over upper half of left lung one heard moist crackling rales. The cervical lymphatic glands at the top of the apex of left lung were indurated and distinctly "feelable." He weighed 5st. 4lbs. The vaccination scars were on the left arm, and the glands over the apex of right lung were indurated. Induration of the lymphatics on the left side of the neck the vaccination being performed on that side), is the rule after vaccination, as any one may observe for himself if he will take the trouble to examine *healthy* child just before vaccination and any time thereafter. I say : *any time thereafter*, for the thing generally persists for a very long time unless cured by medical art.

$R_x$ *Thuja* 30 M. ii. Sac. lac. q. s. Fiat. pulv. Tales. xxiv. One, three times a day.

Aug. 27th — Is well of cough, but the sweats continue. To take no medicine.

Sept. 6th — The most careful examination of chest reveals no rale; there is no cough; the sweats have quite ceased; the said cervical lymphatics can *not* be found. The boy now weighs 5 st. 8 lbs., so that he has gained 4 lbs. in weight since he got the *Thuja*.

Discharged cured.

The boy had been at school, and was sent home to his parents by the school physician on account of his obstinate cough, and because his general symptoms excited alarm. To me it appeared to be the first stage of phthisis. That the boy should increase in weight at home just after returning from school is, of course, not necessarily due to the medicine; home life, too, would improve his nutrition generally, and would perhaps also account for the disappearance of the apex-catarrh, cough, and perspirations. But what is to account for the disappearance of the induration of the cervical glands?

Of course, this case offers but little evidence of the existence of vaccinosis or of its cure by *Thuja*; so I will ask the reader to wade through yet a few more observations which I transcribe from my case books. For if there be such a disease as vaccinosis, in other words, if vaccination have any ill-effects beyond those commonly epitomized under the name vaccinia is clearly important that it should be recognised, and its existence being demonstrated. It is desirable that we know how to cure it. (XIX 45)

## 402. HAIRLESS PATCHES ON CHIN

Mr. __, a London merchant, came under my care on July 27th, 1882, to be treated for some roundish hairless patches on either side of his chin, which began four months ago. The larger patch on right side about the size of a florin. Had also an old hordeolum on his right lower eyelid.

Has been twice vaccinated; the second time twelve years ago; did not "take."

$R_x$ *Thuja occidentalis* 30 (4 in 24) To take one dry on the tongue at bedtime.

Sept. 7th — The bald patches are smaller, the one on the left side nearly gone. Has, apparently, a very bad coryza — ? — organismic reaction? *Rep.*

Oct. 17th — The bald patches are gone; the old hordeolum also gone. The closely-shaven beard is now uniform, the previously existing white bald patches being completely covered with hair.

I give this as an interesting cure by *Thuja,* but I am not very sure that the disease was really due to vaccinosis because of other points in his clinical history. Still it might have been so, as the hair is very powerfully influenced by the vaccine poisoning. Thus Kunkel observed both a very weak growth of hair, and an excessive growing, especially in wrong places, as effects, he believed of vaccination. Therefore let it stand as a doubtful case of vaccinosis for what it may be worth, — but there can hardly be any reasonable doubt as to the cure of the case by *Thuja.*

Here it might not be amiss to observe casually that the presence of sties on the eyelids is often, in my opinion a symptom of vaccinosis. This case is not without practical importance, inasmuch as hodiernal medicine hands over a sty to the chirugeon's art; and all the time, poor old dame, weens herself so very much superior to scientific therapeutics usually called homoeopathy. The conceit of the orthodoxly ignorant is truly sickening. (XIX 48)

### 403. HABITUAL INFLUENZAS, GENERAL ILL-HEALTH AND HEADACHE

Mr. ___, a city gentleman, came under my observation on December 28th, 1882, complaining that he was suffering from a series of neglected colds. He is costive; gets boils and pimples; has a number of warts, both flat and pedunculated; never had gonorrhoea; has severe frontal headache these three months; much pain across chest; and feels so out of health that he can no longer attend to his work, which is only light office work. He especially asks for a preventive for his frequent influenza colds. Flesh is flabby and skin spotted with pimples. The *habitual influenza*, the *chronic frontal headache*, the *pimply skin*, the *feeling of general melaise* point according to my experience, to vaccinosis. But had patient been vaccinated? Yes. Four times, and did *not* "take" the last *three* times. I do not expect many to agree with my theory that, when an individual is unsuccessfully vaccinated, he may have been seriously affected in his health by the reactionless vaccination, perhaps more so than as if it had "taken." But it is a *settled* point with me, and in these cases I find *Thuja* as promptly efficacious as in the ordinary forms of vaccinosis.

$R_x$ *Thuja occidentalis* 30 (4 in 24). One at bedtime and on rising.

January 10th, 1883 — Wonderful improvement already in the first week; the headaches gone (had had them three months); pain in chest gone; and the bowels are less costive. What a change in twelve days!

$R_x$ *Thuja occidentalis* 100, as before.

February 8th — Well; he complains of nothing, and merely calls to thank me.

This case made a considerable sensation in the gentleman's large office circle, partly because the change in his condition was so sudden and complete, and partly because he came to homoeopathy demonstratively unwillingly, and in consequence of the earnest solicitations of his *chef de bureau*. (XIX 50)

### 404. ACNE OF FACE AND NOSE AND NASAL DERMATITIS

A young lady, about twenty years of age, was brought by her mother to me on October 28th, 1882. Patient had a very red pimply nose — not like the red nose of the elderly bibber, or like that due to dyspepsia or to tightlacing — but a pimply, scaly nasal dermatitis, which extended from the cutaneous covering of the nose to that of the cheeks, but appearing here more as facial acne. The nasal dermatitis was, roughly, in the form of a saddle. Of course, this state of things in an otherwise pretty girl of twenty was painfully and humiliatingly unpleasant to her and to her friends; in fact it was likely to mar her future prospects very materially, more especially as it had already existed for six years, and was making no signs of departing. She also complained of obstinate constipation. The pimples of the nose and face used to get little white mattery heads. In trying to trace the skin-affection back to its real origin. I ascertained that the patient was revaccinated six years ago, but she could not remember whether the nose was previously affected or not. This re-vaccination was unsuccessful — *i.e.*, it did *not* "take."

$R_x$ *Thuja Occidentalis* 30 :

November 30th — Pimples of face decidedly better. Nose less red. Constipation no better.

$R_x$ *Thuja Occidentalis* 100 :

January 3rd, 1883 — The face is free. Her mother gratefully exclaims, "She is wonderfully better." I ask the young lady which powders did her *most* good; she says, "The *last*." The skin of the nose is normal, but the constipation is no better, and for this she remains under treatment. That *Thuja* cured this case is incontrovertible; but that it was a case of vaccinosis is not quite so certain, though it is far from improbable. The re-vaccination and inflammation of the skin of the nose were referred both to six years ago, when she was in Switzerland at school; but patient could not remember which was the first — the bad nose or the vaccination. (XIX 53)

## 405. NEURALGIA OF RIGHT EYE

Mr. ___, a gentleman of position and means, about fifty years of age, came to consult me on 28th June, 1882, for a neuralgia of the right eye. He had come in consequence of the cure of a similar case (Case 412).

He complained of almost constant pain in the right eye ever since Christmas 1881, *i.e.*, just about six months. Had had neuralgia in head and shoulders in 1866, and so much morphia had been injected in his shoulders by a doctor in Scotland that it almost killed him : for seven or eight hours it was doubtful if he would recover.

Has a brown, eczematous itchy (at night), eruption on both shins and between the toes. The neuralgia of right eye, and for which he comes to me, is bad both by day and night, but rather worse at night. Mr. (now Sir William) Bowman had examined the eye and declared it to be neuralgia, the eye being normal. Mr. White Cooper had done the same.

On my inquiring when he was last vaccinated, he seemed completely frightened, and stammered out rapidly. "I should not like to be vaccinated again."

"Why?"

"I was very seedy the last time. I was vaccinated — in fact I felt awfully ill for about a month;" and he again hurriedly protested that he would not like to be vaccinated again. The vaccination that had made him so ill was either in 1852 or 1853.

This seemed to me to be a case of vaccinial neuralgia, and therefore I ordered *Thuja* 30, in infrequent dose. This was on the 28th of June, 1882.

July 8th. — But very little pain after the first powder. To have the same medicine again.

The cure proved permanent, and is interesting as proof of the rapidity with which the *most like* remedy can cure a neuralgia. And, considering how "Awfully ill" he had been after his last vaccination, I think it rather probable that this case is an example of vaccinosis. (XIX 55)

## 406. DISEASED FINGER-NAILS

On December 22nd, 1882, a young lady of 26 came under my care for an ugly state of the nails of her fingers. Naturally a lady of her age would not be indifferent to the state of her nails. These nails are indented rather deeply, and in addition to these indentations there are black patches on the under surfaces of the nails, reaching into the quick. Very slight leucorrhoea occasionally. She had chicken-pox as a child of eleven. On her shoulders there is an eruption of roundish patches, forming mattery heads. Has been vaccinated three different times; the last time two years ago, and the nails have become diseased *since* this last vaccination. The black patches have existed these eighteen months.

Looking upon the diseased condition of the nails as evidence of chronic vaccinosis, I ordered her *Thuja* 30 (one in 6).

March 19th, 1883 — Has continued the *Thuja* 30 for just about three months, with the result that within a fortnight from commencing with it the black patches under the nails began to disappear, and there is now no trace of them. The indentations are notably better. The eruption on the back has not been modified, and for this she remains under treatment; but I thought this much of a case of nail disease would be of some interest, and the more so as it is not easy to demonstrate drug-action on nail-growth at all.

We will now go back to the head and the central nervous system. (XIX 58)

## 407. PTOSIS

A young lady of about 25 years of age came to me in May, 1881, telling me that she had had some tooth stumps extracted in November, 1880, whereafter there was haemorrhage for eight or nine hours. Two very able men in the homoeopathic ranks had treated her for some time with much benefit, but she still remained ill. *Conium* had been of greatest use. She still complained of ptosis of left side, sleeplessness; reeling to the right when walking out of doors, tendency to fall to the right. I gave her *Equisetum hyemale* (3 degree), because her tongue cracked. (Clinicians may note this valuable little wrinkle — i.e., cracked tongue — *Equisetum*, of which I first saw an account in the *Therapeutic Gazette.*) It was continued for months with very great benefit, and was followed by *Bellis per.*, and then by *Juglans regia*, etc. Then came *Avena sativa* Q, *Cadmium* 6 and 12, and *Psorinum* 30, and finally *Titanium* 30.

These more or less well-chosen remedies wrought a great change in the patient, but on the 29th July, 1882, she still complained that the left eye was wrong. It made her feel sea-sick when she read; pains in left eye, worse in the early morn; some ptosis of left upper lid; eyeball stiff, and an aching across it and right across the forehead, and she was giddy in walking about.

The case having thus come to a standstill. I cast about for some aetiologico-therapeutic *appui*, and in so doing, learned that she had been vaccinated four times in all; the last time, three years ago, took but faintly.

*Thuja* 30 soon cured the ptosis and the other described symptoms. (XIX 60)

## 408. PARESIS

Mr. —, a private gentleman, married, and one who had always led a healthful life, but too great a traveller, came under my observation early in the year 1882, in a very weak condition. He had had slight hemiplegia of the right side, and still shewed some symptoms of paralysis, *e.g.*, weakness of right arm, occasional dragging of the legs, loss of memory, impaired vision, and loss of power generally. His effective virility was extinct, and had been so for two or three years, and naturally this did not tend to raise his spirits. I treated him for a few months with but slight benefit. When one day he complained of a frontal headache that once reminded me of the *Thuja* headache. I gave him *Thuja occidentalis* 30 (4 in 24), and within a few days he remarked a very notable improvement, feeling better than he had for three years. Getting this report at his next visit, I fell to questioning him about vaccination, which I had previously not done : and what was the answer?

Feb. 24th, 1883 — "How many times have you been vaccinated?"

"I have been vaccinated six or seven times."

"Did it take every time?"

"No, never."

And from close questioning I satified myself that this gentleman had been *six* times *unsuccessfully* vaccinated, and this suggested to me that he was really suffering from that vaccinial blight which I have ventured to call vaccinosis.

Patient had received only four doses of the *Thuja* 30 in the early part of January, 1883, just to cure his headache, and which resulted, *inter alia*, in a hypopubic resurrection of great importance; and the headache having simultaneously left him, he then took the constitutional remedy I had prescribed, viz., *Titanium*, and continued it until a few days ago. I had instructed him to take the *Thuja* only for a few days, till his headache disappeared.

Now, thought I, we will saturate him with *Thuja*, and extinguish the vaccinosis; so I gave him this prescription :

$R_x$ Tc. *Thuja Occidentalis*, 3, 3 iv. To take four drops in water night and morning, and report in a month.

The result was quite satisfactory, and he became — in his wife's words — "quite a different man"; all paralytic symptoms having disappeared, and the old headache had not returned at the end of 1883, when I last saw him. (XIX 63)

## 409. SPINAL IRRITATION

Miss ___, aet 29, came under my care in November, 1882, complaining of owning a spine. She had been under the best physicians and surgeons of London. Had derived a little benefit from many — most, she thought, from the movement cure, under Mr. Roth, of Wimpole Street. She also alleged that mesmeric passes had eased her a good deal.

Her symptoms were legion; she was bent forward, could scarcely walk, her spine very tender and painful; twitchings; pain all down the back; and chilliness, worse at night. Her liver was decidedly enlarged, and there was pain in the right side. This hepatic disturbance was righted by *Chelidonium majus* 1; five drops, in water, twice a day. Then, on December 19th, I gave her *Cedron* 1, which certainly eased the cephalagia and chilliness a good deal, and it was therefore continued till.

February 9th, 1883 — When I went into her case a little more thoroughly as to its annamnesis. She had been vaccinated four times successfully; once it did *not* take.

R$_x$ *Thuja occidentalis* 30.

March 8th — Patient exclaimed . . . "that is capital stuff; I am *very* much better; my back is very much better; the coldness is gone; I am so much stronger altogether."

*Rep.*

March 31st — Back "wonderfully better."

She needed several other remedies, but practically her cure was effected by *Thuja*.

On May 17th she had *Thuja* 100, and soon afterwards began to play at lawn-tennis.

On June 12th she reported herself thus — "I have not been so well for three or four years; I feel strong, and can do anything."

I do not know whether anyone will admit that this was a case of vaccinosis; certain it is that she had been vaccinated five times, and was very ill — practically and invalid — till I gave her *Thuja*, and then she mended, and is now well and comparatively vigorous. (XIX 66)

## 410. SCRIVENER'S CRAMP; CEPHALALGIA, AND ENLARGED SPLEEN

Miss __, aet. 29, a city clerk, came under my observation on May 7th, 1883, complaining of much epigastric beating, pain in left side, great chilliness, and wrtiter's cramp of the right side. An examination shewed an enlargement of the spleen, and a swelling of the left ovary of about the size of a hen's egg. Her breath is heavy, and she gets *giddiness*. She has *frontal headache* of a severe kind, almost every day for a long time.

R$_x$ *Ceanothus Americanus*. 1. Five drops, in water, three times a day.

May 30th — Side is much better; the chilliness is better; the feet warmer; the beating less.

*Rep. et Cup. acet.* 1.

July 30th — Side nearly well; paining every alternate day or so. Pain in the back no better; giddiness better. Complains especially of the severe frontal headache, and the cramps in the right arm are so bad that she has had to give up office work.

Has been vaccinated three times, but the last time it did *not* take.

R$_x$ Tc. *Thuja Occidentalis* 30, night and morning.

August 16th — Headache and writer's cramp well. She returns to work.

November 16th — Continues at office work with comfort; no return of either headache or cramps. Continues under treatment for ovarian tumour and gets *Silicea* 6. (XIX 68)

## 411. ARRESTED DEVELOPMENT AND HEMIPARESIS

Miss __, aet. 16, was brought to me on May 16th, 1883. This was her state : roof of mouth very much arched; left side of face drawn to the left, so that her mouth is awry. She speaks very badly; cannot articulate properly; and is very deaf. Has always been so. Has a polypus in left nostril; the tonsils are enormously hypertrophied; breathes very loudly. Left mamma smaller than the right; left side of throax generally smaller than the right. Tongue is cracked; pain in left side for years; frontal headache for twelve months. Menses normal, having begun six months ago. She was vaccinated at the age of three months; it did not take and so she was done a second time in both arms, when it took fairly well.

Patient is the child of healthy parents, and there did not appear to be anything to account for the extraordinary backwardness. I reasoned that the child had evidently been blighted by the vaccination *for she did not readily take* (the organism resisted and then did take — organism overcome).

$R_x$ *Thuja Occidentalis* 30. Two drops daily, for four weeks.

Now note the sequel, not forgeting that the child's condition had been as described, *nearly all her life*.

June 13th — On this day her mother brought her and reported — this is the note in my case-book : "On the whole very much better; can certainly articulate better!! and the head and face are not so one-sided, and she hears better!!"

Both parents were agreed that the changes had been wrought since the medicine had been taken. The father is an unusually gifted professional man, and the mother an educated lady.

*Rep.*

July 11th — Headache well; side pain better; and the whole state is better. Considering the vaccinial blight removed. I gave *Ceanothus Americanus* 1, five drops, in water, night and morning, for two months. I gave this because the spleen was enlarged, *and I thought its specific influence on the left side generally* might be beneficial. I was not disappointed, but very much gratified to see that the left side of thorax began to *grow*, and also the left mamma. The little play of the imagination here as to the left-sidedness of the action of *Ceanothus* was fruitful.

September 7th — The increased dullness on percussion in the left hypochondrium having disappeared, and the left side having been manifestly bettered, and that considerably, I reverted to the *Thuja*, and this time gave it in the hundredth centesimal dilution.

October 7th — Under this date I read in my case-book — "Side remains well, but she seems to have suffered a good deal generally while taking the *Thuja* 100. She articulates *decidedly* better, speaks now so that I can understand her, and her hearing is greatly improved." She remains under treatment, and will receive other constitutional remedies, but the influence of the *Thuja* upon her has been most marked and remarkable. I have myself no doubt that the child's condition of hemiparesis arose from the vaccinial blight — *i.e.*, from *vaccinosis*, she being originally delicate, particularly her nervous system. (XIX 70)

## 412. NEURALGIA OF EYES OF NINE YEARS' STANDING

Miss ___, aet. 20, came to me on january 18th, 1883, with various ills. The constipation for which I treated her had been cured by *Nux* 30 and *Sulphur* 30, but the *fluor albus* was no better. "But the," said she, "there is the neuraliga in my eyes, which I have had for nine years — nothing has ever touched that." The neuralgia complained of was worse in the morning and at the menstrual period.

*Thuja* 30 (4 in 24). One at night.

I saw her no more till the 8th of December 1883, when she called, complaining of too frequent and too profuse emnstruation.

"What about the neuraligia?"

"Oh ! that is cured; I have not had it since those powders."

Was this a case of vaccinosis?

Patient had been twice vaccinated and the second time was when she was 15 years old, when it did *not take*. I do not feel so sure that this was a case of vaccinosis, because patient was re vaccinated unsuccessfully *after* this neuralgia began, and besides, her mother died of epithelioma, so it may have been merely a case of *sycosis Hahnemanni*. The only certain thing about it is that the neuralgia had lasted nine years, and disappeared after the giving of the *Thuja*. (XIX 74)

## 413. HEADACHE

On January 25th, 1884, I was requested to see a lady in a well-known London Square. She is a trifle over fifty, healthy looking, and enjoying good health except for her *headaches*. These headaches were the bane of her life as any extra exertion, worry, or work put her out and brought them on or exacerbated them. A few visitors at her house, her ordinary social duties a dinner, an evening at the theatre, a little meeting for benevolent purposes, an uncivil servant — each and all put her *hors de combat* with her headache. She had had them "every few days, and ever since she could remember, but greatly increased in severity during the past three years." She did not expect to be cured; "at my age, and after

so many years," said this lady. Moreover, she did *not* believe in homoeopathy, "no, not in the least, but I have tried all the best doctors and they have failed, and hearing from Lady —, that you were specially good at headaches, I determined to send for you."
"Vaccinated?" "Oh ! yes, five or six times; has not taken for years; do you think I had better be done again?"
*Thuja occidentalis* 30.
On Feb. 9th I called. — "Oh, I am better, I have only had one headache — two days after I began with your powders — and I am very much less nervous." To continue the medicine.
March 2nd. — "I have not had any headache at all, though I have been doing just the very things that always bring them on. I have the greatest confidence in homoeopathy." (XIX 77)

## 414. RINGWORM

Said a very well-known homoeopathic practitioner to me in a letter at the beginning of the year. "I have been giving a little girl suffering from ringworm your treatment by *Bacillinum*, but it's no good.
"Have you gone on with it steadily, in infrequent doses, and for several months?"
"Yes, I have, and I tell you it gets no better."
The little child was brought to me, when I found the usual manifestations of rignworm, viz., large patches, originally circular but now covered with scabs. I further ascertained that this child had been under the local homoeopathic chemist before coming to the practitioner, who had given *Bacillinum* a three months' trial.
Any phthisic taint in her?
Both her maternal grandparents died of phthisis.
Here it seemed to me that vaccinosis barred the way. Simple ringworm does not become pustular and encaked with mattery scabs as in this case. Vaccinosis is a filthy pustular art disease that is put into the blood by force. I therefore put the little forty-four month old maiden on *Thuja* 30, when great scabs were still seen on the scalp, but they were drier.
Then after two months under *Bacillinum* 30 (in infrequent doses), the scabs had all fallen off, and the circular patches were covered with young hair. Said her mother, "Oh, she is so much better in every way, and her hair is growing so much that I really hardly know what to do with it."
After another two months of treatment by *Bacillinum* 30, the cure was complete.

And here we see that my colleague, who condemned my views in regard to ringworm, and claimed that they would not hold water, was mistaken in that *Bacillinum* is not homoeopathic to vaccinosis but to ringworm, only — *the vaccinosis barred the way, and when this was removed by Thuja, the tuberculosic mycosis yielded to Bacillinum.* (XIX 80)

# CURABILITY OF TUMOURS

## 415 ABDOMINAL TUMOUR

On November 17th, 1887, I was requested to see a gentleman resident in London who was said to have a very large tumour in the abdomen, and no efforts to cure it had been spared, but they were quite unavailing. As six medical men — including the consulting surgeon and the consulting physician at Guy's Hospital — had seen him and done their best to no purpose, I did not much care to go as a seventh medical man, merely to say ditto to the dictum of the other six. There seemed no chance of a cure, and an operation had been declared to be impossible, evidently because of the position and size of the tumour, and its probable adhesions to adjacent parts and organs. The tumour presumably had its origin in a fall, then eight years ago, on the left side, which fractured the ribs; that is to say, the side had never been comfortable since and for many months this large mass had been growing larger and larger, at first incommoding locomotion and finally rendering it impossible. Patient was not only bedridden, but was not even able to turn over in bed, partly from weakness and partly because of the bulking mass. And patient being a long way past sixty years of age did not make the prospect any brighter.

However, two days later, I did go to see the patient, and found a slender-built man crouched up on his back and a little to the right. As he could not turn over himself his wife and I had to aid him for the purposes of a proper physical examination, which disclosed a huge mass in his left side almost from the nipple to the pelvic rim. There were brown patches on the skin of the abdomen, and inside of the left Poupart's ligament were a number of lumps to be felt like little potatoes, presumably indurated and hypertrophied lymphatic glands. Add to this a quite cachectic look and rather severe adynamia, and the picture of hopeless malignant disease is complete.

I made close enquiry as to the opinions of my six doctorial predecessors in regard to the seat of origin of the tumour, and found that their two family advisers (the same firm) had always held it be connected with the left kidney. And, when they failed to do it any good they called in a physician of repute who thought it could be cured, but when his efforts had also failed a good surgeon was called and he thought it quite incurable. Then came a consulting physician and surgeon respectively from Guy's and the final outcome of all the deliberations was that it was cancer, or at any rate a tumour connected with the spleen which was or had become malignant in its nature, and that the result must necessarily be fatal; a mere matter of time, in fact. The most careful examination did not enable me to say whether it was connected with spleen or kidney or with both : the tumour practically occupied the left half of the abdomen, and,not considering its history, was apparently connected with the spleen. Was there *any* chance of cure? There had been quite enough diagnosing from the stand-point of mere diagnostics, but I found the medicinal treatment had been confined to general tonic and quasi-absorbent measures, probably quinine, iron, mercury, and certainly iodine.

I think any practical physician or surgeon will concede that a more hopeless case to *cure* by medicines is hardly to be found.

To begin with, how are we to choose medicines for such a case allopathically, homoeopathically, or anyhow?

My own plan in difficult cases that seem so hopeless is to lay firmly hold of *some point* that may serve as a reasonable therapeutic starting point whence to carry out a cure.

As a start there is here the traumatic element in the case, that is positive, and my own favourite and well-tried anti-traumatic is *Bellis perennis*; then the proving of this drug, communicated by myself, shews a decided affinity for the left hypochondrium, and finally *Bellis* has already in my hands cured a few tumours.

This plan in the face of desperate odds, to lay hold of any help-promising remedy, is at least a stay for further reflection. *Bellis perennis* as an anti-traumatic and also *Ceanothus Americanus* as a splenic presented themselves to my mind, but which? Candidly confessed I thought the good man doomed, but determined to *try* and save him, and not knowing which of my two remedies was the more likely to do something *quickly* (for the case was urgent — patient's friends had already taken a last look at him as they thought). I gave the two in alternation, and much did I subsequently regret this double shot, for the use of two medicines at one time teaches next to nothing. However *Bellis* Q and *Ceanothus* 1x were given in five drop doses every four hours in alternation; this was on Nov. 12th, 1887, I find, and not the 17th, which was the date of my second visit.

The result of this medication was that after a while patient could turn over in bed, then he could get in and out of bed by himself, and in 17 days from beginning the medicine, viz : on Nov. 29th, patient came to my Westend rooms in a cab with his wife.

The effects of the medicines were great diminution in the swelling (patient had lost much flesh and was still losing flesh) the passage of vast quantities of urine — "it literally pours from me." The skin of the palms of his hands is black but the lines strikingly white in contrast. And the tumour itself was not only much smaller, but more defined. But patient's weakness was terrible; evidently his coming to me was partly ***bravour*** and more an effort of will than real physical power, I therefore stopped the two remedies and gave *Nux-v.* 1x and *Calc. hypophos.* 3x as an indicated all-round pick-me-up.

Dec. 16th — He is much stronger; can walk upstairs, but his tumour is not quite so well. The skin of his hands, etc., is peeling off. Urine sp. gr. 15, containing mucus and phosphates in great quantities.

Repeat first prescription.

16th — He is still getting thinner but he is stronger; tongue very much coated; has to strain much at stool; eats well; he has walked here from the end of the street. Has a cold on the chest and cough, and this shakes him and hurts his side very much.

$R_x$ *Bryonia alb.* 1x and *Phos.* 3x in alternation.

27th — The cough is worse on going to bed and seems to be a spleen-cough.

$R_x$ *Scilla maritima Q* — Five drops in water three times a day.

He did not need any subsequent treatment and he came to say goodbye on Jan. 24th, 1888 — He had lost the tumour and the enlargement and induration of the lymphatic in the left side, and he was rapidly gaining flesh and strength.

All things considered, it was clearly a tumour of the spleen, and I am disposed to think the lymphatics were irritated to enlargement either by the iodic and other irritant topics that had been applied, or else by the pressure of the tumour.

Still, the entire case remains a little puzzling, and others being in possession of its main features can judge as well as myself. At least it teaches — ***nil desperandum*** !

The cure was complete and permanent, which I know, patient turns up in my rooms every few months for his own and my satisfaction. Such a case is an oasis in the desert of a physician's hard life. (XX 100)

## 416. TUMOUR IN THE THROAT

A married lady of fifty-four came on the eighth of August, 1883, to consult me about a lump in her throat. In the left side of the top of the neck here was a hard body about the size of a hen's egg, but flatter. The tumour had been there for a very long time, and with it she had had much throat irritation. It was situated to the left and behind the larynx, but whether actually connected with the oesophagus or larynx I could never quite satisfy myself. It moved up and down with the act of deglutition.

$R_x$ Trit. 3x *Sul. iod.*, 3iv., gr. vj. ter die.

August 22nd — No change.

$R_x$ *Psor.* 30.

October 5th — The throat — *i.e.*, the fulness, uneasiness, pain and distress in the throat — is very much better, and the tumour has sensibly diminished in size.

$R_x$ *Thuja occid.* 30.

Nov. 1st. — The tumour is about half gone.

$R_x$ *Psor.* 30.

29th — The tumour about two-thirds gone; general health good.

$R_x$ *Thuja* 30.

Dec. 21st — There is some tickling in the throat. The tumour is larger again, and the patient feels choky.

$R_x$ *Psor.* 30.

January 14th, 1884 — The tumour has again sensibly diminished in size.

$R_x$ *Psor.-c.*

Feb. 8th — Tumour still swollen.

$R_x$ *Merc. viv.* 5.

March 3 — "I feel the lump very much less, about half its original size," said the lady. She has much rheumatism in ankles and knees.

$R_x$ *Silicea* 6 trit., in frequently repeated doses.

31st — Has been visiting a friend suffering from consumption, and since then has spit a little blood-streaked phlegm; has a good deal of tickling in the throat.

$R_x$ *Psor.* 30.

April 16th — No coloured expectoration for a week, and then very trifling : the tickling in the throat is better, but the throat feels very rough. The tumour is rather smaller.

$R_x$ *Sul. iod.* 3x six grains three times a day.

30th — No coloured expectoration for the past week; the tickling in the throat is very much better, but talking brings it on. The tumour has lately not altered sensibly in size, but it is more self-contained and one can now demonstrate that it is not connected with the larynx, being the areolar tissue behind and to its left. Has a good deal of rheumatism.

$R_x$ Tc. *Cundurango* 1, 3iv. Five drops in water three times a day.

May 21st — Thinks it is not so well; the tickling sensation in the throat is worse. Feels the spring. The throat is worse in the morning and when tired.

$R_x$ *Thuja* 30.

June 16th — Throat rather better; has only had the coloured expectoration once, but the voice is hoarse, and she feels her throat weak. Has rheumatism in ankles and knees worse after motion. The tumour is a trifle smaller.

$R_x$ *Urea* 6.

July 11th — More blood-coloured expectoration. Has had all the symptoms of a cold : aching all over with tingling and feeling giddy and ill; aphonia; much tenderness in the neck; rheumatism better; urine *thick* (unusual); violent tickling in the throat with scraping; and dryness; *the tumour is nearly gone.*

The throat symptoms are worse night and morning, and when she is tried.

$R_x$ Tc. *Phytolacca decandra* 1, Ziv., gtt. v., n. m.

August 6th — Better in every way; the tumour is barely to be found.

$R_x$ *Rep.*

Sept. 3rd — Feels practically well. I can find the small remains of the tumour only with great difficulty.

$R_x$ *Rep.* (at night only.)

Nov. 13th — Still a little uneasiness in the throat.

$R_x$ Trit. 3x *Sul. iod.*

28th — Nearly well.

$R_x$ *Rep.*

Dec. 31st — The tumour cannot be found, but she still complains of a husky voice.

$R_x$ Trit. 4. *Kali brom.*

I did not see the patient again for some months, as the tumour had quite disappeared, and she herself felt quite well, but she came to me again on.

April 10th, 1880 — Complaining of tickling and irritation in the old spot.

$R_x$ *Psor.* C.

May 11th — She feels easier in the throat, but the tumour is returning.

$R_x$ Trit. 3x *Sul. iod.*

Nov. 25th — The lump is still increasing.

$R_x$ *Psor-c.*

This lady came again on February 15th, 1886, and for the last time on the 30th April, 1886, when I discharged her cured. I see her son occasionally on his own account, and thus know that she continues quite well, and has a very healthy general appearance.

February 23rd, 1892 — I happened to see this lady to-day and am glad to say she continues quite well.

*It is no use to urge against the medicinal cure of tumours that so many remedies are often needful : if one remedy will not cure, we must use as many as will and no fewer; such is our art... difficult and too often complex ...* (XX 114)

## 417. WARTY GROWTH IN MOUTH

An officer in the army brought his twelve year-old daughter to me on the thirteenth of November, 1886, telling me that she had something growing in her mouth. A similar growth had come a year ago, when his family surgeon excised it; in six months from the time of the operation it had grown again, making it difficult for the child to eat her food, as it caught the tongue and teeth, and then bled. This time the doctor ligatured it off thoroughly, leaving a hole, and informed the father that this time he hoped its roots were got rid of. Now, it had grown again at the side of the said hole.

On examining the mouth I find in its left side, just to the left of the *fraenulum linguae*, a warty fleshy excrescence, of the shape of a cock's comb, about a quarter of an inch broad at its base, and nearly a quarter of an inch high. Patient has normal teeth : the tongue is coated, and she is very pale. I ordered *Thuja occidentalis* 30 internally in infrequent dose, and a mouth wash of *Thuja* Q, two drops in a dessert spoonful of water night and morning; to keep it bathing the growth as long as possible, and then expectorate.

As this brought the growth down to the size of a pea, treatment was discontinued, but she then bit it on three successive occasions, whereupon it again took to growing, and in January, 1887, when I saw it, it was about as big as a horse bean. This time I ordered *Sabina*, just as I had previously ordered *Thuja*. Under the *Sabina* patient took on a healthy look but a small piece of the growth still persisted, when I ordered *Cupressus Lawsoniana* in like manner as the *Thuja* and *Sabina* had been used. That was in March, 1887, and I did not see her again. But I met her father in October on another matter, when I enquired about the case, and he replied, "Oh, she is quite well; the lump has been gone a long time, but the hole is still there."

So, if you ever get a little cock's comb growth in your mouth, take my advice and have it treated homoeopathically, for it is, as you see, much better than either excision or ligature, and you will thereafter have no "hole" to mark the *locus in quo*.

Any one who is acquainted with the literature of sycosis will not expect me to enter upon so vast a subject here; those who are not are recommended to study it in the writings of Hahnemann, Boenninghausen, Wolf, H. Goullon, and Grauvogl. As, however, I am, so far as I am aware, the first and still the only practitioner to use *Cupressus Lawsoniana,* I may be permitted just to state that I base my use of it upon a fragmentary proving made by myself with the berries and leaves, and from which I conclude that it acts very like *Thuja;* I could not go on with my proving because of the terrible pains it caused in the stomach. I shall refer to it again.

Finally, it might be asked : Why did you not stick to the *Thuja* rather than follow it up with *Sabina,* and then with *Cupressus*? Because *I have found from practical experience that ringing the changes on like-acting remedies conduces more quickly to a cure than going on with the same.* (XX 122)

## 418. CYST OF RIGHT UPPER EYELID

A married lady just under 30 got a swelling in her right upper eyelid in the spring of 1887 and called in the 'homoeopathic' adviser of the family, taking herself, in the meantime, *Pulsatilla* with transitory benefit. This gentleman informed the lady that medicines could *not* cure it, and he advised its removal by operation, which was declined. This family — like many others — are divided in their medical views and proclivities, some being allopathically and some homoeopathically inclined. When their usual 'allopathic' adviser "happened to call to see papa" his advice was also sought as to the possibility of curing the tumour with medicines, and he said, "No! It is quite impossible to cure it with medicines; it is only a little cyst and must be cut out."

The lady had formerly been a patient of mine for enlargement of the left ovary which medicines had cured. Hence she returned to me to see if medicines would cure the little lump on the eyelid — about the size of a pea — wherein she was not disappointed. *Platanus occidentalis* Q was the remedy that cured it.

(Q Gtt. v. nocte maneque.)

I did not mean to give empiric cases of this kind, and I mention this one merely as a further protest against the self-sufficiency of medical ignorance — our grand medical art not even able to cure a little cyst as big as a pea! But this case, though cured empirically, will serve to introduce another new remedy — *Platanus occidentalis* that thrives so beautifully in our London streets. I have found it a remedy of some value in psoriasis and in cystic formations arising from occlusions of the mouths of the outlets of ducts and glands. Whether it has ever before been used in medicine I do not know : I was led to use it purely *ex-hypothesi* and may have more to say about it another time. Here it is mentioned parenthetically and by the way. Certainly it acts upon epithelial structures, and notably on the outlets of the little glands of the skin.

As only one remedy was used the case is proof-affording that at least a little cyst can be removed gently, medicinally *cured in fact*, in the sense of John Hunter.

How do I know that the cure is a Hunterian one?

Five years have elapsed since the little cystoma was cured and there has been no return, and patient continues otherwise in good health. (XX 130)

## 419. OVARIAN TUMOUR

A clergyman's wife, thirty-one years of age, mother of seven children, came to me on May 13th, 1886, for treatment for a tumour within the abdomen. The lady's husband had accompanied their family doctor with her to an eminent gynecological specialist, who had pronounced the tumour a cyst, and both family doctors and the gynecologist had strongly urged an immediate operation.

Of the children born, the most of them were cross births and one was still-born. The baby was two years old. No genesiac fraud.

Patient suffers badly from leucorrhoea for years; she menstruates now every ten days or so; dysmenorrhoea; dreadul dysuria; frequent and most difficult micturition; palpitation of the heart on the least exertion; peculiar tingling sensation down the left side and hand; spleen very notably enlarged; patient often goes faint; fearfully constipated; twice vaccinated; she is always cold; feet and hands go dead white; all her pains are worse at night. On examination I find a tumour of the left ovary of the size of my fist.

Patient was treated with great care and perseverance till September 29th, 1887, when she was discharged cured.

She had a number of remedies, amongst which I will name *Aconitum, Bryonia, Sulphur, Nux vomica, Bovista* and several nosodes. But the remedies that were evidently, obviously, and promptly curative were *Bovista* 3x and *Aurum mur. nat.* 3x.

When I last saw the lady in September no trace of the tumour could be found.

April 25th, 1888. — On this day I again very carefully examined the lady but could find no trace of any tumour whatsoever.

I should add that as a necessary part of the treatment all marital rights and privileges were temporarily prohibited; this is important.

Beginning of 1889. — I again examined the lady but could find no tumour.

January 30th, 1890. — Saw the lady's husband and learned that she continues well.

February, 1892. — Patient brought her daughters to see me. She continues quite well.

April, 1898. — Still quite well. (XX 134)

## 420. ABDOMINAL TUMOUR

A married lady of 40, mother of five children, came to me on August 9th, 1886, for an abdominal tumour situated deep in behind the bowels on a level with the navel. She had been under many able men who had made various diagnostic guesses which, however, did not lessen the tumour, which was the size of a small baby's head : my own diagnosis was retroperitoneal fibroid, which I judged it to be from its position and hardness, and possibly connected with the pancreas or circumpancreatic areolar tissue.

The most distressing symptom of the case was the severe vomiting — at times so bad that she had to keep her couch for weeks together. Patient had not had much to complain of in her 40 years' career beyond severe confinements and occipital neuralgia.

She had not suckled her children. Had been, she said, six times vaccinated, the last three times unsuccessfully. She suffered very much from whites and dysmenorrhoea.

$R_x$ *Thuja.*

September 3rd — Menses much less painful; whites better; has only had one night of vomiting; she is very fond of salt and takes a great deal of it.

$R_x$ *Hecla Montis lava* 3 trit. in eight-grain doses.

October 8th — Whites much better, as also the last menstruation; much neuralgia at the back of eyes, most towards evening. No vomiting, tumour decidedly smaller.

*Psor.* 30 in infrequent doses.

November 22nd — Whites continue better, also the menses; neuralgia nearly gone; much dyspepsia. Tumour about the same.

$R_x$ *Thuja occ.* 30 in infrequent doses.

December 6th — Cannot go on with the powders on account of the dyspepsia; all food gives pain within five minutes, only comfortable when the stomach is quite empty; no neuralgia; whites not quite well; percussion shews the tumour to be very much smaller, but she has a

good deal of backache.
$R_x$ Tc. *Cundurango* 1. Five drops in water three times a day.
January 17th, 1887 — Did her a vast amount of good, notably for her indigestion; whites still continue; backache better, and has felt wonderfully strong and well, though she vomited a good deal last Wednesday. Menses normal; tumour, perhaps, a trifle smaller.
Patient had some nosodes, *Silicea* 6, *Thuja* 30 and then again *Cundurango* 1, and was discharged quite cured on November 21st, 1887; no vestige of tumour left.
I saw patient's sister on April 17th, 1888, and learned that the cure was permanent. Nearly a year later I met the lady at an evening party and during the music in the drawing room she told me — what her looks certainly confirmed — that she continued quite well.
January, 1890 — Continues well. (XX 137)

## 421. TUMOUR IN UTERINE REGION

An unmarried woman, thirty-seven years of age, came to me on August 3rd, 1885, complaining of a swelling in the lower part of her abdomen, and which had been there for some years. It appeared to me to be seated in the broad ligament of the left side near to the uterus. It was hard and about the size of a baby's head. She complained of dreadful pains in the uterus and its region. Seven months before she had a fall from a chair, from which time on the pain had been very severe. For the past two years sensation of *pins and needles* in the hands and arms *on awaking* in the night and *towards morning*.
Patient is a faithful old servant of the parents of the mistress of the woman whose case is narrated in "Tumours of the Breast," and she comes to me in consequence thereof. Her master had lately died, and she had lifted him a great deal during his last illness.
$R_x$ *Med.* C. Six in twenty-four, one at bedtime.
Sept. Ist. — Feels much better; the sensation of formication much less; the tumour is clearly a mural fibroid. Less pain in the uterus.
$R_x$ *Med.* C. 1b.
Oct. 1st — The formication has entirely gone and she declares herself wonderfully better.
$R_x$ Tc. *Bellis per.* 1. Five drops in water night and morning.
Nov. 5th — The tumour is a trifle smaller; gets a pain in it after she has been in bed a few minutes.
$R_x$ *Syph.* CC. Six in twenty-four, one dry on the tongue at bedtime.
Dec. 3rd — The pain is gone, but has the pins and needles on awaking again. The tumour is smaller.

$R_x$ *Med.* CC.
January 12th, 1886 — Pins and needles gone; hands are still numb; no pain; the uterus feels now through the abdominal parietes like one about three months' gravid. There is not, and never has been, any leucorrhoea.
$R_x$ Trit. 6, *Lapis alb.* (Grauvogl's) gr. vj. n. m.
February 16th — Better all round; menses normal; tumour undoubtedly smaller.
Rep.
March 16th — Getting on very well she says. The uterus can be ballooned about just under the umbilicus, and is still tumid.
April 15th — Better; no numbness; no pain; very much smaller; now there is some leucorrhoea.
Rep.
May 20th — Better; no leucorrhoea; no pain; no formication; she feels well, no tumour can be found, and the womb is no longer to be felt or found (as heretofore) through the abdominal parietes.
Rep., but only one six-grain powder at bedtime.
July 6th — "I am getting on very well, thank God." — The tumour has left no trace of itself. Everything normal.
Rep.
Sep. 6th — Well; and long there-after her mistress informed me that patient continued quite well; and, oddly enough, also grateful.
I shall here interpolate the observation that the nosodes are remedies of which I shall hope to treat on a future occasion. I am here treating of the amenability of tumours to remedies, and in the great field of medicine it is much better to take one thing at a time. Any well read homoeopathic practitioner will see probably indications for them in Lux, Gross, Hering, Swan, Berridge, Skinner, and others, notably in the pages of the "Homoeopathic Physician" and of the "North American Journal of Homoeopathy." Whether they are chosen on the isopathic principle of Lux, according to the law of similars, or otherwise, I will not here discuss. (XX 141)

## 422. TUMOUR OF LEFT OVARY

**A Complex Case** — A married lady placed herself under my care on May 26th, 1882, for a tumour of the parts for whose cure she had been advised an operation. She was in a state of great nerve exhaustion, very largely, I think, from observing the course of the case of a friend of hers, who had been operated on for a similar affection and who had undergone great suffering. Patient was at this date thirty-five years of age; had

had two children; was much emaciated, and had a very dusky skin. Her sufferings were extreme, being much intensified by the assiduous marital claims made upon her.

Patient's face was much disfigured with very numerous pimples — large angry inflamed follicles, some as large as peas; she had thus suffered, she said, for six years.

A month before her last baby was born, twelve years before, she was occupied "pettering about" in her green-house, and had uterine haemorrhage.

Uterus very much enlarged : so much so that it appears as a hard ridge above the pubes, and three or four times a week patient has much yellow mattery discharge from the vagina. Burning pain in the rectum and in the tumour, extending at times all over the left side of the abdomen; worse at night. The burning pain and bearing down on micturating, she describes as dreadful; and the womb is the seat of a burning so intense that she says is as if she were on fire. Menses regular but painful at first. She has been vaccinated three times; has used very many vaginal injections. Cannot stand erect.

Liver is painful, and she suffers much from dyspepsia.

$R_x$ *Thuja occidentalis* 30.

June 18th — Less leucorrhoea; she can now stand up straight; the skin of the left side of the abdomen is much darker than that of the right.

$R_x$ *Viscum album* 30.

July 3rd — Very great amelioration of the facial acne, but the pain in the ovarian tumour is dreadful, and hot and burning; worse at night; she complains of constant thirst.

$R_x$ *Arsenicum album* 30.

19th — Is always thirsty; the pain in the tumour is very bad, "burning worse at night."

$R_x$ *Aurum metallicum* 4 trit.

August 31st — There was some improvement (in the pain) at first, but she has gone back, except that the skin of the face continues better, the uterus is rather smaller, and the tumour is more defined.

$R_x$ *Mer. cor.* C.

September 29th — Pain in side decidedly better, but she caught a cold and had a bad cough, the severe dragging from which brought the pain back, though in a less degree. She can now stand up straight and walk about with comparative comfort. Face much improved. The cough is very distressing.

$R_x$ *Dulcamara* Ix.

November 9th — Still some cough that she thinks comes up from the stomach. The tumour is smaller. The cough shakes her a good deal.

$R_x$ *Lycopod.* 4 trit.

24th — The side-pain is worse, in fact, unbearable.

*Que faire?* Fall back on Hypodermic injections, and so get at any rate some temporary relief from pain? No. I *know* that road leads to the bad. *Magis venenum magis remedium* must be true, or there is no science in therapeutics worth the having, and again *aux grands maux les grands remedes*. Finally the dusky coloration, the nocturnal exacerbation, the temporary yielding to *Merc.*

$R_x$ *Syph.* CC.

December 20th — The face is vastly improved; pain in the side better; is getting much fatter, particularly in arms and breasts, and she now weighs 8st. 11lbs. Less discharge.

$R_x$ Trit. 6 *Kali chlor.*

January 24th, 1883 — Pain in the side worse; worse by night; tumour smaller, less discharge, which is now pale yellow.

March 1st — After taking the last mentioned remedy the pain was better, and then I gave *Kali chlor.* again, as the tumour had previously diminished under its use. The burning pain has again returned; she feels sick and is thirsty.

$R_x$ *Syph.* CC.

May 9th — The discharge is *much* diminished; the tumour, though smaller than formerly, is still very evident and very painful, particularly at night.

$R_x$ *Bovista* 3x trit.

June — No change.

$R_x$ Trit. 4 *Lapis alb.*

July 23rd — The pain in the tumour is dreadful.

$R_x$ *Syph.* CC.

August 24th — There is still a good deal of pain, worse at night, but the discharge is less.

$R_x$ *Tinct. Ceanothus Americanus.* Five drops in water three times a day.

October 20th — Better altogether; less discharge; not nearly so distended.

$R_x$ *Merc. mel.* 4.

And one of my reasons for giving this was because I had observed in several cases, that patients taking it in moderate triturations (2—6) have put on a good deal of flesh.

November 21st — Patient has fattened considerably on this prescription, and now weighs nine stone one pound. To continue the same remedy, but in fifth trituration.

January 16th, 1884.

$R_x$ *Tarentula Cubensis* 30.

February 4th — Seems to have set up violent inflammatory symptoms in the tumour.

$R_x$ *Liquor. Sodae chlor.* Two drops in water twice a day.

February 25th — The pain at night is dreadful; the discharge is much worse, but the tumour is much smaller.

$R_x$ *Variolinum* 30.

March 28th — The leucorrhoea is very bad and contains some blood; face is much better.

$R_x$ *Liquor. Sod. Chlor.* in 2-drop doses.

May 12th— Face quite clear; she is very much better, and the tumour has gone down a good deal.

$R_x$ *Merc. Met.* 6 trit.

June 11th — The skin of face is now normal; but there is still a good deal of burning in the swelling, which, however, is again much smaller.

$R_x$ *Thuja* 30.

August 11th — Considering herself quite well, she stayed away last month, and comes now because there are a few more pimples and some pain.

$R_x$ *Liquor. Sod. Chlor.*

January 11th. 1885 — Being so much better, has become irregular in attendance, but since last August she has had *Variolinum* from me with much advantage. The tumour has quite disappeared, and she now comes for a cough.

$R_x$ Tc. *Causticum* 6.

February 9th — Cough gone; now the side pains again, and feels raw; on very close examination, one still finds a rest of the old tumour at its lowest part near the groin.

$R_x$ *Syph.* CC.

March 6th — Wheezy; cough worse in the evening.

$R_x$ *Psor.* CC.

June 12th — The cough went away, and patient has also stayed away till now. The left ovary still troubles her, and the pain is very bad again, and is now *worse after sleep*. When she urinates she passes stringy whites.

$R_x$ *Med.* 30.

July 17th — Has hay-fever (never had it before, she avers); much sneezing; gets an hour of sneezing on rising, and washing brings it on. She is very much better in the hypogastric region, the after-sleep pain particularly.

$R_x$ *Rep.* (C.)

October 19th — The symptoms of hay-fever still persist.

$R_x$ *Psor.* C.

November 14th — Comes for a loud, noisy cough, beginning at 4 A.M., with severe sneezing fit.

$R_x$ *Osmium* 6.

February 12th, 1886 — Cough soon went away after beginning with the *Osmium*.

Patient has called upon me a few times since this day, for colds and pains in the side, but these yielded to treatment of precisely the same nature as already described, and she has had no return of the tumour, and the womb has long since returned to its normal size.

Middle of 1890 — Saw patient, and learned that she continued well.

August, 1892 — Patient continues well and I can find no trace of tumour. She came at this date to me for "flushes" and at my request allowed me to examine for the long-treated and finally-cured tumour. Thus it will be seen that my observation of this case extends over ten years and three months.

Of course, a case of tumour that takes four years to cure, and needs a number of remedies to effect that cure, is, particularly to the uninitiated, of no great interest unless the subject is thought out somewhat, but if this be done, it becomes more and more interesting to the student, and the more interesting the more he knows of drugs, drug-action, the phases and causations of disease and of doctrinal pharmacology. A difficult game of chess can only be understood by one who knows chess well, and only a man well grounded in the science can appreciate a finely played game; to the man who cannot play chess, the grandest game ever played means ... nothing.

To the majority of medical men the just narrated case will mean no more than just this : "Oh, he had a case of tumour; the patient stuck to him. He gave her a lot of different medicines, and after a long time the tumour had disappeared." For all that, the truly competent will see that the game was not only won but at the same time was well-played — and the cure is a Hunterian one, for patient remains well.

I dwell thus on these points not vain - gloriously, but to make it quite clear to those who will sit in judgement on my tumour-curing with medicines, that unless they understand the subject, their opinion of my work is worthless, though they may be doctors of medicines, masters in surgery, licentiates in midwifery and editors of journals : if they cannot play the game they are no judges; if they can they will be delighted in studying the points of a good game well won.

The analogy between the cure of a complex case like this, by divers and diverse remedies, and playing a difficult complicated game of chess is not so very far-fetched, and enables the mind to grasp the mode of procedure.

I always feel that unless we can use a series of remedies in very difficult complex cases, such cases will remain forever uncured or, as people usually say, incurable. And the complaint raised against "using so many medicines in a case" is really on a par with a complaint against a difficult game of skill such as chess that it "takes so many moves to win."

No doubt some of my cases might have been got well much more quickly, but it must be remembered that I was then treading an almost unknown way; the same case now would, I imagine, not take me half the time; but in this I may be wrong. (XX 146)

## 123. UTERINE FIBROID : CHRONIC OOPHORITIS

An unmarried lady, forty-five years of age, came under my observation on February 11th, 1882, suffering, as a gynaecologist and several other doctors had told her, from a fibrous tumour of the womb. Her general appearance was that of a lady at about the sixth month of pregnancy. She had been dissuaded from an operation by two medical men of good repute. Father and brother had died of consumption. Her irides are blue with dark rings round their circumferences. There is a tumour in the right wall of the womb, the size of which I cannot readily determine, but it must be as big as my fist. The left ovary very painful and enlarged a good deal; is tender at menstrual period and most painful then. No leucorrhoea. Patient has a gouty tongue. Has been three times vaccinated and had small-pox twice. Two years ago had eczema which she cured (?) with Turkish baths.

℞ Tc. *Thuja occid.* 30.

March 7th — Slight discharge from vagina — which is most unusual. Slight shew of eczema on her hands.

℞ *Psor.* 30.

April 1st — Last menses excessive; painful motions.

℞ *Merc. viv.* C.

25th — Her knees are very bad — painful and swelled — worse at rest, better moving about. Has small purulent spots about the pubes.

℞ Tc. *Rhus tox.* 3.

March 22nd — *Psor.* 30.

April 5th — Has done her a great deal of good — the swelling is decreasing.

℞ *Thuja* 30.

19th — Better.

℞ Trit. 4. *Lapis alb.*

May 15th — Better.

R$_x$ *Silicea* (6 trituration).
June 7th — Trit. 4 *Plat.*
14th — *Stannum* (cough).
19th — Comes and begs to have the prescription of May 15th : it did her so much good.
R$_x$ *Silicea* 6.
July 10th — Much better.
R$_x$ Rep.
August 7th — R$_x$ *Syph.* CC.
21st — Much cutaneous irritation.
R$_x$ Tc. *Lappa major.*
Then follow *Hepar, Silicea, Ceanothus, Ferrum, Helonias, Tarentula Cub., Sul.* and *Thuja*, etc., when on May Ist, 1884, I prescribed *Chelid. maj.* Q; and on the 20th of the same month the tumour had so diminished in size that I could find it only with great difficulty. But it required more than another year's treatment before the tumour was quite gone, and during this time the changes were rung on the already mentioned remedies and some others, of which two seemed particularly of advantage, viz. : *Urea* (6-12) and *Hecla,* both of which have more than once done me good service in stubborn cases of tumours, the former particularly in gouty persons.
The cure holds good, for I saw the lady quite lately and enquired.
This case was rather instructive to me, more particularly from a pathoaetiological stand-point.
May 1st — Knees are much better — much pain in the back.
R$_x$ *Viscum album* 30.
June 10th — Not so well — menorrhagia and leucorrhoea; haemorrhoids and constipation.
R$_x$ *Nux-v.* 30 and *Sul.* 30.
July 11th — The tumour (from external palpation) seems rather smaller; patient can walk with more ease.
R$_x$ *Sedum acre* 30.
22nd — Has a cold and gets *Bry.* Ix and *Phos.* 6.
August 8th — The vagina has become very irritable, requiring frequent ablutions and lubrications. The left ovary is not so tender as formerly.
R$_x$ *Sempervivum tectorum* 30.
Sept. 5th — Is better decidedly; much sore throat; has always been subject to quinsies and sore throats. Very constipated.
R$_x$ *Merc. viv.* C.
Sept. 30th — Has had globus hystericus; a good deal of pain in the rectum.
R$_x$ *Persicaria urens* 30.

Nov. 2nd — Has "worked wonders" i.e. the bowels act better; the tumour is smaller; has some irritation of the skin, and she looks much healthier.

$R_x$ Rep.

Decem. 14th — Bowels act freely; much pain in vagina, worse at night.

$R_x$ *Syph.* CC.

January 9th, 1883 — It seems that night really means early morning.

$R_x$ *Merc. viv.*

February 1st — Thinks she is worse; the pains cause her to swell out.

$R_x$ *Bovista* 4x.

13th — Feels better; it has done her good.

$R_x$ Rep.

March 6th — *Bovista* 6.

Eczema had preceded the tumour-formation and when the eczema had been got rid of by external means the uterine fibroid began to grow; moreover, after the tumour had quite gone, eczema broke out again. *Quite a number of cases of tumour have their starting point in silenced cutaneous discharges; this is no vague theroretical statement, but a fact in nature which I have oft verified and which is clinically verifiable any day. Many cases of chronic skin-diseases are no more and no less than chronic diffuse cancerosis.*

This is one reason why cancer is more common now than formerly, while skin diseases are less common. The ordinary dermatologist works, unwittingly, great evil; and when driving along the Thames Embankment one day, and gazing at Cleopatra's Needle, I said to myself — How much mischief did good old Sir Erasmus Wilson work in getting together the money that went to fetch and erect that?

A persisting skin disease in a really healthy taintless person is a sight I have myself never seen, just as I am not acquainted with any other causeless effect. (XX 160)

## 424. OVARIAN TUMOUR

On November 14th, 1884, a childless married lady of thirty years of age came to me for a swelling in the left side of the abdomen that had been slowly growing about a year. Patient suffered most severely at the menstrual period, and, for many years, from most severe and distressing leucorrhoea. She also suffers somewhat from haemorrhoids.

In the recumbent position, with relaxed muscles, one feels in the left iliac region a hard tender circumscribed mass of the size of an orange. It came gradually, subsequently to a fall she had about a year before. There are furfuraceous patches on the pubes and skin of the neck.

$R_x$ Tc. *Bellis p.* 3x. Five drops in water three times a day.
Dec. 4th — Did much good, at first particularly; decidedly better; the piles bleed; profuse menorrhagia; leucorrhoea sanguineous and severe. Tumour not perceptibly smaller.
$R_x$ Tc. *Thuja* 30.
Jan. 6th. 1885 — Very much better in her general feelings; only very little pain in left ovarian region; whites better; last period less excessive; the tumour is about the same size but very much less tender.
$R_x$ Rep.
Feb. 5th — Leucorrhoea worse; tumour much smaller; last period much less painful. Complains of a good deal of pain in the left eye and left temple.
$R_x$ Tc. *Bellis-p.* 1. ziv. Five drops in water three times a day. (XX 168)
March 3rd — Leucorrhoea better; tumour about half of its original size; but still tender, and when she hurries it drops. Last period less painful.
$R_x$ *Psor.* C.
24th — Some of her relatives have been paralysed; she gets nightmare; hands go dead; leucorrhoea worse; much dragging down.
$R_x$ *Syph.* CC.
May 22nd — Says she feels well, so much good has she felt from the powders; tumour nearly gone, whites also. Is costive.
$R_x$ *Med.* 30.
June 9th — Tumour rather larger; whites nearly well.
$R_x$ *Syph.* CC.
20th — Tumour much better; whites also.
$R_x$ Trit. 6 *Silicea.*
July 4th — Leucorrhoea again bad; piles bleeding.
16th — The leucorrhoea is less bad; the left ovarian region is again very tender; pains in the eyes in the morning on awaking.
$R_x$ *Med.* C.
August 22nd — Pains in the eyes gone; left side much less tender.
$R_x$ *Med.* CC.
Sept. 3rd — No trace of the tumour can be found either by palpation or percussion. All she now complains about is that she so easily catches cold. She now dances and runs and bends herself at will without feeling the side at all.
$R_x$ *Psor.* C.
Oct. 27th — Well. Discharged.
On two subsequent occasions patient came with a little tenderness at the old ending in a satisfactory enceinture, shews the cure to have been a truly Hunterian one. As to the remedies used, I must say that the bulk of the prescriptions were untried, a few here and there purely empirical,

some on purely homoeopathic symptomatology, some on tradition, and the nosodes on the same line of thought as will be found set forth, to some extent, in my "Five years" Experience in the New Cure of Consumption by its Own Virus," and later on in these pages if time and space permit. If not, the therapeutic principles I believe in I have already sufficiently explained.

By the way, the great objectors to the use of *Bacillinum* and the like for the most part declare that the higher dilutions contain *none of the drug*; but as I use these zoic medicines *only* in high dilutions they are objecting to . . . nothing, and this on their own shewing ! Either the higher dilutions contain of the essence of the drug, or they do not; if they do not the names they go by must be a matter of total indifference. If higher dilutions contain none of the original drug it must follow that *Pulsatilla* CC., *Bacillinum* CC., and *Syphilinum* CC., and *Broomhandle* CC. are one and the same thing, viz. : a wee quantity of sugar of milk.

In what university did these sapient objectors learn their logic? (XX 168)

## 425. OVARIAN TUMOUR

*By Dr. Gilchrist,*
*Lecturer on Surgery in the Homoeopathic Medical College of the University of Michigan.*

A young woman twenty-five years of age had been suffering for five years as follows — Extreme weakness and lassitude; cannot walk much on account of the weakness and trembling of the legs, especially in the open air, when, however, the other symptoms are better; worse, in every respect, from heat and in warm weather; walks bent over, with the hand applied to the right side; sallow complexion, and an expression of suffering in the face; occasionally has a sharp pain, like a stab, in the right pelvic region, obliging her to bend double, causing her to scream and toss about in agony; difficulty in breathing during the catamenia; is confined to the bed during the whole period; always several days recovering from these attacks. During the menstrual interval has yellow thick, offensive leucorrhoea; bowels originally slightly constipated; now, after some years' use of cathartics, immovably so; a well-defined tumour in the right iliac fossa, about the size of a coconut, elastic feel, but hard and immovable, and the seat of an occasional severe cutting pain. During the attacks of colic, I should have said, there was bilious vomiting; uterus prolapsed, inclined to the left side, and owing to the pressure of the tumour directly upon it, could not be moved by any safe or usual exertion of force; has been under allopathic treatment for four years; has been twice tapped, with temporary subsidence of the tumour; has had no treatment for over a year. During an interval of five months, gave her *Coloc.* in varying potencies — never lower than the 200th — resulting in a complete cure. One year afterwards she remained well.

Dr. Dunham likewise cured, by the use of *Coloc.*, a similar case.

Personally, I have an idea that *Colocynth* is an ovary-medicine in the Rademacherian sense. But both Gilchrist and Dunham cured their cases simply by considering the totality of the symptoms, and as these distinguished men cannot do the impossible, it must follow that tumours can be cured symptomatically. Dunham, the gentle scholar, the humble-minded christian physician, is now in heaven, smiling down encouragement upon us who labour on; may his earth-ward smiles strengthen us in our heavenward strivings.

There are a good many simple cases of cure of tumours by medicines strewn about in the very large homoeopathic literature of America : however, they for the most part are very isolated and solitary; taken singly they are curious, interesting, and not infrequently somewhat of the nature of flukes; collectively they are instructive. None of these cures seem to have caused the curing physician to go on steadily and perseveringly at medicinal tumour-curing : in almost every case — perhaps in every one — nothing more came of it : in the end the surgeon alone remained in the field.

Well, it is very difficult; and *symptoms alone do not commonly suffice, and I fancy this is the rock on which they stranded, and still do strand.*

*I wish to say nothing that is unkind to the absolutely-nothing -but -symptoms men, but their self-sufficiency, when they fondle the symptoms as the in-all and be-all of medicine,* is only paralleled by their vulgar imputations of base motives to those who decline to admit that symptoms are other than a means to the end. A grand means, but still only a means : never the goal.

When I brought out my "New Cure of Consumption" I did it because Koch forced my hand, which I had held back for years; my wife often urging me to publish my experience with *Bacillinum* two or three years before Koch's Cure was heard of, but I hesitated, because I felt the world was not ripe for it, and a man with a very large family has no right to court ruin — so I held back. When I did come forward, because of the Koch fever, to vindicate the rights of the homoeopathic school to priority (myself included), I was accused by certain journalistic symptom-hunters of yapping for Kochian loaves and fishes!!!

When I shewed the review to my wife she exclaimed, "What a cruel shame!" But this is only by the way, and only brought in as a parenthesis.

*Que voulez-vous*? think of the inquisition in the name of the gentle Jesus of Nazareth.

Our sufferings are but microscopic specks by the side of mountains. And Paracelsus they actually battered to pieces with cudgels, and then made fun of him because, having written on longevity, he died (!) early! At the same time it is very important to not under-value symptoms as we cannot get on without them; and the more is the pity. I say this advisedly, because symptomatic equations are very time-devouring, and working at them too much is apt to become stultifying, and, I have at times thought, narrows the medical mind — turning it slowly into something very like a machine. When homoeopathy casts off its swaddling clothes, the subjective symptoms will be to Higher Homoeopathy what spelling is to reading. (XX 175)

## 437. CASE OF VERY LARGE FIBROID TUMOUR OF THE WOMB

This case is interesting. An unmarried lady, fifty-one years of age, was sent to me on April 10th, 1883, by the Countess of X. For the past eight years patient had been suffering from a uterine tumour with occasional bleeding, and which had been diagnosed by eminent gynaecologists as uterine fibroid. In external appearance patient appeared to be in the family way at about the eighth month or the beginning of the ninth, when the onus lies well in the meso-gastrium.

The tumour was as hard as a board. Patient also had a fatty tumour under her left clavicle, size of an orange. She was very anaemic and washed-out looking, and had latterly been taking the quack remedies of Count Mattei, with no advantage. Patient's mother died of consumption.

The most prominent subjective symptom was her "blown out" feeling. Objectively she was anaemic and her gait waddling.

I seized hold of the only available point — the *'blownoutness,'* and prescribed *Bovista* 3x six grains dry on the tongue night and morning.

May 3rd, 1883 — She has apparently menstruated, and does not feel anything like so much blown-out in the abdomen. Her feet, which had been much swelled for some time past, were considerably easier; she felt better.

Repeated the *Bovista*.

June 16th — On the whole not any further diminution, and there is some haemorrhage.
$R_x$ Trit. 4, *Lapis alb.*
September 6th — Better; smaller in the body; can now eat vegetables; no vaginal discharge.
Repeated the *Lapis alb.*
October 18th — Well in herself but size of the tumour is not less. Complains of flushes and fullness in the head.
$R_x$ *Psorinum* 30.
November 17th — Worse; larger; very uncomfortable in the body; her eyes are swollen; urine scanty, the feet are swelling.
$R_x$ Tc. *Platina mur.* 3. Five drops in water night and morning.
January 1st, 1884 — Has lost the palpitation; the fibroid is smaller in size; but the lipoma is larger and she has no appetite.
$R_x$ *Psorinum* 100.
February 2nd — Pains in the chest gone; fearful metrorrhagia.
$R_x$ *Variolinum* 30.
March 1st — Looks cachetic; the lipoma is much larger.
$R_x$ *Calcium fluoricum* 6, and also the third decimal of the Pyrophosphate of iron.
15th — No better; feet swell; has much rheumatism. Is always worse in the spring. The unfortunate lady's size is truly frightful.
$R_x$ Tc. *Aur. mur. nat.* 3x, three drops in water three times a day.
April 8th — There is much discharge *per vaginam*, but it is more watery and she can walk better, and the feet are less swelled. Heart beats uncomfortably, and there is a well-pronounced murmur best heard at the base, and no doubt of haemic nature. She has a cough, and there is much distressing aching in the lower part of the abdomen.
$R_x$ Repeated the *Aurum.*
29th — Gouty inflammation of the right foot and ankle; the vaginal discharge has ceased; is smaller certainly.
$R_x$ Repeat.
May 27th — Foot and ankle well except that the ankle bones still ache; the tumour is much smaller, so that patient is relatively comfortable. The old brown discolouration of the skin of the forehead is nearly gone; she is rather restless at night; the fatty tumour remains about the same.
$R_x$ Repeat.
June 29th — Slight vaginal discharge as if a monthly period, but it continued for three weeks; the size of tumour about the same; the lipoma a trifle larger.
$R_x$ *Psorinum* 30.

July 12th — No bleeding; less uncomfortable; soles of feet tender and painful.
$R_x$ Tc. *Urea* 6. ziv. Five drops in water night and morning.
January 5th, 1885 — Tumour a good deal smaller and patient's health is greatly improved.
$R_x$ *Psor.* 100.
April 21st — Did her much good; no bleeding for long; the tumour is diminishing.
$R_x$ *Urea* 6. as before.
June 18th — No bleeding at all; is much smaller; she is quite losing her cachetic look; the lipoma is no smaller; has had another attack of gouty inflammation in the feet.
$R_x$ Trit. 5. *Lapis alb.*
July 16th — Has grown much larger and is not so well in herself; some leucorrhoea; cannot rest at night; goes to sleep for two or three hours and wakes up, remains awake and restless and cannot get off again.
$R_x$ *Urea* 6.
September 1st — Still large.
$R_x$ *Psor.* 100.
18th — Much inflammation in eyelids. Tumour distinctly larger.
$R_x$ *Medorrh.* 100.
March 25th, 1886 — Did her so much good that she has had no medicine since, and she now comes to ask if she need take any more. The tumour has gone down so much that patient has become shapely like any other lady; still gets occasional periods; and as nearly as I can judge the tumour is about two-thirds gone, but the fatty tumour remains pretty much as it was.
$R_x$ *Medorrh.* 30.
April 22nd — Tumour again much diminished in size; no bleeding or other discharge; there is still some rheumatism and left-sided conjunctivitis.
$R_x$ *Urea* 12.
June 17th — Eye well; rheumatism well; no discharge, not much of the tumour left.
$R_x$ Trit. 3x *Hecla leva.*
This ends the treatment, which, it will be observed, began in April, 1883, and terminated in June, 1886, in complete cure of the tumour and restoration of patient to good health.
It will be observed that there are considerable gaps in the clinical narration, and these were due to the fact that the patient is addicted to travelling about a good deal, and so would often absent herself for months.

**Five Years Afterwards. July, 1891** — I am pleased to be able to add that though I have not seen this lady since June, 1886, she sent me word in July, 1891, that she had had no return of her tumour of the womb, and continued in capital health; the occasion of this message was her sending a friend of hers to me to be also treated for a tumour; but for this happy circumstance I should have continued in complete ignorance of the sequel to the termination of the cure.

Of the lady's ungraciousness in not even informing me before I will say nothing, suffice for me that the huge fibroid tumour was radically and permanently cured by medicines, and that fully five years of subsequent good health testify thereto.

Hence I think we may fairly reckon this a truly Hunterian cure. (XX 181)

## 427. TUMOUR OF THE RIGHT BREAST

An unmarried lady of thirty-nine came under my observation, brought by her mother, on May 2nd, 1889. Spinal deformity all her life, and wearing instruments since she was twelve; the lateral curvature being very considerable. Her father died of phthisis; of her *Geschwister* two brothers and two sisters died of phthisis, and one brother died of typhoid.

I have often noticed a proneness to typhoid in those disposed to phthisis, rheumatism, neuralgia, measles and whooping cough, comprise the list of her own previous ailments. Her tongue is pippy in its anterior half; in the outer upper aspect of her right breast, between it and the axilla, there is a tumour of about the size of my (pretty big) fist. Patient complains of being subject to frightful headaches of the right side coming on at midnight and going off at daybreak, very severe dysmenorrhoea all her menstrual life *till the last six months*, when it has been a good deal less severe. She thinks herself that the tumour started from the pressure of the fingers of the person who fits on her mechanical arrangements to support her spine. A very eminent London surgeon who has advised her these fifteen years is of opinion that the tumour is fibrous, and he accordingly advises excision; the local Kensington surgeon agreed, but wished for the further opinion of Dr. — who said the tumour was not fibrous, but strumous, and required to be lanced. The opinions being thus divergent, the advice of another eminent surgeon was taken, and he thought it was spinal, but declined to give a very positive opinion. At this point her mother brings her to me. Patient, I should say, was a huge salt eater. Many blotches in her skin. To my mind the constitutional crasis of the lady was tuberculous, and hence I ordered *Bacillinum C.* in rather infrequent repetition.

May 28th — Pus has evidently formed in the outermost part of the previously hard tumour, where over the skin is red; the lingual papillae (pips) are much less red; headaches are worse (at night — towards morning); there are fewer cutaneous blotches. She tells me she is liable to severe pain in ball of the left foot, worse on approach of damp weather; last period more than usually painful. She retches a good deal. The local surgeon is very angry at patient being under the care of a homoeopath, and begs to be allowed to watch the case as a friend, to which request patient accedes. The good man's conceit does not desert him, and he sends me word that "he awaits the result with calmness," whatever that might mean.

℞ Tc. *Silicea* 6. Five drops in water three times a day.

June 27th — Patient feels much better; headaches better; no pips; no retching; tumour smaller, not so active, and no longer looks so red, but the tissue in its inside has evidently softened, and the contents will clearly have to be voided.

I repeat the first prescription.

July 13th — The tumour has burst and has discharged enormously. The bad nights, want of rest, and the nocturnal headahces led me to give *Syph.* CC. I should have said that patient's friends declare she looks ten years younger, indeed she has a freshness of tint and healthfulness of face that no one remembers to have ever observed in her before. The local surgeon has given up "calling as a friend."

July 27th — The tumour is practically gone and patient is well of herself, but I again ordered *Silicea* to rid her of the hardened tissue around where the abscess broke.

Patient made a complete recovery, the tumour totally disappeared, and for the first time in her life she feels in capital health. This cure made a very deep impression in patient's social circle.

Of what nature was the swelling?

Clearly strumous, and not an organized neoplasm. (XX 190)

## 428. THICKENING OF CARDIA

Lady ____, mother of nine children, came under my observation on March 26th, 1886, for a tumour at the top of the stomach and much vomiting. She was at the time fifty-three years of age, and in a very sad state indeed — hopeless, so every one thought.

That would also have been my view, had my weapons of cure been of the traditional sort. And here I will pause a moment to say that *I do not advocate the use of zoic remedies in simple ailments, just as a general would not fire a big cannon to knock over half a dozen brick-bats.* As I often say . . . *aux grands maux les grands remedes.* Such pop-guns as *Nux vomica* or *Pulsatilla* or *Subnitrate of Bismuth* will not cure tumours of the stomach, and hence if they are to be cured we must bring out bigger guns, and the zoic remedies are the very biggest guns of all beyond compare.

Some ailings are like sparrows : very small arms will suffice to kill them — say hydropathy, or homoeopathic simples, but tumours generally resist small arms.

As Lady ___'s mother died of an internal tumour, naturally her ladyship regarded her own state with all the greater apprehension.

There was pain at the pit of the stomach, constant, gnawing; painful on pressure. Very weak; great thirst; no saliva; she passes a great quantity of pale urine, and must rise four or five times every night to micturate; much heat and irritation in urinary passage.

Head aches at top and back. Violent vomiting. At midnight is always roused by feverishness for the past four years. In the epigastrium is a hard tender mass, corresponding in position to the cardia. She is very chilly. Twice vaccinated. Recounting her health history, she tells me she has had dysentery, ague, piles, anaemia, smallpox, puerperal fever, boils, styes, whites, and was once salivated.

$R_x$ *Medorrh.* 30. One dose evey seven days.

April 14th — The pain at the pit of the stomach is gone; thirst now mostly an hour-and-half after breakfast; more saliva; passes less water; no headaches; no vomiting; still has the "ghost fever;" less chilly; less tenderness at epigastrium, and the mass is seemingly a little smaller.

She begs for an aperient, as there is total inertia of bowels.

$R_x$ *Plumbum* 12, and *Opium* 12, in alternation.

May 7th — Is suddenly plunged into acute grief by the death of her husband of angina pectoris.

$R_x$ Tc. *Ignatia am.* 3x. Five drops in water three times a day.

And thereafter we had recourse to the previously mentioned prescriptions, and then followed some of the remedies I have ventured to term pop-guns (quoad the tumours), and patient was discharged cured — or rather she discharged herself. The case passed out of my mind for several years.

**Five Years Later** — At the end of 1891 and again in the spring of 1892, her ladyship came to bring a grandchild of hers, and hence I know that she has never looked back. She has now a much healthier look than she had six years ago; and, considering what she has gone through, her condition — being in her sixtieth year — must be termed eminently satisfactory.

"Any trouble from your stomach now, my lady?" "Oh! no thank you none at all." (XX 195)

### 429. ATHEROMA OF SCALP — WEN-SEBACEOUS CYST

On June 30th, 1888, a lady of sixty or thereabouts came to consult me for a large wen at the back of her scalp a couple of inches or so behind the left ear.
Had had it for many years but smaller; it is now enlarging. Patient is subject to intermittent erysipelas and much giddiness and swimming in the head.
R$_x$ *Bellis per.* Q.
July 10th — No better; giddiness is much worse with certain movements of the head; there is a sensation in the left hypochondrium as if it swelled up, and then follows giddiness ; also, for years whenever she puts her hands into cold water she gets a thrill under the left ribs. So this is probably spleen — Grauvogl's hydrogenoid constituion — she feels draughts which make her chilly; there is some epigastric throbbing. Patient tells me she once had suppressed measles and suppressed small-pox, and also typhoid.
R$_x$ *Spiritus Glandium Quercus* Q.
17th — Complains of a tender fulness in the left hypochondrium; the left cheek flushes.
R$_x$ Rep.
19th — No better. *Ceanothus am.* 1.
August 4th — Swimming in head and the side much the same; she feels weaker; no pains in the shoulder; side however less swollen.
R$_x$ *Variol.* 30 in very infrequent doses in powder form.
15th — "Since I have been taking the last medicine I have gradually become much better; the dizziness and swimming in the head, and swelling in the side, have been much less."
R$_x$ *Variol.* C. in very infrequent dose.
25th — Nearly well; she is very positive that the powders have done her so much good; the last (C.) even more than the former (30). She has lost her pallor, has quite a fresh colour, and is really quite a different woman. The wen is easier.
R$_x$ *Bellis-per.* Q.
October 20th — Had to give up the *Bellis-p.* and had some more *Variol.* powders, when no further progress being appreciable I gave *Morbillin.* 30 in very infrequent dose (December) when patient passed a round worm and (January) I ordered her *Rubia tinctoria* simply as a spleen medicine, whereupon the atherome broke and discharged a good deal

at times and off and on till it healed and there was an end of it. I might add that *Cuprum, Terebinth, Thuja,* and *Sulphur* were used in the interim, and, on April 6th — I could scarcely find where the tumour had been. The containing membrane was one day pulled away by the lady's friend while dressing the suppurating wen. A good many poultices were used by the lady *while* it was discharging, but *not* before.

It might very naturally be urged by surgery-loving friends : What is the advantage of all this medicating for a bit of wen? Why not just slit it up and pull out the whole thing and have done with it?

Well, in the first place, good and thoughtful practitioners had maintained that operations for wens are at times followed by Bright's Disease, and as Bright's Disease at any rate cannot be operated upon, it is just as well to let the wens alone, since they are a lesser evil than *Morbus Brightii*. Furthermore, *the lady was not well, and it was by treating her ill-health that I succeeded in getting rid of the wen.*

I might add that the *Quercus* will *cause* giddiness, and it is, moreover, a mild, yet powerful spleen medicine.

*The* remedy in the case was evidently the *Variolinum,* and I have no doubt that it cured homoeopathically.

I have known the lady for seventeen years, off and on, as a patient, but had never seen her with a good colour till after the *Var*. She continues very well to date.

At the beginning of the narration of the foregoing case, I said that homoeopathy, organopathy and zoic medicines all helped in its cure; I do not mean that these are distinct from one another, but I mention them thus separately by name because many homoeopaths do not admit organopathy as an integral part of homoeopathy, while many others pooh-pooh or turn up their superior noses at the use of zoic medicines such as *Bacillinum, Morbillinum, Variolinum*. Whereas I maintain that organopathy is basic elementary homoeopathy leading up to symptomatic differentiation, and the zoic medicines begin where the ordinary symptomatic differentiation leaves off. In regard to tumour-curing I find that organopathy is very helpful indeed, and with it I often succeed alone without the serious expenditure of time called for in truly differential symptomatic treatment. It saves the physician's time and preserves his mental strength. *Its weak point is the relatively uncertain power of organ-medicines over the disposition, it gets rid of the product more effectively than it does with the diathesis*. This same weak point, however, exists likewise in purely homoeopathic symptom-covering; in neither case is the neoplastic diathesis materially influenced *unless the degree of homoeopathicity* in the drug chosen be very considerable : for looking deeply into the thing makes us aware that it is *not* the mode of choosing a remedy that is of greatest import, *but the degree of likeness existing between drug-pathogenesy and the natural history of the malady in its anatomical and physiological essence.*

This is where the zoic medication *begins* : it hits the diathetic quality as well as the product. *Here only higher dilutions at longer intervals are any good,* or fuel is added to the flames; whereas in organopathy small material doses act well and suffice, and the doses are repeatedly given with advantage — *the greater the degree of homoeopathicity the higher the dilution and the longer the interval between the doses.* This I have before pointed out in my "Fifty Reasons for Being a Homoeopath," and although it has apparently attracted no notice from critical pens, still herein lies the real solution of the "question of the dose."

Let any clear-headed unprejudiced physician think this matter over and then put the idea to the clinical test and he will find it is true in nature and capable of exact scientific clinical demonstration. It is this idea also that gives a real explanation of homoeopathic "aggravations" that are very real to those who often spot the simillimum, but mere moonshine to those who do not.

Said Dr. Robert Cooper to me one day, in regard to chronic deafness more particularly ...

"Well, I find I cure best if I get an aggravation, so that if I do not get any aggravation I conclude I have not got the right remedy for the case; they may laugh at it as much as they like, *but that's what I find."*

*We do not often get aggravations in organopathic practice, because the degree of drug-likeness to the disease is small*; but they do occur at times when there happens to be a great degree of homoeopathicity existing between drug-action and morbid state; and in reading the literature of the organopaths one is struck with the curious fact that the more experienced they became in applying organ-remedies to organ diseases *the smaller became their doses* : thus Rademacher slowly came down from twenty-five or thirty drops of the ordinary strong tincture to 15, to 12, to 10; aye, even to "one drop well diluted in water!"

If anyone wants an absolutely conclusive ready-made proof that the degree of homoeopathicity regulates the dose, let him compare the results obtained with *Tuberculinum* in Kochian practice and those obtained by myself and others, with practically the same drug, but given in high dilution in very infrequent doses.

Moreover, Koch himself proves the high degree of homoeopathicity of his *Tuberculinum* by getting aggravation *where there is tubercular disease only,* but *his aggravation is very apt to be lethal, but homoeopathic all the same in its nature; and it is lethal because the dose is too great.*

Dr. Kroner, of Potsdam, in the *Zeitschrift des Berliner Vereines homoeopathischer Aerzte,* Vol. xi, part ii p. 191 in his review of *Die Koch' sche Tuberculose-Behandlung auf Grund von Beobachtungen in der evangelischen Diakonissenanstalf zu Stuttgart von Obermedizinalrath Sick;* Stuttgart, 1892 — thus remarks :—

"In some cases I am struck with the fact that after a severe aggravation, calling for the stopping of all further injections, there occurs, sooner or later, not only a return to the *status quo ante,* but decided improvement was observable. And in connection with this, who does not think of examples of such in homoeopathic practice?"

It is but fitting that State Medicine in the German fatherland should thus give a scientific demonstration of the truth of Hahnemann's "aggravation!"

The German Hahnemann is indeed avenged in his own home-land ! (XX 201)

## 430. TUMOUR IN LEFT HYPOCHONDRIUM

A city gentleman, fifty-eight years of age, came to consult me in the month of April, 1888, for a tumour in the left side of his abdomen, reaching from just below the apex beat of the heart to the left as far as the spinal column; from above downwards as far as a transverse line drawn through the navel and to the right to about an inch beyond the mesian perpendicular.

His doctors had given him up, particularly as he had lost flesh and strength; and his aspect shewed that they were right.

To his knowledge he had had the tumour for two years, but he believes it may have been there much longer, and it is slowly growing. The swelling is very painful, and the pain extends to and is also felt in the epigastrium. A deep scar over his left eyebrow dates back 50 years, when he was kicked in that region by his father's horse. He vomits a good deal.

The essential points, therefore, were : the swelling, the pain, the vomiting, the loss of flesh, and the weakness.

As the patient was a very chilly mortal, and worse in wet weather, I concluded that the tumid mass was either a very large spleen or a tumour growing out of it. But which? That could not be determined on the hither side of the *post-mortem* table, and then it would be too late. The exact nature of internal tumours is very frequently simply unknown and unknowable; even puncturing will not always disclose it, and this is often dangerous, and in any case objectionable.

Besides the before-mentioned kick over his left eye, I elicited that he had never been vaccinated, having had variola fully 40 years ago.

Now the effect of acute diseases on the economy are known to last a very long time; how long does not appear to be determinable. I therefore thought that perhaps that might have morbidly impressed the organism, and so be the causal start, improbable as it may appear.

Wherefore I ordered (see my "Natrum Muriaticum" and "New Cure of Consumption" for doctrinal reasons), *Variol.* 30, six globules every eighth day. This was on the 9th of April and on the 12th of May, he reported himself very much better, and the tumour had slightly decreased.

In another six weeks — June 22 — patient had lost all the pain; the vomiting had ceased, and he had gained flesh and strength. But the tumour was *larger* [Aggravation?]

Now thinking that the pyrexia accompanying the variola may have acted causally in the matter (hypothetical again) I gave him *Pyrogenium* 5.

July 18th — He thinks the lump is smaller; has gained flesh, and looks quite healthy. I ordered *Bellis per.* Q, both because of the old blow over left eye, and because *Bellis* has an affinity for the left hypochondrium, and also because it has already cured tumours in my hands. He took thereof six drops night and morning till he had used four drachms.

August 24th — In the perpendicular, as also in the transverse, the tumour has diminished by fully an inch both ways. In himself he is now quite well. It being clearly splenic .

℞ *Ceanothus Am.* 1. Five drops in water night and morning.

October 10th — The swelling is much smaller. He then had *Spirit glandium quercus* Q, and finally *Variol.* C., and in the beginning of 1889 was quite well and ceased attending.

Not long since I saw the gentleman again, and learned that he continues well.

It will be useful to dwell for a few moments upon this case, principally because it shews — what I often notice — that the primary start may indicate the remedy, and this seem to remove the obstacle, or bar to drug action, just as Hahnemann noticed and taught in regard to his *aetiologic homoeopathy* : the *Coethen phase* of homoeopathy.

To bring the treatment down to John Hunter's conception of a real cure of tumour must be our constant aim, and the idea that is worked out in my *"Natrum Muriaticum,"* viz :— a hair of the dog that bit you — seems, strangely, to be helpful.

This idea really lies very deep and bears thinking about and underlies the labours of the isopaths, of Pasteur, Koch, Swan, Ameke. And the line of demarcation appears to me to be what I have given expression to in my "New Cure of Consumption," viz.: "where homoeopathicity merges into identity." In other words the double and opposite actions of large and small doses, as I think "Natrum Muriaticum as Test of the Doctrine of Drug Dynamisation" fully proves in regard to Sodium Chloride at any rate. Working out that thesis turned my mind in the direction of "the remedy in the disease" where it certainly is sometimes, and, perhaps, under conditions. (XX 213)

## 431. LUMP

On June 19th, 1889. This day Mr. ___ called upon me to say he had sadly run down in health owing to domestic affliction and much night watching, and he had begun to find out that he had a left side again, in fact the old lump was again, in fact the old lump.

$R_x$ Tc. *Urtica urens* Q. Five drops in water night and morning.

July 24th — The tumour has gone down; he says : "I can feel it not so large." He feels very well in himself. To continue with the Urtica, which was done till December 18th, 1889, when the most careful examination failed to reveal the smallest remains of the lump.

And how do you feel, said I to him?

"First-rate."

By the way, *Urtica urens* is a splendid splenic, whose clinical history I propose to relate another time.

Patient, I believe, continues well to date.

Was this a genuine neoplasm, a tumour in the strict sense?

Well, the leading allopathic surgeons of London said so, and if their diagnostic powers are vain *what* is their *raison d'etre*? They cannot cure anything.

By the way not so long ago they were very great at blood-corpuscle counting in splenic tumefaction; strange to say that also did not cure anybody, and the blood-cell counting is going ... out of fashion; in fact *is* almost as much out of date as the crinoline. (XX 219)

## 432. ABDOMINAL TUMOUR

The subject of this chapter is an abdominal tumour of special interest, not only on account of its fully successful treatment, but because the case was throughout watched and periodically examined by an allopathic surgeon of repute, who himself advised his patient to make the necessary long sea voyage from a distant hot country to London, to seek further skilled advice in regard to her abdominal tumour.

The surgeon, of course, did not even dream of its cure by remedies, and in sending her home this was not in his mind. But years before I had cured a child of the patient of lymphatic tumours, and so once arrived in London the lady sought my opinion : I found in the upper part of the abdomen a tumour that was of considerable size, having its seat of origin, so far as I could tell, at the left end of the pancreas, but extending across to the right a good way towards the liver. In size it may be said to be about that of a big man's fist, and seemingly a fibroid. For a year past there has been much dyspepsia. The pancreas I considered much enlarged, and the spleen was also increased in size.

Of eight children, five had died in infancy; there was a large brown patch on the forehead almost co-extensive with it; she had formerly had sore throats; her hair has fallen out and is still in the process of falling out, and her nights were bad. Patient was a large salt-eater; had been three times vaccinated, and had had typhoid and ague, as also hypogastric neuralgia; costive.

August 4th, 1886 —

℞ *Sepia* 5. Five drops in water three times a day.

18th — Urine rather slimy; hair falls out rather less. Complains very much of sleepless nights.

℞ *Syph.* CC. in very infrequent dose.

September 15th — The remedy did her constipation much good; the hair ceased falling out; the forehead less brown. The tumour certainly smaller.

℞ The same remedy enough to last two months.

November 15th — The first ten days I took the powders I had a good deal of pain and diarrhoea followed by constipation and bad piles with much smarting rawness. The tumour is without doubt a good deal smaller and much softer.

℞ Rep.

January 31st, 1887 — "I stopped taking the powders and have only just finished them; and I have had to have the doctor here for piles and fissure; he examined my tumour about five or six weeks ago, and said it was half its previous size, and since then I think it is smaller still and I have a difficulty in finding it — it seems much further away from the surface."

℞ *Iris versicolor* 30.

March 12th — "I am glad to be able to report further good progress; I have had my doctor here to see how the tumour was getting on; he says it is much smaller than when he saw it two or three months ago, and is now not longer than a very small hen's egg; I am feeling well in myself and suffer very much less from constipation, and have taken no Cascara."

$R_x$ *Syph*. CC.

May 10th — "The last time the doctor was here. He could not feel any lump, but I am two months gone in the family way. The brown marks on the forehead have gone. I have had dysenteric diarrhoea and am weak."

$R_x$ *Arsenicum* 3 trit. Six grains twice a day.

July 1st —

$R_x$ *Aurum mur. nat*. 3x. Six drops twice a day.

August 12th — Has returned to England, and comes to me worn out with dysentery. *Simaruba* cured it.

$R_x$ *Calc. Hypophos*. 3x, gr. viij. Three times a day.

Sept. 7th — Quite recovered her strength. Returns to her distant home across the sea.

$R_x$ *Aur. mur. nat*. 3x. As before.

Nov. 7th — Feels quite well. Has finished the medicine.

$R_x$ *Syph*. CC.

Feb. 20th 1888 — "I have sent for my doctor to examine my tumour, and he says it is sausage-shaped, but much smaller and flatter. My lady is very fine and healthy, and I am well."

$R_x$ Tc. *Iris versicolor* 3x.

And then followed *Aurum* again as before; when the doctor again examined patient for the tumour, and declared it to have quite disappeared. The cure holds good.

I am very especially pleased to record this case, as its course was carefully watched by an unbiased highly qualified general practitioner (a British graduate), who took no part in the treatment, remaining just an onlooking expert, and who had not consulted at all with me, does not know me personally, and has never even communicated with me, nor has he the faintest idea of what remedies have been used.

He is an allopath, and seemingly, is content so to be and so to remain. How this can possibly be I do not pretend to comprehend. I have often observed this sort of quasi-interest in homoeopathic work go hand in hand with practical and life-long indifference.

I suppose the quasi-interest is no really scientific concern at all, but rather curiosity and a kindly sort of feeling for their clients' fads. The Spanish generals behaved in pretty much the same sort of superior way to one Arthur Wellesley in the Peninsular campaign. But history has squared the accounts pretty fairly.

The following letter from the lady shall end this chapter, to wit :

January 12th, 1889.

Dear Dr. Burnett,

It is six months since I received the last medicine you ordered me.

Shortly after its arrival I had an attack of fever which lasted a long time — over two months; it was simple fever without any complications, but I became very weak with it and was some time getting up my strength again. It is only quite lately I finished your medicine, and two days ago I had Dr. — to see me. He searched long and carefully for the tumour, and I am delighted to say, could not find any trace of it; he says the left lobe of my liver is still slightly enlarged as it has been for a long time. In spite of this enlargement of liver, I have no unpleasant symptoms with it, and feel in perfect health and stength, and am up to dancing and playing tennis, which latter I always do regularly and always feel the better for it. I feel very grateful for all you have done for me. My baby also is well, strong and rosy. May I consider myself out of your hands now? I suppose the only thing for my liver is a change out of the country, but that I doubt if I shall get this year as times are so bad.
With kind regards and good wishes to you for the New Year,
I remain,
Your Sincerely.
**Years Later** — In the Summer of 1892, I saw this lady, and thus know from personal examination that the cure holds good. (XX 222)

## 433. TUMOUR OF TONGUE — PRESUMABLY CANCEROUS

Some five years since a lady, sixty odd years of age, came under my observation for tumour of the tongue for which she had already once undergone a successful operation, i.e. the then existing tumour was a fresh one that had come at the old spot, viz. : the left side of the tongue, and was about the size of a walnut. On the recommendation and homoeopathic, the operation had been performed by a well-known London surgeon. But, as first stated, the tumour recurred. Three homoeopathic physicians strongly urged the imperative necessity of a new operation.

The case was complicated with a fatty heart, atheroma of the arteries, numerous symptoms of paresis, profound adynamia, scrrow and worry without end, and hence very numerous remedies have been called to the rescue, and right well they have responded, for the tumour has long since gone and the lady is still bravely to the fore.

By reason of the extraordinary complexity of this case it would serve no useful purpose to narrate the case in detail, but I might name *Cundurango, Var., Barium, Iodium, Ferrum aceticum, Variolinum, Oleum succini nonrect., Ceanothus, Rubia tinct., Lycopodium* and *Aurum* as remedies that did sound service. At the date of which I am writing these notes — June,

1889, the lady is in fair health and the tongue is well, and it is with the tumour of the tongue that we are here concerned.

January 14th, 1890 — I heard from the lady a few days ago and so can say the tumour continues well. Of course the tongue is not exactly a normal tongue inasmuch as a piece of it was cut away, so it always remains somewhat odd-looking and puckered laterally by the scar tissue.

A number of the homoeopathic practitioners of Great Britain have seen this case and they will readily recognize it by this description of the hard tried lady, who is the widow of an Anglican clergyman on the East Coast.

February, 1892 — At this date I saw this lady and found the tongue still healthy. This lapse of time justifies my calling this a really Hunterian cure. (XX 231)

## 434. POSTAURAL LYMPHOMA — VACCINOSIS AND PSORA

On the first of April, 1886, a little girl of nine years of age was brought to me for advice in regard to her general health, and specially for a small glandular tumour behind the left ear. Delicate as a baby, then got strong; subsequently went thin and deaf — now two years ago — was taken to an aurist who removed portions of the tonsils and thereafter totally excised them. Deafness was better, but patient herself became very ill, was sent to the seaside and recovered.

Now she has bad broken chilblains "and everything with her gets mattery." There is a little lump — presumably glandular — behind the left ear, of the size of a large hazel nut. Acne of skin. Anorexia. Once vaccinated.

Rx. *Thuja* 30, infrequently.

May 11th. — Lump behind ear smaller; flesh very unhealing, but not quite so mattery.

$R_x$ *Psor.* 30, infrequently.

September 30th — Well; no lump and she is bonny.

That the indurated gland behind the ear was of a piece with the tonsillar disease will hardly be disputed, and that the excision of the tonsils was an eminently silly proceeding, must be equally manifest.

Still, of course, vaccinosis is nonsense and psora nothing but moonshine. But, banter apart, will any medical man, of *any* pathy, tell me a shorter and better way to cure a tumour, great or small, than I am here trying to set forth?

I claim that this is a real — a Hunterian — cure, for the disease is cured

in its effect and, I truly believe, in its disposition. Whether a small glandular enlargement may quite rightfully be called a tumour I will leave an open question. (XX 234)
AS this chapter is very short I will add one more case of :

## 435. SEBACEOUS TUMOUR OF SCALP

A married lady, mother of three children, came under my observation at the end of the year 1887, for a number of ailments. She was verging on fifty years of age and had double cataract.
When I say that she came for a number of ailments that is not quite what I mean : I ought rather to say that, though suffering from a number of ailments, she came to me for double cataract and seemed almost afraid lest I might, as it were incidentally, or accidently, cure something else. There was a good-sized wen in the lady's scalp that finally yielded to my treatment. She had taken a great many remedies from me; her constitution slowly improved; she became much stronger; her hair, which had been very thin, grew again, and in the autumn of 1889, while taking *Acidum uricum* 5, the wen disappeared; having burst and discharged.
These wens are very curious things, and to me biologically decidedly puzzling. For instance, why does kidney-disease follow their forcible removal? Why are their owners so prone to pains, and paresis? At present I am studying a number of them with much interest; and although I not infrequently cure them, still I cannot say I understand them. Sebaceous cysts from occluded outlets of the sebaceous follicles are only the dry bones of the things. (XX 236)

## 436. TUMOUR OF LEFT BREAST

On April 16th, 1888, Mrs. X., a young widow, twenty-six years of age, mother of two children, both of whom have, hwoever, died, came telling me she had been under treatment at St. Thomas's Hospital and elsewhere, for a tumour of the breast.
Menses regular, but painful; the tumour is more painful at the monthly time. She had a knock on the left breast 15 months ago. Mr. —, the hospital surgeon, and the surgeons at St. Thomas's, and also the surgeons at the country town whence she hails, all recommended operation.
"Do those gentlemen all recommend an operation?"
"Yes, sir, all of them."
In the outer aspect of the left breast I found a very painful swelling, the

corresponding part of the right breast being also tender to the touch but not the seat of any tumour.

Patient was of opinion that the tumour in the left breast was a trifle smaller than it had been, but much more painful. Anorexia, anosmia. Has been twice vaccinated; had bad measles, a weak chest, pneumonia, bronchitis, low fever and much grief. The first two very obvious points in this case were the grief — fancy a young woman of delicate health, who had lost her two babes and her husband, and who had been recommended by half-a-dozen surgeons of repute to have one of her breasts ablated — then there was, probably, some blow; in fact she dated the whole thing to blow.

Therefore I gave her *Ignatia amara* 1x (dear old Hahnemann, thou hadst not lived in vain if thou hadst left us nought but this one thrice-blessed therapeutic legacy!) and *Bellis perennis* Q.

May 16th — Patient is brighter and better in her self; the tumour is very painful and more defined.

$R_x$ *Thuja occid.* 30.

June 13th — Better in health; very bilious and many headaches.

$R_x$ *Psor.* 30.

July 16th — At first the lump swelled a good deal and then went down again. Patient is very yellow and bilious; the tumour very tender.

$R_x$ *Hydrastis Can.* Q.

August 27th — She does not think there is any real improvement.

$R_x$ *Fer. picric.* 3x ziv, three drops in water night and morning.

October 15th — Nearly well, but she suffers fearfully from neuralgia of the jaw.

$R_x$ *Bacill.* 30.

November — Very bad bilious attack and the tumour has increased in size somewhat.

$R_x$ *Hydrastis Can.* Q.

January 14th, 1889 — The tumour is nearly gone, she says, and I have difficulty in finding its remnant. She is very pale and bilious.

$R_x$ *Rubia tinctoria* Q.

March 11th — The little bit of the tumour that remains is now more evidenced by pains than by bulk.

$R_x$ *Morbill.* 30.

April 8th — Pain is nearly gone, but she will have it that the tumour has grown again a little.

$R_x$ Rep. (C.)

June 5th — The tumour is quite gone; patient is still pale and there is still a little pleurodynia.

$R_x$ *Sabina* 30.

This ended the matter, patient continues well and has no tumour — Saint Thomas's prognosis notwithstanding. (XX 240)

## 437. SMALL VASCULAR GROWTH INSIDE THE LEFT LOWER EYELID NEAR THE INTERNAL CANTHUS

An unmarried lady of some seven-and-twenty summers consulted me on July 25th, 1888, for a small vascular tumour inside the left lower eyelid near the inner canthus, and separated from the caruncula by about the eighth of an inch. What really troubled her was the lachrymation or rather the stillicidium.

She had been aware of this growth some six months, and has been under "proper" treatment for the same, and the treating surgeon has very improperly cauterised it, so of course the surface of the tumour is somewhat cicatricial.

$R_x$ Tc. *Cupress, Law.* 3, ziv. Five drops in water night and morning.

August 22nd — It is rather smaller, but not much. She herself has always been well, but thus far has never had a healthy look.

The *Cupress* drops have, however, brought a healthy hue to her face — "and I never had a healthy colour in my face before in my life!"

She now tells me that she had a similar vascular tumour on the right lower eyelid, but on its outside, but it disappeared herefrom at the time it appeared on the corresponding *internal* spot of the left side. And *yet* the surgeon cauterised it! Patient is curiously affected by the moon, and that in this wise — at full moon her brain seems excited and worried, and she cannot sleep, but if she sleeps, dreams; this has been the case for the past twenty years. Her teeth are greenish and her gums unhealthy.

$R_x$ *Argent. met.* 5. Five drops in water night and morning.

October 8th — The eye has ceased watering and the wee growth is less red.

$R_x$ *Selenium* 5, zic. Five drops in water night and morning.

And under its use the tumour waned and went, but the cicatricial surface due to the surgeon's cauterising of course remains.

October 18th, 1889 — "The last medicine cured it."

January 24th, 1890 — The eye continues well. (XX 245)

## 438. OVARIAN TUMOURS : BEARING ON MARRIAGE — OF THEIR MODES OF CURE

The treatment of tumours in young women has a very vital bearing on the future life, happiness and family life of the subjects. This now following case well exemplifies the point.

In the year 1882 I was requested to meet Dr. M. ___ in consultation in regard to the state of health of Miss X. ___ then just thirty years of age. I found the left half of the hypogastrinum occupied by a large tumour roughly about the size of a big man's fist. It had been much larger and had been reduced to the just-stated size by curative manipulations in which Dr. M. ___ is very expert, but below its man's-fist size the tumour would not go by the curative movement.

Questioned as to the time she had had it patient said many years; it had been subject of treatment during the past four years, and now it was my task to recommend an operation, or to undertake the case to see if remedies could cure it. Although the tumour was not so very large, it appeared very unsightly by reason of the lithe build of the patient, and this unsightliness caused her near relatives to greatly favour an operation, and when I stated that I thought medicines would cure it I fear no one believed me except the patient herself and Dr. M. ____.

It is astonishing with what light-heartedness the belongings of a patient ____ particularly a number of women ____ discuss such operations on *women other than themselves*! In the end my view was accepted. The patient had had yellow leucorrhoea; the menses were very painful and therewith a good deal of vomiting.

My treatment was regularly begun on November 6th, 1882, and my first prescription was *Thuja occidentalis* 30, not only because of the leucorrhoea, but for the vaccinosis, viz.; she had been in all three times vaccinated; the second time was nine years previously, when she was ill for nine weeks with it, and in the winter before (1881) she had fourteen boils. There was also much flatulence, and her constipation she described as "fearful;" subject also to bilious attacks every ten days or so, and the whites of her eyes were dirty-yellow to a degree but rarely seen except in the aged. The *Thuja* seemed to cause a great deal of pain in the tumour : she had one dose every day for a month.

*Psorin*. 30 followed the *Thuja*, and hereupon I find this note in my casebook :

Dec. 13th, 1882 — At first the pain went better and she felt better : now in every way worse than ever; also severe pain in the top of the head; conjunctivae very yellow.

$R_x$ *Thuja* C.

January 1st, 1883 — Her head is very bad; insomnia; starts a good deal on going off to sleep.

$R_x$ *Nat sul*. 4. Six grains in water every three hours.

February 28th — The *Natrum sul*. has seemingly greatly upset her, so much so that she is afraid to go on with it. The initiated will see that the prescription was Grauvoglian. Patient is very bilious.

$R_x$ *Syph.* CC.

March 21st — No obvious improvement.

$R_x$ *Medorrh.* 30.

No change worth naming in the tumour, but the constipation became so bad that it became for the time the substantive complaint. For this *Podophyllin* 2x and *Euonymin* 3x were used, the latter with much satisfaction and general improvement, and under it the conjunctivae cleaned a good deal and the tumour slightly diminished in size.

As she was so *cold*, and had pains in the left side, she received from me *Ceanothus Americanus* 1, and so the treatment went on till August, 1885, when she was discharged quite cured; the remedies used after the *Ceanothus* were, in order named, with intervals of from one to six weeks between the remedies : *Merc. met.* 3, *Variol* C, *Bellis per.* I, *Medorrh.* C., and *Chionanthus* Q.

I several times saw and examined patient and can state that she continued quite well; the whites of her eyes are long since clean.

She has since happily married, and apropos hereof I may say that she *very* greatly improved in good looks under the treatment. Nor is this strange, for so long as the ovary was the seat of a tumour so long was it quite impossible for her to be other than plain : healthy ovaries are absolutely essential to good looks. How hideous those whose ovaries have been operated upon frequently become.

November, 1889 — She continues quite well, so she tells me in a chatty letter. (XX 248)

## 439. TUMOUR OF LEFT BREAST

A married lady, forty-two years of age, mother of seven children, was brought to me by her husband in the month of November, 1886, for a swelling in one of her breasts, which had been hurt. I found in the lowest third of her left breast a hardish tumour, of the size of a hen's egg, which was at times painful. Her menses were always too profuse, so that for many years she had never been able to get over the anaemia due to one period before another was there. Had leucorrhoea badly for many years. On the skin, in various regions, a number of wart-like excrescences. She had had measles, scarlatina and mumps, each twice, she informed me. Had also had variola, and besides this, she had been vaccinated four times, the last three times without success. This fact, together with some of the other already narrated morbid phenomena, viz. : the leucorrhoea, the wart-like excrescences, caused me to regard the case as one of vaccinosis, respectively sycosis.

*Thuja* 30 and *Mag. sul.* 3x enabled me to discharge her quite cured in four months.

Long afterwards she accompanied a near relation to consult me in his regard, when I took the opportunity of examining the breast, but could find no tumour.

The reason why the tumour yielded so promptly lay evidently in the fact that it was merely a hardened mass of normal tissue, and this hardening from infiltration only, I had intended following with *Bellis*, but the lump having disappeared no further treatment was needed.

That the *Thuja* was here the curative agent, I infer from the fact that I first prescribed it with palpable effect; *Mag. sulph.* was the second prescription, and when it was finished patient herself *asked for* the first-given remedy, i.e., the *Thuja*, because it had so much alleviated her menstrual inconveniences.

Patient did *not* know what remedies were given, so the value of her testimony is manifested.

I regarded the tumour as mammary infiltration from ovarian irritation started by trauma. (XX 255)

## 440. TUMOUR OF LEFT HIP

A strong powerfully built maiden lady, about fifty years of age, came under my observation on April 25th, 1889, telling me that she was very anxious about a tumour of her left hip.

An examination disclosed an inflamed hardened nearly circular patch of about the size of a florin depressed in the centre and scaly near its rim. She had spent the winter at the seaside in charge of an invalid, and having for some six months or so noticed a red mulberry-like growth at the above-mentioned spot, she sought to set her mind at rest by shewing said growth to the doctor when he came one day to see her ward. "You had better let me burn that away, or it might give you trouble some day," said he, and at a number of his subsequent visits he took a turn at the burning away proceeding.

The result was that he not only succeeded in burning away the growth, but went on "burning" till he had created a concavity about four times the size of the original growth and about as much below the cutaneous surface as the mulberry growth had been above it.

When the lady went home to Surrey with her charge the doctor urged her to return to him for a continuance of the cauterisation as soon as she could.

Happily better counsels prevailed and after several weeks of fruitless waiting to see if it would heal up, the patient came to me as the holder of a more gentle faith than *burning*.

In five months nothing remained but the hole to mark the *locus in quo*.

The remedies used were *Hydrastis canad.* Q and *Morbillin.* 30, each by itself month about. The use of the former was empirical tradition, of the latter the fact that she had had the measles badly as a child and had suffered much from "lungs." While taking the *Morbillin.* in infrequent dose, in powder-form, the place scaled off several times, and thus the thickening was got rid of.

Afterwards I enquired of her : Which did you more good, the powders or the drops? "Oh ! the powders; I have felt *so* much better ever since I had the powders."

When I reflect upon this case I say to myself thus :

The small tumid mass on the buttock was produced from within the patient, being thus produced from the interior of patient's organism, it is qualitatively and potentially only to be killed from within, *i.e.*, in its vital self; you can no more cure the thing by burning away the excrescence than you can cure the gout by cutting off the gouty toe.

*The growth is a vital product; the growing is a vital process proceeding centrifugally and towards a fixed point on the cutaneous periphery.* (XX 259)

## 441. TUMOUR OF LEFT BREAST

A lady of forty-four, married, but without children, and who had formerly been under my care for neuralgia and recurrent iritis, presented herself to me at the end of the year 1888, with a very hard tumour of the left breast about the size of her fist. The menopause was evidently there as there had been no period since October. Of course, the tumour caused great anxiety, but when I informed the lady that remedies would cure it, she simply accepted my statement and the sequel confirmed it.

The tumour had been as it were quiescent for nine years; that is to say, nine years previously patient had the ague (malarial fever) at San Sebastian, and it was this fever that was said to have caused a lump to come in the breast and which the doctors at the time thought would gather and discharge, but it did not and remained pretty much the same, till the period stopped in October, when it began all at once to grow, and that pretty fast.

Thinking the matter over it seemed manifest that if a lump would stay for nine years, there must be an internal cause — disposition — *ever operative*, for if it had not been *continuous* in its operativeness, the lump must have long since disappeared : a causeless lump cannot be.

Patient had long ago had congestion of the lungs and, moreover, her mother died of phthisis.

I regarded the general state as from the mother's phthisis, and therefore gave *Tuberculinum-C.* in very infrequent dose for several months and this greatly reduced the tumour in size, but it became *more* defined notwithstanding the decrease in size, and this rather struck me. The converse is commonly the case.

I then went back to the time of its origin and found that patient had had much quinine at that period, *i.e.* nine years previously. Now knowing that effects of quinine are long-lasting and at times antidoted by *Natrum mur.* I gave this latter in eight-grain doses of the sixth centesimal trituration three times a day.

March 19th, 1889 — Tumour well defined; size of a child's fist and hard.

$R_x$ Repeat the *Tubercul.* C.

April 1st — Tumour certainly smaller; the pips are numerous but not so florid.

$R_x$ *Fragaria vesca* Q (a very good mamma medicine in the Rademacherian sense, though not one of his medicines), ten drops in water night and morning.

April 23rd — Tumour about half gone. Patient much praises this medicine.

$R_x$ Repeat the *Tubercul.* C.

May 21st — The lump is smaller.

$R_x$ *Fragaria vesca* Q

June 25th — Lump about the same.

$R_x$ *Silicea* 6. Eight drops night and morning.

August 6th — "The lump in my breast is smaller but it is still there."

$R_x$ *Silicea* 12.

August 28th — "The lump in my breast is smaller; my skin is very spotty."

Rep.

November 20th — Tumour not quite gone.

$R_x$ Tc. *Pulsatilla nig.* Q. Four drops in water three times a day.

December 12th — Tc. *Hydrastis canadensis* Q.

January 17th, 1890 — Tumour qite gone.

February 6th — No trace of tumour.

18th — Discharged cured.

My conception of the actions of the remedies in this case may be thus stated. In the first place the *Tuberculinum* cured the maternal taint of tuberculosis; the *Natrum mur.* antidoted the long-lasting effects of the quinine; the *Fragaria vesca* acted upon the mammary organ as a gentle stimulant and woke its life up a little; the Silicea, Pulsatilla and *Hydrastis*

are homoeopathic remedies that may be termed standard polychrests. Let my theories go for just as much as they are worth, but *not* less than . . . The *tumour was cured* and patient remains well.
December, 1892 — Bringing a niece to me for a skin eruption, patient said : "You have never quite cured my spots."
What about the tumour?
"Oh! that's alright." (XX 263)

## 442. SMALL TUMOUR OF RIGHT TESTIS

In the early part of the year 1885, a gentleman came under my observation for a tiny tumour at the bottom of the right testis and about which he had consulted five medical men, of whom three are eminent surgeons of general renown. Opinions were divided as to whether it was of a specific nature of not.
As patient had had it over a year and as he had been very actively treated for it with the usual specifics; and, moreover, as the metal has an admitted affinity for the testis, I gave *Aurum metallicum* fourth trituration, and thereof six grains night and morning. This reduced the little lump about one-fourth.
*Hydrastis canadensis*, fifteen drops a day, in three doses, also did a little and lessened it still further.
There subsequently followed *Syph.* CC., *Psor.* 30, and *Bellis perennis* 1, and in the middle of the summer the tiny tumour had quite gone. It was only about the size of a small nut, but was very hard, irritating, and at times painful.
I saw the patient in 1887 and ascertained that the tumour had not returned.
October 9th, 1889 — The tumour has not returned and patient has continued in splended health.
"Not needed a doctor for years." (XX 270)

## 443. TUMOUR IN THE SHAFT OF THE PENIS

A gentleman, age 52, came under my observation on May 12, 1885, for a tumour of the penis of recent origin — practically recently recognized — and to which his attention had been forced by the fact that when in a state of orgasmic plethora it "looked round the corner." The thing was I thought a kind of bone-like deposit, as the feeling of it gave that impression. It was about two or three lines thick and of the size of a sixpenny piece. Patient had "gone the pace," and had been *blesse par V'enus* in every way known to M. Ricord : of course, lang syne.

He had a number of remedies, and was completely well of the tumour when I examined him on December 9th, 1886, and in the erect position of the member, the direction was straight or very nearly so. Oddly enough, his wife had been formerly cured by me of a tumour of a distinctly ugly character.

He had from me, in the order named, *Chelidonium majus* Q, *Med.* 30; *Urea* 6, *Chionanthus Virgin.* Q; *Med.* C.; *Syph.* CC.; *Stigmata maidis Fl. Ext.*; *Acid. nit.* 3x; *Stillingia sylvat.* Q; *Urea* 6; *Psor.* C.; *Acid. oxalic.* 3x, and *Acid. mur.* 6.

The greatest ameliorations followed *Syph.* and *Urea*, the former seeming to cure the disposition, while the latter very evidently cleared away the product of that disposition.

**Five Years Later** — In April, 1892, I saw him incidentally, when he brought a member of his family to me, and on my enquiry how this old trouble had behaved he said, "Oh! I have been first-rate ever since, it has never returned." (XX 272)

## 444. SWELLING OF THE BREAST AND THYROID

AT the end of the year 1885, a lady of sixty odd years of age came under my observation for a tumour in her neck. Examination showed it to be, seemingly, hypertrophy of the right side of the thyroid gland, which latterly had begun to encroach upon the left one. She had a good deal of salivation, worse towards morning. She says she has usually her ailings in her left side.

In addition to the tumour in the neck, there was also a circumscribed swelling in the outer half of the right breast, which caused her great alarm. She feels very chilly, and has many sensations as of pins and needles. She is also very twitchy.

$R_x$ *Med.* C. in infrequent dose.

December 30th, 1885 — The thyroid tumour, much to my amazement, is distinctly smaller.

Treatment was continued at irregular intervals, and patient was discharged cured on February 27th, 1889, and continues well of the two tumours, and in the enjoyment of capital health.

A good many remedies were of course used, such as *Bellis perennis* Q, *Hydrastis Canadensis* Q, *Baptisia tinctoria* 1, *Tubercul.* C., which did her more good, perhaps, than any remedy she ever took.

In my judgement the two nosodes were essentially the curative agents in this case, and the intercurrent remedies, though needfully helpful, were still not other than empirically indicated on lines already amply dwelt upon. (XX 274)

## 445. SMALL TUMOUR OF LEFT BREAST LYMPHOMATOUS TUMOURS OF NECK

A young lady of 17 years of age was brought by her mother to me on February 25th, 1890, for a small tumour in the left breast that had already been reduced in size by homoeopathic treatment, and also, and principally, for large strumous glands all round her neck under the jaw, giving the young lady an almost hideous aspect, she being very full in the face. She had never been ill till she had the measles at the age of two; the next summer pertussis, thereafter scarlatina, then the glands of the neck became very large, after this she had varicella and typhoid, all very badly; convulsions with nearly all of them. One sees a scar of ancient date in the neck.

After *Scarlatina* C. the tumour in breast — a very small affair — could no longer be found. The glands under the jaw were not altered much, if any.

Under *Bacill.* C., the glands began to lessen in size materially, but a visit to the seaside made them worse again.

July 20th — *Thuja occid.* 30.

October 31st — The contour of the lower jaw can now be readily distinguished, whereas when I first saw the patient, her face and neck ran into one another, the flesh of both being on the same level. "But," said the young lady's mother, "it was not the last powders that did that, but the ones before."

$R_x$ *Bacill.* C.

December 11th, 1890 — The swelling of the glands has about three-fourths gone. Then followed two or three other remedies, and finally the *Bacillinum* again.

Patient paid me her last visit just a year ago. The young lady has come out and been to a number of balls, and is highly delighted. Her mother sent me a photograph of the young lady taken after the cure, and though the neck looks to me still a little full, others do not notice it, nor do the ladies themselves.

This case must be taken side by side with the subject of tuberculosis generally; and in regard to tubercular or strumous glands, it must be remembered that strumous glands may be tubercular, and nothing else, or they may be tubercular *and* . . .

And that is why an indiscriminatingly routine treatment with the zoic specific *must* often fail inasmuch as remedies — at any rate highly dynamized remedies can never cure anything other than that to which they are homoeopathic.

I am here and there struck with the fact that, for instance, *Bacill.* will not act till *Thuja* has been given and then it will act beautifully : the vaccinosis evidently barring the way, much as Hahnemann teaches in regard to psora and the use of *Sulphur* intercurrently. (XX 278)

## 446. CANCER OF THE BREAST

A married lady, 35 years of age, was brought by her husband to me on December 17th, 1888. She had four children, baby being four years old. She had been operated on for cancer of the left breast, some months previously the whole breast — a very large one — being totally ablated, and now a tumour has come again in the right breast, and the old scar has become very painful.

Patient was totally wrecked in her nerves, could not sleep and swayed to and fro in awful dread and fear, exclaiming oh! and ah! being willing and anxious to go anywhere and do anything.

Her hurrying up and down hither and thither I could compare only to the way a hyaena hurries up and down in its cage, and it is almost pathognomonic of the very worst type of cancer, and therefore a symptom I much dislike. An aunt of hers has cancer she tells me, but otherwise her family history is good. She has been twice vaccinated and has had scarlatina and "nerves."

She has a good deal of acne here and there, some of the little inflammatory nodules getting large and very angry.

The cure took just two years, and I could declare her quite cured at the end of the year 1890.

At my special request she resumed ordinary married life again with her husband, she promising me that should she ever have another child she would suckle it with the one remaining breast. There followed cessation of the period in February, 1891, she was safely delivered of a very sweet, healthy little boy in September, and she has very successfully suckled the little mannie with her one breast; and there is now nothing very unusual about this lady, except that she looks *very* thriving, and possesses only one breast.

And the treatment?

Patient received from me in the order named — *Urtica urens* Q, *Psor.* 30, *Hydrastis Can.* Q, *Bellis perennis* Q, *Bacill.* C., *Thuja* 30, *Acid. hippuric.* 5, *Helonias* Q, *Ignatia am.* 1, *Rhus tox.* 3x, *Bacillin.* CC., *Cypripedin.* 3x, and one or two others, and I must leave the case now, which I can do all the more willingly as *the competent can see the reasons for them; for the incompetent I am not writing.*

Very notable surgeons, fellows of the Royal Society, and others are at times condescendingly hopeful that we look forward to the day when "a *remedy* for cancer will be discovered." Whatever knowledge such people possess, or do not possess, there are two things of which they know nothing real, viz., cancer, and the modes of action of remedies in cancer and cancerous diseases.

People may be so eminent that they reach to the topmost heaven, but a concatenation of morbid complexities, each one of which is a vital process, *never* can in the very nature of things be cured by "one" anything.

You might as well try to grow potatoes in a field consisting of *one* chemical element instead of ordinary humus' or live in the hope of some day being able to win a long and very difficult game of chess by making "one" move all by itself.

*This running after a remedy for any disease of a complex nature is simple ignorance of fundamental principles, and bars the road of progress. Cancer is a chain of links, and each kind has links of different nature and each link is a biological process. And you are going to alter all that with "A" remedy*? It is absolutely unthinkable, and has no parallel in pharmaco-biological phenomena. (XX 282)

## 447. SMALL TUMOUR OF PENIS

An unmarried gentleman, member of a learned profession, 46 years of age, came under my professional care on Nov. 14, 1882, for a hard lump on the middle of the shaft of the penis that had been there some months and that was probably of a specific nature. The treatment lasted 13 months, when there was no trace of it left. Patient had *Aur. met.* 4 trituration, and 3, *Aur. mur.* 3, *Thuja* 30, *Platinum* 5 trit., *Kali chlor.* 4x, *Chelid. maj.* Q, *Liquor sode chlor.*, three drops in water night and morning; *Syp.* 200, *Hepar* 3x, and *Sepia* 3x.

**Three Years Later** — In 1886 I saw this gentleman, and ascertained from inspection and palpation that there had been no return of the tumour. The nature of the tumour appeared to me to have been cartilaginous. (XX 288)

## 448. OSTEOMA PENIS

A married gentleman, verging on fifty years of age, came under my observation on November 23, 1888, for certain eye and heart symptoms, acne, and principally for a bony tumour in the shaft of the virile member. He had *Thuja* 30, *Strophanthus* 1, *Ceanothus Am.* 1, and *Bellis perennis* Q, and then *Vaccinin*. C. and thus a year or so passed without patient having mustered courage enough to tell me of his bony tumour; in fact he did not tell me till the month of September, 1890.

In the shaft, a little below the dorsal surface, I found a plate of bone an inch and a half long, and about three-quarters of an inch broad. Its edge felt sharp and of course the organ was held out at an angle to the body, and slightly to the left.

Patient informed me that he had not been fully aware of its presence till three months previously, and then because of its inconvenience on particular occasions, and on account of his clothes. The organ was not the seat of any actual pain, but it ached intensely and persistently; bending himself somewhat forward patient would often distort his face slightly and say, "It aches."

There is absolutely no history or soupcon of any thing specific; and patient is a teetotaler and a nonsmoker, and otherwise a man of irreproachable history and life.

I therefore took, as therapeutic basis, the one elementary and undoubted fact that there was a bony tumour, and prescribed *Hecla lava* 30, five drops in water night and morning. This was on September 17, 1890. And, lest I forget it, I will just add that patient lived then (and lives now) on the chalk whence his drinking water is habitually obtained, but latterly he boils it beforehand.

October 29th, 1890 — The osseous plate is distinctly smaller and thinner, but copulation continues to be very painful.

$R_x$ Rep.

December 3rd — The bone is rather smaller; copulation not quite so painful or awkward, but the organ aches very much.

$R_x$ *Aurum metallicum*, 4th trituration, in eight grain doses at bedtime. And in support of this prescription there was also long-standing diplopia of the auric kind.

January 5th, 1891 — The osteoma penis is about three-fourths gone, but patient complains a good deal of indigestion.

Rep.

January 30th — The eye is better, but there is no further improvement in the bony mass.

$R_x$ *Hecla lava* 12, ten drops in water at bedtime.

March 6th — The eye is not quite so well, but the bony tumour has further diminished in size.

$R_x$ *Aurum met.*, 4 trit. Eight grains at bedtime.

April 29th — The bony tumour is now reduced to a gristly cord, all its boniness having gone; at first it was a longitudinal oblong plate, with a bony feel and sharp edges; now it feels like a tiny rope, but laterally not quite so defined as a rope would be.

$R_x$ *Sodium silico-fluoride* 6; ten drops in water at bedtime.

June 19th — Although the plate of bone has gone, the ridge of hard cord still exists from end to end, but not quite so cord-like.

$R_x$ *Aur. met.*, 3 trit. Eight grains dry on the tongue at bedtime.

August 7th — Patient feels well, but there is still the gristly rope-like remains of the old bony plate.

$R_x$ *Silicate of Sodium* . Five drops in water night and morning.

Nov. 6th — It is gone. *Arnica* 1.

January 29th, 1892 — There is no return of the tumour, but we can just feel a little gristly node in the shaft, and when erect the organ turns aside somewhat.

$R_x$ *Aurum met.* 12.

April 11th, 1892 — Quite well of the part, except that when erect the axis deviates somewhat, so he says. No doubt the tumour overstretched or destroyed some of the fibres, so that although all the tumour has disappeared, the tissue of its seat has lost some of its contractility; in other words the tissue within puckers slightly.

December, 1892 — Cure holds good.

Easter, 1898 — Still quite well; I examined the part 3 days ago. (XX 289)

## 449. KELOID OF FACE

A foreign gentleman, 32 years of age, unmarried, came under my observation on January 22nd, 1886. His flat-backed nose made me think of syphilis. His right ear and the skin in front of it were the seat of a new formation of scar-tissue, in extent about that of a child's palm, but with irregular contour; it was red in part, and portions were shiny and contracted with certain bridles of tissue produced by the contraction, the portion on the concha itself was not so distinctly cicatricial. It was very evidently on the increase.

There were little spots from which a circumscribed inflammatory process seemed to start and finally these ended in scar. I am not very sure that it could be called true Keloid, but it was a new formation of scar-tissue, and I do not know what else to term it.

Besides this he had eczema marginatum on the inner surface of the left thigh. But patient did not really come for this primarily, but rather for an inveterate gonorrhoea of six months' standing that had defied treatment by old school and new, low dilutions and high potencies. The scarring process in the face arrested my attention as being very unsightly and of more interest than a common urethrorrhoea.

In view of his *nez camus* I began the treatment with *Syp*. CC. Slight improvement in both keloid and gonorrhoea. *Medorrh*. 30 also improved both processes a little, but neither had done anything worth while. It turned out that he had had his first gonorrhoea ten years previously, which had been silenced by injections without much trouble. At the end of March I ordered *Thuja occid*. 30 which increased the flow from the urethra very much, but vastly improved the keloid. I then tried *Med*. C. and thereafter *Kali chl*. 6 but with no advantage. The discharge was much more free in the evening and the keloidal dermatitis was very sore when he was lying down. Then for several months patient treated himself with *Sulphur* and *Mercurius* 3x, but no further improvement followed. He had given up my treatment because the last remedy which I gave him in July, viz., *Vaccininum* 30, had made his gonorrhoea flux more profuse and more yellow, and caused great activity in the keloid. I went over his case afresh and noted that his lips were constantly peeling, and he was in the habit of biting off the lose bits of skin. Here I gave *Malandrinum* CC., this was on December 8, 1886. In eight days he returned stating that this remedy had given a new start to his gleet and turned it into a gonorrhoea of the first water, and in examining the parts there was every appearance of a gonorrhoea with profuse yellow discharge. I told him to continue with his *Malandrinum* CC.

January 5th, 1887 — Has had a gathering in his prepuce which discharged for 10 days; the urethral discharge has much diminished. The keloid greatly improved.

*Sepia* 6 then finished the gleet, but the keloid, though slowly improving, for a long time under the different remedies still lingered on.

In March he had *Sabina* 30 for about a month, and thereafter *Cupressus Lawsoniana* 30 for a number of weeks, which finished the cure, and when he showed himself to me in the summer of 1887, I could certainly tell where the keloidal process had been, but its activity was quite extinct, the scar had lost all redness and the remains gave me the impression that he might at one time have had a small burn at the part. Long afterwards his brother consulted me and told me that the cure had proved permanent. (XX 295)

## 450. TWO TUMOURS

A gentleman, twenty-four years of age, unmarried, and following a literary occupation, came under my observation on October 31, 1881, complaining of two tumours. One was very hard, and he had noticed it about two months; it was about the size of a walnut, and seated on the ribs behind on a level with the top of the liver; anteriorly to this a fatty tumour of the size of a half-penny bun; has had this lipoma all his life, and it is now distinctly growing.

$R_x$ *Psorinum* 30; one pilule at bedtime.

November 28th — Both tumours are smaller, the lipoma being also softer.

$R_x$ Rep.

January 9th, 1882 — The hard tumour is gone; the lipoma softer.

$R_x$ Rep.

February 10th — The fatty tumour is still softening.

$R_x$ Rep.

March 6th — The lipoma is still getting softer, and in its upper half is also flatter.

$R_x$ Rep.

April 3rd — $R_x$ Rep.

June 12th — The lipoma is smaller, flatter and softer.

$R_x$ Nil.

July 3rd — Still diminishing.

$R_x$ Nil.

August 2nd — At a standstill.

$R_x$ *Psorinum* 30; one pilule at bedtime.

September 4th — Smaller.

$R_x$ Nil.

September 25th — still smaller.

$R_x$ Nil.

October 23rd — Smaller still, and notably flatter.

December 15th — The tumour very slowly is becoming smaller and softer.

$R_x$ Nil.

February 5th, 1883 — Standstill.

$R_x$ *Psorinum* 30; one pilule dry on the tongue at bedtime.

July 13th — Still diminishing.

$R_x$ Rep.

May 5th, 1884 — There is now only a vestige of the lipoma left, and patient discharged himself.

This case is remarkable as having been treated by one remedy only during the whole time, and one dilution of that one remedy, viz., the 30th; and always the same dose, viz., one pilule.

The remedy was here and there omitted, and when the progress seemed to stop it was again renewed. On the ribs at the back of the liver is a favourite site of these bun-shaped lip-omata.

*P.S.* — About three years before I saw him, this gentleman suffered from a pustular eruption of his hands, for which Dr. A. C. Pope prescribed

*Silicea* 30; but as he only prescribed once, I suspect someone's ointment followed. But I have no positive information on this point. (XX 300)

## 451. LIPOMA CRURIS

A married lady, childless, came under my care on August 1, 1888 for a fatty tumour of the right thigh, near the vulva. Or rather she came under my care really for severe piles, "to avoid an operation," she having heard that I did not think highly of operations. The piles having been cured, her husband enquired whether the fatty tumour could be likewise got rid of by medicines. I replied that I would try, saying that I would at any rate do her no harm.

Patient had often miscarried, and had had a polypus removed from the edge of *os uteri* in former years by operation. She remained long under my treatment, and finally gave it up from weariness; and she did this the more readily as, though the lipoma is not gone, it is very greatly reduced in size. When I took her in hand the tumour, coming exactly between the thickest part of thighs, rendered ordinary walking very difficult. This it no longer does, walking being now comfortable.

Has been four times vaccinated. Is liable to cystitis, which she has had three times. She has also had rheumatic fever and severe sciatica. *Cupressus Lawsonianna, Thuja occid.* and *Sabina* are the remedies that did her good.

Of all tumours, ivory osteomata and lipomata, and certain cystomata, I find the most difficult to touch.

The fatty tumours seem very indolent, and though I generally get them down about one-half or two-thirds, I do not succeed beyond that. Fatty tumours appear to arise from friction, as in this case from the rubbing of the fleshy thighs against one another — as witness the *lipoma professionale* of certain Russian women. Of course, the friction is only the exciting cause, there is the neoplastic disposition behind. They are more common in women than in men, and I know several cases where the exciting cause is evidently due to the friction of the corsets.

I have sometimes thought that the disposition is of a sycotic nature, but I have still an open mind on the subject, and await "more light." (XX 304)

## 452. SMALL LIPOMATOUS CYST

A young lady of ten years of age was brought to me by her mother on March 22, 1889, to be treated for a tumour in the wall of the left side of the abdomen, which had been probed and poulticed by two homoeopathic practitioners. The lump would not go notwithstanding the homoeopathic poulticing and the homoeopathic probing, and then the help of a consultant from St. B's Hospital was obtained, but the tumour would not yield.

After a month under *Thuja occidentalis* 30, the tumour was well on the wane, and without any other treatment slowly withered and disappeared altogether.

**Two Years Later** — There has been no return of the tumour. (XX 306)

## 435. OVARIAN TUMOUR

September 29th, 1886 — On this date a gentleman brought his wife to me for my opinion in regard to a pretty large tumour situate in the region of the right ovary, and which the local doctors had decided, with their permission, to excise.

Patient is forty-five years of age, childless; many years married. The tumour had been coming for seven years, it felt very tense, but whether it was a cyst or fibrous, or what, opinions were divided. In size it is about as big as a baby's head and globular in shape. The lump had only really obtruded itself much upon her notice for the past four months. Leucorrhoea for many years, which diminishes as the tumour gets larger.

Much sinking at the stomach, dyspepsia (long treated as nervous), severe stomachic pains; no pains in the tumour proper; costive; very nervous; once vaccinated; she is very weak, and tired, skin tawny and in parts were brown. "I have always had good, but delicate health; I am bilious but never had any disease, but I once had 'inflammation in the side.'" She is the only child of a father who died at twenty-five years of age of phthisis, and her mother died at sixty-five, of bronchitis.

The treatment lasted over *five years*, in fact nearly six, as I began to treat her in the month of September, 1886, and did not discharge her as absolutely well till September, 1891, when I very carefully examined the lady and could not find any remains of the tumour whatever.

There were three reasons that conduced to rendering the duration of the cure very long, and they were these. First of all the patient was diseased all over, her original crasis was bad, and hence it was not merely a question of curing a tumour as a morbid product and the constitutional disposition thereto, but quite apart from the tumour the patient was ill throughout anteriorly to the neoplastic development, and in this case at any rate it is fair to assume that though the operation had been safely and successfully performed, still that would not have touched the previously-existing diseasedness of the lady's tissues.

In the second place the cure was interrupted and much retarded by a bad carriage accident that happened during its course. And finally the patient lived a very long way off and I only saw her about five times during the whole time; and I might add that the treatment was often interrupted by domestic circumstances, so that though six years elapsed, I find I prescribed altogether about thirty different times, mostly by letter on patient's own reports.

She had from me in the order named — *Sulph.* 30, *Syph.* CC., *Med.* C., *Sepia* 6, *Bryonia* 3x, *Bellis peren.* I, *Cundurango* I, *Aurum* mur. *nat.* 3x, *Platin. mur.* 3x, *Nux* 1x, *Syph.* CC., *Bacill.* C., *Hepar* 3x, *Iodoformum* 3x, *Nux vom.* 1x, *Bryonia* Q, *Salufer.* 5, *Viscum album* 3x, *Fucus vesiculosus* Q, *Hepar* 30, *Trifolium prat.* Q, and *Aur. brom.* 3.

Looking back on the case I am of opinion that it is one of inflammatory cystoma, having its first start in the inflammation in the side.

Patient is now in excellent health, and wrote me a graceful and grateful letter not many days ago quite of her own accord, merely that I might know that my labour of years had not been thrown away. (XX 308)

## 454. RIGHT OVARIAN TUMOUR

A childless married lady, twenty-seven years of age, came to consult me on March 17th, 1885, for a lump in the right side of the abdomen and severe leucorrhoea.

She had been married three years. She complained of feeling tired on awaking in the morning, with a nasty bitter taste in her mouth; severe frontal headaches; had backache low down; feels sick now and again; face spotty; chin pimply on the left side. The size of the "lump in the right side" I find I did not note, but it was readily felt and pointed out by the patient herself. Womb thickened, heavy and lying very low down.

She had been once vaccinated and had had measles, scarlatina and varicella. The origin of the tumour is referred by the patient to falling against, or off a stile. About this time I had been reading of the good results obtained, by a New York gynecologist, in uterine and ovarian tumours and indurations, from medicated sponges placed within a vagina and left there, and which were used in this case, the medication being with Mercurius cor. 6.

These sponges "acted very severely, causing copious discharge of a most offensive kind."

$R_x$ *Psor.* 30.

April 14th — "The appearance of the sponges is now entirely different; now the discharge is yellow and there is no blood, but very offensive;

difficulty in passing water" *in the early morning*.

$R_x$ *Med*. 30, and continue the sponges.

May 30th — "For eight or nine days the pain in the back continued to be very troublesome, some mornings I could scarcely breathe without causing a very sharp pain; this passed off after I had been up an hour; frequent headaches, feeling of sickness whenever I sat up or walked about."

Here I discontinued the use of the sponges as I found not only in this, but in other cases, that their use was fraught with so much discomfort and suffering to the patient, and after all was only local messing and could, in the nature of things, only affect the product of the disposition, and not the disposition itself. Moreover, although the same piece of sponge was only used once, the discharge was rendered very foul and most unpleasant to the lady herself.

*The fact is, the vagina is self-cleansing, and the less it is mechanically interfered with the better*. All these modern difficulty-producing disinfecting injections are irrational, nasty and hurtful, except where there are lesions of continuity of extraneous origin, i.e., not a part of the disease-process itself.

$R_x$ *Med*. C.

July 23rd — The tumour is more than half gone; the chin is covered with hard indolent pimples : whites nearly well; is now much freer from pain at the menstrual period than she has ever been in her life. Very much better all round.

$R_x$ *Bellis*. *p*. 1.

August 23rd — Back very bad, she has retrograded.

$R_x$ *Med*. C.

This did her so much good that I did not hear of her for six months, when I found only a small rest of the tumour, but the uterus itself was stll enlarged.

Here followed *Helonin* 3x in eight-grain doses a day, for a month; then *Aletris farinosa* Q, fifteen drops a day, as an organ remedy, until patient had taken a fluid ounce, and finally, two months of *Aurum muriaticum nat*. 3x.

This brought us to the fall of 1886.

March 18th, 1890 — "I am quite well and walk eight miles a day." (XX 312)

### 455. OVARIAN TUMOUR

I. A lady of thirty years of age, mother of one child, was brought by her husband to me on January 14, 1891, to know whether it was absolutely necessary that she be operated on for the lump in her right side; sad lump was in the position of the right ovary, and about the size of a large orange, and not very well defined.

Its exact nature I could not determine, the examination not being facilitated by very sufficient adipose layers. The tumour *ached* a great deal, and there was leucorrhoea. There; being , certainly rather vague, history of trauma, I ordered *Bellis per.* Q. Ten drops in water night and morning.

February 11th — *Sodium Bromide* 3x. Eight grains night and morning.

March 11th — Last period seven days too soon; thereafter leucorrhoea. The tumour aches.

$R_x$ *Apis* 6. Ten drops in water night and morning.

April 27th — The tumour is smaller; an irritable tongue.

$R_x$ *Colocynth* 12. Ten drops at bedtime.

May 25th — Very much better; sides of tongue frothy.

$R_x$ *Sodium bromide* 3x trit. eight grains at bedtime.

June 22nd — Well; tumour no longer to be found. Discharged cured.

In cases of this sort which yeld in a few months to remedies, their very amenability to the remedies destroys the diagnosis, hence it can only be with the aid of very large experience that we shall be able to construct a therapy of tumours with something like positive differential indications. All being well, I shall, by and by, attempt a few differentiations, but at present I do not feel I have quite sufficient data to go upon. (XX 317)

**II.** March 11th, 1885. — On this date a married lady, forty-two years of age, mother of six children, came to me for an abdominal tumour, situated in the region of the left ovary, with pretty severe concomitant vaginal haemorrhage and slight leucorrhoea. She had been twice vaccinated, and also had had variola. The tumour was long from side to side, *i. e.*, it lay transversely seemingly from the uterus to some six inches to the left, to where the left-hand end of an ovarian tumour would very likely be. The bleeding was at any time and in any position. The tumour had been there, and the bleeding, for about ten months, and were supposed to have had their origin in a fright. Previous to the fright the menses had always been regular, but scanty. Much pain in the tumour.

$R_x$ *Thuja occidentalis* 30.

This cured the bleeding, and the period became normal. But the pain in the tumid mass was worse; the abdomen became more distended; and patient complained very much that when once awake in the very early morning she could not get off again.

$R_x$ *Bellis perennis* 1.

April 15th — No haemorrhage; period normal, except that it is very painful in the left side. Patient feels very ill, faint, and fidgety, and has dreadful backache.

℞ *Variol.* 30.

After this patient felt somewhat better, but tumour was no smaller.

Sepember 3rd — *Psor.* 30.

October 3rd — She is very much better, but bad leucorrhoea has set in, and it now transpires that patient formerly suffered very much from leucorrhoea, which had yielded to suppressive treatment, and after *Variol.* C. there was vaginal haemorrhage which lasted twenty-five days, the period having previously missed. There are many flat warts on the body; much pain in the left side.

November 10th — *Med.* C.

February 2nd, 1886 — This remedy produced a very violent aggravation lasting several weeks, when health returned, the side was practically well, and the tumour was gone.

After this a little swelling of the spleen and liver had to be righted, as also some indigestion, and this *Myrica cerifera* 3x and *Ceanothus am.* I speedily affected, when patient happily passed her change of life.

**Six Years Later** — April 19th, 1892 — I this day carefully examined the patient — as I have done several times during the six years that have elapsed since the tumour was cured — but find no trace of any tumour, and patient is in good health and condition; I claim, therefore, that the cure is a Hunterian one, as not only is the tumour got rid of — the product of the disposition — but the disposition itself is likewise cured. (XX 320)

**III.** An unmarried lady, 48 years of age, whose mother and grandmother died of cancer, as also did one of her mother's sisters, and one of her own sisters has been cured by me of two small tumours, came to me on December 20, 1884, for tumour of the left ovary, almost exactly like the one I have just described; I therefore need not describe it. This lady's most urgent symptoms were leucorrhoea and severe bleeding from the vagina, lasting for weeks at a time. Her period has always been profuse, but formerly lasted only five days, but now it has continued for three weeks. She has been three times vaccinated, and has suffered severely from left-sided neuralgia; the treatment lasted uninterruptedly till August 7th, 1886, but the notes are so volunminous that I forbear to transcribe them, so I will just pick out the salient therapeutic features only.

*Thuja occid.* 30 very materially lessened the leucorrhoea; she had it at intervals for several months.

*Phosphorus* C. completely controlled the haemorrhage for some time; but did not cure it; it recurred. The real cure of the tumour was effected by *Med*. 30, *Sepia* 3x, *Med.* C, and *Psor.* C; the *Kal. chlor.* helped.
The only other interesting point was the fact that *Sanguisuga* off. 3x trituration (a capital and genuinely homoeopathic styptic) given after the *Phosphorus* had ceased to act, stopped the haemorrhage for good and all; it never returned, and that is over six years ago. *Phosphorus* C. was, however, twice given afterwards for little "shows," after which the change of life was established, and patient continues in excellent health to this day, with the sole exception of some nerve twitchings of long standing, and which I have never succeeded in touching.
As five years and a half testify to the cure, I think it fulfils John Hunter's conditions. (XX 323)

## 456. HARD MAMMARY TUMOUR

An unmmarried lady, resident in London, thirty-eight years of age, came to consult me on January 13th, 1890 for a hard tumour on the left side of her chest, that had been growing for the past three years, and is now about the size of an orange.
In the left breast there is a hard tumour, moveable, lying between the mammilla and the manubrium sterni; the left nipple is scabby; left arm aches and feels weak, left breast itself aches. Patient's parents were cousins; father died at 46 of typhoid; mother still living and well, although she had had an ovarian tumour taken away by operation when 21 years of age; patient's only brother is alive.
Three years ago patient knocked her left breast against a post, and she thinks her hard stays have had something to do with it; she is of full figure.
She had been twice vaccinated on the left arm, and her mother says that the first time "her arm was so bad she thought it would come off."
She has had varicella.
The tumour gets larger in wet weather, and before the menses. Her left ear gathers off and on for years.
$R_x$ *Vaccinin* C.
February 14th — Better; less tired and less weariness; the left ear gathers less; tumour rather smaller, but it is very hard, and nodulated; nipple less incrusted; the left arm is now comfortable; she asks for the same powders again.
Patient is dusky and tawny, *ergo, Bacill.* C.
March 17th — Lump is smaller; she looks better : "it was the first powders that took away the weariness."
$R_x$ *Vaccin*. C.
(The nipple is less incrusted.)

April 23rd — The nipple is cleaner.
$R_x$ *Bellis per.* Q; ten drops in water night and morning.
June 4th — Says she is not so well; her complexion is much clearer.
$R_x$ *Thuja occid.* 30.
July 9th — Better; the tumour is not so defined and not so hard, and the nodules are less distinct. There is now no incrustation of the nipples.
$R_x$ *Sabina* 30.
October 15th — The lump is very much better, and now is barely more than hardened milk-ducts. The left nipple is scabby again. The left ear gathers more; the breast is no longer influenced by wet.
$R_x$ *Cupressus Lawson.* 30.
January 7th, 1891 — The tumour has not quite gone.
$R_x$ *Bursa pastoris* 1x; five drops in water night and morning.
December 20th, 1891 — Discharged cured of the tumour, and in excellent health. (XX 327)

## 457. CONGENITAL VASCULAR TUMOUR

Mrs. K. brought her one-year-old baby-girl to me on July 28, 1881. I found on the girlie's back, just to right of the spinal column and below the angle of the scapula, a red vascular tumour of the size of half a walnut, but flatter and more spread out; it was there at birth, and had been growing a good deal lately.

At birth it was not quite so large as a six-penny piece, and it was flat; now it is almost three-quarters of an inch above the niveau. On the outside of the right thigh there had been a similar growth but much smaller, but that has gone all but a few little blood-vessels; the wee patient is in good health, ails nothing, and is fat; has nine teeth, and is beginning to walk.

The family doctor very strongly urged its removal by operation because it had taken to grow so much, but being of opinion that the vascular tumour must have an internal cause of some kind, and as I can, personally, not see how a knife could possibly modify that, I advised its careful medicinal treatment, to the end that a truly Hunterian cure might be effected.

Having nothing to guide me I went on hypotheses, and gave in succession *Thuja* 30, *Ferr. phos.* 6 trit., Q; *Phos.* 1000, whereupon it shrank somewhat. Thereupon came *Psor.* 30, *Sul.* 30, *Chenopodium* 3x, *Lycopod.* CC., *Merc. Met.* C. and CC., *Syph.* CC., and here I see the note "vastly improved," and after *Merc.* "decidedly smaller."

*Thuja* 30 and C., *Aur. met.* 12, *Fragaria vesca* 12, 1x, and *Syph.* CC., finished the treatment and the cure.

It is over ten years since this little lady was brought to me, and the tumour was years before it finally withered and went. I saw patient's mother not many days since, and was informed, on enquiry, that the tumour had never shown any sign of returning since the year 1884 or 1885; and the young lady's back is quite normal in all respects.
I have cured several such vascular tumours on the same lines, but this was the largest of all and the most difficult to cure; the smaller ones need therefore not be further referred to. (XX 330)

## GOUT AND ITS CURE

### 458. GOUT

I. Two years since a middle-aged gentleman of position was down with an attack of gout that had relapsed over and over again, and he had then been in and out of these attacks for nearly six months. He had been swamped with alkalies and *Colchicum*, and mercilessly purged and lulled with narcotics most alarmingly. He thought he would "try homoeopathy," and sent for the writer. I put him on *Urtica urens* as already described, and he was out and about in a fortnight. In a couple of days of the treatment his urine became dark, plentiful, and loaded with uric acid gravel. His enthusiasm knew no bound, and he declared that no remedy he had ever taken (and he had had attacks of gout over and over again, and had taken pretty well all known gout medicines) had really touched his gout like the *Urtica*. With him and his club intimates I became known as Dr. Urtica. (XXI 43)
II. A gentleman of 50 odd years of age, now resident in London, consulted me for gout in the fall of the year 1890. He had long lived in India and suffered much from malaria. After a few weeks of *Urtica*, 10 drops in a wineglassful of water night and morning, he was free from gout, and "My diarrhoea has gone, my gout also; my digestion is better than for long, and my skin is much cleaner." (XXI 45)
III. At the end of the year 1893 the wife of a country squire in Nothunberland wrote me in great haste that her goodman was down with a severe bout of gout, and would I send him medicine forthwith. I ordered him ten drops of the tincture (*Urtica urens*) three times a day, and this rather large dose as he is a very big man, of a somewhat thirsty disposition. I heard no more of the matter; but three or four months later the lady consulted me on her own account here in London, and incidentally remarked, "That medicine soon cured my husband's gout, and he

has not had any since," As before remarked, there is fever with the gouty attack, and a remedy to meet it homoeopathically should show its power of producing fever. *Urtica urens*, in my hands, has produced fever over and over again. In most cases in which its administration was followed by febrile symptoms there was, at least, an antecedent history of malarialism, or actually of recent or remote ague, but this was not invariably the case. Moreover the same thing obtains in regard to *China*. Hahnemann had had ague before he proved the bark on himself and found out its fever-producing power, on which such a huge superstructure has been so solidly erected, — *i. e.*, homoeopathy. (XXI 45)

### 459. THE PATHOGENETIC FEVER OF *URTICA URENS*

On October 3, 1893, a mother of a family, pretty strong, 42 years of age, came under my care for flatulent dyspepsia. No history of ague or malaria. She complained of left sided pain, with coldness and chilli ness, which led me to prescribe *Urtica urens* Q, 10 drops in water, night morning. She reported: "I cannot go on with his medicine; it sets all my pulses beating, makes me terribly giddy, makes me feel as if I were going to topple (forwards) in my bed, and then a bad headache comes on, and when I take it at night it makes me very feverish, so I am leaving it off."

Just nine months later I saw this lady, and inquired if she remembered the very first remedy I gave her. "Oh! yes; it made me terribly giddy, and when I took it at night it brought on fever, so I could not go on with it; and, indeed, I still have some of it left at home now." When she took the *Urtica* in the morning she did not observe that it caused any feverish symptoms, only when she took it at night. The fever of gout generally comes on at night. (XXI 47)

### 460. BOILS

A middle-aged Indian officer suffering from scinde boils consulted me at the end of September, 1893 for said boils, that were growing worse rather than better, although he had been home on their account on leave for five months. He received from me *Urtica* Q, 12 drops in water night and morning, because I regarded it as of malarial nature, for he had had ague years ago, and was still in the habit of taking quinine off and on for fear of its returning, since almost any cold would bring it back. The taking of the *Urtica* was followed by a furious outburst of fever, so severe that patient's condition caused his friends considerable anxiety. He however, made a quick and complete recovery. (XXI 49)

## 461. MALARIALISM

Another case was also that of an officer invalided home from India suffering from "liver" and malarialism, and to whom I gave 10 drops of *Urtica urens* twice a day for his general condition. This, too, was followed with very severe fever with unusually long stages, from which he recovered under *Natrum muriaticum*, 6 trituration, 6 grains every two hours. The subsequent report being — "Those powders cured the fever, but he was very much pulled down."

It is distinctly curious to note the remarkable effects of *Natrum muriaticum* and *Urtica urens* in gout, as well as in ague and malarialism. (XXI 50)

## 462. NEPHRITIC CALCULI

*By S. W. C. Brown, Surgeon to Trindad Hospital, Colorado.*

"The author having been a sufferer from nephritic calculi during the past seven years, and helped at last by *Piperazine* after all other remedies had been tried without relief, brings his own case before the profession in the somewhat deficient state of literature.

"His trouble commenced about seven years ago with a sudden attack of nephritic colic, accompanied by the passage of urate crystals, so sharply defined and so numerous that the mucous membrane was cut by them. They increased in number until half a teaspoonful was passed with each evacuation of the bladder, generally accompanied by haematuria. The body-weight at this time was 260 lbs., urine of normal specific gravity, containing pus corpuscles, blood, and epithelial cells. Shortly after this attack eight calculi were passed, five being unusually large, and all exceedingly painful, unconsciousness supervening in the case of four from three to fifteen hours.

"During the past seven years every sudden jar or jolt produced intense pain over the region of the left kidney, and although eighteen months ago the symptoms suddenly ceased for a time on taking *Herba delvey*, a local remedy of great repute amongst the Mexicans, they return again within three months, whilst during the treatment an enlarged prostate and exceedingly irritable bladder were probably due to the remedy.

"In October last a very violent haemorrhage took place from the bladder or kidney, continuing for four weeks with intense pain, constant catheterisation being required. The incessant pain was localised over the left kidney, and necessitated a hypodermic injection of 8 grains *morphia* daily.

"About this time the author's attention was called to *Piperazine*, although having been on all sorts of treatment without relief, he was rather sceptic as to its value, and did not take to it very readily. The condition was then — weight 170 lbs., pulse 60, profuse diaphoresis, very feeble, confined to bed; examination of urine showed pus, albumen, blood, only 9 ounces daily, which required to be drawn off by catheter, and large amounts of urates.

"The author commenced taking 15 grains *Piperazine* daily in one quart of water. On the third day the urine had increased to 39 ounces, and continued to gain in quantity until the normal quantity was reached, which has continued to the present time. The most satisfaction was, however, afforded by the fact that on the fourth day the intense pain began to grow less, and continued to do so until it entirely ceased. The *Morphia* was gradually decreased, and *Phenocoll hydrochloride* in 10-grain doses taken in the place. At the present time weight is increasing at the rate of 4 lbs. per week, appetite is very good, urine perfectly normal, and business capability restored. The urine examined from time to time whilst under *Piperazine* treatment showed the passage of excessive quantities of urates, but they were always in solution and gave no trouble in voiding.

"In conclusion, *Piperazine* has certainly shown itself in this case a very prompt and powerful solvent of uric acid calculi, and one of very great value in those cases where the knife has hitherto been of doubtful value. (*Notes on New Remedies*)." (XXI 53)

## 463. GOUT

Dr. Mordhorst is himself very gouty, and he gives his own case as one cured by the Wiesbaden *Gichtwasser* (pp. 48-49), and he thus describes his own case :—

"I belong to a very gouty family. My father suffered, my three sisters still suffer from gout. An elder brother of mine died at the age of 46 years of uric acid renal calculi. Already four or five years ago I at times felt a painful sensation on pressure in my left leg along the course of the sciatic nerve. About a year and a half ago I discovered on the inner side of my left knee several small tophi, which at times pain on pressure, and inconvenience me in walking. I have also discovered gouty nodes in several other parts of my body, but these are but seldom in evidence. Whenever I get pains in these affected parts, I drink, for four or five days, two to three bottles of *Gichtwasser* every day, to get rid of them.

The urine becomes strongly, and the cutaneous secretions faintly, alkaline. A small gouty tophus in the flexor pollicis longus of my left thumb, that remained from a slight acute attack, disappeared, all but slight traces, after a prolonged course of the *Gichtwasser*."
Note well that this is the cured state. (XXI 63)

## 464. ATTACK OF GOUT

Lord X. had an attack of gout three years ago, and it fell to my lot to treat him for it. It was the classic podagra. I gave *Urtica urens* Q, five drops in a wineglassful of warm water, every three hours, and his lordship was about as usual in ten days. In another attack since then the same remedy acted with equal promptitude, and to the patient's great satisfaction. His lordship has had quite a number of attacks of gout, and has had the advantage of the services of the very greatest authorities on gout, in London, and, moreover, he has been to the leading spas for gout, and hence his opinion is of value, and this runs thus — "I have never taken any remedy that has done so much for me as *Urtica*; there is no doubt about that." (XXI 73)

## 465. GOUTY OPHTHALMIA

A very gouty city gentleman, just turned 50 years of age, came on 21st October, 1892, to consult me for a slight attack of gouty ophthalmia of his left eye. I ordered *Urtica urens* Q ten drops in water, night and morning, and this cured the ophthalmia within a week, ameliorations setting in already within twenty-four hours. I have been in the habit of seeing this gentleman for a number of years for gouty manifestations, amongst which was a very obstinate gouty eczema. (XXI 74)

## 466. THE *SPIRITUS GLANDIUM QUERCUS*

**Homoeopathically Antidotal To The III Effects of Alcohol.**

**Case 1. Observation.** Colonel X., aged 64, came under my observation on January 15th, 1889, broken down with gout and chronic alcoholism, and pretty severe bronchitis. Heart's action irregular; liver and spleen both enlarged; and he complained bitterly of a gnawing in the pit of the stomach. His gait was unsteady and tottering, his hands quivered, and altogether he was in a sorry plight. The poor fellow had lost his wife, and had for a good while tried to rub along with the aid of a little Dutch courage, in the shape of nips of spirits, for which he was always craving.

Severe windy spasms; no sugar, no albumen.

$R_x$ *Spiritus glandium quercus* Q, 10 drops in water, three times a day.

January 22 — On this day — a week from his first visit — he walked briskly into my consulting room, and brightly exclaimed, "Well, I think you have worked a miracle;" and the curious thing was that his craving for spirits was notably less, he having consumed only one-third of a bottle of whisky in the week, instead of two bottles, which was his usual allowance. The windy spasms had ceased, and his foul breath had become sweet; and finally, his spleen had gone down in size very notably. To leave off the *Quercus*.

February 5 — So little craving for whisky that he offers to leave it off; much less phlegm in chest; no spasms; altogether quite a different man, but is depressed.

$R_x$ *Spiritus glandium quercus* Q, 7 drops in water, three times a day.

February 19 — He is chirpy again, and has no craving for whisky.

The remedy was repeated in May, and I learned some months afterwards, from his daughter, that the colonel contined in fair health, and partook of stimulants "like other people," and without any "craving." (XXI 83)

**Case II. Observation.** A London merchant, 57 years of age, came under my care on October 16, 1888, for necrosis of all the nails of his right hand, and most of those of the left hand, and of nearly all his toe-nails; severe arcus senilis, rushes of blood to the head, buzzing in both ears. I discharged him cured at the end of the summer of 1891, so that he was under my very careful treatment for nearly three years. He was a candid, dutiful patient, and had his reward in being really and radically cured. He first had *Vanadium* 5, 5 drops in water, night and morning, and after one month of this his arcus senilis had notably diminished, and "I do not get so tired, and my hands do not tremble so much." The *Vanadium* was continued for a second month. "Much better in himself; can now do a day's work; trembling all gone; noises nearly well of the left ear, no better of the right." *Thuja* and many remedies followed, with steady amelioration, but something seemed to bar the way to a perfect cure, when he confessed that he thought he took too much sherry in nips. Like the colonel, he was never intoxicated, — never, in fact, *morally* intoxicated, but still never free from the effects of his nips.

$R_x$ *Spiritus glandium quercus* Q, 10 drops in water, night and morning.

This brought out a good deal of gouty eczema of scalp, poll, and backs of hands. It took me ten months to really cure this eczema, and then I had him back to the *Quercus*, which he took, altogether, for three months; and then I find, at the end of my record of his case in my case-book the word . . . *well*. (XXI 86)

**Case 3.** The wife of an officer of position wrote to me some two years ago — " . . . I am not at all satisfied with my husband's appearance. We have had a shooting party, and I am sure he drinks too much. I can always tell by the look of his eyes; they are so yellow, and puffy underneath. I wish you would send him something to put him right : he says he is all right, but I am sure he is not, from his breath.

After a month of *Quercus*, I heard this " ". . . My husband looks wonderfully well." (XXI 89)

**Case 4.** A noble Nimrod, about 40 years of age, a very free liver, and plagued with attacks of gout, came under my observation in the spring of 1891 for varicose veins of the lower extremities, starting originally, it seemed to me, from an enlarged spleen, which was seemingly left after typhoid fever. Knowing his mode of life, and on account of the spleen, I gave him *Quercus* for a month, 10 drops at bedtime, and then noted : "He likes his medicine, as it keeps his bowels very regular."

May 15. 1891. — Veins better; fewer rings under his eyes.

$R_x$ *Petroleum* 5.

July 22 — "He feels his feet hot, and would like the first medicine (*Quercus*), as it seemed to make him feel so well.

$R_x$ *Spiritus glandium quercus* Q, 10 drops in water, at bedtime.

September 8 — In rude health. (XXI 90)

**Case 5.** The following case is very striking, and greatly impressed me : A country squire, from the shire of Moonrakers, bachelor, 60 years of age, was accompanied to me on October 3, 1893, by his brother, resident in London. This gentleman was so very ill that his case was regarded as quite hopeless. He was not capable of stating his own case, and hence his brother did it for him. Patient was flushed, and in much pain over the eyes and in both rib regions. Stooping caused very great pain, worse in the left hypochondrium. Both liver and spleen notably enlarged. He is exceedingly nervous, very depressed, glum, taciturn, and moved to tears by almost anything, He could not walk without support, on account of his great giddiness. His breath was in the highest degree disgustingly stercoraceous (*merdeux*), so much so that I very nearly vomited when examining him. He was personally unknown to me, and I had no history of him, but that smell of breath is an unmistakable sign of the chronic tippler. I subsequently ascertained that he was quite a sober-living man, but took frequent nips, particularly when confined to the house by wet weather. But quite apart from this, the *Quercus* was manifestly homoeopathic to the case.

1. Pain in the left side.
2. Giddiness.

3. Flushed state.

So I ordered *Spiritus glandium quercus* Q, 10 drops in water, three times a day.

October 10 — Less fluttering; giddiness a little better; the tenderness of the rib region much diminished; *breath normal*!

He returned home in six weeks perfectly well. A prettier direct art cure I think I have never seen. (XXI 91)

**Case 6.** Three months ago a city magnate, about 70 years of age, came to me for giddiness, flatulent dyspepsia, depression of spirits. a flushed face, and "altogether below par." His conjunctivae were yellowish, his tongue foul, and his breath the same as in the last-narrated case — stercoraceous and nauseous. Under the *Quercus* the patient made a rapid recovery. his breath becoming sweet within four days. This stercoraceous smell is pathognomonic of undigested alcohol in the *primoectoe*, and is readily perceived two yards away from the patient's mouth, and quite unbearable within a foot or two. Where this smell is present, there is no need to make irritating inquiries as to the imbibitionary habits of the individual, — *Quercus* is indicated. It does not, of course, follow that the *Quercus* is indicated only in the alcoholic state. (XXI 94)

**Case 7.** In regard to the question as to whether and how far the *Spiritus glandium quercus* reaches the craving for drink, the following letter from the wife of a gentleman to whom I had sent the remedy, is of a certain interest :

"Dear Dr. Burnett. — To begin with my husband. He took the drops for a week, and then, as he caught a chill and was very poorly, and in the doctor's hand. I stopped the drops until he was a little better. He has now finished them about three weeks. He says his feet are not half so tender, and he can walk with more ease and comfort. He has not been feeling very well, rather limp, and tired easily. He has, however, slept well and quietly, and while he was taking the drops he drank less, both with and before his meals. The last week or so he is again taking sherry before meals and beer at meal time, so I fully expect a bilious attack, especially as he is not as sweet-tempered as usual. He has been eating better and has come to bed earlier. He has had B. and S. in the morning before breakfast. So please do give him something to stop this craving for pick-me-ups. Air and exercise he has in plenty, so if only his craving, sinking feelings for something can be stopped, he would be as well as possible. I think his hands look less swollen; they were decidedly swollen a little while ago. He looks a little yellow in the eyes, and the skin a little dry and wrinkled. We all notice that he drinks less than he used to, and are all thankful for that; so in time, perhaps, he will be quite right." (XXI 102)

## 467. GOUTY GASTRALGIA OF THIRTEEN YEARS' DURATION

Not long since a gentleman of 60 years of age, who had lived many years in a sub-tropical country, came under my observation for gastralgia extending right up through the chest. Although he had lived in parts where ague is very common, he is not aware that he has ever had ague himself. He has many gouty deposits all over his body, mostly in the neighbourhood of the joints. His throat is gouty, and also his left conjunctiva. There is a good deal of bronchial catarrh. The gastralgia yielded quickly and completely to *Uritca urens*, much to the amazement of the patient, who has been under fully a score of physicians in different parts of the world for this gastralgia, but in vain; and when I first saw him he was just back from Aix-les-Bains, which had also done his gastralgia no good. (XXI 123)

## 468. CASE OF CHRONIC GOUT IN THE FEET AND ANKLES

In the spring of 1891 I was requested to go some distance into Surrey to see a lady of 60 years of age who was bedridden for many months from gout in her feet and ankles. It had started, so it was said, from a chill caught while sitting at a railway station waiting for a train. The feet were swelled, very hot, reddish, stiff, and so painful that the patient swooned when I pressed them but gently. There was persistent insomnia and great depression of spirits. After a year's treatment she was discharged quite well, and has since so remained, and with rather unusual activity of limb. The fact is, having been for a time deprived of the use of her feet, and recovered the same only by slow degrees, she set greater value on her power of locomotion then ever before in her life. She had the following remedies, in the order named — *Urtica urens* Q, *Cypripedium pub.* Q, *Apis mel.* 3x, *Menyanthes trifoliata* 3x, *Bellis perennis* Q, and *Viscum album* 1, and after the use of the last named, patient walked from two or four miles a day, with comfort, pleasure, and satisfaction. And the cure holds good to date. (XXI 142)

## 469. GOUTY INSOMNIA

A gentleman, 80 years of age, formerly in the army, came under my observation on February 17, 1893, for insomnia, distinctly due to his being full of gout. "I cannot get any sleep without chloral; as soon as I lie down at night I get hot, burning, and itchy." His gouty eczema he had got a little under with the aid of sulphur baths. I ordered him *Urtica urens* Q, 10 drops in water, three times a day.

March 3 — "This medicine has done me an immensity of good, but has given me nettle-rash!"

And *apropos* of nettle-rash, everybody knows that the name of the rash is due to the power of the nettle to produce just this kind of rash; those who question this can readily put into the test of practical scientific experiment by handing a few nettles with gloveless hands. I have very often cured nettle-rash with the nettle-tincture, as so many others have done before me.

It seems to me that if any honest enquirer is really desirous of putting the truth of homoeopathy roughly, yet readily, to the test, he needs only handle a few nice nettles with gloveless hands, when he will find that nettles really *do* produce nettle-rash; and then if he will treat a few cases of nettle-rash, occurring as a disease, with some nettle-tea or tincture, he will find that the nettle really does cure the disease nettle-rash; . . . and, if that is not homoeopathy, pray what is it? (XXI 144)

## 470. GOUTY FISTULA

Although fistula is not frequently primarily due to gout, still I have met with some cases of fistula distinctly of gouty nature.

In the month of January, 1893, a gentleman, 30 odd years of age, sought my advice in regard to a fistula in ano — external and incomplete — that had started with an abscess about a year before. After treating him for some time on the same lines which I commonly follow in the treatment of fistula, I found there was a something present barring progress towards a proper constitutional cure. And just when I thought we were at the end of our task, the fistula suddenly inflamed, and it was not until patient had had a course of *Urtica* for a while, and finally, after taking *Spiritus glandium quercus* for some six months with interruptions, that he reported himself as quite cured. He had what might very properly be called fistulitis from indulgence in drink, and each time it yielded very speedily to *Quercus*. Patient himself soon found out which of the remedies did the good, for on one occasion, being at a distance, he telegraphed for this particular medicine. The fact is, the bouts of acute fistulitis followed immediately on certain champagne breakfasts and lobster suppers.

The *Spiritus glandium quercus* has helped me promptly in several other cases of fistula in which the fistulas had become constitutional issues for the excess of alcohol taken into the economy. There are certain cases of fistula that are due almost solely to alcoholism, and these fistulas are simply issues. Woe to the patients if these fistular issues are cured (?) by operation. (XXI 146)

# DELICATE,BACKWARD, PUNY AND STUNTED CHILDREN

## 471. UNILATERAL ARREST OF DEVELOPMENT — LOPSIDEDNESS — ONE-BREASTEDNESS : ILLUSTRATING POST-NATURAL GROWTH

On the 16h May 1883, a young lady, 16 years of age, was brought to me by her father, a clergyman, then residing in Kent. He did so because I had been mentioning to him some interesting curative work I had done in the medicinal treatment of backwardnesses.

The most salient point in the case was the fact that while the right half of her trunk was very nicely developed and the right breast normal and perfect in form, the left breast was only rudimentary, like a boy's, the left arm not much more than half its proper size. The roof of her mouth was very much arched, the left side of her face drawn to one side, so that her mouth was awry. Her speech very imperfect indeed, she being unable to articulate, and her sense of hearing bad, being clearly in a similar state of arrested development. She began to menstruate at 15, and is regular; suffers from frontal headaches, her tongue deeply cracked (chopped, fuissured). On going over this case very carefully, nothing seemed to offer any therapeutic cue : her parents are well and normal, so are her brothers and sisters, and, moreover, all well and well-bred. Vaccinated? Yes; she was vaccinated at three months of age, but it did not take well, and hence she was done again. At this point I must refer to my little book entitled "Vaccinosis and its Cure by *Thuja*", which I beg my readers to peruse, and then return to this narration.

$R_x$ *Thuja* 30.

June 13 — On the whole very much better; can certainly articulate better; and the head is not so much out of the perpendicular.

$R_x$ Rep.

July 11 — The pain in the left side is better; she has threadworms; frontal headache gone; seems very weak.

$R_x$ *Ceanothus Am.* 1x ℥ss., five drops in water night and morning.

*Ceanothus* is a left-sided medicine, — i.e., it acts electively more on the left side of the body, and specifically on the spleen.

August 22 — Pain in the side (a dull sensation really) is gone; she is said to pass shreads from the bowels. All agree that she articulates distinctly better.

$R_x$ Rep.

September 7 — *Thuja occid.* C.

October 17 — Although her side continues comfortable, she seems to have been ailing more generally in herself, AND HAS HAD SOME BOILS. Speaks and articulates decidedly better. The lopsidedness is much less apparent, *the left side having grown.* Hears very much better.

$R_x$ *Psorinum* 30.

November 23 — Left side feels comfortable; further great improvement in her articulation; less lopsidedness; breathing very rough; tonsils are of enormous size; small polypus in the left nostril.

$R_x$ *Euonymin* 3x

January 9, 1884 — Has run down; a crack in left angle of mouth; piles, and has passed thread-worms in great numbers.

$R_x$ Tc. *Sanguinaria* 1x, and a *Teucrium* snuff.

February 8 — Lopsidedness still noticeable; many seat-worms.

$R_x$ *Vaccinin* 30.

March 7 — Much backache; the medicine seems to have completely upset her; hands and feet very cold.

$R_x$ *Ceanothus* 1 and *Hepar* 3x.

April 16 — Side better; hands and feet no warmer. HAS HAD SEVERAL LITTLE BOILS. Still some frontal headache; sick in the 'back'; breathing is better; hearing a little better.

$R_x$ *Psorinum* 30 and *Thuja* 30.

May 16 — On the whole better; complains again much of frontal headache; is not so straight as she was; in the night complains of a lump in the side, and the side is said to swell in the posterior aspect of the spleen region. Talks and hears better.

$R_x$ *Leuticum* CC.

July 11 — Better than ever before; the *nocturnal* swelling gone; tonsils still very large; is again very deaf; her breathing is quite changed, and is now almost normal; she talks away, and evinces an interest in everything; the polypus is smaller.

$R_x$ Rep.

October 17 — Complains of pain in the left breast, and on examining I find shingles just developing in the left side, involving the left mamma.

$R_x$ *Variolin* C.

29 — Cured the pain in the left mamma and blighted the shingles straightaway, and she has been wonderfully well altogether.

$R_x$ Rep.

November 28, 1884 — Is like one of the rest for all practical purposes : her left breast has grown, is well formed, and fit for its natural function.

**Ten Years Later.** The cure holds good. I had not seen the patient during the past ten years until a few days since. It cannot be maintained that patient is absolutely normal, because there is some hesitancy and splutter in her speech, and she holds her head a little on one side, but that is all. *Very* close inspection shows that the left breast is a very little smaller than the right one, but so very slight that no one would notice it unless attention were specially called to the matter, and the less so as the two breasts are very rarely of exactly the same size in anybody.

I call the attention of my readers to the breaking out of boils, and to the shingles, both of which phenomena I regard as constitutional strivings, due to the actions of the remedies administered.

Let us remember that cow-pox is a vesiculo-pustular disease. The arrest of development in this case was due, I believe, to vaccinosic blight, latent, pent-up vaccinosis.

When I speak of *constitutional strivings*, I mean that cutaneous eruptions are very commonly curative in their tendency. (XXII 17)

## 472. PARALYSIS OF LOWER EXTREMITIES

On August 15, 1881, a little bundle of yelling humanity was brought to me on a pillow, and I was told that her father was very ill of locomotor ataxy (whereof he sometime therafter died), and that she was paralyzed of her lower extremities, she being then nine months old. Her gums were livid and very greatly swelled. There was a history of a fall three months before. The child was said to have fallen on the lower part of her spine, where one sees a considerable swelling, bulging in appearance and very red. The special feature of the case lay in the fact that whenever the lower limbs were moved, even the slightest degree, the poor wee mite yelled terribly. I ordered *Thuja* 3x and *Arsenicum* 3 internally, gave the third trituration of *Heclae lava* with its food, and applied very weak *Arnica* to the swelling.

September 16 — Cries and yells as much as ever; takes her food well; ankles are puffy and swelled; gums purple, fleshy, and swelled; the dorsal swelling is clearly *bone*; perspires much in her head; very restless at night.

$R_x$ *Calcarea carbonica* 30 and *Mercurius* 30 internally in alternation, and *Liquor calcis* P.B. to be applied locally.

September 29 — Continues to cry very much; the gums where the new teeth should be are bluish, and look like bags; the sternal ends of the clavicles are very much swelled, as big as large walnuts, — in fact, all her epiphyses are more or less swelled.

$R_x$ *Thuja* 30 and *Calc. sul.* 3x.

October 10 — Mending decidedly.

$R_x$ Rep., and to be taught to eat one ripe pear every day, and to be taken to the seaside, and this because I regarded the case partly as one of land scurvy.

October 26 — Very great amelioration. No longer cries when moved; she stretches herself comfortably; the swelling at the bottom of her back is diminishing; and also that of the epiphyses; the deep purple aspect of the gums has gone.

$R_x$ Rep.

November 26 — The back is nearly well, so are the clavicles, and she has grown five teeth.

$R_x$ *Pulsatilla* 1, and go on also with the *Calc. sulph*.

December 30 — The child is well, ruddy and healthy, but its legs are still very weak. Has now seven teeth. She had during the next four months *Silicea* 30, *Nux* 6, *Psorin*. 30, and *Lathyrus sativus* 3, which last was prescribed on May 8, 1882. I saw her no more for ten years.

**Ten Years Later.** On Oct. 24, 1892 — On this day a nicely-grown, normal girl, seemingly about twelve years of age, was brought to me by her mother to be treated for *stuttering*. It was my former paralysed baby patient!

I ought to mention that, on my ad . ice, this child spent the ten years during which I did not see her at a very healthy seaside resort. She is now at school in London, and bears the climate quite well. (XXII 26)

## 473. PUNY GROWTH; MESENTERIC DISEASE — HYDROCEPHALISM

A puny little boy of 9 years of age was brought to me on February 24, 1891, by his parents, who were in a very anxious frame of mind on account of their little son, inasmuch as his next brother had just died of tuberculosis of the brain coverings.

Patient was puny, old-mannish, pot-bellied, sick, sicky; bad headaches, worse of the frontal region; head swelled, face too small-looking, teeth dirty; glands everywhere feel like nuts; he feels most sick on awakening, better as the day wears on; sleeps badly, dreams of falling.

$R_x$ *Bacill*. C.

March 24 — Has not been actually sick since, but still feels sicky; appetite better, yet still variable; sleeps much better, but he starts. He had then in succession *Calc. phos*. 3x, *Trifolium pratense* Q, *Bacill*. 1000, *Chelid*. 1, *Puls*. 1, etc., till the end of the first year of treatment, when, after *Levico* and *Calc. hypophos*., he is noted in my case-book as doing well.

During the year 1892 the treatment was steadily continued on the same lines, with very slow, gradual, and yet steady improvement.

Likewise during the year 1893, in the autumn of which he had a gastric attack when he was a month under *Baptisia*, and after that he was very weakly in his abdomen; notably were the testicles noticed to be very small, and the boy had no go; a month under *Aurum metallicum* in the third centesimal trituration gave his whole economy a wonderful start.

And now, nearly at the end of 1894, he is almost a normal boy, wildly roughing it with others in a school preparatory for Eton or Harrow.

That this boy's life was saved by the treatment is, humanly speaking, certain, and that his physical and mental state has been very notably ameliorated is willingly conceded by all his relatives, one of whom is the headmaster of one of our public schools, who, in consequence of the course of this case, has placed his own very delicate children under my treatment.

In this case three remedies acted with very striking power — viz., *Bacill.*, *Aurum*, and *Fragaria vesca* Q. The last-named greatly improved his mesenteric glands and his digestion.

Midsummer 1895 — Is now a fine lad, and quite well.

I will add that *Levico*, in 5 to 10 drop doses, is a valuable inter-current help in grave cases where there is much debility, notably after the searching remedies such as *Bacillinum*. (XXII 31)

## 474. CONSTITUTIONAL BLIGHT DUE TO VACCINATION; ECZEMA AND ASTHMA

A boy of 9 was brought to me in the month of June 1892 to be treated for asthma and eczema, both of a severe type. His cough and dyspnoea were dreadful, and his eczema very distressing. "He ails every week, and has tobe kept in and nursed." His teeth were rudimentary, imbedded in tartar; his tonsils much enlarged; and noticing that his cervical glands on the left side were so much worse than on the right, the left side being where he had vaccination marks, I enquired how said vaccination had run its course. "Oh, it did not seem to take, and the skin came out all over with eczema, and he has never got rid of it."

The boy is bent forward, and generally ill-grown.

$R_x$ *Thuja occid*. 30.

July 8 — Much better; cough much better; skin very rough; very moist eczema of left ring-finger. Many pips; glands of both sides of the neck now equally indurated and enlarged.

$R_x$ *Bacill*. CC.

August 8 — "Oh, his teeth look so much better, much of the tartar has fallen off them; * tonsils swelled."

$R_x$ *Acid. nit*. 30.

September 5 — Glands nearly well; eczema about the same; pretty bad of both ring-fingers.

And thus the treatment went on till the fall of 1893, when patient ceased attending. He had up to that date several nosodes, *Thuja* 30, and for months a course of *Bacillin*. (C., CC., and 1000).

In regard to the accumulation of tartar on the teeth, already in my own first proving of *bacillin*., I thereafter noticed the falling-off of two or three cakes of tratar from my lower incisors (never before or since); and in many of my published cases this curious influence of *Bacillin*., has been noticed. (XXII 35)

## 475. DEAFNESS

A stunted little maid of 12 years was brought to me on June 27, 1892, because she was undersized and deaf. The glands under the right ear are indurated and enlarged; her tongue pippy; she is dusky in the neck. Patient had had ringworm for two years, and when that was cured (?), she went deaf. She has been twice vaccinated.
$R_x$ *Bacill.* 30.
July 25 — She has begun to grow.
$R_x$ Rep.
August 26 — Her teeth are clearing.
*Ib.* Cc.
September 26 — Is growing; hearing much better; teeth getting cleaner and of a better colour.
*Ib.* C.
And thus the treatment was continued till the summer of 1893, at which date I find in my case-records the following note : — " Has grown enormously; her glands are better; still deaf;" since when I have not seen her, but quite lately I heard from her mother that patient is in good health and away at school at the seaside, but she is still hard of hearing. (XXII 39)

## 476. PUNY GROWTH, NOCTURNAL FRIGHT, AND DEAFNESS

On February 21, 1887, Edwin was brought to me for his puny growth, deafness, and habitual alarming fright at night. In aspect he was thin, very bony, flat-chested, and his skin "nothing but veins," so to speak. In both groins and in both sides of his neck very numerous hypertrophied glands were discernible; and, as if to be quite certain of physical destruction, he was the slave of a certain secret habit. He was brought to me about every month for three years, and was then discharged cured, and he has since taken, and still maintains, a very high position in his chosen profession. He had from me during the first year — *Lueticum* CC., *Thuja* 30, and then *Aurum muriaticum natronatum* 3x, *Pyrogenium* 6, *Psorin*. 30, and *Bacillinum* 30; and by this time he had improved in every way, — his nights were good, the frights disappeared, he began to be less veiny and to grow, and his deafness had disappeared. He had fought manfully against his evil habit with partial success.
In the second year he had several months of *Bacill.* C., *Sabina* 30, *Platina* 30, *Fragaria vesca* Q, and at the end of it his physique and morale were much improved, and I find in his case-record at this date the significant word, *clean*. Some of the same remedies were repeated during the third year, until he was discharged, as above stated, cured. *Pyrogenium* 6, three drops in water night and morning, continued until a two-drachm bottle

was taken, appeared to cause his nose to bleed. Edwin continues to thrive to date, but is still shy and taciturn, but so is his mother. As to the habit of self-abuse, which was a great obstacle in this case, I shall refer to that later on, under a separate headline. Here I would just remark that, according to my experience, the thing is most commonly physical disease, — evil rather than vice or sinfulness. In fact, it is an aberration purely in the animal sphere rather than sin on the spiritual plane. (XXII 41)

## 477. GLUMNESS : A TACITURN BOY

There is a certain type of child — more frequently boys than girls — who hang their heads and who will not willingly answer questions put to them, and who will not talk if they can help it. The boy in question was brought to me on May 21, 1892, and although reputedly in good health, he hung his head habitually and refused to talk. In asylums this kind of individual is a familiar sight. Such people will sit for hours together bent forward and looking steadfastly at nothing, and when spoken to they vouchsafe no reply, — they are just mum; though if irritated will fly at you. Although fifteen years of age he still had a lady to accompany him everywhere, and to whom he was greatly attached. he gave no answers to my various questions, only assenting very decidedly to the lady's statement that he suffered greatly from headaches. At his school he was considered a dullard, and no one ever heard of his even wishing to distinguish himself or get a prize. The headaches were over his eyes; his tongue was white, with many red pips imbedded in the thick coating. He had been twice vaccinated, he tanned unduly in the sun, and his superficial inguinal glands were hypertropied; testicles small.

℞ Tc. *Fragaria vesca* 1x, ten drops in water night and morning. This was given on account of the state of the tongue, and with such a tongue the *Fragaria* is a very notable stomachic, the headache being evidently from the state of the abdominal glands. Under its influence the boy visibly improved in every way : his headaches became much less severe, and he looked brighter; moreover, he held himself better, and would answer questions sometimes.

This was followed by *Thuja occid.* 30, and after this he had no more headaches at all.

After that he had *Bacill.* CC., *Puls.* 1, and finally, on account of his poor testicular development, he was a month under *Aurum metallicum,* third trituration, which effectively righted that wrong, and he forthwith took a proper position in his school, and at the next prize distribution he greatly astonished those who had known him by carrying off several prizes. He afterwards called to say good-bye to me, and gleefully told me of his triumphs. He had ceased to be mum or peculiar.

A year later his father accosted me at London Bridge Railway Station, and expressed his great satisfaction at Tom's capital condition. (XXII 44)

## 478. SPINAL CURVATURE : STUNTED GROWTH

In the spring of 1894, a boy of ten years and a half of age, of fairly good weight viz., 4 st. 8 lb., but in height only 4 feet 3 inches, was brought to me by his mother (herself for many years a sufferer from spinal disease), on account of slight spinal curvature and stunted growth, or perhaps, I should rather say backward growth. He had the too-wide and too-stodgy aspect of such a condition. An examination revealed indurated and hypertrophied glands in both sides of the neck and in both groins, and very small testes indeed. This boy had a somewhat pleasing but peculiar aspect and manner that I have occasionally seen in boys whose testicular development is backward. I first noticed it in such a boy in a Continental hospital many years ago, and have never forgotten it : once seen always remembered, but very difficult to describe. I would say that there is an unusual openness and frankness in their gaze and approach, too much *empressement*, a full-of-confidence, jump-down-your-throat, meaningless, laughing unconsciousness that is very striking, and not entirely pleasant.

This boy had from me, in a six months course of treatment, *Tub. test.* C; *Bacill.* 30; *Thuja* 30; and *Aurum metallicum*, third trituration; and during that time he had taken to growing, and the following letter from his mother tells the rest :-

"Sept. 5th.

"DEAR DR BURNETT, — My little boy's school opens on September 25. I suppose he is now well enough to return to his work? He continues to grow and look well, and the difference in the appearance of his back is perfectly magical to me, to whom this weakness has always been a trouble. You certainly have given him exactly the help needed, and I am truly grateful. The other two boys are both benefiting, the younger more especially. The neck gland is not visible to *me* now. I say *to me*, because I seem to notice these things more than the others, and realize their importance. — Believe me, with many thanks."

And, again, in June 25, 1895, the mother writes me :

"I was at Eastbourne for a school festivity, and saw L., who looks splendid, so much so, that I think you need scarcely see him before his holidays; but he has no more powders, and I wondered if you would kindly send him another box to go on with. I do not want him to stand still, but to an ordinary eye he is in perfect health.

"I shall see G. at Harrow on the 3rd July.

"I remain, with many grateful thanks." (XXII 48)

## 479. PUNY GROWTH, SPINAL CURVATURE AND ACNE

A young lady, 22 years of age, was brought by her mother to me on May 6, 1890, for her spine, and what might be termed general puniness, and for which there seemed no assignable reason. In her face we saw a large spider naevus, and the skin of her shoulders was the seat of a fair crop of acne pustules. Her spine was curved, but it was that kind which ought, I think, to be called lopsidedness, and which is in reality an undue preponderance of the right half of the body over the left; and the spinal curvature is due to the pulling over of the muscles of the stronger side. It is not really a *spine* affection at all : the great bulk of the "spines" of young ladies are of this nature. Patient stoops a good deal, and squints a very little. This case is the type of very many, and they arise from malnutrition of the (commonly) left half of the body. In observing the mode of growth of children, I have often remarked that their strong parts, so to speak, grab the nourishment first, and thus, if too little is absorbed and assimilated, the weaker parts go short. I will narrate a case that bears this out by-and-by.

As this young lady's left side was at fault, and as she had been vaccinated on the left side, and was suffering from squint and acne, and her spleen being, moreover, swelled, I began with *Thuja* 30, and then continued with *Bellis perennis* Q, of which latter she took altogether an ounce. She was under these two remedies for about a year.

Then followed, in the order named, *Viscum album* 1, *Fragaria vesca* Q, *Bryonia alba* Q, *Saw Palmetto* Q (with vast benefit), and I shortly afterwards heard that she was engaged to be married. (XXII 52)

* Spider naevi generally disappear under *Thuja* 30, long used and *in*frequently repeated.

## 480. STUNTED GIRL

An anaemic, dusky, undersized mite of a girl was brought by her mother to me on August 29, 1888, for *debility*. She had had hepatitis; her incisors were markedly notched, she suffered much from toothache and croup, and her superficial glands were greatly hypertrophied, and finally, she was much plagued with oxyures. During the first nine months she had *Lueticum* CC., *Bacillinum* C., *Cundurango* 1, *Sabina* 3, and *Thuja* 30, and during that period gained 7 lbs. in weight, and she looked much better and was notably brighter.

Then followed *Pulsatilla* 1, *Ferrum picricum* 3x, *Psorin* 30, *Nux vomica* 1, when a further increase of a pound in weight was noted, and the seat-worms had ceased from troubling. Some other remedies were then given, notably *Rubia tinctoria* Q and *Hydrastis canadensis* Q, and my last note of her case is dated February 26, 1890, and runs thus: "Vastly improved, and now weighs 4 st. 6 lbs."

By the way, *Rubia tinctoria* is an excellent remedy in splenic anaemia. I usually give 10 drops of the strong tincture three times a day. (XXII 55)

## 481. ARRESTED GROWTH ; CHRONIC SWELLING OF THE SPLEEN ; PERITONITIS AND DROPSY

An extremely freckled, dusky, dropsical lad of 16 years of age was brought by his father to me on October 7, 1881, to be treated for .... "He is in a very bad way, and has dropsy in his stomach." As a babe he nearly died from the bottle, his mother being unable to suckle him, when a good wet nurse was obtained, and he grew fatter and stronger than his brothers and sisters, and was doing well until two years ago, when he was at school at the sea-side, and there one day was caught in a storm, and ran home a distance of two miles, thereby hurting his left side, from which he has never really recovered; it has pained him ever since. He has ascites, his micturition is painful, there is a kind of chronic diarrhoea, and although sixteen years of age there is not the faintest sign of pubescence. His spleen and liver notably enlarged, his face thin, his chest bony and very veiny, teeth notched, tongue thin and cracked, abdomen distended with water, the skin dirty-looking and earthy, glands in the groins enlarged, and legs thin, almost like long sticks.

Clearly abdominal glands were diseased, and the outlook was very gloomy.

In such a case one hardly knows where to begin. What struck me was the enormous number of freckles on his face, and as I had a few times succeeded in ameliorating that condition with *Badiaga*, I put patient on that remedy for two months (1 and 3x each for one month), with the result that his freckled state lessened, and patient, who had weighed 6 st. 9• lbs., came down to 6 st. 4 lbs.; but whether this diminution was a good sign or a bad one we could not readily determine, because it might have been from loss of flesh or from less water within the abdominal cavity. Damp weather made his diarrhoea worse, and he had now taken to wetting his bed. As he was distainctly worse in the wet and damp, I gave him the fourth trituration of *Nat. sul.*, and of that 6 grains three times a day. After this, on January 4, 1882, his weight was 6 st. 3 lbs., and he had ceased wetting his bed. Still very distinct ascites.

$R_x$ *Ceanothus* 1.

January 12 — Weight, 6 st. 1 lb.

$R_x$ *Thuja* 30.

January 20 — He is worse; the dropsy is increased, and the whole of the belly is very tender.

$R_x$ *Psorinum* 30.

February 1 — The diarrhoea has ceased; weight, 5 st. 13 lbs.; belly so very tender that he can no longer bear the jolting of the carriage. During this month he had *Calc. carb.* 30, *Colocynth* 6, and the second trituration of the *Iodide of Arsenic*, and at its end weighed just 6 stones.

He went on all March, April, and May under *Berberis vulgaris* 3x, *Ammon. carb.* 3, *Dioscorin* 3x, *Dioscorea* 3x, *Argentum nitricum* 1, *Nux vomica* 3x, and then *Merc.iod.* cum *Kali iod.*, 3x trit., and on June 5 the body-weight was 5 st. 6 lbs., and patient was still almost as ill as ever. And what rendered it so very difficult to really gauge out patient was the diminution in his weight, viz., whether was that less flesh or less dropsy.

$R_x$ *Lueticum* CC. was at last determined upon, and straightway improvement set in.

June 26 — Much better all round. Weight, 5 st. 5 lbs.; measures 24 in. round the belly; sleeps better.

$R_x$ Rep.

July 12 — Weight, 5 st. 5 lbs. He looks cleaner, whiter (less brown). The change in the colouration of his abdomen is marvellous; it is now not very much too dusky, and the belly is very much less tender; glands less prominent.

$R_x$ Rep., et *Hepar sul.* 3x.

He was discharged as being in a normal condition on February 8, 1883. On September 12, 1883, he saw the late Dr Dunn, formerly of Doncaster, who was then acting for me during my holiday, for "Enlarged inguinal glands, painful; *Hepar sulph.*," which words I see in my case-book in dear old Dunn's handwriting.

**Eleven Years Later.** Patient is now a busy city man in good health and condition, and just on the point of getting married : "As soon as business gets a bit better," in his own words.

This young man's mother had water on the brain as a child, whereof the shape of her head still bears eloquent testimony. (XXII 57)

## 482. PUNY GROWTH; RINGWORM OF SHOULDER AND CHRONIC INSOMNIA.

A little lassie of 8 years of age was brought by her mother to me on November 21, 1892, because she was weedy, pale, non-thriving, sleepless and restless at night, grinding her teeth, etc. The delicacy appeared to date from chronic diarrhoea from which she suffered a good deal as a baby. Her teeth were not growing properly, and her lymphatic glands were indurated and feelable in neck and groins.

*Bacillinum* CC., C., and 30, *Thuja* 30, and *Tub. test*. C., were the principal remedies I employed in the case, and after a few months much improvement set in. Patient sleeps well. After two years the young patient was quite a fine girl, although in my judgment still too pale, which I ascribe to the state of the air of the neighbourhood in greater London, where she resides. What the child now really requires is a few years residence at the seaside, by preference the first year or so at Worthing, the second at Brighton, and then, a year or two at Eastbourne or Folkestone.

The grandest results in the treatment of backward children are obtainable when the constitutional bars to physical and mental completion are medicinally removed, and THEN the full effects of food and air crown the edifice. I do not mean that food and fresh air are at any time unimportant, but *what I do maintain is that disease taints in children are NOT curable by ANY AIR or ANY DIET whatever*. The power of the organism to resist them may, however, be much increased. I will, later on, exemplify what I mean by narrating the case of a toothless boy at Eastbourne.

When I name certain places as suitable for delicate children, it is to be borne in mind that I am writing in London, whence said places are readily accessible. (XXII 64)

## 483. TOOTHLESSNESS, RICKETS, RINGWORM, PUNY GROWTH AND UGLINESS

By toothlessness I mean that the patient, a little girl of 7 years of age, who was brought to me in the winter of 1893, had only very rudimentary bits of something imbedded in tartar where the teeth ought to have been. Her hair, too, was very, very weak, thin, dry, and she had patches of ringworm, with areas of "Diffuse Ringworm" (Alder Smith) here and there on her scalp, worse on the left side. Numerous superficial glands, indurated and enlarged. In general aspect the child was puny and very ugly. I put her on the treatment set forth in my little work on "Ringworm," and a year later (she was on the remedy a full year, and on no other, but at longish intervals between the doses, and all of the thirtieth centesimal potency) her mouth was full of teeth, her hair had grown, and the little maid looked positively pretty, as one would expect from her young and good-looking parents. Her teeth are *not* yet white, and only poorly covered with dentine, but still she has a mouthful of teeth, and they will certainly go on improving in quality. No trace of ringworm or scrofula left, but the hair is still lacking in gloss.

Midsummer 1895. — Continues very thriving. (XXII 67)

## 484. RUDIMENTARY TEETH IN A BOY OF ELEVEN YEARS OF AGE; DIURNAL AND NOCTURNAL ENURESIS AND PIGEON-BREASTEDNESS

A rather fine-grown boy of 11 years of age was brought to me on October 3, 1893, because of his teeth, and for life-long enuresis. "The dentist says he can do nothing, as his teeth have not properly grown, and what little of the teeth is above the gums is almost all covered with tartar." So it was; moreover, the nose and naso-pharynx were crammed full of adenoids, and his tonsils were large, hence no one will be surprised to learn that he was also slightly pigeon-breasted.

This kind of rudimentary teeth one meets with pretty commonly in delicate children. The teeth have really not grown properly, and the little tips of teeth do not look like proper teeth at all, but like little spikes of tartar; they do not appear to have any enamel at all. I have already related cases of cure of this miserable state, so I need not unduly dwell upon this one. I last saw patient in April 1894, when he could breathe comfortably through his nose, the pigeon-breastedness was almost a thing of the past, the tonsils had gone down a good deal, and his mouth was full of teeth — perfectly good? No, not perfectly good, but still very passable. The young man had *Thuja* 30, *Bacill.* 30, *Tub. test. c.*, and then two others. I may see him again before this goes to press, and if I do I will add a note of any further progress he may have made since from the effects of the stock of medicines which I ordered for him when they went abroad in the summer. But probably I shall not see him further unless he goes back in his health in some way. I should have stated that the patient no longer wets his bed or his clothes, — which he had been in the habit of doing all his life to his own intense mortification. By the way, some parents chastise or scold their children for wetting their garments and bed . . . why not scold and chastise them for getting the measles? There was another point in this case that was very dreadful - viz., the boy's motions stank horribly : this soon disappeared under the treatment which I have just detailed. I will now narrate another case similar in some respects to the foregoing, and yet quite different, and which clearly shows that fresh air and ample feeding are *not* of themselves capable of *curing disease* or disease-taints which bar development : FRESH AIR CANNOT CURE DISEASE. (XXII 69)

## 485. CASE OF TOTAL ABSENCE OF FRONT UPPER INCISOR TEETH

On July 27, 1893, a small, thin, narrow-chested, drum-bellied, stunted boy of 8 years of age, son of a staff officer, was brought to me for his pining delicate state; he had no upper incisors at all, though one could see them shaped in the gums; his lips peeled very readily and constantly (so did the lips in the just narrated case!); his motions stank dreadfully; he wet his clothes by day and his bed by night, and he was a ravenous eater.

At the moment at which I am writing he has been just eighteen months under my care, and he is now the happy possessor of *good* teeth; and he is in all respects about normal, except that he still wets himself, and the glands in his groins are still feelably indurated and enlarged. The treatment was the same as the last, except that he was also two months under *Mal.* 30 and C.

His teeth are now very good, and of an excellent colour. The foul-smelling motions of delicate children are so distressing for those in charge of them that this alone urgently needs curing; but the cure must be vital and constitutional : using deodorants and disinfectants to the dejecta does not cure the unfortunate patients.

This boy had been sent to East bourne to reside, but his teeth did not grow till the disease-taint had been cured by medicines.(XXII 73)

## 486. IMPERFECT SENSE OF SMELL, DANGEROUS PERIODICAL NOSE-BLEED IN AN UNDERSIZED GIRL OF ELEVEN YEARS OF AGE

A stumpy, undersized girl of 11 years of age, of good parentage, was brought to me on June 19, 1889, for periodical epistaxis of three years' duration, that had latterly become alarming in extent, necessitating nose-plugging. "She loses a great deal of blood, and the doctor says that her life is in danger, and that an operation on the nose is the only hope of a cure." The child had had diarrhoea, varicella, measles, whooping-cough, and sore throats, and had been once vaccinated. She resides with her parents in a notedly healthy country place.

Patient was naturally anaemic from the haemorrhages; her nose ached; incisors slightly notched; there is pretty severe nasal catarrh, and she gets rid of a good deal of "thick yellow stuff" from the nostrils.

$R_x$ *Thuja occid.* 30.

July 15— Less bleeding; bad croupy cough. A slight "Shew."

$R_x$ *Bacill.* C.

August 2 — No bleeding at all, and patient is very well.

$R_x$ Rep.

September 16 — No bleeding, but has a taste of blood in her mouth, particularly when she sneezs. No cough. Her teeth are of a bad colour.

$R_x$ *Luet.* CC.

October 25 —Epistaxis twice, but much less profuse than formerly; her tongue is very long and very pippy.

$R_x$ *Bacill.* CC.

November 22—No epistaxis, but a prickling in the nose, as if it were going to come on. A bad cough.

$R_x$ *Calc. phos.* 3x

February 12, 1890 — She has grown and spread out in size; no cough; no nose bleed. Practically well, but still rather stunted.

$R_x$ *Pulsatilla* 2.

October 29 — Has greatly grown; one or two attacks of bleeding; right nostril very sore.
December 17 — Well.
February 29, 1892 — Well. The medical men who treated this case before I did, and who very loudly proclaimed the impossibility of its cure by any means whatsoever except an operation on the nose of a rather severe nature, and who, moreover, ridiculed any attempt to cure the same with medicines — these medical men have *not* been converted to homoeopathy by my success, but many of their neighbours have. Allopathy is in an advanced stage of senile decay, from which there is no recovery, and the sooner the general break-up comes the better for mankind. Thus, here is a young girl with dangerous nose-bleed of long standing slowly getting worse till her, very life is threatened; allopathy plugs the nares, and afterwards administers tonics, and finally, in the despair of the debility of senile decay, gives the case over to the surgeons, who propose waging war upon the poor nose according to the principles of rhinology (one of the occult sciences of modern medicine), while all the time it is a constitutional disease that causes the haemorrhage, and it is not a nasal disease at all!
**Three Years Later.** Patient continues quite well. (XXII 75)

## 487. MISSHAPEN HEAD ; ADULT MENTAL INFANCY OF A MAN TWENTY-SEVEN YEARS OF AGE

A big-grown man, 27 years of age, was put under my treatment in May 1889 by his relatives on the strength of my opinion that he might be rendered more or less normal by medicinal treatment, notwithstanding the fact that he was 27 years of age and still mentally infantile. Looking at him full in the face, one noticed his forehead was very bulging; no eyelashes; a dull expression; general headform abnormal. The history is that of "water in the head as a child," and that he has never been like others"; his sisters say "he is soft," and call him "daft." Being unable to do any head-work, he has had none to do, but has remained mentally fallow, and hence, though the son of gentle folks, is quite illiterate. The skin of his head seems to him to be very *tight**, whereof he complains a good deal; also of pain both in his forehead and at the back; his skin is very dusky; a number of his symptoms are aggravated at night. I examined him very closely, and roused his interest in his own case. He was in no sense insane, but clearly had plenty of mind; but it was hidden behind a cloud. He would seize his scalp in his hands and tell me impressively that it was *too tight*, and he complained of being such a heavy sleeper, and of not being able to do anything at figures or any "head-work."

* Most probably a physical fact primarily due to the watery state of the encephalon.

I call very special attention to this case, because it fully illustrates my contention that *lying mentally fallow* is not the proper treatment for juvenile cephalic invalids. This young man, being the son of gentlefolks of means, position, and intelligence, was allowed to lie mentally fallow all his life on medical advice, and he certainly grew up all right except for his dunderheadedness. Not only so, but he had an outdoor life, and when a full grown man he was, on advice, sent out to a colony with a very bracing, invigorating climate to rough it, and he carried out the thing so completely that he worked for long at heavy, rough outdoor work, quite getting his own living at felling timber and heavy farm work; it considerably strengthened his body, but he, at the time of which I am writing, had just returned from his long absence "roughing it," as dunderheaded as he ever was. Now, note the effect of treatment.

The first remedy was *Luet*. CC., which was followed by "an irritation of hands and face that keeps him awake *by night*; it burns; does not trouble him by day."

His head is better !

*Thuja* 30 followed, and seemed to try him a good deal. He had been twice vaccinated.

He then had *Nux vomica*, and after that *Bacill*. C., and here he began to learn arithmetic, his head being so much better; and in September the first prescription was repeated.

October 23 — Getting quite strong; pigeon breastedness much less pronounced. He is getting on well with his learning "the three R's."

$R_x$ *Morbillin*. 30.

November 27 — Is now enjoying his learning, principally writing and arithmetic.

$R_x$ *Bacill*. C., *Zincum aceticum* 3x, *Thuja* 30, *Calc phos* 3x, etc., carried us on to the year 1891, when patient had so far progressed in his learning that he obtained a berth in a city financier's office, where he still continues earning his living *at head work* entirely.

The foregoing case very aptly illustrates the thesis which I am here trying to maintain, viz., *that it does not suffice* to leave the delicate and backward in a fallow condition, trusting to their "growing out" of their maladive conditions, for they are nearly as likely to grow into them as to grow out of them. This young man remained mentally fallow so far as learning was concerned, and he made no mental progress His muscles were used, for these were well exercised,; his brain did not improve, for it lay fallow. It was allowed to lie fallow because it was unfit to work, and no doubt it was wise not to work it in its unfit state; but that did not suffice.

You cannot grow a good biceps by carrying your arm in a sling, neither can you cultivate brain-power by leaving the brain idle. *Muscle-power is gained by muscular exercise; brain power is gained by brain exercise*. And if the brain is in a morbid state, the malady from which it is suffering must be cured, whereafter the brain may be safely exercised and thereby strengthened. Muscle-exercise does not directly strengthen the brain; neither does brain-exercise strengthen the muscles : due exercise of each duly develops each; over-exercise of either is at the cost of the other. A given organism can produce only so much and no more. Great brain-workers are not muscular; great muscle-workers are not at the same time capable of great brain work; it is impossible, all cackle to the contrary notwithstanding.

It is of prime importance to keep the foregoing lesson well in mind. I say *great* brain-workers cannot at the same time be *great* muscle-workers. It is not maintained that an individual of great muscular power may not at the same time be a big-brained, highly-intellectual person. What I maintain is, that I never yet met a person who excelled in both. Gladstone is a great brain-worker, and can fell a tree; but I do not believe that Gladstone would ever have taken a high position in a competition with wood-choppers or woodmen of eminence on their own lines; and half a glance at his structure shows that he was never particularly muscular.

A given organism can only produce a given amount of energy and no more. Dr. Grace, the great cricketer, will not go down to posterity as a great physician, just as light-weights do not make good coal-heavers, nor do the best coal-heavers excel in light and elegant movement of body or swiftness of foot. To each his own excellence. (XXII 80)

## 487. HUNCHBACK

A lady brought her 11-year old, greatly-deformed son to me on January 29, 1886. I noted that patient was frightfully deformed : at his birth both his collar-bones were broken, and had united without ever having been set. His mother had taken this, her only son, to many doctors — surgeons and physicians — of the highest repute. She says 200! He was strapped up in a very formidable and efficient iron jacket, and he has had all the advantages of our best orthopaedic hospitals.

His belly is like a bulging pot. His spine is bent from side to side, the left scapular region forming the hunch.

Patient is very thin; liver much enlarged; macrocephalic head; skin, notably at certain points, very dusky; many indurated glands in the usual places; teeth literally rotten.

$R_x$ *Luet*. CC.

March 12 — Has been very much relaxed in his bowels from the powders; complexion already much cleaner, and the skin of his body less dusky. Belly has gone down.

$R_x$ Rep.

April 16—Better; skin less dusky; suffers very much from hiccup, lasting at times half an hour.
$R_x$ *Med*. 30.
July 12—Hiccup cured; the lad stronger and less crooked. Anorexia. *Nux vomica* 3x.
October 20 — Has grown very much; the skin of his body is till very "browny," though less so than formerly. No hiccup.
$R_x$ *Luet*. CC.
December 3 — No return of the hiccup; skin very much less dusky; is growing much straighter; but his glands are still visible, and like chains of kernels.
$R_x$ *Psor*. 30.
January 12, 1887 — Has a cold; strawberry tongue; but generally he is thriving.
$R_x$ *Puls*. 3x.
February 16 — Tongue is better; has hiccup twice a day, but has had a better appetite.
$R_x$ *Med*. CC.
April 4 — Still has hiccup; he is pale.
$R_x$ *Luet*. CC.
May 20 — No hiccup; has had toothache. Strawberry tongue.
$R_x$ Tc. *Fragaria vesca* Q, zij, five drops in water night and morning.
August 5 — A little hiccup; anorexia; tongue normal in aspect; still very swarthy.
$R_x$ *Luet*. CC.
October 21 — His skin is getting quite a clear English colour; still has hiccup a little; he is straighter, fatter, and slightly ruddy.
$R_x$ *Cyclamen Europ*. 1, five drops in water night and morning.
December 6 — Has had an accident.
$R_x$ Trit. 3 *Aurum metallicum*, four grains every morning.
January 27, 1888 — During the time he was taking the *Aurum* he was poorly; since then he is better, and he is now clean and white-skinned. Very bad teeth.
$R_x$ *Bacill*. C.
June 29 — He has been so much better that he has neglected to report himself. The number of feelably indurated glands in the sides of his neck is smaller, but still there are a goodish many of them.
$R_x$ *Luet*. CC.
September 5 — Greatly improved; skin still too dusky; many dark mother's marks.
$R_x$ Tc. *Cundurango* 1x, ziv., five drops in a little water at bedtime.
March 8, 1889 — Comes and exclaims, "I am getting on finely." He has practically become like any one else in colour; though, of course, his bones are still, as they must ever remain, crooked; but though so remaining, they

are fixed and strong, and the lad is above the average intellectually.

I saw him infrequently in 1889, and a few times in 1890 — once for a cough, and once for a bilious attack.

He is now grown up, and articled to a professional man in the city, and a bright future seems in store for him; and, moreover, if he in due course should marry and have offspring, there is no reason why such offspring should be other than healthy and normal in structure.

Such a result from medicinal treatment must be considered eminently satisfactory, for although the individual's back continues crooked, his *quality* is now almost, if not quite, normal; and it is this *quality* which would be propagaged, and not the crookedly fixed bones of his back, which would not be transmissible. (XXII 93)

## 489. ASTIGMATISM DUE TO MALNUTRITION — TREAT THE PATIENT AS A WHOLE

Some years since the younger son of the headmaster of one of our well-known public schools was sent to me; he was under an eminent oculist for his eyes, and wore spectacles for his astigmatism and headaches. The spectacles were, from the quasi-scientific standpoint, well adapted for the purpose, and they were praised by the boy as being a great comfort to him, and his mother was distinctly of opinion that he was less subject to headaches and could see much better with his spectacles than without them.

That the treatment was scientific in its adaptation I do not deny; that it was really the right treatment I absolutely deny; it was only quasi-scientific because it did not take due congnisance of all the facts of the case. Let me state my thesis : — The boy was only half grown; he was about nine years of age; the true object to be aimed at was not a palliative temporary one, but one of the organic mending, *to the end that his eyes might become of themselves efficient organs of sight* to last during the natural life of the individual. Do spectacles effect such organic mending? No, they do not, but rather tend to prevent it.

If you want to make a weak arm strong, do you order it to be carried in a sling? The boy's general nutrition was poor, his hands were indurated and enlarged, his limbs thin, his abdomen distended, and the state of his eyes was of a piece with that of the rest of his organism. I ordered his spectacles to be removed, and treated his entire being with remedies, and in time he improved in health, he grew stronger in *all* his organs and parts, and his eyes grew and improved in like manner, so that now he has no need of spectacles whatever, and I see no reason to suppose that he ever will need any.

It is not enough that the means be scientifically adapted to the case; we must be sure that the object aimed at is the right one. Artificial teeth are useful for those who have lost their natural ones, but artificial teeth do not help backward teeth to grow and get strong; a wig may usefully take the place of lost hair, but a wig does not help weak hair to grow.

In like manner, weak, imperfect eyes are not mended with spectacles. The eyes are living organs of the body, and as such can be vitally improved by proper internal treatment. Only failing this is the aid of scientifically adapted spectacles to be invoked.

Is it not a sad thought that the great army of eye-doctors are to a man nothing but mechanicians; and what is still sadder, they do not even aim at being anything else. (XXII 103)

## 490. ARRESTED DEVELOPMENT OF EYES AND TEETH

A frail, undersized, almost toothless girl of 16 was brought to me on November 11, 1887, principally for her eyes. She had been at the ophthalmic hospitals, and also under the best ophthalmic surgeons, for "inflammation of the nerve of the sight," and was informed that she would probably go blind. However, she had mended under their own care till the present time so far that spectacles were of some slight service. She suffers much from headaches, which are worse in bed at night. Her teeth are indented in dots, notched, and imbedded more or less in tartar. Much toothache.

$R_x$ *Luet*. CC.

December 9 — Headache better; toothache gone.

$R_x$ Tc. *Geranium Robertianum* 3x, ziv., five drops in a tablespoonful of water night and morning.

January 4, 1888 — Headache much worse, also toothache.

$R_x$ *Luet*. CC.

February 1 — About the same; tuberculous teeth.

$R_x$ *Bacill* 30.

March 9 — Much pain in the right side of the face; worse on getting warm in bed.

$R_x$ Trit. 3 *Aurum met*., four grains dry on the tongue at bed-time.

May 9 — Very drowsy; pains now worse after food.

$R_x$ *Thuja occid*. 30.

June 17, 1891 — Been going the round of the oculists again. Typically tuberculous teeth; much frontal headache.

$R_x$ *Bacill* CC.

July 15 — Headaches worse; eyes ache very much; teeth beginning to clean a little.

$R_x$ Rep. (1000).

And thus the treatment went on till the summer of 1893, when patient's teeth and general physique were notably improved, inclusive of her eyes; but just as the teeth are still imperfect though very much improved, so are her eyes; and I have now ordered the mechanical dentist for her teeth and the mechanical oculist for her eyes, as further *organic* improvement is not to be expected.

Spectacles come in for the organically irremediable; but to start children in life with spectacles without first trying to mend their ocular defects virtually is hardly worthy of really scientific physicians.

A truism?

Quite so, but bespectacled children are all over the place nevertheless, and practically no one ever tries to cure eyes. (XXII 107)

## 491. ASTHENOPIA IN A BOY OF NINE

A little boy, 9 years of age, born at Lucknow, came under my observation in the fall of 1891 for asthenopia. He was brought so that I might give my approval of spectacles ordered, or to be ordered, by an eminent eye surgeon. As I thought remedies would cure the asthenopia, I forbade the spectacles. The first remedy given was *Urtica urens* Q, for his spleen, which was enlarged, and clearly of malarial origin. This bettered the spleen, and the lad was in many respects much better.

After being two months under the *Urtica*, the symptoms that remained were —

1. His eyes felt cold.
2. Then they felt hot.
3. And then they watered a good deal.

These symptoms seemed to me to be of a malarial nature and sequence corresponding to the cold and hot stage and the stage of sweating, and hence I ordered *Natrum muriaticum*, 6 trit. This was followed by so much amelioration that I did not see him till the following spring, when the same remedy was repeated.

In the fall of 1892, I again saw the lad, and thought I would look away from the asthenopia and photophobia altogether, and *treat the patient*. His tongue was very pippy, and his cervical glands were enlarged and indurated. After a few months of *Bacillin*. CC., patient was quite well of himself and of his eyes. Once in June 1893 I gave him a short course of infrequent doses of *Sulphur* 30, because his eyes troubled him a little in the evening, since when he has continued quite well in all respects.

In this case two pathological elements are distinctly traceable. 1stly, The basic hereditary tubercular tendency, evidenced by the state of his cervical glands; and 2ndly, the acquired malarial impress on the organism. *Urtica urens* and *Nat. mur* met the latter homoeopathically, but still a really permanent cure was not attained. Then the basic constitutional taint was cured by the *Bacillin*., and the last faint flicker of the asthenopia was got rid of by *Sulphur* in dynamic dose; and *Sulphur* is, as shown by Dr. Robert

T. Cooper, a very notable remedy for ague, and we all know it as a classic antipsoric of almost ancient renown. (XXII 111)

## 492. DEFECTIVE DEVELOPMENT OF EYES AND BRAIN

A little girl, 5 years of age, was placed under my professional care on December 11, 1884, for defective development of eyes and brain, apparently from constitutional delicacy, and then originating from the effects of a fall. It is not easy to gauge the effects of a fall; usually the point is really this : What is the *quality* of the person who falls? In this case the patient is the coal-black variety of the strumous; her forehead was low and projecting; she was blind from double cataract, due probably to shock in the first instance, and then the lenses gradually silted up. The child was dull, nervous, readily frightened by the least noise, and she had been vaccinated in the usual way successfully. I proceeded first against the vaccinosis with *Thuja* 30, and this seemingly caused a bout of vomiting, whereupon improvement in the vision set in.

January 5, 1885 — Grinds her teeth at night.

℞ *Luet*. CC.

February 1 — Pupils less dilated; decided general amelioration, and notably in the state of her nerves; she is less irritable, and much more amenable to reason. *Thuja* C. then followed, but apparently did no good, when *Luet*. CC. was repeated.

March 24 — Sight and temper better; sleeps well; she has, and has had for long, ill-smelling footsweats; she can now see large capital letters, as well as at a greater distance; and, for the first time in her life, her bowels act well of themselves.

The treatment was continued very irregularly till June 1888, since when I have no further information, and the condition then reported to me (I did not see her) was thus described by her father, — "She sees better, and walks about with increased confidence."

The principal point of interest to me in this case was the very decided good effects of *Platanus occidentalis* Q, which was given for a number of months with very evident benefit to the nutrition of the child's lenses, and consequent improvement in her vision. The dose was five drops night and morning.

The treatment of this case was carried on in a very irregular manner, owing to a variety of circumstances, and as patient lived at a great distance I was not able to see her. (XXII 119)

## 493. EMANSIONAL TROUBLES IN YOUNG GIRLS

These are many, and so readily remedied by our medicines, that I will only shortly narrate one case.

Miss E., in her seventeenth year, of full habit, was brought by her mother to me from Ireland on December 16, 1884, because of her inability to pass the Rubicon of young womanhood. Her skin was blotchy and pimply; leucorrhoea pretty bad; weight on the top of the head, frontal headache, and swelled feet and legs. *Pulsatilla* was given, but failed.

Then, in January 1885, I gave *Bellis perennis* 1, ten drops in water night and morning, because of her tired feeling and acne.

February 14 — Has duly menstruated, and is not so tired, but her feet are much swelled.

$R_x$ Trit. 3x *Helonin*.

March 21 — Menstruated four weeks ago; feet well; head well.

$R_x$ *Bellis per*. 1, as before.

April 18 — Well, except that there is the least bit of swelling of the right foot, and still suffers from acne. She had been vaccinated, and hence I gave *Thuja* 30.

**Five Years Later.** September 1, 1890. — She has continued quite well, but she is now anaemic; her feet swell again, the menses are very scanty, and she gets fainty attacks.

$R_x$ Trit. 3x *Trillium*.

October 6 — "A capital change," and she continues, I believe, well.

There is no very special interest in this case, that I merely relate it to show that the delayed passage into womanhood is readily remedied by gentle innocuous medicines, and in a manner worthy of our advanced civilisation and refined culture. (XXII 122)

## 494. INCONTINENCE OF URINE CONSIDERED AS RETARDED DEVELOPMENT

For some time now I have regarded wetting the bed in children who have attained a certain age as *retarded* or arrested development about the sphincter region of the bladder.

A lad of 17 years of age was brought to me on March 28, 1890, for life-long nocturnal incontinence of urine.

$R_x$ *Thuja* 30.

May 26 — Very much better; has wet his bed only three times since commencing the *Thuja* powders.

$R_x$ Rep.

June 20 — No better; and has hay-fever and some emphysema.

$R_x$ *Lobelia acet*. Q, five drops in water night and morning.

July 30 — Better much all round, though the incontinence is not much better.

$R_x$ *Brachyglottis repens*. 3x, five drops in water night and morning.

October 30 — Did him so much good that his parents thought him cured; latterly he wet his bed again.

$R_x$ Tc. *Jaborandi* 3x.
February 11, 1891 — He is much better than formerly, but he still wets his bed.
$R_x$ *Med.* CC.
May 20 — Did not wet his bed at all while taking his medicine; but does it again now.
$R_x$ Rep.
July 24 — Quite cured; he wet his bed for the last time on May 26.
The cure has proved permanent.
The question of bed-wetting in children is very much more important than the inexperienced might imagine; the unfortunate sufferes feel very much humiliated, and their moral tone is distinctly lowered by the habit. A few cases are very easily cured with almost any well-chosen remedy, but where the case withstands domestic allopathy, domestic homoeopathy, local allopathy, and local homoeopathy and consultants of all sorts (as in this case), it is best to take a wide aetiological survey of the case, and treat it as arrested or retarded development. (XXII 125)

## 495. AN EPILEPTIC, HOPELESSLY-DISEASED BABY TWENTY MONTHS OF AGE

There are cases which at times are brought to one that are so bad that almost blank despair takes possession of one's mind at the merest contemplation of them. Such a case was presented to me in the month of February 1885. The wee girlie had been declared by two competent physicians of Leeds to be "an incurable epileptic, and hopelessly diseased."
She had always been much constipated, but fairly well till her double teeth began to come; with them came convulsions, "and one doctor said they were epileptic when he saw them." When she was about eleven months old the fits first appeared, seven fits in one day, and then on some subsequent occasions, when as soon as the symptoms of a fit set in the gums were lanced, and that generally stopped them. The breath smells sour, the tongue coats, and the stomach gets out of order when these attcks come. Now the teeth are beginning to decay. She is a cheerful, sturdy-looking child, large for her age; sleepless, and immediately after food a bright red flush appears in one cheek.
After two months of treatment (*Var.* 30 the first month, and *Luet.* CC. the second), comes this note in my case record : —
April 1 — Has cut a tooth with a fit, but *no foaming at the mouth* as on all previous occasions.
$R_x$ *Var.* C.
May 19 — Has been a fortnight without medicine; two attempts at fits, but they passed off.

$R_x$ Rep.
June 16 — No fit; has cut a double tooth; sleeps badly.
$R_x$ *Luet*. CC.
July 16 — No fit; has cut another double tooth. — only one more to come.
And now for the kernel of the homoeopathic nut — the child's father wrote : . . .
July 15, 1885. — "A rash appeared in the bend of the right arm about three weeks ago that looked almost like ringworm, but it certainly is not that; the rash has appeared also under the chin, and lately on one leg; sometimes it is much inflamed and irritated, at other times there are only a number of very small dark spots, which seem to be drying up."
$R_x$ *Luet*. CC.
The appearance of an eruption in the course of truly constitutional treatment is, in my judgement, a sure sign of a thoroughly radical constitutional cure; and so it proved here : the eruption gradually died away and that child never looked back.
Two years later I felt curious to know whether the cure held good, for we cannot ever reckon upon a case of epilepsy being cured, unless after years of waiting, and the reply came — "These powders quite cured her, and she is still quite well, although the two doctors gave her up to die as 'hopelessly diseased."
The explanation of the cure is merely that the case was one of pent-up syphilitic taint (possibly in the second generation), which the child's nature was battling with, and when this was cast out on to the external surface of the body in the form of a rash, the bar to the child's growth was removed. And this case, therefore, beautifully illustrates and amply justifies my contention. (XXII 130)

## 496. A PARTIALLY DEAF AND DUMB CHILD

On October 25, 1882, a lady brought her 7 year old daughter to me because she could neither hear nor talk properly; she hears a little, and jabbers something, but it is not articulate. The child is almost mindless, incapable of thinking; she does not know her own name. On my asking her where the fire is, she . . . puts out her tongue! Presumably she had an idea that I was a doctor, and that such a person looks at tongues. Then she repeated the word *"fire"*. She is described as dreadfully passionate and irritable. Had abscesses as a baby, and has ringworm for years : has it on her head now. The mother's idea of the origin of the child's life-long delicacy is that it started when the mother was carrying her *in utero,* when she on a certain occasion was severely chilled in cold water. Patient's right pupil is smaller than the left; right side of her chest is sunken; she has thread-worms; lids of left eye apt to be contracted, especially in the morning.

I ordered the child to be oiled night and morning in the manner I have already described, and prescribed *Bellis perennis* 1, five drops in water night and morning.

November 23 — The mother fancies patient is a wee bit sharper.

$R_x$ *Psorin*. 30.

December 29 — Is thought by her friends to be a little quicker, and, cried the mother, "The ringworm on her head is gone!" And she had had it for two years.

$R_x$ *Thuja* 30.

January 30. 1883 — She is beginning to speak better, but her temper is described as violent.

$R_x$ *Psor*. C.

February 26 — Speaks a little better; she makes greater effort to articulate; there is no sign of ringworm.

$R_x$ *Thuja* C.

April 7 — She is bright; there is improvement all round; she is better tempered and less irritable.

$R_x$ *Luet*. CC.

May 2 — Is better altogether.

$R_x$ Trit. 3 *Cuprum sul.*

June 15 — Still improving; less cross; less excitable; talks more hears better.

$R_x$ Rep.

July 13 — Great improvement articulates a little; thinks better.

$R_x$ *Bellis per*. 1.

October 8 — Talks, and her intellect is developing.

$R_x$ *Silica* 6.

I have not since heard of the case, but up to this point the child had very greatly improved in every way. (XXII 130)

## 497. BACKWARD GROWTH, MESENTERIC DISEASE AND EVIL HABITS

I am strongly of opinion that evil habits in the young are of physical origin and nature, and that they can be cured by medicines, if physicians will take the trouble. The subject of this narration was brought to me on November 8, 1883, because he was small for his age (11 years); had a drum-belly, very tender; indurated mesenteric and other glands; "and I am sorry to say he has a very wicked habit, and constantly plays with his private parts," "he also has constant diarrhoea."

Is he a naughty boy in any other respects?

Oh, no, he is a dear, good boy; but for that one dirty, wicked habit his father vows he will kill him if he does not leave it off.

Does his father consider that the diarrhoea is also sinful?

Of course not, what do you mean?

What I mean is simply this — Your son, is diseased, and his diarrhoea, his drum-belly, his dirty habit of masturbation are all of a piece, and all from his diseased glands; cure his disease, get him well and healthy, and he will leave of his dirty habit of masturbation, just as he will cease to have the diarrhoea.

So it happened; in a very few months the boy was cured, and got healthy in body, healthy in mind, and healthy in habits! When he was vaccinated he had a very bad arm.

On December 8 his body-weight being 4 st. 5 lbs., he was ordered to be rubbed with oil night and morning, and to have 6 grains of *Ars. iod.*, 4 trit., four times a day.

December 13 — Weight, 4 st. 8 lbs., so he has put on 3 lbs. in weight, and his diarrhoea is rather better. His feet are ill-smelling and sweaty.

$R_x$ *Silicea* C.

January 13, 1883 — Weight, 4 st. 8• lbs. Bowels better; belly less tender, but there is still tenderness at the sides. The boy is very much improved all round; feet sweat as much as ever.

$R_x$ *Thuja* 30.

February 16 — Weight, 4 st. 9• lbs. Feet dry, bowels regular, but he has pain in his abdomen pretty badly when he gets warm in bed at night.

$R_x$ *Luet*. CC.

This practically completed the cure, for after it was finished in March, *Psor.* 30 was ordered for a month, and then no further treatment was needed, and the lad was physically and morally healthy and clean : his evil practice was entirely given up, and apparently forgotten. (XXII 134)

## 498. BLIGHTED BY AGUE.

A stunted, forward-bent, asthmatic girl, 17 years of age, was brought over from the United States of America and placed under my professional care in the month of April 1886. The unfortunate child had had ague on and off ever since she was eleven months old, and in addition to that she had had pneumonia three times, as well as measles, whooping-cough, chicken-pox, and German measles. Her mother is under me for asthma, and two of her cousins for acne and comedones, and her mother's mother died of phthisis. Patient's skin was very dry, she perspired but very little, made water very frequently, had moderately bad leucorrhoea, and suffered much from dysmenorrhoea. Had also a good deal of anginal pain down the sternum; spleen very large; apex of right lung dull on percussion.

She remained under my care nearly three years, and then returned home practically well.

The remedies that cured the spleen were *Oleum succini non rectificatum* Q, which she took in five-drop doses twice a day for three months, and *Med*.

CC., *Bacill.* 30, and *Bellis perennis*, and also *Cenothus Am.* 1x, and *Nux vomica*.
Two or three months of *Luet.* CC. wrought a great change in her constitution, and after three or four months under the influence of *Psorinum* 30, her asthma was so far well that she could lie down in bed and sleep all night like other people.
The special point in her case is the very remarkable improvement in her bodily development and carriage, quite apart from the cure of her asthma and of the chronic enlargement of her spleen. Her father, a well-known public man in America, was greatly pleased with the remarkable change in his daughter. (XXII 138)

## 499. SEXUAL ABUSE & DIARRHOEA DUE TO ENLARGED INDURATED GLANDS

I was sent for some fourteen years ago into Surrey to see a girl of 9 years of age, who was guilty of self-sexual gratification to a dreadful degree, occupying herself hours at a time thereat till she was quite exhausted. Her parents were in a sad state of mind, and communicated the fact to me with much embarrassement, and then volubly anathematizing the poor child as vile, and given over to sinful depravity. Due investigation into the case showed that she had enlarged indurated glands in her groins and pelvis generally — the ovaries, no doubt, being in a like morbid state. The child also suffered from spells of diarrhoea, and I explained to the distressed parents that the supposedly wicked habit of the patient was as a matter of fact not wickedness at all any more than her diarrhoea, both being due to the state of the various glands respectively involved. This took a great load off the parents' minds, and I set about proving the correctness of my diagnosis by curing both the naughty habit and the diarrhoea, and the morbid state of the glands, and in less than two years the girl's glands were normal, her diarrhoea had quite disappeared, and the habit in question had also been quite given up, and apparently forgotten! That little girl is now a grown woman, and as sweet and pure as any parents could wish, and has seemingly not even any recollection of the past at all.
The chief remedies used in this case were *Thuja, Sabina, Bacill.*, and *Platina*, all in the higher dilutions, and infrequently repeated. (XXII 143)

## 500. MASTURBATION WITH ENLARGED GLANDS

Several years since a greatly distressed mother brought her four-year-old boy to me, telling me, after much hesitation, that he was hopelessly given over to self-pollution, from which he would not desist, notwithstanding the most severe chastisements administered by both father and mother, the father often declaring in extreme anger that he would kill him if he did not leave off; but leave off he would not, and whenever he could hide or creep under the table unobserved, he would give himself over to furious masturbation.

I explained to the mother my views of the true nature of the case, which greatly relieved her mind, for she had become fully persuaded that she was the mother of a moral monster.

Due examination showed that his abdomen was greatly distended, and his inguinal glands were enlarged and indurated.

After a few months' treatment, the mother ceased to bring him, and when she subsequently came on another matter concerning her own health, and I enquired about little Jack, she exclaimed, "Oh, he has quite given that up, and seems to have forgotten all about it."

A few months later she brought little Jack again : "He has begun with his old habit again, but nothing like so badly as before."

I put him under a further course of treatment, and then lost sight of him. Quite lately his father came to me on his own account for a cough, when I enquired about Jack : "Oh, he is quite well, and I don't think he remembers anything about it; I can not understand a child at that age, etc."

I had very great difficulty in convincing this gentleman that poor little Jack's "dirty trick" was physical disease merely and only, and in no sense moral obliquity; indeed, I did not quite succeed, for he shook his head and said, "I hope it is so, for I would have killed him if he had not left off."

This subject is of vast importance to mankind, and I trust most sincerely that the time is dawning for us to thoroughly grip the true nature of things, and not imagine that we can whip away this habit when due — as it mostly is at the start — to physical disease. For it were quite as rational to whip or otherwise chastise our children because they get diarrhoea or the measles. (XXII 145)

## 501. EFFECTS OF VACCINATION

A little girl of 3 years of age was brought to me some time since for this same thing, — the wee mite would "work with crossed legs" in a manner I will stop short of describing. Notwithstanding her tender age, the habit had become inveterate, and she would continue at it almost by the hour. Eminent medical men had declared the case to be one of disease of the spinal marrow that was incurable, and would end in paralysis. The aspect of the child was peculiar, inasmuch as there was, for her age, notable enlargement of the breasts. There were no indurated glands anywhere to be found, and the child was fat and well formed, excepting, that the mammary enlargement gave her the aspect almost of a wee pigmy woman. Not finding anything whatever in her physical state to account for the said naughty habit, I enquired closely into her history, and found that she had been vaccinated on the leg in lieu of the arm, and that not long after the vaccination — done when the child was about a year old — she began to work about with her legs, and gradually formed the habit in question.

Those who care to learn my views in regard to the effects of vaccination will find them expressed in my small work entitled "Vaccinosis and its Cure by *Thuja*."

I used in this case not only *Thuja*, but almost all our great anti-sycotics before a cure was permanently effected; in the end I did, however, succeed. Vaccinosis is in the very deed a very real disease. (XXII 148)

## DISEASES OF WOMEN

### 502. ABOUT SEPIA

I was not very long after this driving one day into the country accompanied by an eminent clergyman, a grand old man, and a staunch old homoeopath, whose benign smile of pity for all non-homoeopaths very much impressed me, who spoke to me during the drive thus : . . . "I took my daughter Julia to Dr. X. (an eminent gynecologist), because she complained of a pain across her back and local catarrh, and he examined her and told me the womb was enlarged, and that she must wear a support."

"But surely, doctor, you do not suggest that for a young woman like my daughter Julia; can you not cure that condition with medicines?"

"No, there is no cure for it except wearing a support."

"Well, doctor, I cannot consent to such a thing, I must find something better than that; what do you think of homoeopathic medicines?"

"Homoeopathic medicines! what nonsense."

"Poor man," concluded my venerable friend, "we must pray for the Lord to open the eyes of his understanding that he may see the truth; I gave Julia *Sepia* for some time, and quite cured her." (XXIII 10)

### 503. RECURRENT ABORTION

A childless lady, nine years married and who, though childless, had yet had seven miscarriages, with all their attendant miseries of floodings, grief, and disappointment, placed herself frankly under my care on January 26, 1880, for the purpose of putting a stop to these habitual mishaps, and in the hope of having living children. The late Dr. Smith was of opinion that one-half of this lady's womb was ossified : the curious thing was that patient regularly aborted at 5 months, and the placenta was always adherent. Period normal; some neuralgia of *right* ovary. The uterus itself was thick and heavy, and one side of it much more rigid than the other. After *Alnuin.* 3x, and *Kali chlor.* 6, each for a month, she fell pregnant, and with a view of trying to lessen the unilateral hardening of the womb, so that it might properly expand at the right time, I put patient on an exclusively fruit and vegetable diet; but she appeared unable to stand it, and so I allowed her one meat meal a day — one o'clock — but nothing else night and morning save fruit and soft vegetables at will. Big baby boy born May 22, 1881, and since then she has had five others, all hale and hearty, so she told me the other day (August 1893). Of course, patient had a number of medicines to prevent abortion and for her very troublesome piles — *Ferrum* 6, *Aesculus* 12, *Silicea* 12, and *Sulphur* 30 — but the principal lesson teachable that stands out is the elementary fact, that the organ diseases of women are amenable to drug action, and that diet can be made to play a part in abortion. I kept this lady on very low diet, and on several occasions with her first three children, when abortion or miscarriage was very imminent, I stopped nearly all food and all drink, allowing only fresh fruit for days together, till the hypogastric tumult had been starved out. With her last three children no treatment and no dietetic precautions were needed or taken. One has not often an opportunity of narriating such a long history as is here possible. (XXIII 12)

## 504. THE TRAUMATIC UTERUS

One meets with a number of youngish married ladies who are constitutionally sound and are yet great sufferers. In May 1880, such a one came to seek my help : she was 26 years of age, had been married five years, was the mother of one child, which was born at the end of the first year of married life. Applied Malthusianism accounted for the childlessness of the subsequent four years. Patient, from being of bonnie round figure, had become bosomless; her spine had two aches, an up and down rhachialgia and a pain across the back, — the classic uterine backache we all know of. The menses every sixteen days; the womb thick, sappy, and low-lying; leucorrhoeal ooze coming from the os. Patient was a mere wreck of her former self, and all for fear there should be too many people born into the world.

"No, I will not; I do not care; I'd rather die."

I should have said patient suffered much from insomnia, and had frequent attacks of nerve tortures.

I regarded the state as one manifestly from a battered, misused uterus, and so proceeded therapeutically with *Hypericum perf.* 3x, with *Arnica* 2, and concluded with *Bellis per.* 1. There was much improvement in the uterine sphere, and the menses had become less frequent. But the spinal irritation was much to the fore : *Guaco* 3 "did me great good; it stopped all the sickness and relieved the back very much."

Then a long railway journey upset the spine a good deal, and flooding set in; *Kali chlor.* 6 and *Fer. phos.* 6 stopped the bleeding, and *Cuprum acet.* 3x took the pain away from the side.

Then came *Guaco* 3 and *Bellis p.* 1, each a month by itself, with much amelioration.

There finally remained a condition in which almost any excitament brought on the poorly time, and this was cured by *Cedron* 3x, 5 drops in water every three hours. To *Cedron* I was led because patient complained very much of coldness in the abdomen : "Oh, my stomach is so cold." (XXIII 16)

## 505. DISPLACEMENT OF WOMB FROM ACCIDENT : THE ORGAN TWISTED

In dislocation of the uterus from accident the sufferings are frequently very severe indeed. Thus a married lady came under my observation on May 9, describing to me how eight years before she was touring in Switzerland, and had a fall which was followed by much bearing down and terrible pains across the hypogastrium. With this there was much irritation of the bladder. She suffered these horrors for three years before she could summon up courage to go to a doctor. Finally the pains drove her to an eminent London gynecologist of world-wide reputation. This gentleman failing to even relieve her, she consulted a second physician, and he also failed, and considered she would never get well owing to the intricate nature of the complaint. The uterus and everything seemed as if they were being dragged out of her body. Homoeopathy she despised and ridiculed, and it was only after eight years of suffering that she overcame her prejudice and consulted me. In addition, besides the forenamed symptoms, there was a peculiar form of leucorrhoea coming on every four or five days "in little torrents of thick yellow discharge."

*Secale cornutum* 3x cured this case so rapidly and completely that the displacement must be regarded as having been most probably a twist of the parts.

There was no mechanical interference on my part whatever, and the cure proved permanent.

That *Secale* was homoeopathic to the case no competent person will deny, especially if he has ever seen the effects of a full dose of ergot on a parturient person, who had a strong back and plenty of muscle. (XXIII 28)

## 506. POST INFLUENZAL NEUROSES

A married lady, 26 years of age, mother of three children, was brought to me from a distance on May 12, 1893, . . . "My cousin is just a wreck."

Patient was of fine stature — what the French call *large* — of tender fibre, her tissues having large meshes. Such people look much more healthy than they really are, and very commonly they are the product of a cross between a powerful individual and a consumptive one; the dash of consumptiveness is shown in their growth-largeness; they are large-celled and lacking in toughness. It was so in this case : her father died at 29, of phthisis; her mother is well and strong. Patient had had measles twice; influenza twice; and had been three times vaccinated; and only last year had had scarlatina. At her first confinement she was fearfully lacerated, and was subsequently sutured in five places. The case being very complicated, let us take it in sections from above downwards :—

1. Complete aphonia for some weeks, cannot produce any sound beyond a very slight indistinct whisper.
2. Left lobe of liver considerably enlarged and very tender.
3. Tongue mapped and very pippy; by mapped tongue I mean the so-called *lingua geographica*.
4. Spleen moderately swelled.
5. Very constipated, and much pain in back and sides.
6. Pretty bad haemorrhoids.
7. The uterus is enlarged.
8. The right ovarian region is the seat of a tumid mass rather bigger than my fist; the left one also, which is very painful.
9. There is severe but intermittent leucorrhoea.
10. The period is too frequent and excessive.
11. And the crowning misery of this unfortunate lady was total inability to pass water for the past two months, being obliged to use the catheter.
12. Many nerve-symptoms more or less distressing; and as these seemed to be largely due to her overcome two attacks of influenza, I started my therapeutic campaign with *Cypripedin* 3x, 6 grains three times a day.

*Cypripedium pubescens, Cypripedin,* and *Scutellaria lat.,* and *Scutellarin,* have long been my sheet-anchors in post-influenzal neuroses.

This bettered the neurotic part of the aphonia, and also the constipation, and patient was altogether brighter in her nerve life.

The spleen being swelled, and patient having at times some intermittent febrile movement, I followed with *Urtica urens* (gtt. xx. *in die*), and the more readily because of the retention of urine. This started a critical curative diarrhoea, under which the spleen became normal and the piles disappeared, and the aphonia lessened somewhat further. The retention of urine no better.

The retention being due, at any rate in part, to a swelling of the circum-urethral tissue, which I have at times reduced with the aid of *Saw palmetto* Q, I gave this in 5-drop doses four times a day, but it did no particular good; and hence I studied the case somewhat further, and because patient woke up with the pain between 3 and 4 A.M., the tongue being mapped in the centre, I gave *Mal.* 30 in infrequent dose.

The mappiness of the tongue disappeared under *Mal.* 30, but the pips stood out very prominently, and she now stated that she was worse in the evening. This was June 9, 1893, and under July 3 I find this note : . . . "Has twice lost her voice; tongue very much furred of a morning; constipation quite gone; piles gone."

$R_x$ *Arnica* 1, 10 drops in water night and morning.

August 14 — Voice quite well these four weeks; bowels normal; still inability to pass water, though the pain at the time of passing it is much less, the quantity more natural. Very severe leucorrhoea, causing great inconvenience. Insomnia.

$R_x$ *Med.* 1000.

September 11 — Voice normal; sleeps better; the pain in the side still comes on in the night; very much troubled with the whites; still unable to pass water; left lobe of liver tender.

$R_x$ *Chelone glabra* Q.

October 16 — No great change.

$R_x$ *Zincum acet.* Q.

November 24 — Period scanty; anorexia; breathless; palpitation of the heart; still cannot pass water naturally.

$R_x$ *Hydrastinin. mur.* 3x, 5 drops in water night and morning.

January 22, 1894 — "I have no pain in my side at all, ever; I pass water quite freely at times, but not always; piles and constipation very badly."

$R_x$ *Sulphur* 30 (infrequently).

March 2 — Piles and constipation cured; very bad white; micturition normal.

$R_x$ *Med.* 1000.

This finished the cure. Patient remained well, and in November, 1894, had another baby, and thereafter no trouble. (XXIII 31)

## 504. ENLARGEMENT OF WOMB : DROPSY OF LOWER EXTREMITIES

Mrs. X., 43 years of age, mother of a family, came to me on October 21, 1891, complaining of having frequently aborted, and of "weak heart, considerable swelling of lower abdomen, and dropsy of the lower extremities." She wears a pessary to keep up the heavy womb, as otherwise she cannot walk. Severe leucorrhoea. It seemed to me that the heart was not at fault, but that the entire trouble lay in the enlargement of the womb. She had lost a favourite child — her only boy — and was bowed down with grief, which latter called certainly for *Ignatia*. The pressure of the huge uterus, however, called for *Bellis*.

$R_x$ *Ignatia am.* 1 and *Bellis per.* Q, 20 drops of each daily in alternation.

November 4 — Distinct improvement in every way; leucorrhoea much better; can walk better.

During November and December she had *Helonias* Q and *Arnica* 1, when she was very much better, and exclaimed, "My swelled stomach is as flat as a pancake." Leucorrhoea and dropsy gone. No longer needs any pessary.

*Baccillinum* CC. followed, and under this the left leg swelled again. Early in 1892 she had a few weeks of *Fraxinus Americanus* Q, 10 drops twice a day, and was then in capital health, and functionally regular. (XXIII 39)

## 503. SUBINVOLUTED UTERUS FROM CONSTITUTIONAL CAUSE.

A married lady, 29 years of age, mother of one child two years and nine months old, was brought to me by a lady friend of hers, an old patient of mine, for a sad state of womb disease that had baffled all attempts at cure. The uterus was very much enlarged from subinvolution dating from her only pregnancy, and in which the placenta had been adherent; the rectum was packed full of piles that bled often very severely, and, besides this all, patient often had leucorrhoea and profuse monthly periods; vulvar and rectal regions deeply pigmented; inguinal and cervical glands like so many marbles. Her general condition one of great debility, and, moreover, she was very thin; her 'friends had given her up as a hopeless case. "No hope, I suppose," said her friend to me privately.

It was quite evident that though the case was one of womb enlargement, this enlargement was only a part, and only an insignificant part, of the case.

The prime element in this case was that constitutional state which lay behind the placenta praevia; this became more manifest after *Bellis perennis* Q and *Sepia* 5 had failed to do any great good (during the month of July 1892).

At the beginning of August things were very bad, and patient had again lost flesh. The duskiness of the body, the evening febrile movement, the emaciation, led me to give *Bacillin.* (CC.), under which remedy patient lost her fever and put on flesh. Then under *Thuja* 30 she lost ground, and I went back to *Bacill.* (C.), and kept her under its influence for a number of months — when, thereafter, *Fraxinus Americanus* in small material doses brought the womb back to its right size, and to-day, patient is plump and well, and has again resumed her wifely position, for which she had been so long unfit. The phthisic element in this case could only be met dynamically by a remedy of high similitude, and although the constitutional element in the case had been really and radically cured by the high potency of the pathological simillimum, still the womb remained enlarged. The organ was then met with an organ (i.e., womb) remedy — *Fraxinus Americanus* in small material doses — and the cure was complete, I had the very greatest difficulty to persuade the lady that I thought the organ returned to its normal size. August 1896, patient continues well and is *enceinte*. (XXIII 46)

## 509. EXCESSIVE ENLARGEMENT OF THE WOMB : THE ORGAN TO BE REMOVED BY OPERATION

Two or three years ago — rather more perhaps — a lady resident in London was in the habit of consulting me about her skin and about her children's ailings. We had many friendly chats, and latterly she was often tearful and seemingly in much distress. What is the matter? said I.

Oh! my favourite sister is so very very ill, the doctors have but very little hope of her.

This kind of thing recurred repeatedly, and finally she told me that all the doctors had decided that nothing but a very severe operation would now avail anything, and arrangments had been made to have it carried out forthwith, and rooms had been engaged off Cavendish Square for the purpose.

Great operations on women are common enough, and I did not heed the lady's laments very much, and I should not have done so had she not broken down with grief, and begged me to see whether the terrible operation could not be averted. "They are going to take the whole womb right away, it is so big that the body cannot contain it, and all the five doctors declare that that is the only thing that can be done."

It was arranged that the patient should be brought to me on the following Monday, the operation being fixed for the Tuesday.

Mrs. John X., mother of six children, aet. 38, was brought to me in July 1892. She came — was brought, that is — merely to please her heart-broken sister, and to prove to her that nothing could possibly be of any service save the formidable operation to be performed next day.

Briefly, it was a case of a hugely hypertrophied uterus, that was so much in excess of the space Nature had for its storage, that the unfortunate lady could do nothing whatever, and it was barely possible to even keep the immense mass somewhat propped up with the aid of a very large pessary. The womb had been scraped by one eminent surgeon, systematically curetted by another, and vigorously cauterised by a third, but it seemingly only got bigger.

There had been at one time a severe rent in the womb at one of her confinements; later on there was adherent placenta, and thereupon followed divers floodings, till, when I examined her, the uterus was big, hard, heavy, and thick.

Patient was well preserved in person, and quite free from disease in the ordinary sense, and, in fact, apart from the huge uterus, she was fairly well in herself, except that she was pale and anaemic from her too frequent periods.

medicines would quite cure her, and that such a terrible mutilation of her person was not necessary.

"But the operation is fixed for tomorrow morning!"

"What if it is? Have it put off, at any rate."

"But I have come all across the world for the purpose of having the operation done; it is too late to alter now."

The lady could not be persuaded to have the operation postponed, inasmuch as she had come over on purpose, and she had been terribly tortured with her poor womb, and she had borne the long voyage bravely, in the joyful anticipation of being finally rid of the unbearable burden for good and all.

"How old are you?" said I.

"Thirty-eight."

"And your husband, is he a worn-out old man?"

"Oh dear, no, not at all; he is really a young man still, and very strong."

"And your are going to have yourself thus mutilated, — you with a strong young husband?"

The contemplated operation was abondoned *for a time*, to see whether our medicines would do any good.

I removed the pessary, and ordered the lady 5 drops of the strong tincture of *Fraxinus Americanus* three times a day in water.

In a week already the operation was given up provisionally; in three weeks all idea of an operation was given up as certainly needless; and in seven weeks the patient could, and actually did, go to Scotland, and there took long walks on the moors without even a backache. The womb had simply diminished to about its normal volume, and gravitated back into its proper place, — and this under the sole influence of one medicine only — viz., the *Fraxinus Americanus*, at first in 5, then in 6, and latterly in 10-drops doses.

Patient had formerly had a good deal of *Quinine*, and was very cold and chilly; this was cured by *Nat. mur.*, 6 trit. She had been three times vaccinated, and was sycotic. *Thuja occid.* 30 and *Mal.* (C.) cured this state, and on one occasion I gave her *Ignatia amara* but all this was *subsequent* to the cure of the womb by *Fraxinus Am.* I dwell upon this to make it quite clear that the patient was cured of the uterine hypertrophy, and was running about on the Scottish moors, rejoicing in her new-found liberty, solely from the use of little material doses of one organ remedy — *Fraxinus Americanus*.

More than three years later — December 1895 — an aunt of this lady called upon me on her own account, and on my inquiring after my *Fraxinus* patient, she exclaimed "Oh! she is splendid, and her social duties are very heavy, owing to her husband's official position. Nobody can understand it." (XXIII 50)

## 510. ENLARGED WOMB DISTURBING MICTURITION, WITH SEVERE VOMITING.

The mother of six children, 72 years of age, sister of Sir William X., came under my observation on November 18, 1890, for insomnia and vomiting. The region of the pylorus being tender had led to the diagnosis of cancer of the pylorus, which appeared fully supported by the patient's semi-cachectic appearance. There was also some dullness on percussion in the pyloric region, and cruel attacks of dysepesia came on in the night.

There seemed little doubt as to the diagnosis, particularly as there was at times a very foul uterine discharge.

The womb was very large and anteverted, pressing on the bladder and causing much distress, as patient was often unable to pass water except in the erect position, the body being poised so as to take the pressure off the bladder. From my knowledge of the family constitution I was disposed to attribute most of the lady's symptoms to the bladder and uterus, which certainly were very distressingly to the fore : it seemed to me probable that the flatulence, fermentation, vomiting, and nocturnal attacks of vomiting might very well have their origin in the hypogastrium. This view of the sequence of the symptoms in the case was supported by patient's narration that she had formerly suffered much from leucorrhoea, and that a number of years after her change of life she had a bad discharge from the womb, and which was got rid of with the aid of vaginal injections.

I ordered *Bursa pastoris*, Q, 5 drops in water every four hours, and later on 6 drops night and morning only. Patient was completely restored to health thereby, and no other remedy was needed or given. At first sight such a thing seems next-door to impossible, but when we note that the Shepherd's Purse is a very splendid uterine remedy, we understand how it would be possible, which experience confirms.

This lady remained to my knowledge quite well for years, — indeed, I believe she is still alive. To this case I should have liked to append a few remarks on the suppression of whites by injections as a cause of disease, for this case was clearly of such an origin, but I must leave that for little further on. My choice of *Bursa pastoris* was because it is very apt to set up uterine discharge, and I have before shown, it is most certainly a uterine medicine. Moreover, it seemed to me, from patient's narration, that the nature of the case was gouty rather than cancerous, which the sequel has proved : there had been a gouty catarrh of the endometrium; this was refused outlet as leucorrhoea, and so it was reflected back on to the duodenal region. (XXIII 60)

## 511. BAD LEG — ENLARGED UTERUS —INTERMITTENT LEUCORRHOEA — AGUE CAKE — FRONTAL HEADACHE

An unmarried lady, 48 years of age, came to me in March 1895, for a bad leg. The bad leg consisted of a flat *mass* of quite small varicose veins about the left ankle, constituting a flat tumor raised about a quarter of an inch above the level of the skin. Towards eveing this varicose mass burned a good deal. Patient changed fifteen months before her visit to me, but suffered from intermittent leucorrhoea, and when the leucorrhoeal discharge came on the burning in the varicosic lump was intense. The uterus was moderately enlarged; general health excellent, barring the flushes, which were trying. Patient came bacause she was much concerned about the varicosic mass on her ankle, which would, she had been informed, become a "bad leg." The very moderate enlargement of the womb did not sufficiently account for the mass in question, and the burning in it seemed curious, notably the great burning in it when the leucorrhoeic discharge was active. I have elsewhere maintained that leucorrhoea is frequently connected with the spleen. A distinguished physician has tried to ridicule this, but I am still of the same opinion, and here reiterate the statement that leucorrhoea is frequently connected with the spleen, and this case strongly confirms this view. Finding that patient's spleen was swelled, I enquired if she had ever had ague? "Yes, in India, ten years ago." The leucorrhoea I regarded as from this spleen enlargement, and I also thought the varicosic tumour was likewise due to the state of the spleen.

*Pulsatilla* Q is a most useful organ remedy for the womb after the change of life, when there is no period to be disturbed and when the organ is moderately enlarged. During the menstrual life it is apt to be too disturbing, and must then be used in dilution if homoeopathically indicated. (XXIII 66)

## 512. VARICOSIC SWELLING

Miss X. took *Pulsatilla* Q, 5 drops in water night and morning, for a month, and it did good to the womb, and the whites and flushes were a little improved; but patient complained very much of feeling cold, though the weather was warmer than it had been (April 10). The spleen swelling seemed to me to be the primary seat of the mischief, and hence I ordered *Urtica urens* Q, 5 drops in water night and morning, and it very soon became manifest that the hypothetical diagnosis was correct, for the spleen came down in size, the chills disappeared, the varicosic swelling waned, and patient and physician were both delighted. Subsequently when *Urtica* had seemingly exhausted its action, and something appeared to bar the way to a complete cure, I made further inquiries, and elicited the fact that Miss X. had been four times vaccinated, and that her headache was much worse in the morning. The *Pulsatilla* had much improved the headache at first, but it returned. The *Urtica* did it no good, but *Thuja* 30 in infrequent doses cured the headache right off and completely.

Then *Ceanothus Americanus* 1 was given for some time — several months — and when I last saw patient she was practically well. A very small bit of the varicosic swelling alone remained, for which I ordered some remedy which I have not noted. I often pass Miss X. in the street, and to judge by her looks and pleasant greetings I have no doubt she is well. (XXIII 69)

## 513. PLEURODYNIA OF LEFT SIDE.

I desire here to add a word or two more or less apposite to the question as to whether the spleen stands in any relation to the uterus. I maintain that it does (see my *Diseases of the Spleen*).

The submammary pain — the classic "pain under the left breast," and its equally classic remedy, *Cimicifuga* — indicate a certain relationship between the uterus and upper part of the left side in women. "Pain in the side" is very vague, but many ladies complain to me of it. In this case the pain was located under the left ribs — *i.e.*, in the spleen region (spleen enlarged); the pain was worse periodically (every third day), but never absent. Patient *formerly* suffered from leucorrhoea. From the history of the case I was led to give *Bellis perennis* Q. It did a little good; but the pain returned, and then disappeared under *Tub. t.* C. (patient was losing flesh, had hectic flush of cheeks, worse in the afternoon). All periodicity left, and then followed *Cimicifuga* 1, *Thuja* 30, *Sabina* 30, and finally, *Tub. t.* C. When the pain had gone, the spleen was normal, and Miss C. had gained many pounds in weight, and since continues well. Here the pain in the side came subsequent to the disappearnce of the leucorrhoea, and from the remedies that acted curatively I fell sure it was a case of sycosis (hydrogenoid constitution) and psora mixed. (XXIII 72)

## 514. SUBINVOLUTED UTERUS — HAEMORRHAGE — BACKACHE

A gentleman, resident of South America, formerly a patient of mine, sent his young wife home to be here placed under my care for serious ill-health. This was August 1894. Patient had borne a dead baby in the previous June, and had got very low from haemorrhage, which had never left off since the miscarriage.

The enlargement of the womb is considerable, the backache very bad, the haemorrhage severe, and with this, patient has lost a good deal of flesh; her skin (of covered parts) very deeply pigmented; her inguinal glands enlarged.

The diagnosis here was perfectly clear, viz., a very much enlarged womb. Now, it might be supposed, from my many laudations of organ medicines, that I should forthwith give this patient a good organ remedy, such as *Bursa pastoris, Helonias dioica, Franxinus Am., Aletris farinosa;* but I did not, and this brings me to a very important part of my task. But, perhaps, I had better record the case first, and comment upon it afterwards.

$R_x$ *Tub. t.* C. This was my first prescription on August 31.

September 17 — The haemorrhage has ceased entirely!

$R_x$ *Fraxinus Americanus* Q, 6 drops in water three times a day. This caused a considerable diminution in the size of the womb, with corresponding amelioration in the backache. Then first prescription of the *Tub. t.* C. was repeated, and continued for some time. In the winter *Saw palmetto* Q, and thereafter *Quassia* Q, when in the following June patient returned to her husband restored to comparative health.* (XXIII 74)

## 515. UTERUS ENLARGED — BACKACHE; GREAT DEPRESSION OF SPIRITS.

A maiden lady, aet. 38, came over from Ireland to be under my observation. The chief and most troublesome symptom was depression of spirits of a somewhat severe type. As this lady had been four times vaccinated, and *was much upset by travelling,* I began with *Thuja occid.* 30.

At her next visit she told me she was much less unhappy, but that her backache was very terrible. An examination showed the womb to be thick and heavy, its neck very pulpy, and the backache was worse between 10 to 11 A.M.

The depression of spirits and the thickened state of the womb both seemed to call for *Aurum,* and this I ordered thus : $R_x$ *Aur. met.,* 3 trit., gr. vj., one powder night and morning.

May 12 — The neck of the womb is much less pulpy to the touch, and patient is bright.

$R_x$ Rep.

June 25 — "I am so much better; I can run up and down stairs without my back aching as it used to do;" and as to depression, "I am quite jolly." Said her brother-in-law to me thereafter, . . . . . "You made a fine cure of my wife's sister; we are all very grateful, for we quite expected we should have to put her into an asylum." (XXIII 80)

## 516. CONSUMPTION WITH NIGHT SWEATS FROM SUPPRESSED LEUCORRHOEA DUE TO SUBINVOLUTED UTERUS

I hold very strong opinions on the question of intro-vaginal injections :

* This lady's husband wrote to me in August 1896, saying that my patient continued well and was expecting to be confined very shortly.

they are altogether damnable and pernicious, shallow in conception, wrong in theory, and harmful in practice.

A married lady, about 30 years of age, mother of one child, came to see me on February 5, 1891, for consumption. The case was quite a clear one, offering no difficulties of diagnosis : patient had a bad cough, night sweats, bloody expectoration, a tender spot in the right lung, as nearly as may be where the right bronchus begins to ramify. She has an affectionate, wealthy husband, who had the most eminent lung specialists of Europe to attend his wife; she had wintered in the South of France and in Algeria, and the thing had been kept at bay, but no cure had resulted, and the wasting process went on.

$R_x$ *Bacillinum* C.

March 2 — Was much better, but has a fresh cold and is worse than ever.

$R_x$ *Bacill.* 30.

17 — Urine thick, sedimentous; still coughs; nocturnal perspirations, no better, break out at 3 A.M.; period normal, bowels normal, but she is pale and *cold*.

$R_x$ *Urtica ur.* Q, which seemed to cure her; but on May 14, some slight pulmonary haemorrhage with the expectoration alarmed the family, and I went over the case carefully afresh, and came slowly to the conclusion that the pulmonary affection was from whites, suppressed with intro-vaginal injections, and not primarily a pulmonary case at all. To find the primary starting-point on any ailment is of the highest importance, dency it who may.

$R_x$ *Med.* CC.

In a week the lady wrote telling me that since taking the powders she had got a good deal of pain in her back, lasting for an hour or two each day, viz., from 12 to 2 P.M., and some coloured discharge had come away like shreds of skin. "I had less of the pain to-day, but to-night at dressing time (7-30) a larger piece came away, and I thought it well to send it to you to let you see [it was a piece of fluffy, shreddy tissue covered with mucus and blood, size of a haricot bean]; I had the same sort of thing for some time when I was recovering from my confinement, about eight or ten weeks after it, and was then recommended to syringe with sulphate of zinc and alum, which soon cured (!) it. This time it began after the period had been over for one day; my back feels better to-day." The medicine to be finished.

June 2 — Still coughs; the expectoration is yellow, thick; the tongue white, and the cough worst in the early morning.

$R_x$ *Med.* 1000.

Result, perfect cure.

**Five Years Later.** Patient continues quite well of her lungs, and is indeed in splended health, and has borne two bonnie children since her cure. (XXIII 84)

## 517. UTERUS ENLARGED : INFERTILITY

The case before me now is that of a married lady, 27 years of age, two years married, and childless. I found the uterus enlarged and retroverted, which amply accounted for both dysmenorrhoea and sterility. Patient had numerous little lumps on her scalp, and a lipoma on her left hip, size of an oyster; patient was also troubled with seatworms, and was thin, had evening flushes, and in addition to this she suffered from hay fever. Very scurfy scalp. A good deal of indigestion, and moist palms. I first treated the lady's constitution for a year, during which period she had *Bacill.* CC. (for three months), *Saw palmetto* Q, and *Mal.* CC., when she was much better in a general way, but no sign of a pregnancy. Followed *Aur. met.* 3x, which did the uterus much good; and after *Thuja* 30 and *Saw palmetto* Q she fell pregnant, one year and seven months after coming to me. A fine boy arrived in due course; and two years later a friend of hers exclaimed to me one day, "Oh! Mrs. X has another baby." (XXIII 89)

## 518. STERILITY; MISSHAPEN UTERUS; PERIOD IN ABEYANCE

A married lady, 28 years of age, came to me on February 11, 1891, telling me that she had been married five years, but was childless, to her great regret. Her uterus seemed to have no cervix at all, and although 28 years of age and five years married, she had had only seventeen or eighteen monthly periods *in her life*, and none at all for the past eleven months.

For ten years she had had a fixed pain in the left side of the abdomen, just under the ribs. The pain was constant, and dated from enteritis of ten years ago. Patient had suffered very much from hysteria, and is very thin, pale, washed-out and very depressed.

There being much dulness on percussion in the painful spleen region, I started with *Urtica urens* Q, 10 drops in water twice a day.

February 19 — After beginning with the tincture, the side pain became much worse; but in four days all pain and swelling had gone. . . . "Something seems to have gone down in my left side."

Rep.

March 10 — The pain in the left side now comes and goes, and is relieved by fomentation.

$R_x$ *Thuja* 30.

April 23, 1891 — More pain.

$R_x$ *Bursa Pastoris* Q, 7 drops in water night and morning. This restored the menses, and patient felt herself very stronger.

May 28 — The period continues, but is very painful.

$R_x$ *Pulsatilla* Q, 6 drops in water at bedtime.

July 21 — Has just returned from the continent, and during her absence has had two periods. Her spleen is still very large; she is chilly; her breasts are now "much more natural," and the whole abdomen also.
$R_x$ *Bellis perennis* Q, 10 drops in water in the morning on rising.
August 26 — No period.
The case has no further point of interest beyond the fact that the lady since then has borne two bonnie children; and when her sister came to me on her own account not long since, I sent a reproachful message complaining that the children had not been shown to me, and that I should have been glad to know how the uterus had behaved; but the message the other day came back :... "Tell the doctor my children require all my time and attention; I have no time to spare to come to him!" (XXIII 91)

## 519. STERILITY

A married lady, 28 years of age, came under my observation on January 19, 1893, to be treated for sterility. She bore a dead child two years ago, and there had been no conception since. Patient's husband is a much respected allopathic surgeon, who does "not believe in homoeopathy at all, you know;" but still, "must confess that it seems very good for women and children."
Patient suffers very severely from leucorrhoea, ever since her thirteenth year. Her husband has never had syphilis. The whole uterus is swelled, and the entire fore-uterine region very tender to the touch. Patient once lay on her back for three years on account of her womb.
$R_x$ *Aur. mur.* 3x, ziv., 5 drops in water night and morning.
March 12 — *Enceinte* ! and feels very well and full of joy, for she had already almost given up the hope of having a family; a good deal of nausea.
$R_x$ *Thuja occid.* 30.
April 27 — Doing well, but the morning vomiting is very bad indeed, almost an illness in itself.
$R_x$ *Med.* 1000, which promptly and completely cured the morning sickness.
*Med.* 1000 for this ailing is a grand friend in need and indeed; many a time ladies have written for "those powders that cure morning sickness," and this is the remedy. The dose is not to be lightly repeated; in this case the first dose aggravated, the third was followed by a cure. (XXIII 94)

## 520. ENLARGEMENT AND DISPLACEMENT OF THE UTERUS; PERI-UTERINE HAEMATOCELE

A married lady, 25 years of age, came to me on March 4, 1892. She had been two years married, and was childless. She handed me the following note :

"Mine has been considered a case of tubular pregnancy, but is now called an effusion of blood from the Fallopian tube, left side, and which the doctors have told me could not be cured without an operation; but hearing from Mrs. R. of your successful treatment of her case, I feel anxious to come to you."

[Mrs. R.'s case was one of ovarian tumour of left side, (see Case 422 above) and is narrated in my *Curability of Tumours by Medicines*; and, by the way, Mrs. R. has continued in good health to this day, and quite free from tumour.]

I found a tumid mass in the region of the left ovary, size of man's fist; the uterus enlarged and pulled over to the left, the cervix almost obliterated, and its posterior wall bulging backwards on the rectum, thick and hard. Patient's period was said to be normal, though there was a browny discharged from the vagina between whiles.

There was in this case a very obvious constitutional background to the disease-picture here presented; the state was not merely one of an enlarged womb, and merely displaced by its weight, but the haematocele had also to be reckoned with *in its constitutional causation*.

Now, patient's father died at 48 of fistula, which may fairly be assumed to be of a tubercular nature; a number of her brothers and sisters died in infancy; her tongue was very pippy in its interior half.

Patient was put under *Bacill.* CC. for a month.

April 1 — The lump is much smaller; she feels sick and bilious. Still many pips.

$R_x$ *Fragaria vesca* Q, 5 drops in water night and morning.

April 27 — The brown discharge has ceased.

$R_x$ *Sabina* 30.

May 27 — Period normal; watery whites; lump still there, though smaller.

$R_x$ *Arnica montana* 1x, 5 drops in water night and morning.

June 24 — Less watery whites; many pips.

$R_x$ *Bacill.* CC.

July 22 — Tumour gone, but the womb is still heavy.

$R_x$ *Fraxinus Americanus* Q.

August 27. — Discharged cured. (XXIII 101)

## 521. ENLARGED UTERUS OF CONSTITUTIONAL CAUSE; SPERMATOPHOBIA

On February 6, 1889, a married lady, mother of four children, came under me for pains in the breasts at the period, constipation, enlargement of uterus, palpitations, and great weakness; her horror of child-bearing could only be described as awful, an all-consuming life-paralysing dread. She was very thin, and might be described as having absolutely no breasts, owing to practices arising out of her painfully obstrusive spermatophobia.

Closely regarded, this mental state was probably due to actual disease, and prompted by the instinct of self-preservation. Two brothers had died of phthisis, and she hereself had pneumonia last year. The life-long constipation was practically a substantive disease.

R_x *Bacill.* C.

March 8 — "I am very much better; I feel stronger, able to walk; my appetite is better; but very little pain in the breasts, and . . . will *any one be able to believe it?*"

I confess I hardly like to pen a statement of facts that take so much believing. The life-long constipation — for which she had been almost dosed to death with aperients — was a thing of the past, and the action of the bowels was perfectly normal. She had been three times vaccinated, *ergo, Thuja* 30.

April 8 — Bowels quite regular. "The first powders quite cured my constipation." She is of opinion that the first powders were remarkably good aperients, and says the last powders do not act so well on the bowels as the first.

R_x *Bacill.* C.

May 8 — Bowels costive again; breasts seem slightly increased.

R_x *Sabina* 30.

June 26 — Bowels regular. "I am so much stronger."

The constitutional cause having been got rid of, *Helonin* 3x, *Bellis perennis* Q, and *Hydrastis canadensis* Q followed as organ remedies, and *Bacill.* C. was once repeated; and twenty-six months from the beginning of the treatment patient was well and plump, and was discharged cure. (XXIII 107)

## 522. PROLAPSE UTERUS AND HAEMORRHOIDS

I will just relate one case :— A lady, widow of a notable London physician, suffering from complete *procidentia uteri* and very bad haemorrhoidal bleeding, wrote to me one day from the country to say that she was driven almost mad with painful micturition; the burning and straining were truly awful. *Triticum repens* Q, in 10-drop doses frequently repeated, brought a most grateful letter, with the request, that she might have a supply to keep by her. Cough grass is highly esteemed, and much used by British herbalists as a bladder medicine. I have used it these twenty years, and declare it to be a splendid medicine in dysuria. (XXIII 118)

## 523. THE HAEMORRHOIDAL UTERUS : STERILITY

On October 8, 1889, a married lady, 28 years of age, consulted me for what I sometimes think of as a haemorrhoidal uterus, viz : the period is

disturbed, and the haemorrhoidal veins seem to bleed vicariously for the endometrium, the period itself being scanty. This lady had only one little girl 5 years of age, but she was most desirous of having more family, and her husband very desirous of having an heir, he possessing large estates. I began the treatment with *Nux* 30 and *Sul.* 30 night and morning in alternation. Patient had been to Schwalback to no purpose.
November 14 — Much better; period scanty.
$R_x$ *Bellis per.* Q, 10 drops in a tablespoonful of water night and morning.
January 16. 1890 — Much better. There being some endometric catarrh, and patient having been twice vaccinated, the second time nine years ago unsuccessfully, I now ordered *Thuja* 30.
February 13 — "For the first time in my life my period come on exactly the day four weeks, and although the piles are still there, they do not trouble me." As patient had had typhoid at five years of age, I ordered *Pyrogenium* 5, 3 drops night and morning.
April 20 — Is enceinte.
A little girl came in the course, and all went well.
October 13, 1891 — Patient did not suckle her little girl, and the uterus is now subinvoluted; the piles are again to the fore, and her husband is most anxious for a son and heir. *Nux* 30 and *Sul.* 30 were given, as on the previous occasion.
Jamuary 9, 1892 — Is weak.
$R_x$ *Levico* (strong), 10 drops in water at bedtime.
February 11 — Period four days late.
$R_x$ *Thuja* 30.
March 14 — Period one day late.
May 5 — *Bellis perennis* Q.
September 26 — Piles rather worse. *Nux* 30 and *Sul.* 30.
January 10, 1893 — Patient is depressed, and despairs of ever having her heart's desire, particularly as the period has become very infrequent. I thought it therefore desirable to rouse the parts to greater life, and prescribed *Aurum muriaticum* 3x,. 5 drops in water night and morning.
February 4 — Period much more satisfactory. She is altogether better.
$R_x$ *Fraxinus Americanus*, in the mother tincture, 10 drops in 3j. water night and morning.
March 16 — *Enceinte.*
A fine boy arrived in due course, and all went well.
July 7, 1896. — "Oh! he is a splendid boy; he is nearly three years old, and so well." (XXIII 120)

## 524. ENLARGED UTERUS DUE TO ABORTION

Lady X., well past 40 years of age, and not very long married, aborted at the end of 1891. The uterus was found very heavy, lowlying, and soft and warm to the touch, and bleeding at times.

I began with *Bellis perennis* Q 10 drops in water three times a day. This was continued with much advantage for about three weeks, when *Helonin* 3x followed, and then *Arn. mon*. 3x.

In the fourth month of the treatment *Thuja* 30 was given; in the fifth month *Arnica montana* 1x; and during the last month *Fraxinus Americanus* Q, when Lady X. was discharged in splendid health and entirely normal in the uterine sphere.

Lady X. had received injections from her family doctor, and some of her trouble was due to said injections. (XXIII 124)

## 525. NEURALGIA OF THE BLADDER; STERILITY; WITH ENLARGEMENT OF THE UTERUS AND OF THE SPLEEN

Lady K. sends me Mrs. Y., now home from Africa. She is 35 years of age, has been married for eighteen years, and has had no child for fifteen years, when she was confined of a still-born child. There was last year a bad miscarriage, and since then she has never been well, though all the time under the care of a very eminent gynecologist. This gentleman's diagnosis is neuralgia of the bladder. Patient is obliged constantly to pass water : the pains are burning; very, very small pips; anaemic; dark under eyes; very depressed before the period. The breasts give a good deal of trouble, being the seat of prickly pains.

Patient had had sunstroke,* and was commonly worse in the evening.

$R_x$ *Bacill.* CC. This was August 1892.

September 6 — Pips less distinct; the urinary trouble is much better; less backache; not at all depressed before this period.

$R_x$ *Thuja* 30.

Sept. 23 — Period so much better; the left rib region bulges a good deal and is rather painful.

*Persons with a consumptive strain in their constitutions are very prone to sun-stroke, typhoid fever, and in later life to softening of the brain.

$R_x$ Tc. *Urtical ur*. Q, 7 drops in water night and morning.

November 1 — Tc. *Saw palmetto* Q, 7 drops in water night and morning.

Christmas 1892. — Mrs. Y. is enceinte.

August 10, 1893 — A lady coming; to me on this date told me, "Mrs. Y. is daily expecting to be confined" (in last letter).

This case was one not properly termed sterility, perhaps, but at any rate it was one of childlessness from constitutional diseases.

Mrs. Y. is in an out-of-the-way part of Africa, so I have no knowledge of how things went. (XXIII 126)

## 526. ENLARGEMENT AND DISPLACEMENT OF UTERUS — NEURALGIA OF FIVE YEARS' STANDING — STERILITY

Countess X. came under my observation on January 22, 1887, for neuralgia of the forehead and top of head during the past five years; she suffered also from severe leucorrhoea, and for the same period of five years; and her married life was also of the same duration, viz., five years. She had never been pregnant at all, visits to Schwalbach notwithstanding. The neck of the uterus enormously thickened, the os pointing rectum-wards. Period every three weeks, and lasts a week, and very painful.
$R_x$ *Sabina* 30.
February 9 — Period lasted a week, but was only painful for two days. She feels better.
$R_x$ Rep.
March 23 — Period very painful. $R_x$ Tc. *Fluor. aurant. amar.* Q, 5 drops in water night and morning.
April 21 — Neuralgia gone; the menstrual pain is seemingly in the uter itself.
$R_x$ *Thuja* 30.
May 3 — Uterus much more comfortable; leucorrhoea certainly b
$R_x$ *Helonias dioica* Q.
June 2 — The neck of uterus is very hard; neuralgia b
Patient wonders whether she will ever have a child. Said
only want one boy to succeed to the peerge. We don't want an
we are too poor to keep any more. No, we don't want any girl;
too poor!"
$R_x$ Tc. *Aur. mur. nat.* 3x.
July 26 — No neuralgia; no pain at period; the neck of the uterus is short and softer.
$R_x$ Rep.
August 18 — Rather a sore throat; menses two days only; no pain; whites gone; the elongated hypertrophied cervix is half an inch shorter, and the uterus in an almost normal position.
$R_x$ Rep.
November 1 — No white; uterus still heavy and hard.
$R_x$ *Bellis perennis* Q, 5 drops in water night and morning.
February 11, 1888 — The os points right on to the rectum.
$R_x$ Trit. *Plat. met.* 3, which was continued for some time, till her ladyship had taken sixty 6-grain powders, when she fell *enceinte*, and in due course bore a fine boy, who is the heir-presumptive to the peerage, and a grand little man he is, so I am told. (XXIII 129)

## 527. ENLARGEMENT OF UTERUS — BAD LEUCORRHOEA — STERILITY

Lady X., 24 years of age, has been married several years and is childless. The gynecologist, manipulations and operations, together with syringing and Schwalbach, have not mended matters. Her husband is next heir to a peerage, and "my husband is getting very angry with me because we have no heir, for his uncle comes next after him, and he hates him."
Patient, so good and so willing to do the bidding of her lord, had broken down in her nerve-life, and was getting bad attacks of somewhat grave hysteria.
Uterus enlarged, anteverted; much catarrh of the endometrium. *Bellis perennis* Q, *Ignatia amara* 1x, *Oleum succini* non-rect., and *Fraxinus Americanus* Q, all followed on lines already given, when on September 8, 1892, distinct improvement was noted in the uterine sphere, but her ladyship was getting thin, with circumscribed flush on each cheek of an evening.
R$_x$ *Bacill.* CC.
October 18 — Fearfully swelled around the hypogastric area, and yawns most painfully.
R$_x$ *Aur. mur.* 3.
November 26 — Morning vomiting. Period three weeks overdue. *Viburnum* Q.
A bonnie boy was born in due course, and since then two other children have followed, so I learned when I met her ladyship down by Rotten Row. (XXIII 132)

## 528. FISTULA IN ANO

Early in this year, a married lady, 34 years of age, came under my observation for fistula in ano. In my opinion, fistula, wherever situate, is almost always tubercular alone, or tubercular and something else. It also frequently happens that oophoritis is likewise of tubercular quality, with or without a superadded gleety quality. The lady in question had had ovaritis (or, as I prefer, on philologic grounds, oophoritis), which formed purulent collections in the tissues, and these pointed in the anal region, where they were operated upon. It was finally held that the fistular issues at the anus would not heal because of their connexion with the left ovary certainly, and probably with the right ovary also. So it was determined to perform ovariotomy on this lady, so that she might be rid of the *fons et origo mali*. This was done, both ovaries being removed, and very prettily and neatly it was done. And the result? The lady had no further menstruation, became enormously obese — almost formlessly so. And the fistula? They continued to bother just the same as before, for the simple reason that fistulae commonly are of constitutional nature and origin, and the cutting out of the tuberculous ovaries did not cure the organismic tuberculosis, any more than cutting off a gouty toe will cure the gout.

A brother and a sister of this lady had both died of phthisis, and this lady had phthisis situate in her ovaries and the anal region, in the form of ovarities and fistula respectively. Gout in the eye is as much gout as gout in the big toe, and tuberculosis in the ovaries is as much phthisis as phthisis pulmonalis, and requires the same qualitative treatment as set forth in my *New Cure of Consumption*.

This treatment was adopted for Mrs. R. on March 17, 1896.

June 2 — The 3 year old fistula has healed.

$R_x$ Rep.

September 15, 1896 — The fistula remains healed, and its former canal can be traced by the colour of the skin for fully two inches. (XXIII 136)

## 529. PTHISIS PULMONALIS

Few kinds or forms of disease permit the clear clinical proof of disease-quality better than tuberculosis, for unless the disease-quality be radically cured the treatment goes on and on, not infrequently to a fatal issue. Thus, a few months ago a gentleman came to me from the neighbourhood of Birmingham. He was about 28 years of age, and was the subject of tuberculosis, manifested at the time of his first visit to me as phthisis pulmonalis located in the upper third of the right lung, and as scrotal fistula of the right side. There were frequent blood-spitting, night-sweats, bad cough, moderate loss of flesh, dusky skin, and great weakness. The progressive history of the disease was very instructive, and bears out the views I am at this point trying to lay before my readers. The thing began as tubercular synovitis of the right knee joint (he was puceau, and hence had not had gonorrhoea); and to prevent any spread of the disease to the constitution, his right leg was amputated just above the knee. All went well and patient made a good recovery, and was supposed to have had the primary seat of the disease totally removed and his life saved. After a while, however, tuberculosis broke out in his left testicle, and many consultations of eminent surgeons were held as to what to do next. It was finally decided to remove the diseased testicle to save the constitution, and he was assured that this time the cure would be radical. The left testicle was accordingly removed and patient again made a complete recovery, and returned home and to his business full of hope and gratitude to his surgical benefactors. After a while tuberculosis broke out in the remaining testicle; the organ swelled, inflamed and broke, and discharged bacilli-containing pus. Many more consultations took place, and as there was a bad cough, physicians were called to consult with the surgeons, and then came blood-spitting : nevertheless it was decided to remove the remaining testicle. At this stage patient came under our scientific homoeopathic treatment. He is getting well, but the point that here concerns me is that surgery cannot cure constitutional disease even though expressed only in a part. (XXIII 139)

### 530. RINGWORM : SCALP

A girl of 11, with ringworm on the scalp; the lymphatic glands everywhere palpable, and her ribs very flat; strawberry tongue; a bad cough, worse at night; although 11 years old she had practically no teeth, that is to say, they were rudimentary and not above the level of her gums. *All* her mother's brothers and sisters had died of consumption; after three months' treatment with our ordinary remedies we had made but small progress, and then I kept patient altogether five months under the bacillic virus, with the result that her palpable glands ceased to be palpable; her ringworm disappeared; her ribs took on a better form; her breathing was notably better; and, *mirabile dictu, her teeth had grown.* She is now well, and has a mouthful of teeth which are quite passible. (XXIII 12)

## THE CHANGE OF LIFE IN WOMEN

### 531. ADDISON'S DISEASE FROM SUPPRESSED LEUCORRHOEA

In the month of July 1891, a New York merchant brought his wife to London to place her under my care for vomiting, great debility, weakness and a brown discolouration of the skin. Patient was forty-one years of age, and was still regular, but had no children. That Addison's disease is a branch of the tree known as tuberculosis seems very possible; but although this patient was in a state of debility in her youth which bordered, they said, on consumption, and her own father had succumbed to phthisis, still the most striking symptom was a fearful backache that resisted all treatment, and in the main my remedies did patient but very little good. It did not matter whether the remedies chosen were high, low, or medium, or whether the prescriptions were routine ones, "snap-shot" ones, or laboriously repertorial — they all failed more or less; and although amelioration frequently set in here and there, and patient would begin to get better and to carry a little healthier colour, still more of the spells of improvement was lasting — mine was a variable work of Sisyphus. So passed three years, till one day she exclaimed to me — "I have the whites, and I am now not able to check them like I have been." Further conversation elicited the fact that the *beginning of* patient's ill-health coincided with the cure (?) of her severe leucorrhoea with injections! And during all these three years of my generally pretty close prescribing, as soon as she began to mend a bit the whites appeared, whereupon these were attacked and qualled with injections, and patient went worse again! It was a very different affair as soon as the injections were given up, and in a few months patient was vastly improved, and got into fair health, but never really well, and died of vomiting and debility after a very long railway journey, followed by a long carriage drive in the cold in July 1896, no doubt of Addison's disease, I quote the case here merely to show the part in it played by leucorrhoea, otherwise it does not touch our subject very closely. But it brings home to my mind the fact that in this case, at any rate, the leucorrhoea was an outlet from the economy, and beneficial to it in the same sense as a leaky boat may be kept afloat by adequate baling-out of the water, no matter how laborious the baling-out might be. It is most probable that if this lady's leucorrhoea had been let alone, she would have fared better; and had the causal tuberculosis been first cured, early in life, Addison's disease would never have developed. Leucorrhoea is often a manifestation of a tubercular constitution, and when suppressed leads to graver developments of the same diathesis. And surely if leucorrhoea is sometimes a manifestation of a tubercular diathesis, it is not the leucorrhoea which is primary, but the tuberculosis, which is the real disease, and the leucorrhoea is secondary to it, and its existence constitutes in the main an outlet for morbid matter or disease-stuff of some kind. These are no fanciful pictures, but based on facts from my own experience, and they may be seen in my (and anyone else's) clinical work any day and almost any hour. (XXIV 11)

## 532. CHANGE OF LIFE, FIBROID TUMOUR OF THE UTERUS, HAEMORRHOIDS WITH VERY SEVERE RECURRENT HAEMORRHAGE FROM THE BOWELS

A childless widow, fifty years of age, was brought to me on July 9, 1891, suffering from the above very formidable ailments. She changed a year previously, and ever since gets attacks of bleeding piles every five or six weeks. The fibroid tumour was about the size of a man's fist. Patient was very pale and ill, worse towards evening.

Patient was discharged cured at the end of 1893, she having attended very regularly all the time. The tumour slowly disappeared, the attacks of piles ceased, as also the rectal haemorrhages. I only name the case here because of patient's old, old habit of *using vaginal injections,* which, in my opinion, led up to the formation of the tumour. Leucorrhoea is a catarrh differing very much in pathological quality in different cases; there is not one substantive disease called leucorrhoea, but the thing is commonly of a depurative nature, and stopping it by local measures is a wrong proceeding. Leucorrhoea may in many ways be compared to eczema of the skin, for eczema is also a catarrh, often of a depurative nature, and treating eczema by local remedies, unguents, and lotions is equally a wrong proceeding. (XXIV 12)

## 533. NOTE ON *LYSSINUM*

I do not know where to fling in an odd note on this important remedial agent that I have used for a good many years in here and there a case, and in its own little sphere of influence it is even in erotomania, with me, a tried remedy. And I have extended its use to some of those many cases of spasms and the like, so often met with in clinical life, whose cause is really primarily from unsatisfied sexual longings, often called hysteria. The sufferings of the celibate state, notably in women, are at times amenable to its benign influence, and to this I was partly led by a consideration of the prime cause of rabies, viz., pent-up sexual longings. We will not dwell too much on the subject, but I feel bound to name this, my valuable clinical friend. I use 30 and C. and higher only. And when we reflect on the truly awful sufferings of this lyssic state in the human subject, we must gratefully accept the help which *Lyssinum* can give. Of course, like all homoeopathically used remedies, it fits only certain cases, not by any means all, for *Med.* and *Luet.* (both high) also play a great part in such loveless states.

"I am roused in the night with such fearfully horrible, sinful feelings" calls for *Med.*

"No sooner does night come on than I am a prey to such dreadfully sinful desires that drive me mad" calls for *Luet.* Now are all these sin? I cannot think so; to my mind they are no more sinful than colic or neuralgia; they are just the sufferings of our common humanity, and what sufferings too! Much worse than mere pain. (XXIV 12)

## 534. TUMOUR OF LEFT BREAST AT THE MENOPAUSE

It is very instructive to note the beginnings of tumours principally in the breasts and womb as the change of life *is looming*, but has not yet arrived. I read it thus : The pre-existent constitutional taint that heretofore has overflowed and sailed off in the menstrual flux no longer does so completely, and hence the organism has to deposit what has remained behind somewhere, and this constitutes the beginning of many of the tumours. Of course, the causation may not be *merely* a lack of elimination by way of the period, but it is seemingly so to a large extent.

Miss X., forty-five years of age, came under my observation on 27th October, 1891, for a tumour in her left breast, that had been growing for about a year. We observed an induration of the tissues, about the size of a child's hand, in the outer aspect of the left breast; it was tender to touch and somewhat painful : worse at night. Period painful, regular : whites formerly pretty bad, but they had disappeared for some time, and were now returning slightly. Tongue very frothy, in two rows.

$R_x$ *Viburnum* Q, Ten drops at bedtime.

November 19th — The tumid, indurated mass is nearly gone; much painful indigestion.
$R_x$ Tc. *Bellis p.* Q. Ten drops in water at bedtime.
January 21st, 1892 — No pain last period. Less haemorrhoids.
$R_x$ *Hydrastis Can.* Q. Ten drops in water night and morning.
March 17th — Breast well; whites gone.
December, 1892 — No return of tumour, and patient quite well in herself. (XXIV 15)

## 535. THE PRECANCEROUS BLEEDING WOMB AT THE MENOPAUSE

There are a large number of cases of bleeding from the womb at, and about, *and after* the change of life that come before me, that are almost always considered by me as incipient cancer. That they are cancer in the early stage I have no doubt whatever, but inasmuch as they get well, often very quickly under the use of *Gold* and other remedies, I will content myself with speaking of such as the precancerous bleeding womb.

Mrs. W., forty-four years of age, mother of nine children and had also four miscarriages, came under my observation at the end of the year 1891. She had for the past five or six months considerable bleeding from the parts on and off all the time, but particularly excessive about the period. Some years ago patient vomited a good deal of blood. She is very weak and anaemic, and is, in the opinion of her own doctor, suffering from incipient cancer of the womb. Her mother died of cancer of the womb at seventy-one, and one of her sisters died of internal tumour at fifty.

$R_x$ *Aurum muriaticum* 3x, ziv. Three drops ir. water three times a day.
February 9th, 1892 — Patient is very lavish in her praise of this medicine. "Oh, I am so much better, the bleeding has gone." She feels very much better in herself; the tenderness of the womb has gone, and it is now normal to the touch. To go on with the medicine for some time.

I never beard any further of the case, and I should not have narrated it at all, were it not that it is only one of numerous cases of the kind that have come under my care, and of which many have promptly got well under the action of *Aurum*. (XXIV 16)

## 536. THE PRECANCEROUS BLEEDING WOMB

Some years since, Mrs. E., sixty years of age, was taken suddenly with haemorrhage from the womb, and fainted while on a visit to the house of a patient of mine. The local doctor (a very experienced all-round learned practitioner) was hurriedly sent for, and declared it cancer of uterus. It transpired that attacks of bleeding had been the rule with her for year past, which her anaemic, cachetic look fully corroborated; the bleedings were very ill-smelling, spoken of as "fleshy," like "cold soup." Patient had a large blood bleb on lower lip of long standing. The diagnosis being called in question, a second opinion of the chief surgeon of a well-known cancer hospital was sought, and he fully confirmed it. The lady returned home and had the infirmary doctors of her native city to say what they thought of the case, and they agreed that it was cancer, and recommended immediate operation.

"No," said patient, "I'll not be cut about; I have seen enough of that. If I'm to die, I'll die!"

I put her on *Aurum*, as in the previous case, and in three months she was seemingly quite well.

Three years later she had bleeding again, and the same remedy again put her right.

Two years after this she had another relapse, the smell being very bad. The same remedy was again ordered, and again it put her right and so she continued when I last heard from her. She must now be about seventy years of age.

September 23, 1896 — I happen to have just received a letter this very day from this lady's friend, from whom I enquired about the patient's state last Tuesday. She says :— "Mrs. E. came to see me to-day; she is a good deal better, and seemed in good spirits."

December 23 — She writes :— "I am a good deal better; all discharge has ceased."

Spring of 1898 — On enquiry I hear : "Mrs. E. continues well." (XXIV 17)

## 537. NEURASTHENIA AT THE MENOPAUSE

A maiden lady, forty-three years of age, came under my observation on January 19th, 1892, telling me of her painful nerves and flushes that have troubled her ever since she changed. She gets gouty swellings of the feet, and has whites. Is much given to sleeping draughts. The womb is somewhat large, the pain in the feet considerable depriving her of sleep. On condition that she abjures sleeping draughts once and for all, I undertake her case. This is an invariable condition with me, as it *is quite impossible to really cure people who take hypnotics.*

I gave *Fraxinus Amercicanus* Q. Ten drops in water at bedtime.

March 3 — Has done her much good; womb is lighter, and she is better able to do her work. She sleeps now quite well without any sedative, a sure proof that the neurasthenia was here primarily a womb ailing.

Flushes no better; skin very irritable : costive.

$R_x$ Tc. *Urtica ur*. Q. Five drops in water night and morning.

March 31 — "The first bottle suited me better for nervousness; flushes much better; general health also."

Followed a month of *Fragaria vesca* Q, and then *Fraxinus Americanus* Q, when patient had nothing further to complain of beyond her hard lot in life, for which latter I, however, know no healing herb. (XXIV 18)

## 538. GENERAL BREAK-UP AT THE MENOPAUSE ULCERATED WOMB

Weak constitutions often break up at the change of life, particularly if there is any great trial falling to their lot, which in this life is common enough. Such a case came under my observation in the spring of 1893.

Mrs. X. aged fifty-two, mother of six children, tells me she has been ailing very much ever since the change; the womb is ulcerated : she is "nothing but skin and bones;" chronic cephalalgia, insomnia, ; she retches and vomits; she complains of "whirlings like windmills in her head."

Her physicians have practically given her up, and they all have put her on sleeping draughts and "soothing injections."

"My husband is dead," said she, "and I am, as you see, not far from it, and I do not care to live any longer except for my dear children; my poor darling who has gone home would like me to try and live for our children's sake."

I consented to treat her on conditon that she should give up all narcotics and local messings for the internal ulcerations.

Her grief was the very first point to consider, and this, with the vomiting, more than justified my first prescription, *Ignatia amara* 1x, zss; five drops in water three times a day. This having done good, the primary constitutional blight had to be seen to, as this it was that produced the extreme emaciation; one of her sisters had died of phthisis, and hence I ordered *Bacill.* CC.

Then followed *Puls.* Q, *Nux* 1, *Quassia* Q; and patient's digestion and general condition were much improved. But the nervous symptoms were very distressing : almost complete adynamia. Several months under *Kali phos.*, 6 trit., and then a short course of *Cypripedin* 3x.

September 27 — "I am fatter; my nerves feel better, and altogether I feel stronger."

$R_x$ *Scutellartin* 3x. Six grains dry on the tongue twice a day.

October 25 — Nearly well of all her nerve troubles; sleeps, however, very badly.

$R_x$ *Bacill* C.

After this patient never looked back, and she is to-day in a good, healthy, plump condition, and, humanly speaking, good for another quarter of a century.

In grave, complicated cases it is best to pick out the central points in them and start *from* them. Thus, in the foregoing case, there were — 1. grief; 2.

consumptiveness; 3. neurasthenia — and from these out the therapeutic efforts were directed.

The totality of the symptoms principle was here not the best, because of the several different causations of the symptoms which were thus of different pathological qualities.

At the change of life it is well to keep the fundamentals of the basic constitution of the person well and fixedly before one's mind, and in the second place construct a history of what the individual has gone through, and then separate, mentally, the various groups of symptoms and cure them groupwise and not altogether — only thus is success in grave life threatening cases possible. (XXIV 19)

## 539. RETARDATION OF THE MENOPAUSE

It not infrequently happens that when the time has arrived for the period to cease, it will not do so; that is to say, there is bleeding but no true ovulation, and this is disease. When ladies over fifty years of age say to us chirply — "Oh, I have not changed yet!" the statement is commonly of some gravity. The period due to an ovulation is health; the quasi-period is only haemorrhage of the same nature, as, for instance the bleeding from haemorrhoids or from the lungs, and each kind of haemorrohage has a pathological quality of its own. Thus, when a consumptive person bleeds at one time from the lungs, at another from the haemorrhoidal veins, and at another from the vagina, the haemorrhage is in each case presumably of the same pathological quality.

Mrs. G., fifty years of age, mother of six children, came to me on September 22, 1892, telling me she was still regular, but the flow was very excessive. Close enquiry showed that the thing was not an ovulatory period, but an habitual periodical haemorrhage. With her first child patient had had whiteleg (phlegmasia alba dolens), which left leg still swells and troubles her. Those conversant with this form of leucocytosis will not marvel when I say that after a three months' course of *Thuja* 30, *Sabina* 30, and *Cupressus lawsoniana* 30 (each one month by itself) patient's left leg became comfortable, and her periodic bleedings from the uterus ceased.

When the period is unduly prolonged, in nine cases out of ten it is no longer an ovulation at all, but there is something wrong with the person, which wrong should be set right in lieu of making efforts to stop the bleeding. (XXIV 21)

## 540. CASE OF PRECANCEROUS UTERUS AND ABDOMINAL TUMOUR AFTER THE MENOPAUSE

The name of precancerous uterus is not an accepted nosological entity, and what I really mean is cancer; only as patient has got quite well, some other name must be found, and whatever its nature, certainly it was a case of greatly diseased womb coming after the menopause. So much is quite certain.

In the region of the pancreas there was a swelled mass. Patient is a maiden lady of fifty-two years of age, and came to me in the spring of 1893, saying she had changed several years ago, and now for the past five years has an ill-smelling copious discharge from the vagina, principally thick, mattery, and yellow. After using *Sul.*, *Urtica ur.*, *Trifol.*, etc., I on June 22 prescribed *Aur. mur. nat.* 3x, five drops in water night and morning, which was continued for nearly four months, and the discharge slowly diminished, and in October had ceased. In November the discharge had returned, the right breast swelled up very considerably and was tender, and *Tub. t.* C. was given for several months, and then *Aurum* for a number of months, and patient was discharged cured in April, 1896. Patient's mother died of cancer of the womb, and a sister of cancer between uterus and rectum. (XXIV 22)

## 541. PROLAPSUS UTERI OF MANY YEARS' STANDING

A widow lady, fifty-seven years of age, was conducted to me by her sister on October 9, 1888, suffering from prolapsus uteri of many years' duration; the exact number is not noted. She is obese and scant of breath. Cannot move about without her pessary, which she, however, only wears by day, and places it in position herself. Flushes, leucorrhoea, and occasional bleeding from womb.

$R_x$ Tc. *Helonias dioica* Q. ziv. Five drops in water night and morning.

November 27 — *Thuja*.

December 29 — Can now go about without pessary without any particular inconvenience.

$R_x$ *Helonias dioica* Q.

February 2, 1889 — "I have felt wonderfully easy without any pessary."

$R_x$ Rep.

April 11 — "I can walk quite well without knowing anything is wrong." Leucorrhoea pretty bad at times.

$R_x$ *Aletris farinosa* Q, ziv. Five drops in water night and morning.

May 14 — Was quite well, but has now a little intravaginal pressure again, which she thinks has come from over-stretching.

$R_x$ *Sabina* 3.

September 20 — Complains that the Sabina does not suit her so well as the former drugs; womb coming down on over-exertion, but now when it does it is much softer than it used to be.

$R_x$ *Helonias dioica* Q, which finished the cure.

Seven years later, September 1896; this lady came in to see me the other day, and tells me she continues quite well in all respects, and is very active on her feet, as she now keeps her bachelor son's house in the country. Has never used a pessary since November 1888; but during the whole of the interval I have heard from her at odd times, and have, time and again, repeated the remedies before-named whenever over-exertion, etc., had produced discomfort or slight relapses. (XXIV 22)

## 542. PRURITUS

After the menopause (and also before it), but particularly as the turn of life approaches, and often for many years after it the peculiar irritation known as pruritus or itching is apt to become very troublesome indeed; it is located mostly in the vagina, vulva, or anus, or thereabouts. It is often accompanied by eczema, and may be symptomatic of internal disease. It is usual to order soothing applications for this ailment, and their name is indeed legion.

Is the treatment of pruritus by soothing applications efficacious and rational? It is neither. I grant that a little *Calendula* ointment, lanoline, or vaseline, or the like, do ease for the time, and that, perhaps, harmlessly, and that is no small boon, as it allows patients to get to sleep. But when it comes to forcibly lulling sensation of the parts with active sedatives, I believe such a proceeding to be very harmful.

A proper course of homoeopathic treatment commonly suffices for its cure, but not always; there are some obstinate cases that defy all known efforts at cure. The very largest amount of success is obtained when we obstract ourselves from the name of the ailment and study the constitutional bearings of the case, and treat the woman's organism on general principles. Here the Totality of the Symptoms principle works exceedingly well, particularly where the pruritus seems to exist by itself without any diagnosable anatomical pathological basis.

Taken by itself, the most frequently successful remedy in my hands is *Caladium seguinum*, about the fifth dilution. It almost always does some good. *Sepia* comes next, but personally I generally have recourse to nosodes before I can really and radically cure it.

Sometimes the spleen is at fault in pruritus vulvae, and when the irritation is at the seat the liver may require attention. Some people find that pruritus ani will depart when the usual nightcap on retiring for the night is omitted.

Cases of pruritus vulvae are sometimes due to tight-lacing — in fact this is pretty frequently the case in ladies of full habit and slightly disposed to gout : if such patients happen to lie abed for any trifling indisposition they are not troubled with pruritus, as the viscera are thereby relieved from pressures. A lady consulted me not long since for a tumour in the vagina : it was a vaginocele about the size of a Tangerine orange. "And is it not strange," said she, "the lump goes away very often when I stay in bed for a day or two, but it is generally there soon after I have properly dressed," *i.e.*, when she had put on her stays. I explained the matter to her, and recommended a discontinuance of the lacing; but I hear from her husband that she laces tighter than ever, and, of necessity, the vaginocele persists. Most commonly there is a pathologic quality underlying the pruritus, such as gout, scrofula, eczema, when, of course, we must look away from the symptom pruritus, and attack the said pathological quality. (XXIV 23)

## 543. CLIMACTERIC — CATARACT

A well-preserved, fresh-looking maiden lady, fifty years of age, came under my observation at the beginning of 1895 for incipient cataract, which began when the periods began to wane.

For six months patient took *Pulsatilla* Q, seven drops in water at bedtime. September 3, 1895 — Distinct improvement in her vision; left side of tongue swollen. The same remedy was again ordered and persevered in, with pauses, and the report in June, 1896, was : "Oh! I see very much better." (XXIV 28)

## 544. SEVERE CLIMACTERIC FLUSHINGS

"As medication by various glands is still on its trial, except, perhaps, that of the Thyroid in Myxoedema, individual experiences, if recorded, will help in estimating rightly its value, and in indicating the class of cases in which treatment may be used with benefit. It is with this object I record the following case :

"Miss C., aged fifty-two, for more than three years suffered from severe menorrhagia, and during part of that time from metrorrhagia also. The latter was relieved by the removal of a pedunculated polypus growing from the cervix. The menorrhagia, however, continued, the periods occurring about every three weeks, and lasting a fortnight or even three weeks. The bleeding was very severe, and not influenced much by drugs, though Ergot (both by mouth and hypodermically), *Hydrastis, Liquor Ferri Perchloridi, Potassium Bromide, Hazeline, Arsenic,* and *Thyroid gland* were tried. During the last two periods, however, *Calcium chloride,* in scruple doses, three times a day, seemed to have a good effect, but this might have been due to the natural close of menstruation. Frequent plugging of the vagina, sometimes twice a day, was the only means of controlling the haemorrhage, with iced injections on removal of the plugs. Hot douches were not so effectual as the cold.

"When at last the periods ceased, the patient was much troubled with frequent and violent flushings, which at night, in winter, would wake her up, the face being in a burning heat, while the hands and body were icy cold.

"For these flushings I ordered five-grain doses of *Ovarian Gland three times a day*. For the first day or two there appeared to be no effect, then the flushings rapidly became less frequent and intense, and were nearly cured by the time three dozen doses were taken. The patient now tells me she is free of them, but gets a 'threatening' if she omits the capsules for some days. One dose occasionally keeps her free."

The treatment of the case is bad from our homoeopathic standpoint, and I only quote it as suggestive of the use of Ovary Extract in the flushes when *Lachesis* and other remedies have failed. (XXIV 33)

## 545. CANCEROUSNESS TRACED THROUGH LIFE CLEARLY EVIDENCED AT THE MENOPAUSE

A gentleman brought his wife to me on June 26, 1897, for a painful swelling in her LEFT breast; and as the case brings out one of the chief points of this little treatise, I will narrate it pretty fully.

Mrs. S., aet. forty-three, married these twenty years, but childless. Has pains in her left breast that wake her up in the night and cause her much anxiety. Her father died at sixty-three of diabets; her mother, at fifty-two, *of cancer of the LEFT breast*; her sister, of cancer of the same breast, at forty-three, just after the change; a brother, at forty-five, or rapid phthisis.

The inner half of patient's left breast is the seat of diffused swelling since the change, which occurred at forty years of age, that is three years ago. There is nothing unusual in this history, but let us trace back her *health* history and see how that stands. Soon after marriage she was under treatment for womb trouble — ulcers at the os; these ulcers were cauterized severely and oft, and times daily for weeks together; they were then painted regularly and for long periods. She has been using vaginal injections for pretty bad whites for many years. She injects hot water into the vagina on her physician's advice every day for the past fifteen years, and still the whites — yellow and sticky and corroding — continue the same as ever. "All my life I have never been ill and also never well." Right lobe of thyroid somewhat enlarged for a year past. The breasts often swell. Has had gallstones twice.

We are here not concerned with the treatment of this particular case (moreover, it was only begun yesterday), but it illustrates clearly what I hold and what I should like to teach, viz., that the various ills and ailings of women are not of a local nature, and must therefore not be locally regarded or treated.

I read the phenomena thus : The ulcers at the os, the leucorrhoea, the sterility, were of a cancerous nature (precancerous, as Hutchinson would say), and inherited from her mother, and that the ulcerations and whites should have been treated on constitutional lines from the beginning in lieu of the local measures of cauterizing and painting the seemingly offending parts. And as to the treatment of the case, now it is manifest that we have to deal with a constitutional ailment located primarily in the uterus, and thence reflected on to the breasts, so ablation of the left breast would be useless, inasmuch as the root-ailing is located primarily in the womb. My object in narrating the foregoing is to bring before the reader's mind how the thing appears to my mind — the ulcers and the leucorrhoea were not to be regarded as the ailment to be treated at all, they were only the local expression of the enemy within, and not the enemy himself — rather were they its voice.

What I am trying to say is that silencing the ulcers and leucorrhoea was bad practice, not only doing no good to the woman's organism, but rather harming her. So long as the monthly flow continued, so long did this lady live on in a fair state of health; but since it has stopped she has ailed rather more, the right lobe of her thyroid has become enlarged, and now the left breast is enlarging and hardening, and has already become the seat of a good deal of pain.

The persistence of leucorrhoea after the menopause is of considerable import, and certainly betokens positive disease of the womb (or ovaries), and the same may be said of the swelling of her breasts, for breast is an appendix to the womb, and ever under its influence and domination. Whenever there is anything wrong with the breasts I direct my attention straightway to the womb, for it is in the womb, respectively the ovaries, that the ailing is surely primarily located.

When I speak of leucorrhoea I mean leucorrhoea and not gonorrhoea. This latter is a dirty disease introduced from without and not from the constitution, and should be killed *in situ* the sooner the better, if possible. I hold the same of the acarus disease — the pure itch — the nasty little acari are from without, and should be slain. (XXIV 34)

## 546. RHEUMATOID ARTHRITIS

Rheumatic gout at the change of life is indeed a very large order; a series of remedies are needed to cure the same. A sample of how I get along with them here follows.

Mrs. X., aet. sixty-five, mother of one child, born when she was forty-one (married at forty), since when she had gone very stout and suffered from rheumatic gout ever since her menopause. Right knee and left ankle much swelled; cannot walk; dreads cold water, urine thick; is much distressed by inability to retain her urine; altogether she is in a sorry plight.

*Med.* 1000, in infrequent dose.

July 22 — Urine much clearer, and there is much less difficulty in retaining it.

$R_x$ Rep.
August 12 — Pains and swellings much diminished.
$R_x$ Rep.
September 16 — "Decidedly better," her husband writes, "more like her old self, a good deal better all round."
$R_x$ Rep.
October 19 — Well, except that she is stiff.
$R_x$ *Bellis per*. Q. Ten drops in water in the forenoon.
November 25 — $R_x$ *Bryonia* 0.
December 20 — *Acid. oxalic* 1.
February 2, 1892 *Bacill*. CC.
March 1 — "My wife is quite well of her rheumatic gout, and the water is quite comfortable, but she is weak.
$R_x$ *Fer. Picric* 3x. Three drops in water three times a day.
April 11 — "A few pains here and there, but what can you except in this heat?"
$R_x$ *Salix alb*. Q, zj. ten drops in water twice a day.
Long after, I saw this lady's husband about his varicose veins, when he told me Mrs. X. continued free of her pains and swellings, and in very good general health. And still later, I had the same report from her step-son. (XXIV 39)

## 547. INCONTINENCE OF URINE AT THE MENOPAUSE

After the change of life ladies are not infrequently troubled with inability to hold their water : the causes vary considerably; and where the sweat glands are inactive *Jaborandi* is a good friend, as the following brilliant little cure will show :
Countess G., verging on fifty years of age, consulted me on November 6, 1890, for inability to contain her urine, worse when she had a cold, which was then [illegible] case. The point which struck me most was her dry skin. "I never perspire," said she. I ordered *Jaborandi* 1, ten drops in water three times a day. To the great delight of her ladyship the medicine cured the incontinence right away. (XXIV 40)

## 548. CLIMACTRIC INSANITY

Miss X., thirty-seven years of age, came under my observation on September 10, 1891 : father died at seventy-six; mother and most of her brothers and sisters living. She has had no period since last May, and for six and a half years only here and there a menstruation, not much more than a show; numerous strumous scars under *right* side of jaw. Spleen very large. Had diphtheria in Rome in 1883. Much hypogastric hyperaethesia. *Right* ovary terribly sensitive, the lightest touch in the region causes her seemingly intense pain. Vaginal irritation maddening. She twitches and jumps. Severe frontal headache all her life. Used to have leucorrhoea, for which she had many vaginal injections. Three times vaccinated. Has had the Weir-Mitchell treatment. Has had enlargement of the glands, mumps, varicella, morbilli, pertussis, shingles of right side of trunk. Mentally she is held to be insane by her belongings, wherefore she has been in "Homes," and goes about in charge of a paid "friend." She flushes in conversation, talks incessantly about the evil conduct of — others! — and her own lot. With her, SELF begins, SELF continues and SELF remains the one absorbing subject from sunrise to sunset. She had first *Urticaria* Q as a spleen medicine, and then *Viscum album* 1 an ovary medicine.

October 1 — A period has come on!

$R_x$ *Kali Brom.* 3.

October 21 — Much better. They (i.e., her friends and relations) are bad, it is true, but not altogether devoid of regard for HERSELF.

November 3 — $R_x$ *Bursa pastoris* Q.

November 26 — Her nose has bled four times.

$R_x$ Rep.

December 3 — Great vaginal irritation and whites.

$R_x$ *Viscum alb.* 1x, and then followed *Ignatia* 1 and *Puls.* 1.

January 4, 1892 — Saw patient with a good period, but her hypogastric hyperaresthesia was very distressing : everything that touched the hypogastic region, or even the apprehension that something might touch it, would send patient off into twitches. She was also very excited, and her attendant was almost driven beside herself, hence *Lyssin* 30, twelve globules over a fortnight. The improvement therein was very great; she became much less excited, and the hyperaesthesia greatly diminished. Followed here a course of *Fraxinus Americanus* Q, to bring down the uterine enlargement.

March 1 — Has been wonderfully better, but has had no period for seven weeks. Mindful of the submaxillary strumous scars, I ordered *Bacillin.* CC., and then *Bursa pastoris* Q, which was followed by a period and further general improvement.

After that *Fraxinus Americanus* Q was again given for the heaviness of the uterus, which remedy earned the sufferer's repeated praises.

By the middle of 1892 patient began to go about with almost any lady of her own choice, and went then into society a little, and by the end of the year, the remedies already named being given as called for by their respective indications, and in addition, the sexual excitement was well met by *Salix nigra* Q, prepared, I believe, from the aments, and given in ten-drop doses. The *Salix* was given on several occasions, and mostly with benefit. "*Lyssin.* cures the same symptom, but more in the nerve sphere, whereas *Salix* seems to me to act on the womb itself more.

April 11, 1893 — Still under *Salix nigra* Q, and has had several periods. She is now quite sane, and no longer considers her relations so sinful, and at this period she began to go back in her own case historically; and made it clear to my mind that though she was now having here and there a period, the same was not "like it used to be, for formerly when I was as well as any lady could wish to be, and the joy of my darling father who was different and was *preceded by whites*, and the periods I get now have no whites with them, and they don't do me any good." Thinking of the suppression of leucorrhoea by vaginal injections, and of her three vaccinations, I ordered *Mal.* C. on May 16.

June 29th—Just had a period *preceded by whites*, and mentally she is nearly normal. She goes about by herself when she thinks she will, but generally has now a lady companion like any other well-to-do lone lady. No further period occurred, and it became manifest that she had really changed for good and all. Here a new order of things came to the fore; the patient *had* changed and became mentally normal (from the treatment I believe), but flushes began to worry, and the month was here divided into two parts: during one part she was depressed in a wonderful degree, and during the other she became sexually excited, and it took me over a year to get the mastery over these, for which the remedies were *Salix nigra* Q, and *Bacill.* 30, and this last seemed to finish the cure completely. During the years 1894-5-6 patient ran up to town to see me once in a way for some of the symptoms that recurred, and I see from my notes that *Fraxinus Americanus* Q, *Salix nigra* Q, *Sepia* 30, *Sabina* 30, and *Lyssin.* 30 were the remedies used. The long intervals between the prescriptions led me to infer that each one duly did its work. Patient continues quite well to date, and when I saw her a few months ago she looked in splendid health, and was then off on her own initiative on a tour round the world. "I have never seen the world, but now I am so well I want to do so, and so I am off; I have no one to please but myself." Here came a merry laugh, and "Good-bye, doctor, I am very grateful to you but I shall come and see you again some day."

So we see that *homoeopathy patiently applied can minister to a mind diseased, only there is no specific for an abstraction bearing a name as if it were a tangible entity that had got into a wrong place, and needed only to be seized by "a cure" and ousted from its place.* Strictly speaking we cannot cure diseases at all. We can, however, cure people whose states and conditions bear man-given names, such as insanity, hyperaesthesia, a cold, rheumatism, or what not. It lies in the nature of things that we should think and talk of diseases as entities, and just as every baby gets a name, so does every disease.

The foregoing case I call "Climacteric Insanity," but other nosologists might prefer another name.

"But, doctor, you use such a lot of remedies; who is to know how to cure "Climacteric Insanity?" Quite so. I once played a game of chess all night, and I really could not say which move won the game, or which portion of

the night's work caused the fever that set in next day.
"That's a long ladder you have got there, Carter."
"Yes, sir, it is; but you see your house is so high. (XXIV 42)

## 549. SEVERE NEURALGIA

A married lady, mother of five children, verging on fifty years of age, and just changing, came to me on May 7, 1891, for severe neuralgia of the left side of face, running from left ear to the left angle of mouth, where it remains, preventing her often from opening her mouth. It first came in 1886, when she was in North Devon, and has plagued her ever since. "Nothing does it any good." Of course not! Has not neuralgia been declared incurable by *regular medicine*? Then how dare any self-respecting physician presume to even try to cure it?

There were two distinct rows of froth lengthwise along the tongue, which was white and thickly coated : distressing flatulence and acidity no end. The pain is said to be worst in the evening and when tired; it comes on gradually and disappears gradually, but it has two very characteristic symptoms, viz., it is worse at the seaside and rouses her from her sleep. *Natrum muriaticum* 6 and 30 cleaned her tongue, and caused greeny-browny diarrhoea. Passing wind eased the pain. But after this the neuralgia was worse than ever.

June 9 — "The pain is awful, it roused me twelve or fourteen times last night, and I have fearful acidity."

$R_x$ *Glinicum* 1000, in infrequent doses.

June 23 — Almost well; sleeps quite well and undisturbedly.

$R_x$ Rep.

July 28 — Neuralgia gone, but her digestion is not quite happy. Has been four times vaccinated.

$R_x$ *Thuja* 30.

I believe there has been no return of neuralgia, which I conclude from the fact that patient, who lives quite near me, not been to me since, which I think she certainly would have done had it returned.

***Note On Glinicum***

*Glinicum* is none other than *Medorrhinum*; then why multiply names? Only because I obtained the matrix of this myself from a typical case, and macerated it myself in spirit of wine, and so I *know* what it is and how prepared, and any one else can do the same at anytime and anywhere in the whole wide world. Furthermore, we can use the name *Glinicum* just as we use *Met. alb.*, *Verb. sap.*

In simple georgic and bucolic times our weeds no doubt amply suffice for our ailings; but in these polyandrous days, when late marriages are the rule, and gonococcic fluxes are all over the place, we must need go to the source of the disease for its remedy — for *ubi morbus, ibirremedium* is a blessed fact. Chinchona does not grow in cold wet places, that's where we find the willow.

My indications for *Glinicum* are : roused in the small hours of the morning by the pain, acidity, coated tongue, filthy taste and breath, uncleanably dirty tongue, weakness, pallor, chilliness, worse from cold wet; and moreover *Glin.* is largely a left-sided remedy. *Glin.* wipes out half the cases of sciatica that pass my way. What a record! (XXIV 46)

## 550. NEURALGIA IN A LADY EIGHTY-SIX YEARS OF AGE,

Although this case has no right to be here, I add it next to the *Glinicum* case to show that I do not regard *Gli*[illegible] a a specific for neuralgia. Every case of disease needs its own remedy, though like cases call for like remedies, so that we may nevertheless really claim to have generic specific, if I may use this odd term.

In May 1891, I received the following letter :

"Dear Sir, ___ At the instances of my friend Mr. L. of ___, and with the approval of my regular attendant Mr. ___, I write in the hope that you may possibly be able to give relief to my suffering during many months past, from neuralgia in the left side of my face, etc."

"I am a widow in my eighty-sixth year, etc."

Here the neuralgia did not rouse her in the small hours of the morning, but was almost always bad at bedtime. This *excludes Glinicum*.

Neuralgia worse from eating, talking and laughing. Patient had been twice married, and was a widow for the second time, and in her eighty-sixth year, and could yet laugh! Decidedly a case worth curing!

I did not see the lady, and her regular medical attendant gave me no information (not he), though he magnanimously alluded to the unclean thing; but patient's father died (at eight-two) of asthma, and her mother (at forty two) of pulmonary phthisis, and the aggravation was *in the evening*, so I ordered *Baccill.* CC., three doses in a fortnight.

June 4 — "On the whole I think I have had fewer paroxysms of pain about bedtime."

$R_x$ Rep.

July 7 — Nearly well.

$R_x$ *Bacill.* 1000.

Cured. (XXIV 48)

## 551. FAGGED WOMB

Near the change of life we occasionally come across what I would call a fagged state of the uterus; the organ is weary — fagged.

Such cases are apt to be complicated with disease, but I will shortly narrate a case in which there was no disease — merely fag.

Mrs. P., aet. forty-six, came to me on March 28, 1893. Here are the notes : Fag, suffering; wants to lie down; has done a good deal; husband vigorous; married late; has three children; period regular; backache; womb is thick but high up, no disease."

$R_x$ *Bellis per.* 0, zj. S — Ten drops in water night and morning.

June 8 — "Has done me a world of good."

$R_x$ Rep.

August — Quite well.

This morning (July 11, 1897) I received a letter from a colleague in America, asking me what my indications are for the use of *Bellis per* :

Dear Colleague — *Bellis per.* is our common daisy; it acts very much like *Arnica,* even to the contingent production of erysipelas; it causes pain in the spleen, and generally symptoms of coryza, and of feeling very tired, person (the writer) wanting to lie down. it acts on exudates, swellings, and stasis, and hence in a fagged womb its action is very satisfactory; indeed, in the discomforts of pregnancy and of varicose veins patients are commonly loud in its praise. In the *giddinesses* of elderly people (cerebral stasis) it acts well and does permanent good; likewise, and particularly in fag from masturbation, in old work-men, labourers, and the overworked and fagged, it is a princely remedy. In the head-sufferings of elderly working gardeners its action is very pretty. Its action in the ill-effects from taking cold drinks when one is hot is now well known. It is a grand friend to commercial travellers, and in railway spine of moderate severity it has not any equal so far as my knowledge reaches. I think *stasis* lies at the bottom of all these ailings. — Yours, etc.

P.S. — When given at night *Bellis* is very apt to cause the patient to wake up very early in the morning, hence I order it by preference to be taken not too late in the day. I have often cured with it the symptom "wakes up too early in the morning and cannot get off again," and here the higher dilutions act much more decidedly and lastingly as a rule and without any side-effects, for here the action is purely homoeopathic and not simply deobstruent. (XXIV 49)

## 552. ARTHRITIC PAINS

A married lady, aged fifty-four. Mother of two children, came to consult me on May 24th, 1894, for arthritic pains in the left hip and outside the left thigh, and in the left knee, coming on since the change of life. The condition had so persisted that her case had come to be regarded as not likely to be cured at all. Patient was very chilly, wherefore I began with *Urtica urens* Q, which did not very much good.

June 28th — The pains are no better, they are terrible of the warmth of bed.
$R_x$ *Luet*. CC.
August 14 — There is very great improvement.
$R_x$ Rep.
September 12 — The amelioration is maintained; her nights are no longer so terrible; indeed, "Oh, how nice it is to be able to lie in the bed at night without being wakened with pain."
$R_x$ Rep.
November 22 — "You have done wonders."
$R_x$ Rep.
At the beginning of 1895 patient's husband informed me that the cure was perfect, and long afterwards I heard from him that she continued quite well, and could and did walk miles, and her sleep and rest at night quite normal. Whether the case was really of an arthritic nature may, perhaps, be doubted. Here we have a proof for the ten thousandth time that high dilutions do act curatively, and that a well-defined characteristic symptoms or keynote can lead to most brilliant cures, and the best of such keynotes is that one can remember them and so save time. The time spent with one's nose in a repertory ought to be saved, if possible. Said a well-known gentleman on entering my consulting room one day : "I say what a lot of repertories you have; I am astonished; I have always understood that you never used repertories, and go in mostly for what you call organ remedies. "Ah" said I, the repertory is my haven of refuge to which I fly in case of need; the more I know of the diseases themselves the less I need repertories; I live and move and have my medical being in *behind the symptoms,* where lies the future of Higher Homoeopathy : organ-remedies are only the bottom rung of the ladder. (XXIV 50)

## 553. RHEUMATOID ARTHRITIS AFTER CLIMAXIS

A maiden lady, forty-nine years old, was conducted to me by an old patient on July 23, 1893, when she told me she had been suffering for the past three years from rheumatic gout, crops of red lumps, with stiffness of legs and arms at the joints, accompanied by much pain, worse by day on moving, and in warm weather. The joints are swelled, and crack and grate. Used to have whites, and had influenza seven years ago.
$R_x$ *Med*. 1000.
August 23 — Much better. Knees much less painful they grate less on movement, and the lumps are gone.
No medicine.
September 20 — Well.
No medicine.
October 18 — Well; discharged. (XXIV 51)

## 554. SYCOSIS AT THE CHANGE OF LIFE

Mrs. X., forty-six years of age, childless, came under my observation on May 3, 1897. She was vaccinated at eighteen, and from that time on to this present time she has been subject to "no end of shows." *i.e.*, here and there tiny bleedings from the parts. She is very passive, mentally inert; uterus enlarged.
$R_x$ Tc. *Aur. mur.* 3x. ziv. Five drops in water night and morning.
May 24 — She now consents to have her long worn pessary removed.
$R_x$ *Thuja* 30.
June 2 — Her pessary having been removed causes her no inconvenience, and there has been no show. She is stronger; is worse in the summer than in the winter; she is unable to lie on her left side.
$R_x$ *Tub. test.* C.
July 20 — Complains of muddle headedness.
$R_x$ *Spirit. gland quercus* Q. Ten drops in water night and morning.
August 27 — The pain in her left side rouses her from sleep at night, enabling the wind to pass, and then relieving said pain.
$R_x$ *Fraxinux Am.* Q.
October 21, 1898 — Has done her much good; she has had one proper period, but no "show."
$R_x$ *Thuja* 30.
November 15 — The flatulence wakes her up, and her breath is very foul. *Med.* 1000. After which she was very much better, and no longer roused by flatus.
P.S. — *Roused from sleep* is a thoroughly reliable keynote for Med. I observed it pathogenetically on myself first, and have verified it clinically many times. (XXIV 52)

## 555. SOME PHTHISIC MANIFESTATIONS AT THE CHANGE OF LIFE

There are many cases that baffle the best unless aetiologically regarded. Thus, three weeks ago, a lady who formerly been cured by *Bacillin*, of pulmonary haemorrhage and loss of flesh, sent me an urgent request to cure her incoercible vomiting, saying : "I have been so well, and am expecting to be confined in about a month, but latterly I have been constantly vomiting, until I am now losing flesh, getting so thin, and can keep nothing but a little brandy on my stomach; please send me something to stop my vomiting, for nurse says the baby will be dead if this goes on much longer." The vomiting was worse in the afternoon, and there was some fever and hectic flush.
It seemed to me probable that the intrapelvic congestion had a dash of the consumptive quality about it, and so I dissolved ten globules of *Bacill.* C.

in four drachms of spirit of wine, and directed her to take five drops in water every four hours.

A fortnight later she wrote me — "Oh, that marvellous medicine, I only vomited once after that first dose."

The same idea often helps me in climacteric troubles : thus, Mrs. X., forty-seven years of age, came under my care on July 24th, 1896, telling me — no, that was not the way it came about, for previous to that her husband had visited me telling me his wife's life was despaired of on account of such severe anaemia, due to severe floodings coming on at regular intervals like a period, and lasting from six to seven days. "My wife is drained to death by it, and our family doctor gives very little hope of her; she is now almost always confined to her bed, and iron tonics no longer do her any good."

"Yes, we have had several other medical gentlemen to consult with Dr. C., but they give me but very little hope, and I don't think there is anything more that can be done, she is so short of breath that she cannot even stand." After few months' treatment this lady came to London for some social functions, and after a further year's treatment she was practically well, and away in the Welsh hills with her husband on a holiday. About two-third of the period she was on *Bacill.* or *Tub. test* 30, C., and also had *Med.* C., *Thuja* 30, *Sabina* 30 and each a month of *Urtica urens* Q, *Prunus Virginiana* Q, and *Salix nigra* Q (ten drops of either two or three times a day, for their organopathic effects). Consumptively disposed ladies are very apt to have floodings at any of their congestive functions, and they frequently increase in severity as the time of the change comes on. Thus, this lady was in the habit of menstruating very freely, but after forty years of age it slowly became worse and worse, till the thing could only be termed periodical floodings, resulting in alarming anaemia. The florid. freely menstruating lady of thirty is very apt to be drained almost to death by forty or so, unless the blood-taint be wiped out before, by say *Bacill.* or other such remedies. (XXIV 53)

## 556. THE PESSARY CRAZE

A lady, just over forty years of age came under my observation in November 1896 for enlarged womb, excessive periods, and foul, putrid leucorrhoea. "I am in an awful state, I am going rotten, I am sure I am!" Here we have an example of a very fine, rosy person, exceedingly good-looking (by the way a kind of good-lookingness which I have come to regard as almost pathognomonic of consumptiveness), who had had very free periods from a sappy state of uterus; and now that the change is looming, her troubles are all accentuated; and as her very religious husband has for years been doing *what Onan did*, the womb has become so heavy that most of leading homoeopathic physicians and gynaecological surgeons have been ordering injections, douches, — "Dr. X. ordered me very hot water injections for the whites, and he also put in pessary, but could not get one to fit comfortably then. I have had six or seven and this one hurts terribly."

Now this lady was of the thriving consumptive build (tall and large, lax, rosy, full-bodied, soft-mannered, good-looking, languid, often tired), readily parting with blood, and come now the threshold of the climaxis, her accumulated troubles were threatening to wreck her altogether. She sought the help of homoeopaths, who did not reckon with her constitution, who moreover regarded her "three times vaccinated" as an additional proof of her good health, and whom commended the Onan-like withdrawals (what Onan did, not Onanism so-called), as "so prudent and considerate, you know." My own diagnosis in this case was — 1. Hereditarily consumptive; 2. Vaccinosis; 3. Thickening and enlargement of the womb from genesiac fraud. This poor lady formerly had piles for which she sought the advice of a prominent follower of Hahnemann, who... oh yes! he did, cut them off!

Was your operation for piles successful?

Yes, very.

But I thought you said that you have now bad bleeding piles?

Yes, so I have; they came again two or three years after they were operated on.

And you are constipated, are you not?

Yes, but my doctor has ordered remedies for that.

So here we have in a middle aged lady, still well-nourished and fresh-looking —

a. Operation for piles.
b. *Enemata* for constipation.
c. Hot water and medicated vaginal injections for the whites.
d. A fine choice of pessaries to prop up an enlarged womb, and the result? In the patient's words : "I am going rotten." A little further on such idiotic lines of treatment, and then the diagnosis of cancer of womb would have to be made, and then an operation would be performed, and then the whole crowned by a widower's tears and the regrets of her motherless children.

But was there any alternative?

Yes, that lady is now cured by commonsense homoeopathic treatment. The *Tuberculin* (30, C, CC.) cured the consumptiveness : the antisycotics *Thuja* 30, *Sabina* 30, *Cupress. Law.* 30, *Med.* 1000, cured the whites, and organ-remedies brought down the uterus to its present moderate size and bulk; and Mrs. X. is at this moment spinning about on her bike a free and happy woman.

It was *Fraxinus Am.* Q, ten drops in water night and morning, that reduced the womb in size the most promptly (See my *Organ Diseases of Women*).

Everything is relative and comparative : given an enlarged ulterus, it is better to prop it up with a comfortable pessary than to let it flop down on the floor of the pelvis and protrude ; but inasmuch as the too heavy organ goes down by reason of its bulk and weight, it must follow that if this bulk and weight be sufficiently reduced the organ will rebound to its old place, and need no pessary to prop it up. In addition to this, we have to bear well in mind that the pessary as a foreign body is, as such, highly objectionable in the parts, and is in fact filth-producing, making the poor sufferer shrink from her very self by rendering what should be sacrosanct a veritable cloaca. *Interfaeces et urinas nascimur* is right enough, because natural, but we may fairly stop at that. (XXIV 55)

## 557. POST-CLIMACTERIC DYSPEPSIA

Mrs. N., fifty-two years age, mother of four children, and having had two miscarriages, came under my observation in June, 1897. She has been twice vaccinated, the last time at twenty-one unsuccessfully. Has had dyspepsia for many years, much more severely since she changed. The bowels are very tender to the touch : the urine ill-smelling ("fishy"). Her flushings are distressing and like waves of heat. She is now very thin, but used to weigh 11 st. Suffers much from "yellows" (i.e., yellow leucorrhoea) and has twice had polypoid growths taken from womb.
$R_x$ *Thuja* 30.
July 9 — The right side of tongue is much thicker than the left. Sinking, empty feeling.
$R_x$ *Scirrh*. C.
August 10 — Pretty bad flushes.
$R_x$ Trit. 3x, *Ovary Extract*, gr. vj. One powder at bedtime, which very greatly relieved the flushes.
The influence of the *Thuja* 30 on the dyspepsia, and that of the *Ovary Extract* on the flushes, was marked and incontestable.
Patient remains under treatment. (XXIV 57)

## 558. ECZEMA AND WARTS

A lady of fifty-four years of age consulted me on August 24, 1896, telling me she was suffering from a nasty eruption on the scalp, with great loss of hair, and quite a number of raised warts on her hands, four of which warts were large ones, and these had been there for three years. She changed two years ago.
$R_x$ *Thuja* 30.
October 2 — The warts have quite disappeared; her scalp is a mass of scales, and "all the hair is going."
$R_x$ *Bacill* C.

November 20 — No, warts; scalp is improving; flatus bad.
Rep.
February 1, 1897 — Much better of scalp; no return of warts.
$R_x$ Rep.
May 10 — Rep.
July 2 — Pains in the joints of fingers.
$R_x$ *Thuja* 30.
August 6 — Head better; fingers painful.
$R_x$ *Psor.* CC., which finished the cure.

The remarkable cure of the old-standing warts struck me very forcibly; not that curing warts by *Thuja* is at all new or unusual, but to cause any growth of any kind soever to disappear right away under the influence of any drug whatever in the thirtieth centesimal dilution is a marvellous thing to me, and not the less marvellous becuase it has been done so often by so many for the past two or three generations.

Why did I give *Thuja*? Traditions, and also because the lady in question had been in her day three times vaccinated, the last twice unsuccessfully. And an unsuccessful vaccination means, to me, that the virus has been taken up by the organism and there lies latent for future ill — the organism having failed to react. (XXIV 58)

# ENLARGED TONSILS CURED BY MEDICINES

## 559. TUBERCULOSIS LUNG — FROM T.B. TESTICLE

In October, 1985, I received the following letter :
"10th October, 1895"
"Dear Sir, — Tomorrow, Friday, I intend to bring my brother to you for advice. He has had two operations — removal of leg twenty years ago in consequence of a white swelling at knee, and at Christmas 1894, removal of one testicle, in consequence of a swelling of a tuberculous nature. Since then it has attacked his other testicle, and another operation is advised; we seek your guidance in the matter. — Yours truly."

Patient's father died at sixty of tabes dorsalis, and his mother of apoplexy at forty-five. On examination, I found him in fairish condition, but very dusky; spits blood off and on for years; dulness under right clavicle; right leg amputated above knee; left testicle ablated, its position occupied by ill-healed scar; right testicle swelled, in its lower half solid, and on its outer surface three discharging fistular openings.

This gentleman's medical advisers were of opinion that though the case was hopeless by reason of process having already gravely affected the right lung, still they thought the removal of the remaining testicle might prolong life, inasmuch as the testicle was evidently teeming with bacilli which had already spread to the right lung.

Let us consider this case, which has many points of importance. Now. if the infection had spread from the circumference towards the centre, the reasoning would seem to be sound, but is that here the mode of progress? It appears to me that a bacillary invasion *may be* from without inwards, but in most cases I think the individual becomes qualitatively, potentially tuberculous, and nature, so to speak, picks up the bacillic elements somewhere within the organism where found, and bundles them off, away from the central organs and parts to, or towards, the periphery.

This point is of the highest practical importance as bearing on treatment, for if the process is centrifugal, surgical interference may be quite useless, and even harmful; and so in the case of enlarged tonsils, which is the point I am driving at.

I have thought the matter out, after carefully watching many clinical cases, and I find the trend of vital processes to be from within outwards, and the peripheral manifestations are principally nature's ways of turning the tubercular and other elements out of the economy, *i.e.*, nature's midden-outlets from the more important inside.

If any one will take the trouble to watch nature's ways — say, in skin diseases — he will see that even where the first origin of disease is by infection at a given point of the outside, the disease indeed at first marches inwards; but then in the within great battles are fought and many slain, whereupon the organism reacts centrifugally by carrying the dead and dejected inside the camp to a point at the periphery — *i.e.*, she ejects them.

I determined to act on this view, and began to regard and treat chronic cases dynamically from within.

This case — from October 1895 to the end of the year, all through 1896, all through 1897 and 1898 — was treated steadily and persistently with infrequent doses of *Bacil.* 30, C., *Tub. test.* 30 C., and some half-a-dozen other remedies, and at the moment at which I am writing. March 1900, patient is in good general health and spirits, and so he has been nearly all the time. At first his cough and blood-spitting lessened, and finally disappeared altogether; neither lung has any trace of active disease now for very long, but the place, where the left testicle used to be, *opened and became fistulous,* in even pace with the healing up of the right lung and the disappearance of the cough, and this is still somewhat flickeringly active here and there, thus conclusively proving that the left testicle was the midden of the economy, which being ablated and forcibly healed up, nature then chose the right testicle and the right lung as her next least harmful offal pit. The surgeons who ablated the left testicle to save the organism have watched this case during all this time, urging for many months the terrible danger of delay in operation on the remaining testicle; and now that the patient has been well and sound of wind for very many months, they are of the same opinion still! Thus we see that a case of an admittedly tubercular nature, chronic, steadily progressing deathwards, was steadily left to itself surgically — dynamic doses of *Bacillinum* given at about eight-day intervals for several years, and the patient has slowly got well, and so remains; the healing processes taking place in the inverse order of their appearance.

The tubercular process in the right lung was the last to appear and the first to disappear, then followed the right testicle, and finally the points of severance of the left testis.

I have watched this in a certain number of other chronic tubercular cases, and with the same result. So long as the peripheral opening is free to discharge, patient's life is safe, and if antibacillinic treatment be perserved in for many months, or several years, a genuine cure results. This is beautifully seen in fistula in ano, and in chronic tuberculosis of the tonsils.

Any close observer, if sufficienty patient, can convince himself that in the common chronic tubercular processes having a peripheral manifestation, the natural course which nature follows is centrifugal. (XXV 21)

## 560. TUBERCULOSIS GLANDS

Thus, only two days ago, a young lady, niece of Lord X., was sent to me for treatment. Eight years ago she developed a strumous gland in the right side of the neck, an inch and a half below the ear; said gland was very neatly excised. Six years ago another lump was also equally neatly excised, and now there is another lump come at the side of the very neat scar, also evidently a gland. That the thing is constitutional is thus clearly manifest, and this is made more certain by the fact that menstruation now occurs every fortnight, and the glands in the right groin are found to be indurated.

It therefore follows that the treatment should be from within, and the local peripheral tubercular processes are to be regarded as outlets, and *not* as inlets, wherefore the ordinary surgical treatment of such tubercular processes is wrong and harmful. (XXV 29)

## 561. CHRONIC COUGH. TUBERCULAR DISEASE OF LEFT ELBOW

A single gentleman, thirty-two years of age, came under my observation on March 14, 1899, telling me that he had tubercular disease of his left elbow joint these twelve years. Six operations had been performed on the part, in Germany, during these twelve years, with the view of eradicating the disease, and thus saving the constitution, and with it the patient's life, but the seat of operation would never quite heal. Patient is well nourished,

and I found his left elbow joint almost anchylosed, but an unhealing fistula exists at its side, from which mattery stuff is oozing. He is advised to have the whole joint excised, so as to be rid of the fistula. I advised, on the contrary, that internal treatment was the real thing to do. Patient consented, and placed himself frankly under my care for that purpose.
I began with a month of *Bacill.* C.
April 11 — Less discharge from the fistula.
Rep.
May 8 — I notice that the cough is worst in the morning, and in my experience the exclusively *morning* cough is often vaccinosic, and, moreover, I find patient was vaccinated as an infant, and again at twelve or thirteen for the second time.
*Ergo, Thuja* 30 for a month in infrequent doses.
June 21 — The opening of the fistula is much dryer and shows a tendency to close.
$R_x$ Rep.
July 25 — The fistula has healed, but only with a scab.
$R_x$ *Bacill.* C.
August 22 — Well, save a very little morning cough.
$R_x$ *Thuja* 30.
October — He is quite well, and with friends in Germany.
April 5, 1900. — Remains quite well; no cough, and the elbow has quite healed, and he has increased in weight.
From this case it seems to me that the nature of the ailment was vaccinosis implanted on tuberculosis, and that, moreover, the two existed side by side, each as a separate biosis, working from the centre towards and into the periphery. (XXV 31)

## 562. CHRONIC STRUMOUS GONITIS

A clergyman's son, thirteen years of age, was carried into my consulting room on June 12, 1899.
Rather pale, big for his age, well-grown, but his right knee had long been the seat of strumous disease. The knee three-fourth anchylosed, and at its side a sore place, whence came oozing matter from the diseased joint.
Leading surgeons, seeing no hope of a cure other than by operation, recommended resection, which was about to be performed. Patient had been troubled thus for a number of years, and all concerned were more than willing that an operation should put an end to the wretched thing.
At the end of four months, all the time under *Bacill.* 30, in infrequent doses, all discharge ceased, and in ten months from commencing the treatment, the knee was quite healed, and the lad in every respect in capital condition.

Movements are now being used to see if the amount of motion of the joint can be increased, which seems probable.

My point is, that the disease was of the constitution and from the centre to the outside, in which manner it was also cured. (XXV 34)

## 563. ENLARGED TONSILS

Cecil, aet. eight, was brought to me by his mother on May 20, 1897, for enormously enlarged tonsils, pains in stomach after food, snoring at night, with restless sleep, dull and stupid. He was nearly three years under me, and then discharged in excellent health. After one month under *Thuja* 30, my note is "vast improvement." The improvement continued under *Bacillinum*. "He sleeps quietly and works better at school."

He came to me a few times in 1898 and in 1899, and when his mother brought him to me for my final inspection, I had the great satisfaction of observing a fine healthy lad, with tonsils long since restored to their normal size and functions. The boy has lost his stupid look and takes a good position at his school. (XXV 36)

## 564. ENLARGED TONSILS AND ENURESIS

Whether the tonsils stand in any relationship of a peculiar nature with the root of the bladder or testicles has not been demonstrated.

Prosser James used to teach that the ovaries and the tonsils have vital connections, and we know of the behaviour of the parotid glands and the testicles in cases of mumps. The parotid glands and the tonsils are certainly pretty near physiological relations as well as neighbours anatomically.

A lad of sixteen was brought to me on January 12, 1897, suffering from "he wets his bed sometimes, and his tonsils are enormous." the right one being the larger. Many of his lymphatic glands are indurated, and he also suffers somewhat from eczema. He was discharged cured at the end of 1899, though his enuresis had long been well before then, and also his tonsils, but the eczema persisted till then, and in fact there are traces of it still.

He had a number of remedies, *Luet*. C. and *Thuja* 30 did perhaps the most good.

Where a case is of deep-going constitutional nature, it can only be cured by a series of remedies; and when the thing is cured, it is further of only historic interest. It is very difficult to say exactly how much of the curing was done by each separate medicine; so here. (XXV 38)

## 565. ENLARGED TONSILS AND ADENOID GROWTHS — SOMNAMBULISM

Master X., ten years of age, was brought to me by his mother on October 19, 1899. He had been operated on for adenoids two years ago, but with no benefit. He has a chronic discharge from right ear, of which he is deaf; is stupid, cannot learn his lessons; sleeps very restlessly, and is often found walking in his sleep, causing much alarm and anxiety.

$R_x$ *Thuja* 30.

November 16. — He is better, and his schoolmaster reports him a little less stupid.

To continue with the *Thuja* 30.

January 11, 1900 — His sleep-walking is very bad; the right ear runs very much; his violent outbursts less frequent.

$R_x$ *Luet*. C.

February 8 — The improvement in his powers of learning is reported by his schoolmaster to me personally as wonderful; no longer walks in his sleep.

$R_x$ Rep.

March 17 — The improvement is increasingly manifest; tonsils nearly normal.

$R_x$ Rep.

April 12 — The improved condition is more than maintained, I recommend his mother to keep him under my observation at certain intervals till the cure is consolidated.

I think it may fairly be conceded that the cure of an individual's enlarged tonsils by scientific medicinal treatment is incomparably better that merely ablating them.

Be it noted that not only the boy's tonsils were cured but the boy himself; he became mentally much more active and efficient, his sleep improved, his somnambulism was cured.

Be it also noted that a child with enlarged tonsils is in bad health otherwise; the tonsils are not ill of themselves, but from the organism. (XXV 40)

## 566. DEAFNESS FROM ENLARGED TONSILS

The deafness from enlarged tonsils is often due not only to the obstruction of enlarged tonsils, but to the quality of the lining membrane of the Eustachian tubes, and adenoids in the naso-pharynx, so that the mechanical removal of the tonsils bodily, together with the adenoids, is often of no avail in these cases of deafness, nor does it suffice when the mucosa of the pharynx is hypertrophied.

Thus a boy of ten years of age was brought to me on September 1, 1889. He had been deaf for five years. His tonsils were removed by operation, but his deafness was in nowise improved. The boy was anaemic, readily took cold, and had had ophthalmia.

After *Morbill.* 30 there was some improvement in his hearing, then followed *Scarl.* 30 for a few weeks, and on November 25 I wrote in my notes of the case :

"Hearing quite well; he is altogether different; his teeth are very soft."

$R_x$ *Calcarea fluorica,* 3 trit., tales xxiv. One dry on the tongue at bedtime.

Long afterwards, on January 22, 1898, he was reported as hearing quite well. It seems to me it is vain to expect to change the vital state of the tissues of the body by cutting bits off; at most we can expect only such amelioration as may accrue from the removal of obstacles to normal processes. In the foregoing case the deafness was not due to the obstructing tonsils, and hence their removal had, as to the hearing, no good result. As the quality of the removed tonsils was certainly of the same nature as that of the linings of the pharynx and Eustachian tube, it must follow that most probably the remedies that cured the deafness would also have cured the tonsils of that which caused their enlargement. (XXV 42)

## 567. ENLARGED TONSILS

In the month of December 1896, a chubby little boy of seven years of age was brought to me for enlarged tonsils. His father had years before been a sufferer from fistula in ano, for which he was assured by eminent London surgeons and specialists there was absolutely no cure without operation, one going so far as to say that "any man who tells you he can cure fistula by medicines is a liar." I assured this gentleman that medicines given with much patience would most probably cure his fistula. He put himself under me, and I cured his fistula with medicines.

Now he is told the same story about his son's tonsils, which I entirely deny, and maintain that enlarged tonsils can be cured by medicines alone. This lad was under my care till the end of 1897, when his tonsils were, in his parents' opinion, quite well.

Patient was thus a year under the influence of remedies. First he had *Tub. test.* C.; then a month under *Thuja* 30, then for two or three months under *Tub. test.* C., and finally *Bacillinum* 30 finished the cure. (XXV 45)

## 568. ENLARGED TONSILS — ADENOID GROWTHS — BACKWARD DEVELOPMENT

A thin, puny boy, eleven-and-a-half years of age, was brought to me on November 17, 1898, his father telling me that the patient was in a very unsatisfactory state; was thin, listless, apathetic, could not learn his lessons - - his schoolmaster saying the boy was stupid and incapable of learning. His tonsils very large, bulging out under his jaw; naso-pharynx half filled with adenoids. No one could get an answer from him.

I have seen him every month, and now, after sixteen months' treatment, his tonsils and adenoids are much improved; patient has captured a good position in his school, is much praised by his master, and his father tells me how delighted he is to see the progress in every way.

I might go on and fill a big book with records of cases of enlarged tonsils cured by medicines, but for that I have neither time nor inclination. When I first became convinced by practical experiment of the workability of the law of likes in the cure of disease, I took the trouble to read the history of the good work done by the veteran practitioners in old files of their journals, and I must confess that the present race of homoeopathic practitioners compare very unfavourably with those of twenty, thirty, and forty years ago.

Many years ago *Baryta carb.* 30 or 12 was in very high repute for the cure of enlarged tonsils. Its reputation was well founded, as I can testify. Taken by itself, it is the biggest tonsil medicine we have. Where the tonsils have enlarged from vaccinosis, *Baryta* will not do much until the vaccinosic quality has been got rid of by *Thuja*, or *Silicea*, or what not.

Similarly, where the tuberculosic quality lies behind, *Bacill.* is needed first, and then the *Baryta*, and so on. (XXV 48)

## 569. DEAFNESS DUE TO ENLARGED TONSILS

In the course of the year 1899. Miss E. T., aet. 13, was brought to me by her mother, telling me that patient was deaf from enlarged tonsils, and that her doctor had ordered their removal. I could only find one enlarged lymphatic gland on the left side of the neck. This was her vaccination side, and the lassie being strong and otherwise in good health, I thought we had to do with a simple case of vaccinosic hypertrophy of the tonsils.

In a few weeks the tonsils went down and her hearing was quite restored. The remedy : *Thuja* 30, in infrequent doses.

It is not to be forgotten that a competent (or, at any rate, orthodox and qualified according to law) medical man had declared an operation absolutely necessary. No medicines would, he said, be of the least avail. Still *Thuja* 30 cured the case. (XXV 58)

## 570. ENLARGED TONSILS AND DEAFNESS

On September 23, 1889, a strumous girl of eleven years of age was brought to me by her mother for enlarged tonsils and deafness arising supposedly therefrom. The tonsils met in the middle, so that the uvula was in part invisible.

*Thuja* 30, *Bacill*. C, and one or two other remedies were given, when —
January 17, 1890 — "I do not see much difference in her tonsils yet."
$R_x$ *Vaccinin* C.
March 12 — "Tonsils about the same."
$R_x$ Trit. 3x *Baryta carb*., gr. iv. One dry on the tongue night and morning.
April 19 — The tonsils are distinctly smaller.
$R_x$ Rep.
May 30 — No further diminution in the size of the tonsils.
$R_x$ *Silico-fluoride of Sodium*, 3x trit., gr. vj. One dry on the tongue at bedtime.
July 16 — Tonsils are considerably smaller. The case was cured by the spring of 1890, and the remedies that achieved this result were the foregoing, and then two months of *Phytolaccin* 3x, two months of the third trituration of the *Silico-fluoride of Sodium*, and finally a two months' course of the third decimal trituration of the *Phosphate of Lime*. (XXV 60)

## 571. ENLARGED TONSILS AND ADENOIDS REMOVED BY OPERATION

In 1899 a gentleman brought his nine-year-old son to me for what his physicians term Imperfect Development of the Brain. This was supposedly due to enlarged tonsils and adenoid growths. The boy did not speak till two or three years of age — indeed he cannot articulate properly even now. He wets his bed, and has a piled-up cranium; but the point I wish to bring out is that the influence of the removal of tonsils and adenoids is not an unmixed blessing.

He breathes better since their removal, but since then he is much *more* nervous; he squints, and is very odd in his ways; he gesticulates and assumes odd attitudes, looking idiotic, and yet he seems to me to have ample brain power. He is cryptorchic. He hits his mother on the face and throws tea-cups at his parents, and throws people bits out of window.

These nervous symptoms have come on so very much *worse* since the removal of tonsils, etc.

There appears to be no doubt that there was very great exacerbation in all his nerve symptoms subsequent to the operation, though the breathing was distinctly improved. I may, perhaps, be permitted here to refer to my little work *On Delicate Children* for further particulars on this subject. (XXV 62)

## 572. ENLARGED TONSILS AND INSOMNIA

There are certain cases of enlarged tonsils historically readily diagnosed that will mend rapidly, and by rapidly I mean in a few months. Thus a gentleman brought his little girl of eight years of age to me in the fall of last year. The tonsils were moderaltely enlarged and also many of the lymphatics, but the most distressing thing was the girl's sleep. Here the amelioration was very great — in fact she was practically cured in six months. There was a period of two months under *Luet*. C. to start with, then *Thuja* 30 for a month, and the former prescription then repeated, when patient was discharged cured. (XXV 64)

## 573. ENLARGED TONSILS AFTER REMOVAL OF ADENOID GROWTHS.

A very delicate backward child was brought by her mother to me at the beginning of 1899, suffering from enlarged tonsils. Although the adenoid growths from which she had suffered had been removed by operation, still her eminently silly expression had not improved. She did not breathe nicely, a little phlegm in her throat see-sawed backwards and forwards without seemingly ever being got rid of. Though ten years of age, her eye-teeth are still absent. After three months of *Bacill*. 30. her intelligence very greatly improved; she breathed better, and without the phlegmy nasal state.

She was then a few weeks under *Thuja* 30, and then again another *Bacillinum* 30. Whereupon her eye-teeth at last appeared, and that quite sound.

There afterwards followed the same remedies repeatedly, and also *Sabina* 30.

Now, after thirteen months' persistent treatment by medicines, her tonsils are about the right size, the breathing is good, and patient is somewhat nearing the normal; she articulates now, and answers a question promptly, and her parents and their friends are struck by the very great change that has come over her is to be borne in mind that where the tonsils are enlarged that is not, as a rule, the only abnormality, for very commonly the enlargement is only one of the ailings of the individual. The tonsils are glands, and where one gland is swelled there are often many, and after all is said and done you cannot cut away disease with the surgeon's knife. (XXV 65)

## 574. ENLARGED TONSILS

In the medicinal treatment of enlarged tonsils there are two main lines of procedure, and the first is to cure the cause of the enlargement, which is commonly not only not attempted, but it is not even thought of. For it must be manifest that to get rid of the cause of the enlargement is the prime consideration. If this be done the enlargements usually disappear — this is the best way. When you cut off a tonsil you certainly get rid of it, so you do if you shrivel it with gland tissue-destroyers, but the perfect cure is where the enlargement disappears under the influence of dynamic remedies : here the normal tonsils remain to do the work allotted to them within nature's cycle.

That this is really so may be seen in cases where the tonsils are not bilaterally enlarged, but only on one side, and in such other cases where the tonsils are enlarged at the beginning of the cure, but where only one tonsil will yield to the given remedy. Thus Miss Marjorie X. was put under me on June 26, 1899 for her huge tonsils; they literally held the uvula tightly between them, and breathing was distressing, and swallowing miserable. After the patient had been two months under *Thuja* 30, and then a month under *Bacill.* C., I find the following note in my record of her case.

November 20, 1899 — "The left tonsil is no longer enlarged, but the right one is very large."

So we have here a rather curious find : under *Thuja* and *Bacillinum* one tonsil becomes normal in size while the other is still enlarged.

If we want to be quite successful in the treatment of enlarged tonsils by medicines, we must look away from the mere tonsils, and remember that although the tonsils are the thing complained of, the constitutional cause of their enlargement is the real disease, and this it is that cannot be removed by operation. Those who see the mere enlargement, and give remedies for such enlargement merely — those practitioners will mostly fail to cure enlarged tonsils by medicines, and will have much to say of the advantages of their mechanical removal.

It is not at all a bad plan to begin the course of treatment with *Sulphur* 30; after a while follow with *Calcarea carb.* 30, and in the third place give *Thuja occidentalis* 30. Each remedy should have a month or two to develop its action, to do its work.

As a rule before these have done all their work there is evidence of amelioration in the child's health, and the enlargement has somewhat lessened. (XXV 67)

# INDEX TO REMEDIES